Cosmetic Surgery - Techniques for the Most Popular Aesthetic Surgery Procedures

Edited by Angelo L. Cuzalina

Published in London, United Kingdom

Cosmetic Surgery - Techniques for the Most Popular Aesthetic Surgery Procedures
http://dx.doi.org/10.5772/intechopen.1003449
Edited by Angelo L. Cuzalina

Contributors
Alanna Fostyk, Alicia Sigler, Alicia Sigler-Moreno, Ana C. Weck Roxo, Andrew Sohn, Angelo Cuzalina, Anthony Congiusta, Artem Krutyansky, Brandy Fenwick, Carlos del Pino-Roxo, Chandler Hinson, Chase Nelson, David Borg, Engin Selamioğlu, Hallie Masters, Kristian Bugeja, Kurt Lee Chircop, Manik S. Bedi, Marco Swanson, Maria Jubran-Khoury, Mark A. Foglietti, María M. Cabrera-Cifuentes, Mohammad K. H. B. Abdulaziz, Mohammad Kamal, Morgan L. Fish, Niran Maharjan, Pasquale G. Tolomeo, Pasquale G. Tolomeo, Polly Jasper, Rebecca Kelley, Riekie Smit, Ronald Brooks, Sebastian Gutierrez de Pineres, Sebastian Gutierrez De Pineres, Victoria Bouillon, Víctor M. Whizar-Lugo

First published in London, United Kingdom, 2025 by IntechOpen
IntechOpen is the global imprint of INTECHOPEN LIMITED, registered in England and Wales, registration number: 11086078, 167-169 Great Portland Street, London, W1W 5PF, United Kingdom

For EU product safety concerns: IN TECH d.o.o., Prolaz Marije Krucifikse Kozulić 3, 51000 Rijeka, Croatia, info@intechopen.com or visit our website at intechopen.com.

British Library Cataloguing-in-Publication Data
A catalogue record for this book is available from the British Library

Cosmetic Surgery - Techniques for the Most Popular Aesthetic Surgery Procedures
Edited by Angelo L. Cuzalina
p. cm.
Print ISBN 978-0-85014-999-9
Online ISBN 978-0-85014-998-2
eBook (PDF) ISBN 978-0-85466-013-1

If disposing of this product, please recycle the paper responsibly.

Meet the editor

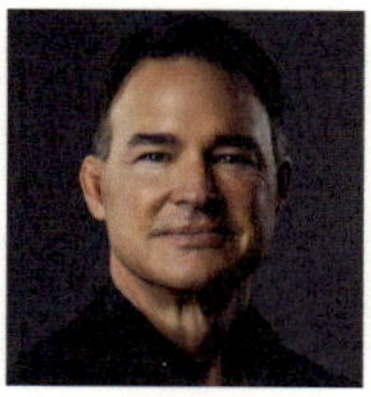

Dr. Angelo Cuzalina is an award-winning cosmetic surgeon known for his artistry, innovation, and leadership in aesthetic surgery. He was board-certified in facial and full-body cosmetic surgery and served as President of the American Academy of Cosmetic Surgery and the American Board of Cosmetic Surgery. He is the founder of Tulsa Surgical Arts, and he has performed over 18,000 procedures. He is internationally recognized for his expertise in complex revisional surgery, achieving dramatic yet natural-looking results. Dr. Cuzalina lectures worldwide, trains fellow surgeons and has authored numerous scientific publications. As a former collegiate wrestler turned accomplished sculptor and surgeon, he brings discipline and passion to his surgical practice and personal life.

Contents

Preface

Cosmetic surgery has become increasingly popular as individuals seek to enhance their appearance, restore confidence, and improve overall quality of life. The decision to undergo cosmetic procedures is deeply personal and influenced by cultural, psychological, and social factors. The list of cosmetic procedures, both surgical and non-surgical, continues to grow, and patients are seeking the best advice and expertise for a wide range of aesthetic problems they want to address.

With advances in surgical techniques and medical technology, cosmetic procedures are now safer, more effective, and offer quicker recovery times than ever before. Surgeons and aesthetic providers are tasked with staying up-to-date with the latest innovations and safest procedures to deliver their clients the desired results.

From facial rejuvenation to body contouring, today's cosmetic surgeries are designed to provide natural-looking results while minimizing downtime and risk. The chapters present a thoughtful perspective, ranging from fundamental or standard basic procedures to complex and revisional cosmetic surgery procedures performed by those with decades of experience.

Patients now have access to a wide array of surgical and non-surgical options tailored to their unique aesthetic goals. Procedures such as breast augmentation, liposuction, facelifts, and rhinoplasty continue to evolve with the integration of new technologies and patient-focused techniques. This book is divided into three easily followed sections. Starting with

The book begins with Section 1, which offers a detailed description of techniques for endoscopic brow lifting, various face and neck lifting (including deep plane facelifts), as well as lip lifts, facial implants, and filler injection techniques. Section 2 focuses on breast and body cosmetic surgery. Exploring various techniques for breast reduction, breast augmentation, simultaneous augmentation and breast lifts, revisional breast surgery, high-definition liposuction, abdominoplasty, as well as body contouring after massive weight loss. Section 3 will review various methods to enhance healing after cosmetic surgery, including lymphatic therapy and the use of hyperbaric oxygen.

This book provides a comprehensive overview of the most commonly performed cosmetic surgery procedures, current best practices, and patient-centered approaches in aesthetic surgery. It also highlights key innovations and perspectives from leading surgeons worldwide.

The contributions of our authors—each an expert in their field—are gratefully acknowledged. Their dedication to advancing aesthetic surgery and sharing their valuable insights is what makes this work possible. I would like to extend my sincere gratitude to all the authors for their valuable contributions, as well as to the reviewers whose insightful feedback has helped refine the content of this book. Special thanks go to the Publishing Process Manager, Mrs. Ivana Barac, for her invaluable support and expertise throughout the editorial process. We hope this text inspires further research and innovation in cosmetic surgery, leading to improved results and enhanced safety.

Dr. Angelo Cuzalina
Tulsa Surgical Arts,
Tulsa, Oklahoma, USA

Section 1

Facial Cosmetic Surgery

Chapter 1

Facelift (Cervicofacial Rhytidectomy) Surgery

Anthony Congiusta, Angelo Cuzalina and Maria Jubran-Khoury

Abstract

This chapter will highlight how facelift surgery has evolved over the course of the last century and describe the current techniques and trends in facelift surgery. As more surgeons become familiar and competent with facelift surgery, different techniques develop to achieve long-lasting esthetic results. Surgeons must balance the risk of complications such as facial nerve injury, sialocele, and unnatural appearance with the potential for superior and longer-lasting results that meet or supersede patient expectations. The facelift techniques described in this chapter will include subcutaneous, deep plane, and extended deep plane facelift surgery. The chapter will also include treatment of the neck, with particular attention to management of the platysma muscle and the submandibular glands.

Keywords: facelift, deep plane facelift, rhytidectomy, submandibular gland reduction, SMAS, platysma, submentoplasty

1. Introduction

The face is one of the earliest areas of the body to appear aged. Thus, the goal of many surgeons, estheticians, and nurse injectors is to remove, decelerate, halt, and reverse the signs of aging in order for patients to appear more youthful.

To address these objectives, a facelift may have more impact than any other surgical procedure [1]. For the majority of the twentieth century, facelift surgery dissection was limited to the subcutaneous plane. Surgeons who performed these procedures were looked down upon by their peers due to taking "unnecessary" risks to satisfy what was considered to be an extremely vain goal of looking younger [2, 3]. With the negative connotation over facial cosmetic surgery at the time came a slow evolution of facelift techniques. Over time, however, the desire for a more rejuvenated physical appearance became more widespread throughout society, leading to increased public demand of the procedure. As facial surgical anatomy became better understood, the quality of anesthesia increased, the number of surgeons increased, and the desire for long-lasting results intensified, different techniques were developed involving manipulation of other facial structures besides the skin and subcutaneous tissue [3].

Within the past few decades, there have been many types facelift surgery dissections described in the literature such as the subcutaneous facelift, biplane facelift, composite facelift, deep-plane facelift, subperiosteal facelift, the endoscopic facelift, and the minimal access cranial suspension (MACS) facelift. Many of these techniques involve management of the platysma muscle and the superficial musculoaponeurotic system (SMAS), which were initially described by Skoog [4] and Mitz and Peyronie, [5] respectively, in the 1970s.

Skoog is the first surgeon who developed a technique where the deep structure was moved as well as the skin [6]. By the 1980s, a combination of complete platysma muscle transection, plication, and lateral pulling was presented as the way to achieve a superior result [1]. It has become common practice for facelift surgeons to manipulate a musculofascial plane to achieve improved and longer-lasting results [2]. It is crucial for surgeons to appreciate and realize the face as a continuous unit, comprised of different subunits, and that to achieve an esthetically balanced "youthful" or "rejuvenated" look may require additional adjunct surgical and nonsurgical procedures.

Facelift discussions in this chapter will focus on the author's preferred technique while offering insight to other methods.

2. Pertinent anatomy

A deep understanding and knowledge of the clinical anatomy and of the etiopathogenesis of facial aging is mandated for facelift surgery, regardless of technique used.

Facial tissue and structures are arranged in layers in a predictable configuration, though the thickness and density of each layer is variable [7]. The face has been traditionally described as having five distinct layers: skin, superficial fat, superficial fascia or SMAS, deep fat and areolar tissue, and periosteum or deep fascia (**Figures 1** and **2**) [1, 7–9].

Skin thickness varies throughout the face. While the thinnest skin is found in the upper and lower eyelids (approximately 400 microns) [7], the thickest skin is found

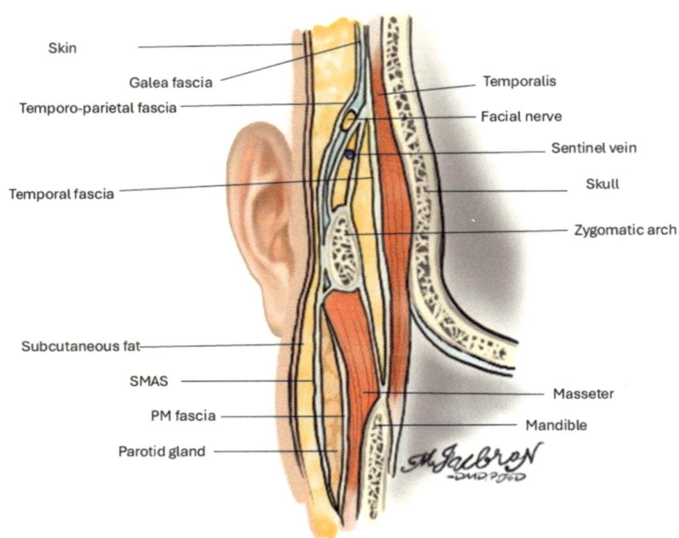

Figure 1.
Cross sectional facial anatomy depicting facial layers and relevant structures for facelift surgery. The facial nerve resides in the layer deep to the temporoparietal fascia and superficial musculoaponeurotic system (SMAS).

DOI: http://dx.doi.org/10.5772/intechopen.1008512

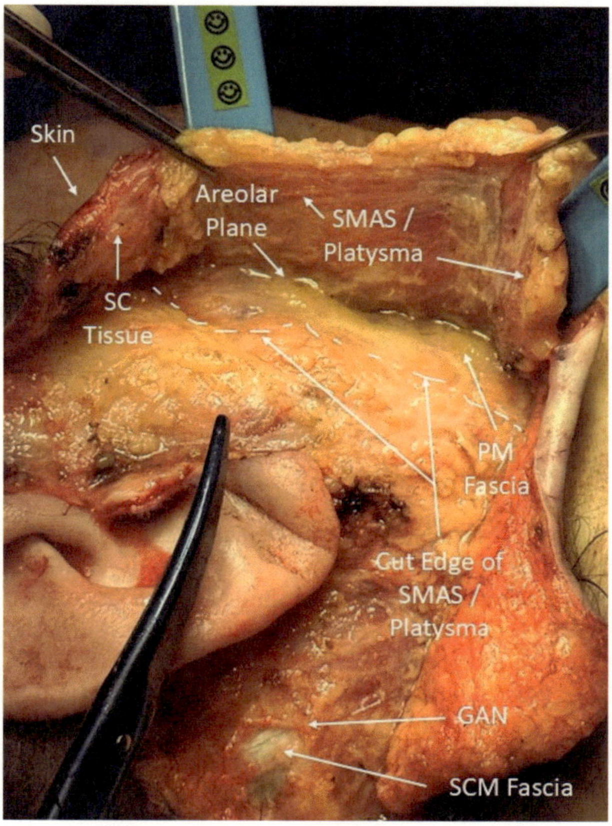

Figure 2.
An intra-operative view of a deep-plane lower face and neck lift depicting the five facial layers: skin, subcutaneous (SC) tissue, superficial musculoaponeurotic system (SMAS), the areolar plane, and the deep fascia, which includes the parotidomasseteric (PM) fascia. The platysma is continuous with the SMAS inferiorly. Posterior to the ear, the fascia of the sternocleidomastoid (SCM) muscle and the greater auricular nerve (GAN) are visualized.

in the forehead and mentum (approximately 2300–2500 microns) [7] and nasal tip (approximately 2900 microns) [10]. The blood supply to the skin comes from the dermal plexus of blood vessels. To ensure maintenance of this blood supply and flap viability, an even layer of several millimeters of fat should be left adherent to the facelift flap. This will also help minimize contour irregularities of the skin once the flap is repositioned.

The subcutaneous layer and superficial fat are located between the dermis and the SMAS. This plane is generally considered as "safe" due to the scarcity of important anatomic structures present in this layer. The subcutaneous tissue is thickest along the cheeks, anterior neck, and nasolabial folds and is thinnest in the eyelids, lips and mastoid regions. Some authors go one step further in saying that it is nonexistent in the lower eyelid [7]. Dissection during facelift surgery over the malar region, in an area called "McGregor's Patch," can be tenuous due to fibrous retaining ligaments attaching this layer to the periosteum. Additionally, "McGregor's Patch" contains blood vessels and nerves that make the dissection more challenging. The retaining ligaments that are present throughout the subcutaneous layer attach dermis to periosteum and are known as the "retinacular cutis" [1].

The third layer is the superficial fascia, which envelopes the facial mimetic muscles and separates the more superficial subcutaneous fat from vital structures such as the parotidomasseteric fascia and facial nerve branches. This layer is continuous from scalp to clavicle and has different names depending on the region of the head it is located (**Figure 3**). The most superior subregion is the galea aponeurotica, which envelopes the frontalis and occipitalis muscles. Over the temporalis muscle is the superficial temporal fascia or the temporoparietal fascia, which is continuous with the galea aponeurotica superiorly and the SMAS inferiorly. The SMAS extends from the temporoparietal fascia to the platysma and superficial cervical fascia. The superficial cervical fascia extends from the inferior border of the mandible to the clavicles and envelopes the platysma muscle.

The SMAS layer was first described as a fibromuscular layer between facial mimetic muscles and the dermis [5]. While its existence was called into question by authors such as Jost and Levet [11], many surgeons at the present time agree that the SMAS separates the subcutaneous fat from the underlying parotidomasseteric fascia and treat this layer frequently during facelift surgery.

The platysma muscle is another important structure in facelift surgery. Anterior neck laxity and platysmal banding are classic signs of aging (**Figure 4**). Platysmal banding occurs as a result of a weakened and redundant muscle fibers and dehiscence of fibers in the midline of the neck [8, 12] Platysma anatomy may vary and can be classified into three types. Type I, the most common variation, consists of platysma muscle fibers that are separated at the suprahyoid region and are interlaced at about 2 cm below the chin. In Type II, the platysma muscle fibers are interlaced at the level of the thyroid cartilage. In Type III, the platysma medial fibers remain separated up to the chin [13].

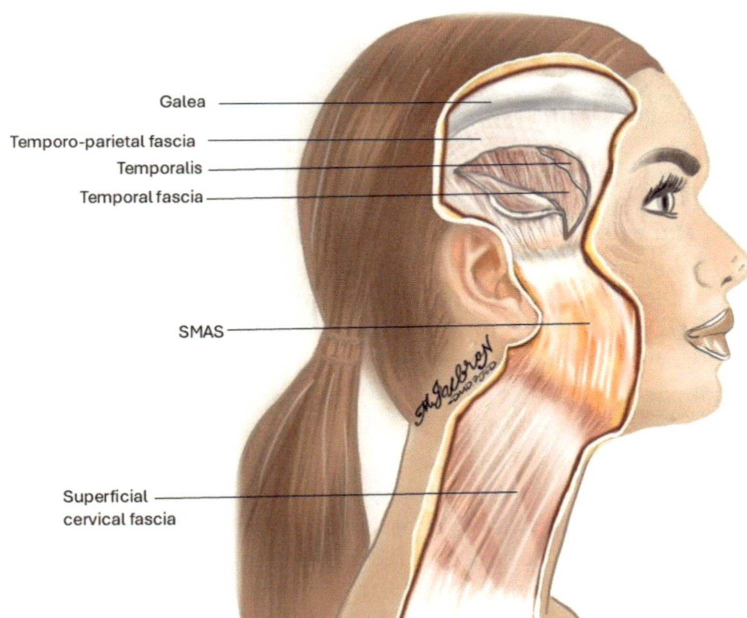

Figure 3.
The SMAS in continuous with the temporoparietal fascia superiorly and the platysma / superficial layer of the deep cervical fascia inferiorly. The galea aponeurotica is continuous with the temporoparietal fascia.

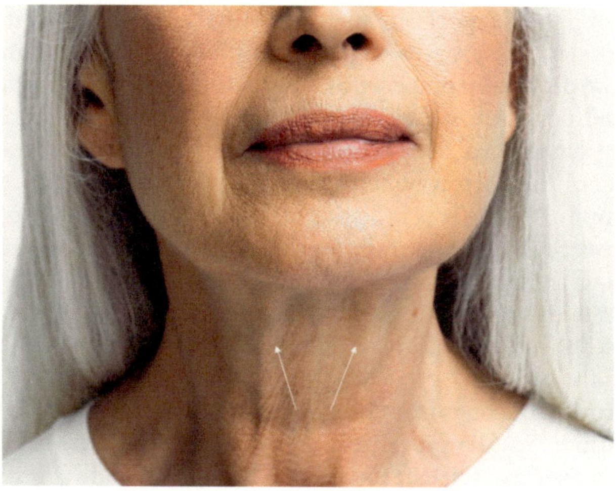

Figure 4.
Platysmal banding (arrows) can be a telltale sign of aging. As a person ages, the platysma muscle may become lax or hyperactive leading to redundant muscle fibers and even an increased cervicomental angle.

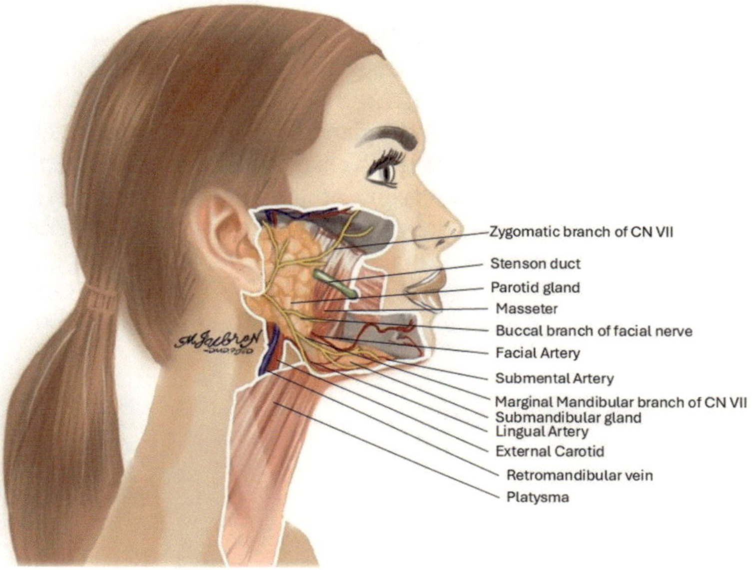

Figure 5.
Deep to the SMAS lies several important anatomic structures that the surgeon must be mindful of while dissecting in this plane.

The deep fascia layer is located deep to the SMAS-platysma layer, separated only by a virtual plane of fascial spaces and retaining ligaments, i.e. the "loose areolar connective tissue layer" [9]. Deep to the SMAS, the surgeon will encounter branches of the facial nerve, the parotid gland and duct, the external jugular vein, the greater auricular nerve, and facial artery and vein (**Figure 5**). The areolar plane separates the superficial fascia from the deep fascia and periosteum. Within this plane are the muscles of facial expression, all of which are innervated by the facial nerve along their deep surfaces, with the exception of the mentalis, buccinator, and levator anguli oris muscles, which are innervated along their superficial surfaces. Minelli et al. write that unless surgically opened, this fourth layer is not present as part of human facial anatomy and that it exists as a potential dissection plane within specialized areas of deep fascia [14].

Deep fascia and periosteum make up the fifth layer of the face. The deep fascia is divided into three subregions: deep temporal fascia, the parotidomasseteric fascia, and the deep layer of the deep cervical fascia [8]. Over bony structures like the zygoma and cranium, this layer is indistinguishable from periosteum [1]. The deep temporal fascial overlies the temporalis muscle and divides into superficial and deep layers at the level of the zygomatic arch. The parotidomasseteric fascia invests the parotid gland and overlies the masseter muscle. The deep layer of the deep cervical fascia encompasses the deep fascial layers, including the pretracheal, prevertebral fascia, and carotid sheath.

It is also important to recognize submandibular gland ptosis because if it goes unnoticed, the esthetic result of facelift surgery will be less than satisfactory as the patient may have a residual bulge in the submandibular triangle (**Figures 6** and 7) [12]. Submandibular gland ptosis may be difficult to detect pre-operatively if excess skin laxity and jowling are present. While it is generally accepted that submandibular gland reduction can improve the neck contour of patients with prominent glands, the procedure remains controversial as it is neither easy to learn nor easy to perform [15]. The capsule of the submandibular gland, formed by the investing deep fascia of the neck, is the key to surgical control of this region [15]. The vessels on the capsule immediately lateral to the gland include a tributary of the facial vein and the facial artery on the deeper aspect, which may extend a branch into the gland (**Figure 8**). A deep perforator artery courses through the substance of the gland from deep to superficial and often goes unnoticed until the superficial part of the gland has been excised [15].

Regarding facial nerve branches (and some other important structures), facelift surgeons must be mindful of three main danger zones: the mid-zygomatic temporal region, the malar eminence, and the area at the mandibular inferior border near the angle [16].

The mid-zygomatic arch area contains the frontotemporal branches of the facial nerve, which cross over the arch anywhere from 10 to 31 mm anterior to the most

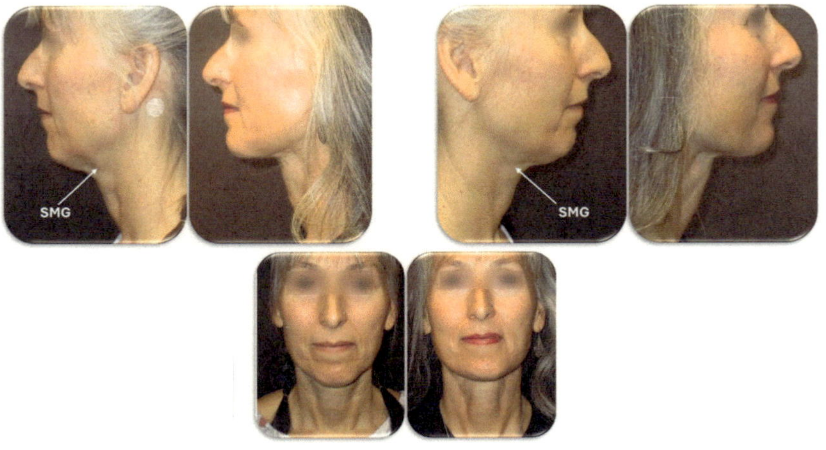

Figure 6.
A 52-year-old white female showing 3 views before and 5 months following a submentoplasty with submandibular gland (SMG) reductions, chin implant and facial fat grafting. The bulge in the submandibular triangle is obvious pre-operatively and would have been more noticeable following a facelift or submentoplasty had the glands not been reduced.

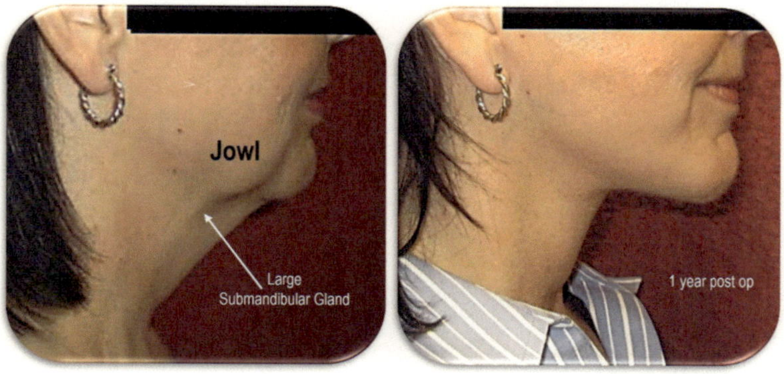

Figure 7.
A female patient before and after a lower face and neck lift that included a submentoplasty and chin implant. The submandibular gland bulge seen in the before (left) photograph would have been more obvious post-operatively had it not been reduced, diminishing the esthetic outcome of the surgery.

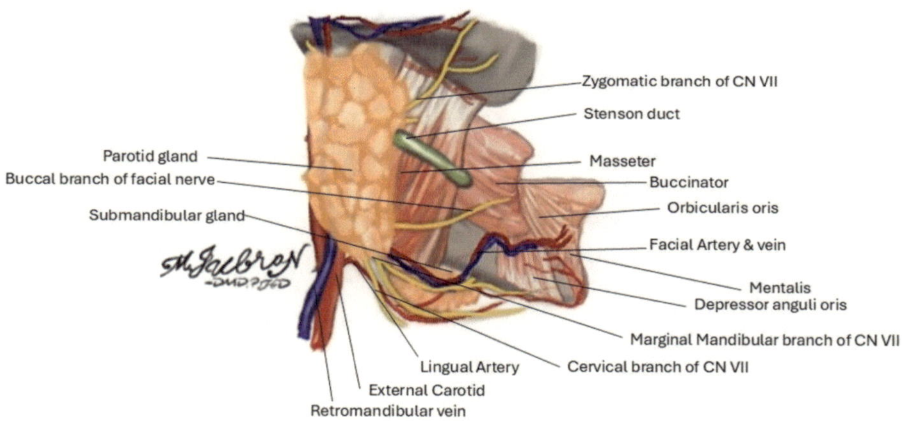

Figure 8.
The facial artery and submandibular gland share an intimate relationship. During submandibular gland reduction, meticulous technique and strict hemostatic control are crucial to avoid excessive bleeding.

anterior point of the tragus [17]. This represents an area at risk because there is less soft tissue present over the bony arch, leaving the nerve more vulnerable to injury [16, 17].

The second danger zone to be aware of is at the malar eminence and is colloquially known as "McGregor's Patch" or "the bloody gulch" [1]. This area contains zygomatic retaining ligaments that perforate the SMAS and adhere to dermis. The zygomatic branch of the facial nerve, which crosses cephalad near the lateral canthus is also within "McGregor's Patch" [16]. The region receives blood supply from the transverse facial, angular and infraorbital arteries and also includes perforating branches of the transverse facial artery and a venous plexus composed of transverse facial and angular veins. This danger zone must be undermined and passive for most patients undergoing facelift surgery as freeing this area separates the zygomatic ligaments [1].

The third danger zone, a short distance anterior to the mandibular angle and below its inferior border, concerns the marginal mandibular branch of the facial nerve. This motor nerve courses just below the inferior border of the mandible in approximately 20–50% of cases and may be found as inferior as 1.5 cm below the inferior border of the mandible. Injury to this nerve denervates the depressor labii

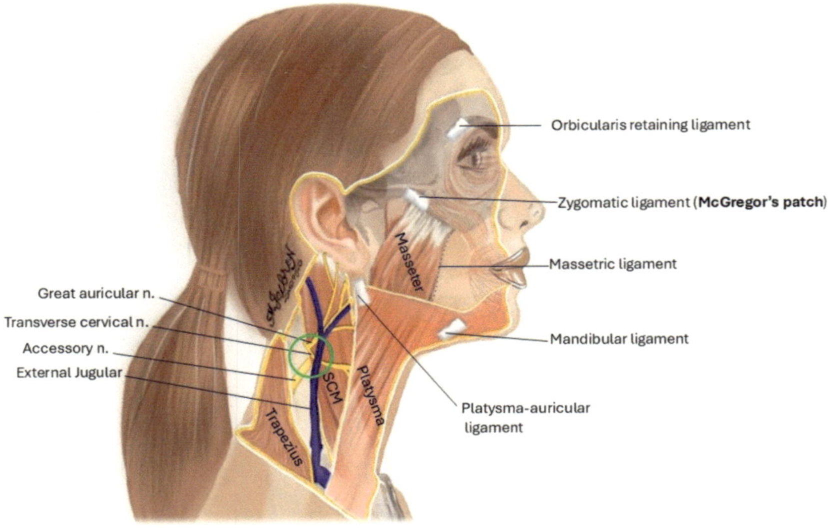

Figure 9.
Erb's point (green circle) is an important anatomic landmark as three important structures can found here: the external jugular vein, great auricular nerve, and spinal accessory nerve.

inferioris and the depressor anguli oris muscles, resulting in the lower lip to drop when speaking or smiling [18].

Another "danger zone" exists in the neck by the name of Erb's point or McKinney's point (**Figure 9**). It is a point approximately 6.5 cm inferior to the external auditory meatus where the greater auricular nerve and other cervical plexus nerves, the spinal accessory nerve, and external jugular vein exit from behind the posterior border of the sternocleidomastoid muscle. The greater auricular nerve provides sensory innervation to the earlobe and lateral cheek. It is the most commonly injured nerve in facelift surgery [1, 19].

3. Patient selection

Indeed, a large part of achieving excellent facelift results is patient selection. A discussion with the individual should center first on his or her desires and motivations for seeking surgical correction [20]. Although patients are becoming more well-educated, most do not have a true understanding of all the factors that contribute to facial aging and their respective surgical remedies, leading them to often present with inaccurate or incomplete conceptions of treatment options [1].

Cosmetic surgeons should be vigilant in their surgical work-up and pre-operative evaluation as patients tend to downplay their medical comorbidities. Based on the medical history, certain laboratory tests and studies may be required. The health and welfare of the patient is always paramount.

When a patient seeking facelift surgery presents to the surgeon's office, it is important to discuss risks, benefits, alternatives, and limitations of the procedure. Additionally, it is crucial to determine if the patient has adequate social support and time off from work to sufficiently recover from surgery.

Patients with unrealistic expectations, with body dysmorphic disorder, with overly narcissistic or immature personalities, who speak negatively about other surgeons, who overreact to small flaws, who "know" more about a procedure than the surgeon, and who complain about financial arrangements should be considered nonsurgical candidates or, at the very least, should be referred elsewhere [21]. Other "red flags" that may be predictive of patient management issues include patients who continuously talk and not listen, unfriendly or impersonal patients, patients who are rude to staff members and nurses, patients motivated to undergo surgery due to a failing marriage, promotion, or some type of loss, patients who are overly impulsive, those obsessed with online cosmetic surgery ads and websites, and young patients who have already had numerous surgeries [21]. Patients with severe systemic diseases, such as heart failure, renal failure, and poorly controlled diabetes are not candidates for facelift surgery. Additionally, patients with skin disorders, such as Ehlers-Danlos Syndrome, progeria and elastoderma can experience severe wound healing issues and, therefore, are not candidates for rhytidectomy [22].

3.1 Patient evaluation

There are many different indications for facelift surgery involving age-related facial changes. Cutis laxa of the jowls and cervical region, deepened nasolabial folds, and plastysmal banding are main complaints that can be targeted by a facelift surgeon [16]. Other complaints such as "age-spots", discoloration, and rhytids in the upper facial third should be addressed with different modalities.

While typical facelift surgery addresses the lower third of the face and neck, it is important that the initial consultation is comprehensive and that the patient understands that other procedures may be indicated for other areas of the face. An excellent facelift result may be compromised by severe facial rhytids and brow ptosis in the upper third of the face that was not addressed. Younger patients with genetically obtuse necks and good skin tone may be candidates for an isolated submentoplasty (**Figure 10**). Preoperative evaluation of the patient's face and neck should involve inspection and palpation of facial structures [22]. The cosmetic surgeon should evaluate the face and neck as a unit and then divide the face into even vertical fifths and horizontal thirds. The patient's Fitzpatrick skin type (**Figure 11**), overall facial fat content, Dedo classification of cervical abnormalities (**Figure 12**), and asymmetries all play a role in treatment planning. Patients with higher Fitzpatrick skin types may be predisposed to hypertrophic scar formation and pigment changes along incision lines [22]. Patients with less facial fat volume at baseline typically demonstrate better

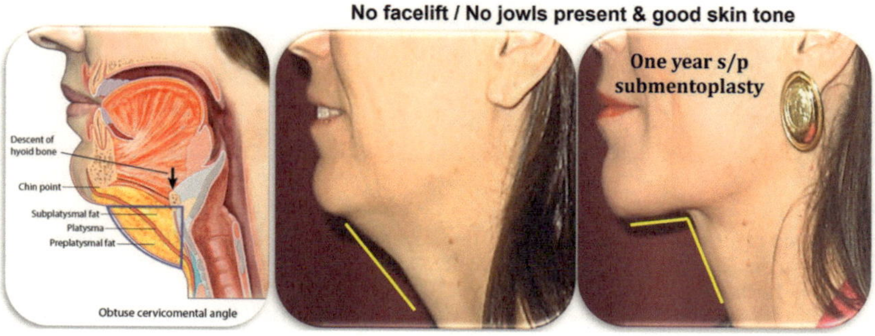

Figure 10.
Patients with a genetically obtuse neck who present without jowling and with good skin tone do not require facelift surgery and can achieve great jawline definition and an acute cervicomental angle with an isolated submentoplasty.

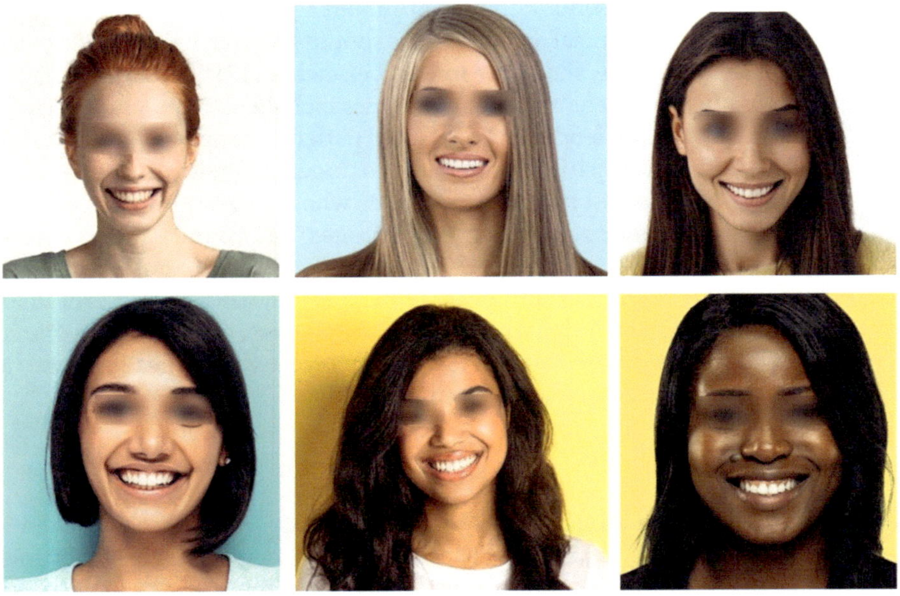

Figure 11.
The Fitzpatrick skin classification generalizes skin types from type 1 (top left) to type 6 (bottom right). The system is based upon skin response to sunlight and generalizations with hair, eye color and the amount of melanin.

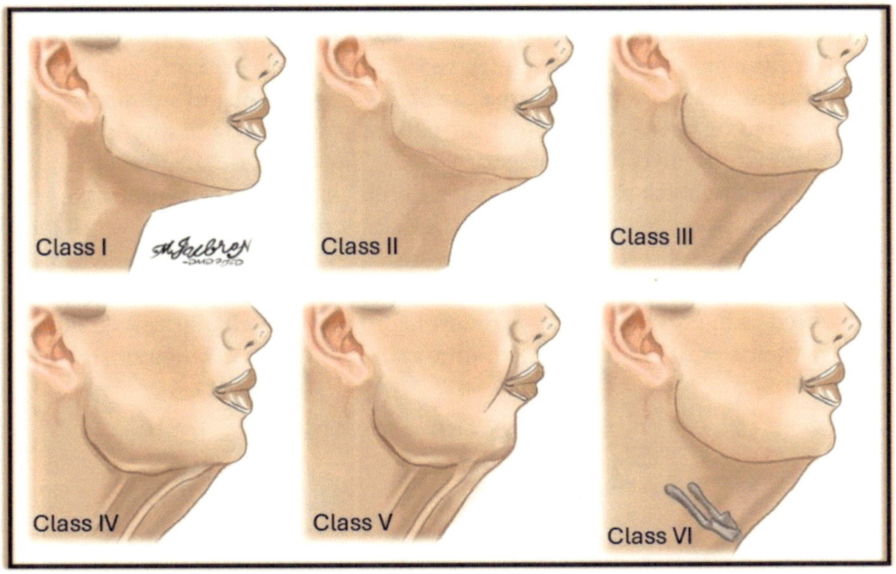

Figure 12.
The Dedo classification for cervical abnormalities. Class I: well-defined cervicomental angle, good muscle tone, minimal submental fat. Class II: Lax skin without fat accumulation and without platysmal weakness. Class III: Excess submandibular and submental adipose tissue. Class IV: Platysmal attenuation. Class V: microgenia/ retrognathia. Class VI: low hyoid.

postoperative contouring when compared with patients with greater facial soft tissue volume [22]. Those with a higher Dedo classifications, i.e. classes V and VI, should be informed of limitations of the postoperative esthetic appearance of the neck if undergoing facelift surgery alone, and should be offered concomitant procedures, such as a chin implant, if indicated.

Obtaining a standardized set of photographs are absolutely essential in any cosmetic practice. Patients undergoing cosmetic facial surgery should have frontal, profile, and three-quarter views taken while the head is in neutral position and the face is in repose. A frontal photograph in full smile is also obtained, as is a worm's eye view. Addressing objective findings, such as facial asymmetries, to the patient during the initial consultation is an important step in setting expectations, limitations and establishing trust. These photographs taken at the initial consultation visit and/or during the preoperative appointment will become invaluable when assessing postoperative results and may be used to remind patients of certain findings that may have been present all along.

3.2 Patient preparation

After the appropriate work-up has been completed and surgical consent has been obtained, the patient is reminded of key pre-operative instructions: avoiding non-steroidal anti-inflammatory medications (NSAID), such as aspirin and ibuprofen, and Vitamin E 2 weeks prior to surgery to minimize platelet dysfunction and unwanted bleeding intra-operatively [16]. The patient is encouraged to refrain from alcohol consumption for 3 days prior to and 2 weeks after surgery. Herbal supplements are also stopped 2–3 weeks preoperatively to avoid adverse reactions intraoperatively or postoperatively: chondroitin, ginko and garlic (bleeding), ephedra (cardiac effects), Echinacea (barbiturate and halothane toxicity, allergic reaction, immunotoxicity), glucosamine (hypoglycemia), goldenseal (photosensitivity, sedation), kava root (sedation), and milk thistle (volume depletion) [22].

Other preoperative measures include a thorough washing of the face and hair with germicidal soap the night before and the morning of surgery. Due to increased anxiety levels, certain patients may benefit from preoperative oral sedation with a mild benzodiazepine the night before and the morning of surgery [16]. The patient should be instructed not to wear any facial makeup on the day of surgery.

On the day of surgery, the patient is marked while in an upright position to ensure proper identification of anatomic landmarks, areas of concern, and boundaries. The hair is taped or braided prior heading to the operating room. Wrapping the patient's hair and head with paper tape can be helpful in avoiding the nuisance of loose hair while attempting to suture [16].

Once the appropriate depth of anesthesia has been achieved, the patient is lightly prepared with alcohol or povidone-iodine just before local anesthesia is infiltrated along the planned incision lines. The surgeon should wait at least 15 minutes before making an incision as it takes that amount of time to achieve maximum benefit of local vasoconstriction. At this time, the patient typically receives a weight-based dose of cefazolin and 8 mg of dexamethasone intravenously [16].

4. Anesthesia

A crucial component of a successful and smooth surgery is profound local anesthesia, whether the patient is undergoing monitored anesthesia care (MAC) or general anesthesia. Regional nerve blocks are helpful to improve pain control, especially if the patient is under MAC.

Tumescent anesthesia consisting of 50 mL of 2% lidocaine and 0.5 mL of 1:1000 epinephrine mixed in a 250 mL bag of 0.9% normal saline is infiltrated throughout the patient's face and neck using a 20- or 22-gauge spinal needle connective to an automatic pump. The resultant solution consists of 0.4% lidocaine and 1:500,000 epinephrine. Alternatively, a 500 mL bag of 0.9% normal saline may be mixed with 50 mL of 1% lidocaine and 1 mL of 1:1000 epinephrine. Tranexamic acid (TXA), an antifibrinolytic that inhibits conversion of plasminogen to plasmin, may be mixed with local anesthetic or into the bag of tumescent anesthesia to reduce the risk of intraoperative bleeding and postoperative drainage [23]. In a prospective study involving 39 patients undergoing facelift surgery, Kochuba et al. demonstrated that the use of subcutaneous TXA injection, in conjunction with local anesthesia with epinephrine, has been shown to be safe, with less bleeding time, operating room time, and drain output when compared with traditional local anesthesia with epinephrine [24].

Another technique of local anesthesia administration is using 50 mL of a 1:1 mixture of 1% lidocaine with 1:100,000 epinephrine with 0.5% bupivacaine with 1:200,000 epinephrine. The resulting epinephrine concentration is 1:150,000, the lidocaine concentration is 0.5%, and the bupivacaine concentration is 0.25%. This solution is injected via standard needles on 10-mL syringes along planned incision lines and in the subcutaneous plane.

5. Technique

Early techniques of facelift surgery focused on small incisions near the hairline in natural skin creases with excision of skin and closure without underminding [3]. The main goal of the subcutaneous facelift is to tighten the loose facial skin and remove the excess without addressing deeper tissues. While relatively straightforward and safe, it fails to address ptosis of the midface and the effects of aging on structures deep to the skin [3].

Facelift surgery begins with a submentoplasty depending on the amount of subplatysmal fat, platysmal laxity, skin quality, and patient goals of treatment. Many facelift surgeons perform midline platysmal plication, which may reduce the amount of laxity of the muscle, but may also compromise some of the elevation that could otherwise be obtained in the jowl region.

A #15 blade is used to create a 2.5 to 3.5 cm curvilinear incision along the submental skin crease, or just posterior to it if a concomitant chin implant is to be inserted (**Figure 13**). The incision is undermined circumferentially in the subcutaneous plane to allow for insertion of facelift scissors. The facelift scissors are used to release the mandibular ligaments bilaterally and to undermine the skin while leaving an even layer of subdermal fat on the underside of the skin flap to maintain its blood supply. With the use of a lighted retractor, supraplatysmal dissection is carried inferiorly to the clavicles, posteriorly to the sternocleidomastoid muscle, and superiorly to the inferior border of the mandible (**Figure 14**). Wide skin undermining is necessary to allow proper skin redraping after treatment of deeper tissues has occurred [16].

Open suction-assisted lipectomy is then performed using a 6 mm spatulated cannula on the fat overlying the platysma muscle. Not only does open liposuction allow for better cervical contouring, but it also allows for better visualization of the platysma muscle and its boundaries.

Next, the medial edges of the platysma are identified and excised from the location of the submental incision inferiorly towards the clavicle using monopolar

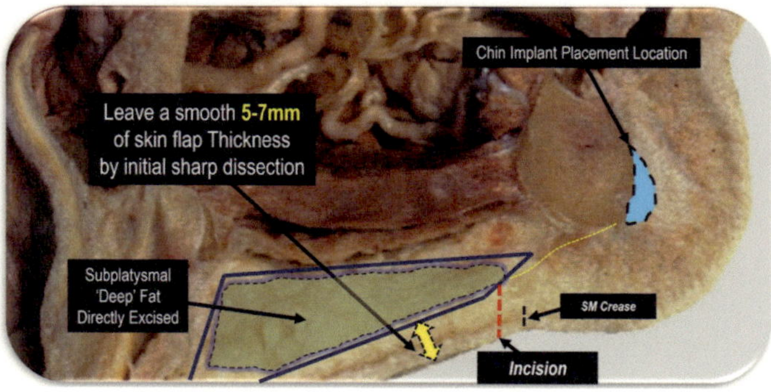

Figure 13.
It is critical to maintain an even healthy later of fat on the skin surface when planning direct excision of deep fat.

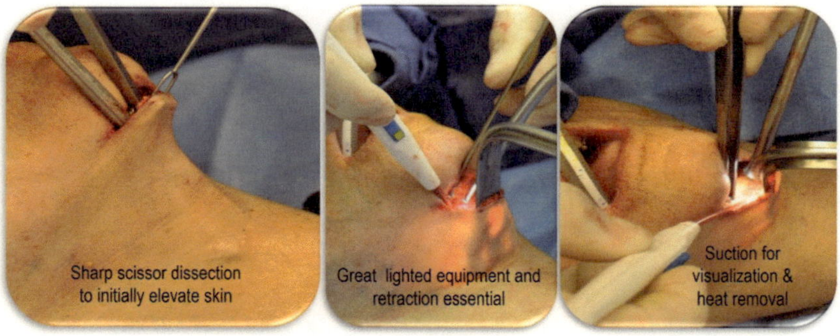

Figure 14.
A submental skin flap is made through a submental crease incision and supraplatysmal undermining is performed sharply using facelift scissors. Electrocautery is used for hemostasis while use of suction is critical in removing heat from the surgical site.

electrocautery. The cut edges of the platysma are identified and then bilateral platysmal myotomies are performed approximately 2 cm inferior to and parallel to the inferior border of the mandible. It is at this point where the bulging of the submandibular gland becomes most evident. Once the superior myotomy is completed, a second and more inferior myotomy is performed and extend to the most posterior end of the superior myotomy, thus creating a wedge of platysma muscle that is to be removed (**Figure 15**). Any associated subplatysmal fat is sharply removed with the platysma muscle.

After the subtotal platysmal excision, the submandibular gland is identified. If indicated for removal, the submandibular gland is exposed by making an incision through the superficial layer of the deep cervical fascia (SLDCF) along the inferior aspect of the bulge, parallel to the inferior border of the mandible. If the incision were placed more superiorly, the marginal mandibular branch of the facial nerve would be at higher risk of injury. Once the incision is made, the ptotic submandibular gland is visualized as it often herniates through the fascia (**Figure 16**). Carefully, the superficial portion of the submandibular gland is excised using monopolar electrocautery. The remaining deep portion of the submandibular gland is cauterized to ensure hemostasis. The SLDCF is then closed using resorbable suture to help reduce the risk of a post-operative sialocele. The submental incision is the packed with moist gauze while the lateral and posterior dissections take place.

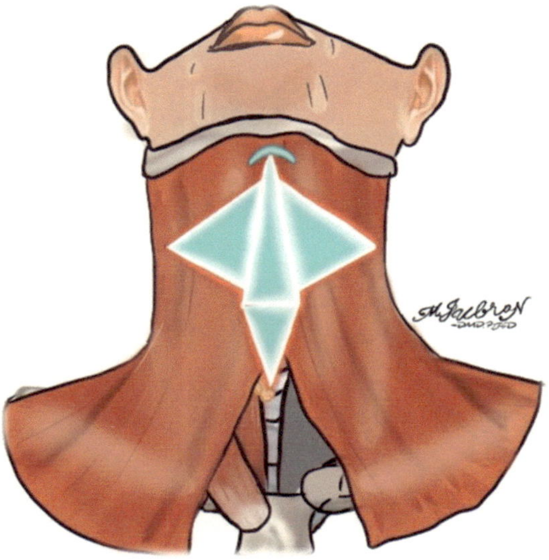

Figure 15.
The platysmal muscle and subplatysmal fat are sharply removed with electrocautery from the level of the curvilinear submental incision (blue curve) inferiorly towards the clavicles. A triangular platysmal wedge is excised laterally (blue triangle), with the superior border of the cut being parallel and approximately 2 cm inferior to the inferior border of the mandible.

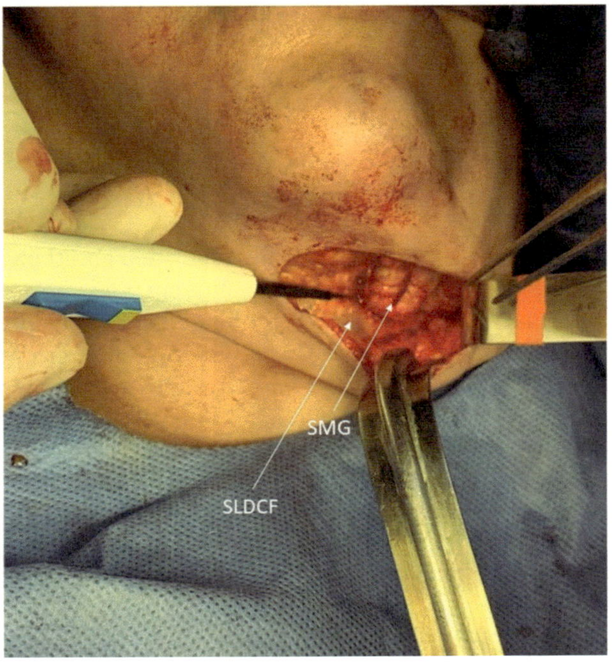

Figure 16.
The left submandibular gland (SMG) is seen herniating through an incision made in the superficial layer of the deep cervical fascia (SLDCF). The surface of the SMG resembles that of a walnut or a human brain.

The subcutaneous lateral dissection begins with a curvilinear beveled incision in the temporal tuft, above the level of the ear. The incision is through skin and into the subcutaneous layer. The incision is extended along the pre-auricular crease, endaural

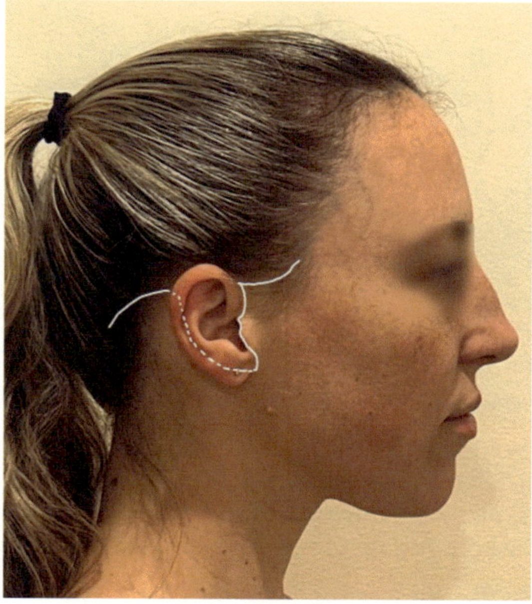

Figure 17.
Planned lateral facelift incisions. Advantages include a posterior scar hidden within the hairline and less risk for tissue ischemia because of thicker flaps. Disadvantages include a more challenging alignment of the posterior hairline.

along the tragus, and then in the crease of the ear lobe. Posteriorly, the incision is made along the ear crease, slightly on the conchal cartilage and extended towards the mastoid prominence within the hairline (**Figure 17**).

Facelift scissors are used to sharply dissect in a subcutaneous plane anteriorly to the area of the nasolabial fold, orbicularis oculi muscle, and about 1 cm lateral to the oral commissure, leaving an even layer of fat on the skin flap approximately 4–6 mm thick (**Figure 18**). The subcutaneous plane is connected with the neck dissection that was performed through the submental incision.

The posterior dissection occurs in the plane deep to the hair follicles to ensure that an adequate amount of fascia remains present for resuspension. Dissection is carried inferiorly to the level of the sternocleidomastoid fascia and extended approximately 2 cm inferiorly and medially. Facelift scissors are then used to connect with the neck dissection and the anterior subcutaneous dissection.

At this point, a decision is made on how to treat the SMAS. The key factor in determining how to treat the SMAS layer is what is required to give the patient the ideal and necessary elevation, making this portion of facelift surgery opportunistic [25].

The SMAS is incised along or just below the zygomatic arch, approximately 1 cm anterior to the helix. Sub-SMAS dissection then extends approximately 2 to 3 cm anteriorly. The SMAS is then undermined inferiorly in front of the ear and to the level of the cut platysma edge, which is about 2 cm inferior to the inferior border of the mandible (**Figure 18**). Care must be taken while in this plane to keep the parotidomasseteric fascia intact and to ensure adequate tissue coverage over the zygomatic arch and facial nerve branches. Once the posterior edge of the SMAS is adequately released, dissection proceeds anteriorly across the anterior border of the parotid gland and may expose the underlying masseteric fascia. At this point, the buccal branch of the facial nerve and Stensen's duct may be identified (**Figure 8**).

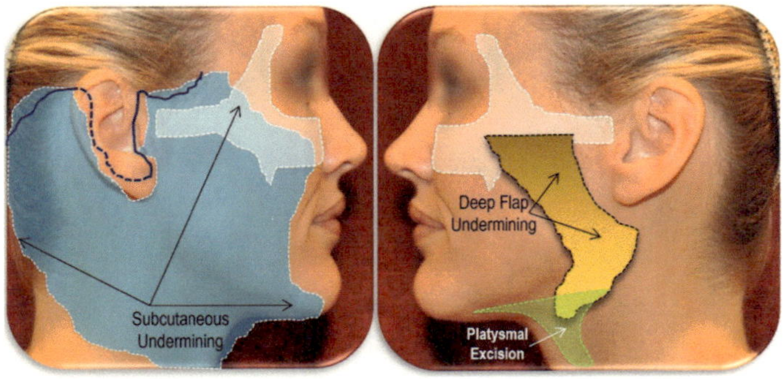

Figure 18.
Average incisions, subcutaneous and deep plane dissection planes.

As dissection approaches the inferior border of the mandible, care is taken to avoid injuring the marginal mandibular branch of the facial nerve. This may be done by clearly visualizing the deep surface of the platysma muscle and keeping the fascia intact over the nerve.

Once hemostasis is achieved and adequate deep plane dissection has occurred based on the patient's tissue quality and retaining ligaments, the vector of elevation is determined. Generally, a posterosuperior vector is chosen for deep plane and skin flap elevation. However, vectors differ slightly anterior to and posterior to the ear in order to provide the most naturally esthetic outcome. The deep plane is lifted more superiorly in front of the ear, whereas the skin is slightly more oblique anteriorly. The opposite is true posterior to the ear, where the skin is re-draped in a more superior vector and the deep plane is more obliquely positioned (**Figure 19**) [25]. In this region, the platysma and SMAS may be manipulated in a number of ways. The cut edge of the platysma may be cut, folded upon itself, and plicated in the region of the mandibular angle to accentuate the gonial angle (**Figure 20**).

Regardless of whether the surgeon is using more conservative SMAS techniques, such as plication or imbrication, or the deep plane approach, key anchoring sutures are crucial to elevating and resuspending the SMAS. The first key suture is placed at the inferior tragus and then the superior tragus. The cut edge of the platysma muscle is then suspended to the mastoid fascia. The temporoparietal fascia and

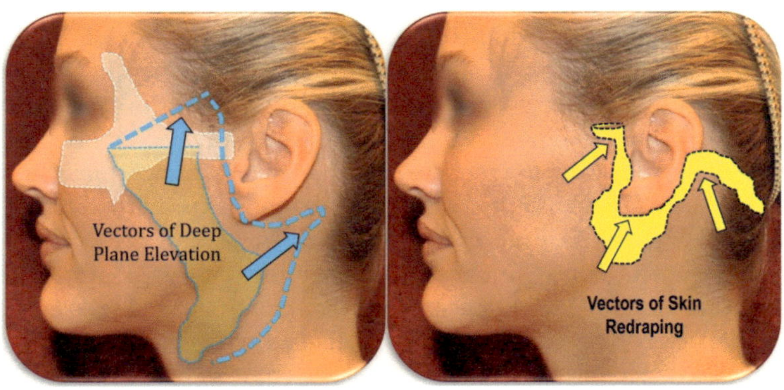

Figure 19.
The vectors of deep plane elevation / lifting shown above are different than those of skin elevation / re-draping. The vectors of skin re-draping prior to excision are passive with minimal tension.

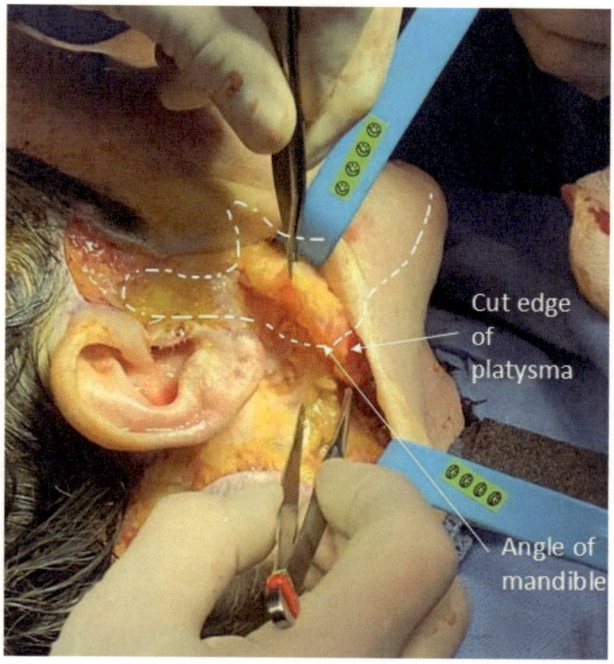

Figure 20.
The cut edge of the platysma can be manipulated and plicated to 'auto-augment' the mandibular angle. The mandible, outlined in white, can be augmented or accentuated in other ways such as the platysmal hammock, in which the platysma is secured to the mastoid fascia and draped under the angle of the mandible, fat grafting, and mandibular angle implants.

SMAS are sutured to the deeper temporalis fascia and the subcutaneous tissue is subsequently closed.

Next, the skin is re-draped. The position of the earlobe base is chosen so as to not apply tension in the inferior direction and result in a pixie ear deformity. The skin is secured to the base of the earlobe. The posterior skin flap is advanced anteriorly towards the ear, ensuring that the hairline is aligned properly. The skin flap is closed in layers as the excess skin is trimmed with facelift scissors to allow for tension-free closure. The skin is closed with resorbable suture.

If indicated, a Jackson-Pratt drain may be placed through the submental incision, exiting the undermined tissue in the postauricular region. The submental incision is closed in layers. Finally, antibiotic ointment or Aquaphor is generously applied to the incisions after suture placement and dressings are placed with minor pressure to avoid vascular compromise to the skin flaps [25].

5.1 SMAS techniques

Soon after the SMAS layer was thoroughly described by Mitz and Peyronie, [5] a major paradigm shift in facelift surgery occurred. The fibrous adhesions of the SMAS to the overlying subcutaneous fat and skin allowed for surgical manipulation of the SMAS to effect changes in the skin [3]. The main methods for addressing the SMAS involve either plication or imbrication [3]. Plication relies on suture suspension alone whereas imbrication consists of an incision within the SMAS layer with resection of a portion of the SMAS followed by suture suspension of the ends to reverse vectors of aging [3]. Richard Webster was one of the first to recommend a "short flap" with

SMAS plication [26]. Imbrication typically involves a limited sub-SMAS dissection to the anterior border of the parotid gland [3].

When performed properly, SMAS plication and imbrication pose minor risk to the facial nerve while achieving good long-term results [3]. However, SMAS plication and imbrication are less effective in rejuvenating the midface and melolabial fold as they are the jaw-neck line [3].

5.2 Deep plane techniques

A glaring weakness of employing SMAS techniques during facelift surgery is its inability to effectively rejuvenate the midface and malar fat pad [3] In 1990, Dr. Hamra described the deep-plane rhytidectomy to address this problem, in which he elevated the soft tissues of the midfacial region between the superficial and deep fascia [27] Dr. Hamra's technique consisted of a subcutaneous dissection in the pre-auricular region that extended anteriorly to a line extended from the lateral canthus to the angle of the mandible, at which point dissection proceeded in the sub-SMAS plane. The sub-SMAS dissection is carried medially over the zygomaticus major and minor muscles to an area lateral to the melolabial fold [3].

The deep-plane technique is meant to improve the nasolabial fold, neck and midface to a greater extent than either SMAS plication or imbrication. However, whether or not it truly does is a matter of debate. Proponents for the deep-plane technique also claim longer lasting improvement, a natural appearance, and decreased incidence of hematoma and flap compromise [3]. The disadvantages of the deep-plane technique include more extensive tissue trauma, longer recovery period, more technical dissection with increased risk of injury to the facial nerve, and longer operative time [3]. Even when performed by experienced surgeons, the deep-plane facelift places facial nerve branches at more risk of injury during dissection than the SMAS techniques [28].

Ivy et al. found no detectable improvements in a side-by-side comparison in patients with SMAS facelifts versus composite rhytidectomies [3, 29]. Becker and Bassichis concluded that for patients under the age of 70 years, the deep-plane facelift did not offer superior results over SMAS plication facelifts [3, 28]. In their small study population, however, they did note that patients aged 50–69 years had a trend towards obtaining better results from SMAS plication facelifts whereas patients aged 70–80 years had a trend towards obtaining better results from a deep-plane facelift [28].

The composite facelift, which addresses the neck, lower face, midface / lower lid junction, and upper face with volume augmentation, is a more comprehensive technique for facial rejuvenation. It involves repositioning of essentially every deep structure whose character influences the topography of the face [6]. This approach, which was first described in 1992, incorporates the orbicularis oculi muscle with the facelift flap so that the orbicularis oculi muscle, malar fat, and platysma muscle would all be left with the skin and their intimate relationship would be maintained [6, 30, 31]. According to Choucair and Hamra, there are four structures that need to be addressed in a composite rhytidectomy: the platysma / SMAS, the meso-mandibularis mesentery, the fat overlying the zygomaticus major and minor muscles, and the lower eyelid fat [6]. The composite facelift vector involves a strong superior medial vector of the upper face and an obligatory medial vector of the forehead lift [6]. Lastly, an arcus marginalis release with preservation of the lower eyelid fat is necessary to create more youthful appearing lower eyelid [6].

5.3 Less invasive techniques

Shortly after the deep-plane facelift became popular, a counter school of thought emerged towards less invasive techniques. Deep-plane facelifts required more operative time, involved more risk, and necessitated longer recovery periods. The minimally invasive techniques offered less downtime, less surgical time, and were often less risky and could be performed under local anesthesia [3]. However, skepticism remains at large as some believe that "short scar" facelifts are much less than a true facelift and provide less result and longevity when compared to a traditional rhytidectomy [21].

One of the "non-surgical" techniques that emerged in the 1990s was the threadlift. This technique involved the placement of barbed threads subcutaneously which were pulled in the appropriate vector to achieve a lifting effect, with excess suture being trimmed at the entry point [3]. A main advantage of this technique was its "non-surgical" nature and instant results. However, the longevity and effectiveness of the procedure was shortly brought into question [3].

In 1999, the "S-lift" was brought back into popularity by Dr. Saylan, who claims the technique was originally developed in the 1960s. This short-scar technique involved an S-shaped skin excision across the non-hair-baring skin at the helical root, skin excision, and vertical and O-shaped purse-string sutures though the SMAS and parotid fascia in small bites. The permanent sutures were secured to posterolateral periosteum of the zygomatic arch to achieve the lift [32]. The most obvious shortcoming of this technique was the inability to improve the cervicomental angle and overall neck laxity [33].

The S-lift technique was later modified by Tonnard et al. who dubbed the procedure the Minimal Access Cranial Suspension Lift (MACS lift). The authors changed the location of the incision to follow the border of the sideburn, excised skin after the lift, and placed purse-string plication sutures to the temporal fascia, rather than the zygomatic arch [3, 34]. The MACS lift was noted to have similar results to SMAS plication and imbrication techniques [35].

5.4 Volumetric techniques

Facial aging does not solely involve the descent of soft tissue as a result of gravity, but other processes such as loss of facial volume and tissue elasticity. It is now understood that deflation is a major component of the complex facial aging phenomenon and cannot be corrected by facelift surgery alone [36]. Contemporary surgeons appreciate that adding volume in the midfacial region, whether by injectables or facial implants, results in greater rejuvenation that facelift surgery alone [21]. Younger-appearing people tend to have fuller cheeks and a more rounded facial contour which eventually give way to a more aged appearance with hollowing, accentuation of bony contours and thin skin. While many surgical techniques focus on addressing the soft tissue descent, they are limited in addressing volumetric changes and skin quality. This is why many cosmetic and plastic surgeons today incorporate volumization into their treatment algorithms while performing facelifts [3].

The idea of soft tissue fillers has been around since the late 1800s. Materials still being used today include autologous fat, silicone, collagen, calcium hydroxyapatite, poly-L-lactic acid, and hyaluronic acid products. Of these, the hyaluronic acid products are most widely used due to their longevity, efficacy, safety, and reversibility [3]. Hyaluronidase is readily available to be injected and breakdown the injected hyaluronic acid filler, which can help reverse rare catastrophic events such as intra-arterial infiltration [3]. The development of longer lasting injectable fillers and the realization of the benefit of adjunctive volume restoration have led surgeons to select simpler facelift techniques [6].

Another option for facial volumization is facial implants. Malar, infraorbital, and nasal implants offer ways to add volume back to the midface whereas chin and mandibular angle implants offer ways to add volume to the lower facial third.

6. Complications

Several factors have been shown to consistently predispose patients to complications after facelift surgery: preoperative intake of aspirin or other anti-platelet or anticoagulant drugs, active smoking, intraoperative use of epinephrine, postoperative emesis, and poorly controlled blood pressure [22]. Male patients also carry a much higher risk of postoperative hematoma due to the more vascular, sebaceous, thicker facial skin compared with females [22].

As patients undergoing facelift surgery are often elderly and may have multi-system disease while being on several medications, it is essential to have patients properly screened, medically optimized by their physician(s), and undergo a proper preoperative work-up. With proper preoperative screening, older patients can undergo rhytidectomy with relatively low risk [19]. One of the surest ways to prevent tragic complications, such as death, is for the surgeon to do his or her due diligence in preparing the patient appropriately.

Complications from facelift surgery can be divided into three broad categories: intraoperative, early postoperative, and late postoperative.

Intraoperative complications include: unexpected bleeding, anesthetic complications, undiagnosed ptotic submandibular glands, cyanotic fap or perforated flap, nerve injury, and irregularities [25].

Submandibular glands tend to descend and become more ptotic with age despite coverage from the superficial layer of the deep cervical fascia. A ptotic gland, however, may go unnoticed preoperatively due to older patients often presenting with skin laxity and jowling. When the SMAS is pulled posterosuperiorly intraoperatively, a ptotic submandibular gland may be recognized as a persistent bulge in the antegonial notch region. To address this issue, some surgeons advocate for a submandibular sling to elevate the gland superiomedially. This technique does not always achieve its intended goal and, thus, a better course of action would be to redirect and manipulate the SMAS layer or perform a submandibular gland reduction [16].

Smokers present well-known surgical and anesthetic risks to facelift surgery. From an anesthetic perspective, smokers tend to have more reactive airways, increased secretions, decreased lung capacity, and oxygenation problems [37].

Early postoperative complications include: hematoma, infection, wound dehiscence, skin flap necrosis, and motor and sensory nerve dysfunction [25].

Preoperative management of baseline hypertension is critical to decrease the risk of hematoma [22]. Indeed, elevated systolic blood pressure is the most common modifiable risk factor for postoperative hematoma [19]. Administering clonidine 0.1 to 0.2 mg before surgery has been useful in stabilizing and lowering blood pressure adequately during the perioperative period to reduce the risk of hemorrhage [16, 22, 37]. Preoperative smoking, a history of aspirin or NSAID intake, and male gender have also been shown to increase the risk of hematoma formation [38].

Early intervention in suspected expanding hematoma is the most reliable measure to prevent devastating complications of the facelift surgery [22] Small, undrained hematomas may lead to skin contour irregularities and pigment changes [12, 19]. An expanding hematoma is a true emergency in facelift surgery and requires expeditious surgical evacuation to prevent airway compromise and skin flap necrosis [19, 37].

Postoperative infection following rhytidectomy is uncommon. In a systematic review of various SMAS facelift techniques, Jacono et al. report an postoperative infection rate of 0.53, 0.77, 0.73, and 1.12% in SMAS plication, SMASecotmy / imbrication, deep plane, and composite facelifts, respectively [39]. The main pathologic offenders of postoperative infection tend to be members of the *Staphylococcus* species. To reduce the incidence of postoperative methicillin-resistant *Staphylococcus aureus* (MRSA) infections, patients who are MRSA carriers should be treated with topical nasal mupirocin ointment, chlorohexidine mouth rinse and full-body chlorohexidine soap for 5 days preoperatively [40]. Additionally, MRSA carriers should be given vancomycin, rather than a first-generation cephalosporin, as a preoperative antibiotic [19].

Active smoking is the most common preoperative risk factor for skin necrosis postoperatively. In a retrospective study, Rees et al. report that smokers were 12.46 times more likely to suffer skin sloughing when compared with nonsmokers and that smokers have a 7.5% chance of developing skin slough after rhytidectomy [41].

Patients undergoing facelift surgery should be counseled preoperatively about some sensory deficits after their procedure, especially in the pre- and postauricular areas [37]. Usually, the altered sensation is temporary and may resolve over a 90-day period. Similarly and fortunately, weakness of the muscles of facial expression, caused by injury to branches of the facial nerve, is typically temporary and resolves over a period of weeks to months. Damage to the facial nerve branches may be caused by direct injury, neuropraxia, thermal injury, compression injury, or other causes [37]. For both sensory and motor nerve injuries, patient should be reassured that the effects are likely temporary. For motor nerve injuries that do not improve over the course of 90 days, consultation with a microneurosurgeon is strongly advised [37].

Late postoperative complications include: abnormal wound healing, earlobe distortion, alopecia, hairline changes, platysmal banding, skin pigment changes, chronic pain, numbness, or facial weakness, sialocele, seroma, and a dissatisfied patient [25].

Incision design plays a vital role in proper healing and preventing distortion of anatomic structures. Patients should be marked while in an upright position and prior to injection of any tumescent or local anesthesia to avoid gravitational changes in skin draping and prevent distortion of anatomical landmarks, respectively. Improper incision placement may lead to unesthetic scarring, transposition of hair-bearing skin to a region normally without hair, increased wound tension, and distortion of anatomic structures.

Due to the nature of a deep-plane facelift, including submentoplasty, the large amount of dead space that is created increases the chance for postoperative fluid accumulation in the form of seroma, sialocele or hematoma. Sources of sialoceles post-facelift surgery may be the parotid or submandibular gland. Although sialoceles rarely require surgical management, treatment often requires serial aspirations, antisialagogue medication, and gentle pressure dressings. Sialoceles from the parotid gland tend to have much higher fluid collections than those from the submandibular gland and may take up to 1 month to fully resolve [12]. If parotid gland injury is detected intraoperatively, the injured tissue may be cauterized and sealed under

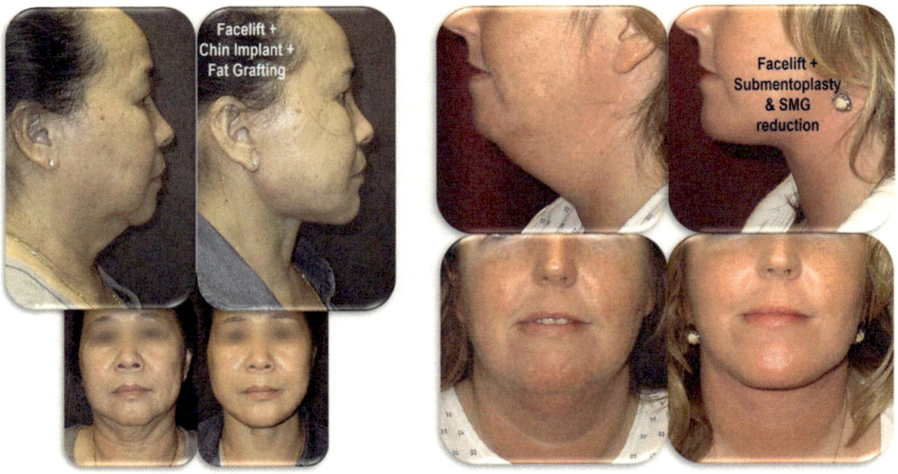

Figure 21.
Patients are shown before and after facelift surgery in conjunction with other facial cosmetic procedures. One of the most drastic areas of improvement for these patients is the cerviomental region which was obtuse preoperatively and is now more acute. Additionally, their jawline is more defined. (SMG – submandibular gland).

SMAS closure to reduce the risk of a parotid sialocele [19]. Similarly, after submandibular gland reduction, the SLDCF may be closed over the submandibular gland to minimize risk of a submandibular gland sialocele. It should be noted that the reliability of these methods is unclear.

Patients who are unhappy or dissatisfied with their results are likely to voice their opinions to the surgeon. The surgeon must be attentive, listen carefully, and not be defensive. Ideally, through the detailed consultation and preoperative evaluation, patients with unrealistic expectations would have been denied surgery or gone elsewhere. The patient must be advised that if a revision surgery is indicated, enough time should pass to allow adequate healing from the initial procedure as this will allow for a better, rather than rushed, result.

7. Conclusion

Facelift surgery has evolved dramatically since its inception. Better understanding of surgical anatomy, advances in technology, and the increase in number of well-trained and qualified surgeons have led to the development of safe, reproducible, long-lasting, and effective techniques. Despite these advances, the surgeon must be patient, understand his or her patients, and develop a comprehensive treatment plan to prevent complications and obtain superior results (**Figure 21**).

Author details

Anthony Congiusta[1*], Angelo Cuzalina[2] and Maria Jubran-Khoury[3]

1 Connecticut Surgical Arts, Norwich, Connecticut, USA

2 Tulsa Surgical Arts, Tulsa, Oklahoma, USA

3 Headandneck Artist, Tel Aviv, Israel

*Address all correspondence to: anthony.congiusta.90@gmail.com

References

[1] Niamtu J. Cosmetic Facial Surgery. 2nd ed. Elsevier: OHCE; 2017. Available from: https://bookshelf.health.elsevier.com/books/9780323394031

[2] Tobin HA, Cuzalina A. Chapter 27 SMAS surgery versus deep-plane rhytidectomy. In: Controversies in Otolaryngology. Stuttgart: Georg Thieme Verlag KG; 2001. Available from: http://www.thieme-connect.de/products/ebooks/lookinside/10.1055/b-0034-50973

[3] Barrett DM, Casanueva FJ, Wang TD. Evolution of the rhytidectomy. World Journal of Otorhinolaryngology Head and Neck Surgery. 2016;**2**(1):38-44. DOI: 10.1016/j.wjorl.2015.12.001

[4] Skoog T. New Methods and Refinements: Plastic Surgery. Philadelphia: WB Saunders; 1974

[5] Mitz V, Peyronie M. The superficial musculo-aponeurotic system (SMAS) in the parotid and cheek area. Plastic and Reconstructive Surgery. 1976;**58**(1):80-88. DOI: 10.1097/00006534-197607000-00013

[6] Choucair RJ, Hamra ST. Extended superficial musculaponeurotic system dissection and composite rhytidectomy. Clinics in Plastic Surgery. 2008;**35**(4):607-622. DOI: 10.1016/j.cps.2008.05.014

[7] Sykes J, Dilger A, Cotofana S. Demystifying the deep plane facelift: What it means anatomically and why it works. Facial Plastic Surgery. 2020;**36**(4):351-357. DOI: 10.1055/s-0040-1714267

[8] Cuzalina AL, Tolomeo PG, Mañón VA. Neck lift with platysma excision. Advances in Cosmetic Surgery. 2022;**5**(1):79-97. DOI: 10.1016/j.yacs.2022.01.003

[9] Minelli L, van der Lei B, Mendelson BC. The deep fascia of the head and neck revisited: Relationship with the facial nerve and implications for Rhytidectomy. Plastic and Reconstructive Surgery. 2024;**153**(6):1273-1288. DOI: 10.1097/PRS.0000000000010556

[10] Cho GS, Kim JH, Yeo NK, Kim SH, Jang YJ. Nasal skin thickness measured using computed tomography and its effect on tip surgery outcomes. Otolaryngology and Head and Neck Surgery. 2011;**144**(4):522-527. DOI: 10.1177/0194599811398936

[11] Jost G, Levet Y. Parotid fascia and face lifting: A critical evaluation of the SMAS concept. Plastic and Reconstructive Surgery. 1984;**74**(1):42-51. DOI: 10.1097/00006534-198407000-00006

[12] Cuzalina LA, Koehler J. Submentoplasty and facial liposuction. Oral and Maxillofacial Surgery Clinics of North America. 2005;**17**(1):85-98. DOI: 10.1016/j.coms.2004.09.008

[13] Cardoso de Castro C. The value of anatomical study of the platysma muscle in cervical lifting. Aesthetic Plastic Surgery. 1984;**8**(1):7-11. DOI: 10.1007/BF01572778

[14] Minelli L, Brown CP, van der Lei B, Mendelson B. Anatomy of the facial Glideplanes, deep plane spaces, and ligaments: Implications for surgical and nonsurgical lifting procedures. Plastic and Reconstructive Surgery. 2024;**154**(1):95-110. DOI: 10.1097/PRS.0000000000011078

[15] Mendelson BC, Tutino R. Submandibular gland reduction in aesthetic surgery of the neck: Review of 112 consecutive cases. Plastic and Reconstructive Surgery. 2015;**136**(3):463-471. DOI: 10.1097/PRS.0000000000001526

[16] Cuzalina A, Copty TV, Ali Khan H. Rhytidectomy (face-lifting). In: Current Therapy in Oral and Maxillofacial Surgery. Philadelphia, PA, USA: Saunders; 2012

[17] Kucukguven A, Ulkir M, Bilgic Kucukguven M, Demiryurek MD, Vargel I. Defining a Preauricular safe zone: A cadaveric study of the frontotemporal branch of the facial nerve. Aesthetic Surgery Journal. 2021;**41**(4):398-407. DOI: 10.1093/asj/sjaa232

[18] Truswell WH. Approaches to reducing risk in Rhytidectomy surgery. Facial Plastic Surgery Clinics of North America. 2020;**28**(3):419-427. DOI: 10.1016/j.fsc.2020.03.008

[19] Sinclair NR, Coombs DM, Kwiecien G, Zins JE. How to prevent and treat complications in facelift surgery, part 1: Short-term complications. Aesthetic surgery journal. Open forum. 2021;**3**(1):ojab007. DOI: 10.1093/asjof/ojab007

[20] Schaner PJ. Evaluation of the esthetic surgery patient. Atlas of the Oral and Maxillofacial Surgery Clinics of North America. 2004;**12**(1):1-30. DOI: 10.1016/j.cxom.2003.10.004

[21] Niamtu J. Evaluation of the facelift patient. Atlas of the Oral and Maxillofacial Surgery Clinics of North America. 2014;**22**(1):1-8. DOI: 10.1016/j.cxom.2013.10.002

[22] Santosa KB, Oliver JD, Thompson G, Beil RJ. Perioperative Management of the Facelift Patient. Clinics in Plastic Surgery. 2019;**46**(4):625-639. DOI: 10.1016/j.cps.2019.06.008

[23] Schroeder RJ, Langsdon PR. Effect of local tranexamic acid on hemostasis in rhytidectomy. Facial Plastic Surgery & Aesthetic Medicine. 2020;**22**(3):195-199. DOI: 10.1089/fpsam.2020.0061

[24] Kochuba AL, Coombs DM, Kwiecien GJ, Sinclair NR, Zins JE. Prospective study assessing the effect of local infiltration of Tranexamic acid on facelift bleeding. Aesthetic Surgery Journal. 2021;**41**(4):391-397. DOI: 10.1093/asj/sjaa198

[25] Cuzalina A, Amoli B. The opportunistic rhytidectomy: The biplane facelift. Atlas of the Oral and Maxillofacial Surgery Clinics of North America. 2014;**22**(1):53-67. DOI: 10.1016/j.cxom.2013.10.003

[26] Webster RC, Davidson TM, White MF, Bush JE, Smith RC. Conservative face lift surgery. Archives of Otolaryngology. 1976;**102**(11):657-662. DOI: 10.1001/archotol.1976.00780160053003

[27] Hamra ST. The deep-plane rhytidectomy. Plastic and Reconstructive Surgery. 1990;**86**(1):53-61

[28] Becker FF, Bassichis BA. Deep-plane face-lift vs superficial musculoaponeurotic system plication face-lift: A comparative study. Archives of Facial Plastic Surgery. 2004;**6**(1):8-13. DOI: 10.1001/archfaci.6.1.8

[29] Ivy EJ, Lorenc ZP, Aston SJ. Is there a difference? A prospective study comparing lateral and standard SMAS face lifts with extended SMAS and composite rhytidectomies. Plastic and Reconstructive Surgery. 1996;**98**(7):1135-1143.

DOI: 10.1097/00006534-199612000-00001

[30] Hamra ST. Composite rhytidectomy. Plastic and Reconstructive Surgery. 1992;**90**(1):1-13. DOI: 10.1097/00006534-199207000-00001

[31] Hamra ST. Repositioning the orbicularis oculi muscle in the composite rhytidectomy. Plastic and Reconstructive Surgery. 1992;**90**(1):14-22. DOI: 10.1097/00006534-199207000-00002

[32] Saylan Z. The S-lift: Less is more. Aesthetic Surgery Journal. 1999;**19**(5):406-409. DOI: 10.1053/aq.1999.v19.101748001

[33] Karam AM, Nayak LM, Lam SM. Short-scar purse-string facelift. Facial Plastic Surgery Clinics of North America. 2009;**17**(4):549-556. DOI: 10.1016/j.fsc.2009.06.007

[34] Tonnard P, Verpaele A, Monstrey S, et al. Minimal access cranial suspension lift: A modified S-lift. Plastic and Reconstructive Surgery. 2002;**109**(6):2074-2086. DOI: 10.1097/00006534-200205000-00046

[35] Prado A, Andrades P, Danilla S, Castillo P, Leniz P. A clinical retrospective study comparing two short-scar face lifts: Minimal access cranial suspension versus lateral SMASectomy. Plastic and Reconstructive Surgery. 2006;**117**(5):1413-1425. DOI: 10.1097/01.prs.0000207402.53411.1e

[36] Rohrich RJ, Durand PD, Dayan E. The lift-and-fill facelift: Superficial musculoaponeurotic system manipulation with fat compartment augmentation. Clinics in Plastic Surgery. 2019;**46**(4):515-522. DOI: 10.1016/j.cps.2019.06.001

[37] Niamtu J. Complications in facelift surgery and their prevention. Oral and Maxillofacial Surgery Clinics of North America. 2009;**21**(1):59-80. DOI: 10.1016/j.coms.2008.10.001

[38] Grover R, Jones BM, Waterhouse N. The prevention of haematoma following rhytidectomy: A review of 1078 consecutive facelifts. British Journal of Plastic Surgery. 2001;**54**(6):481-486. DOI: 10.1054/bjps.2001.3623

[39] Jacono AA, Alemi AS, Russell JL. A meta-analysis of complication rates among different SMAS facelift techniques. Aesthetic Surgery Journal. 2019;**39**(9):927-942. DOI: 10.1093/asj/sjz045

[40] Buehlmann M, Frei R, Fenner L, Dangel M, Fluckiger U, Widmer AF. Highly effective regimen for decolonization of methicillin-resistant *Staphylococcus aureus* carriers. Infection Control and Hospital Epidemiology. 2008;**29**(6):510-516. DOI: 10.1086/588201

[41] Rees TD, Liverett DM, Guy CL. The effect of cigarette smoking on skin-flap survival in the face lift patient. Plastic and Reconstructive Surgery. 1984;**73**(6):911-915. DOI: 10.1097/00006534-198406000-00009

Chapter 2

Endoscopic Forehead and Eyebrow Surgery

Anthony Congiusta, Angelo Cuzalina and Maria Jubran-Khoury

Abstract

Esthetic concerns of the forehead and eyebrow regions affect people within a wide range of age groups. While many facial cosmetic surgical procedures are typically performed on patients in their mid-40s or older, an endoscopic forehead and brow lift, as well as other types of browlifts, may be performed on younger patients because of their genetic predisposition. Additionally, aging does eventually lead to forehead and brow ptosis for nearly all patients. The surgeon must address all problems to achieve optimal results and patient satisfaction. The goal of this chapter is to review relevant facial anatomy, indications and contraindications, surgical technique, and complications as they pertain to eyebrow and forehead cosmetic surgery.

Keywords: browlift, endoscopic browlift, blepharoplasty, forehead lift, minimally invasive

1. Introduction

The forehead, eyebrows and eyes are among the most important determinants of facial expression. They allow people to express a range of emotions. Raised eyebrows and wide-open eyes may indicate surprise whereas scrunched brows and squinted eyes may indicate anger. Indeed, Charles Darwin, in his book *The Expression of the Emotion in Man and Animals*, refers to the corrugators as "grief-muscles" due to their conjoint yet opposed action resulting in the formation of furrows on the forehead and their association with the emotional states of grief and sadness [1, 2]. The upper third of the face plays an integral role in facial harmony and esthetics. As aging occurs, many people experience similar changes, namely tissue descent, in the upper facial third due to gravity, sun exposure, and genetic factors. Heavy forehead and glabellar skin with deep facial rhytids and eyebrow ptosis lead to a tired and aged appearance [3].

Many techniques have been developed to rejuvenate the upper facial third, none more popular than injection of botulinum toxin type A, which is the most common cosmetic procedure globally [4]. When treating the aging face, it is critical to correctly diagnose and identify areas that need to be addressed. There are several types of surgical techniques to address the brows and forehead including the endoscopic, coronal, direct, anterior hairline, posterior hairline, transblepharoplasty, suture suspension, barbed threads, and radiofrequency browlifts [5].

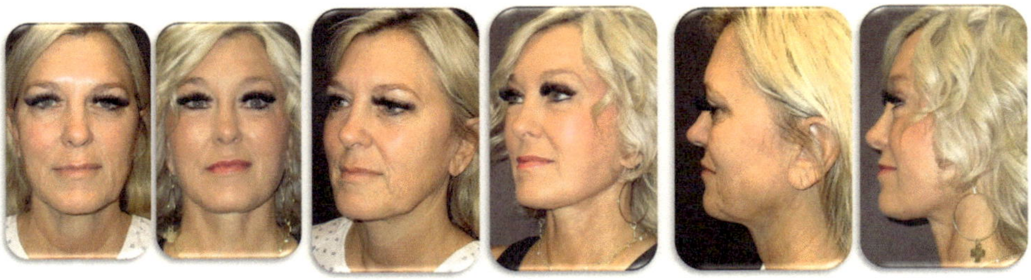

Figure 1.
A 57 year-old woman shown before and 1.5 years following a deep plane facelift, endoscopic forehead and brow lift, and facial laser resurfacing. The outer third of her eyebrow region (hooding) is the defining area improved by a good brow lift.

Unlike the lower third of the face, which may require treatment in many patients older than 40 years, the upper third of the face may be indicated for rejuvenation in patients in their 20s or 30s due to genetic predisposition [6, 7]. Thus, a comprehensive examination of the entire face must be performed by the cosmetic surgeon in order to achieve superior outcomes and patient satisfaction. Failing to address the upper third of the face in a patient who, for example, is presenting for facelift surgery, will lead to suboptimal results.

Due to gravity and time, the aging process causes a descent of soft tissues and typically results in forehead and brow ptosis which, in turn, may lead to lateral hooding and visual field deficits (**Figure 1**) [8]. Patients who present with signs of aging of the upper facial third also typically present with excessive wrinkling, fatigued-appearing eyes, and excess upper eyelid skin laxity [7]. They may also present with facial volume loss and evidence of photodamage. Specific elevation and correction of the upper facial third and lateral eyelid hooding, along with a reduction in wrinkling and treatment of any photodamage can result in a naturally appearing and rejuvenated look that will enhance the patient's overall beauty. The goals of a browlift are to stabilize the brow at an esthetically pleasing height and morphology and to decrease forehead and glabellar rhytids, lateral canthal hooding, and infrabrow skin while concealing scarring and avoiding the stigmata of facial cosmetic surgery, namely an elevated hairline, over elevated brows, and a surprised appearance [8, 9].

The goal of this chapter is to review relevant facial anatomy, indications and contraindications, the author's preferred surgical technique, and complications as they pertain to eyebrow and forehead cosmetic surgery.

2. Anatomy

The face is commonly thought of as being divided into equal horizontal thirds and vertical fifths. The upper facial third is measured from trichion (the midline point of one's normal hairline) to glabella (the smooth prominence between one's brows) [6, 10]. The middle and lower facial thirds are measured from glabella to subnasale (the midline point where the nasal septum meets the upper lip) and from subnasale to menton (the most inferior point of the chin), respectively [6]. The vertical facial fifths are measured from the pinna to the lateral canthus on both sides, the lateral canthus to medial canthus on both sides, and medial canthus to medial canthus centrally (**Figure 2**) [10].

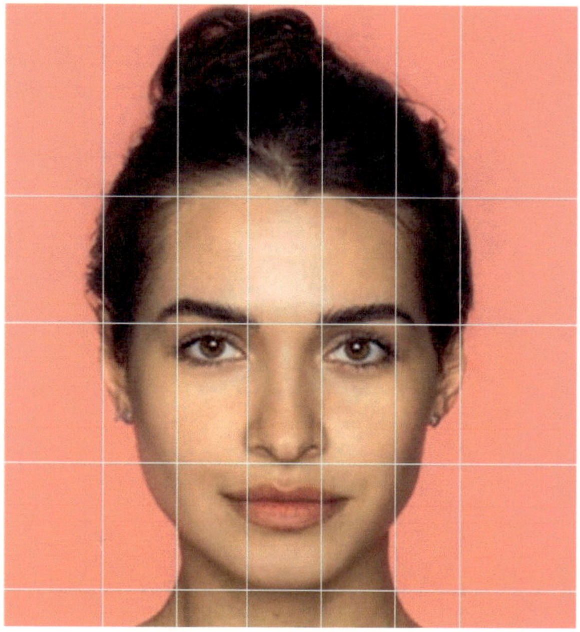

Figure 2.
While no patient's face is perfectly symmetric, understanding the relationship between facial height and width will allow the cosmetic surgeon to better achieve facial harmony.

Generally, in a non-receded hairline, the hairline should be 5 cm from the brow in females and 6 cm from the brow in males [10]. An esthetic female eyebrow is arched and positioned just above the orbital rim with the peak of the brow between the middle and lateral third of the brow. The lateral third of the female brow ideally lies roughly 0.5–1 cm above the orbital rim [6].

Regarding the bony anatomy, the frontal bone comprises much of the upper facial third. Male foreheads are longer, with a vertically oriented slope that increases in projection over the frontal sinus whereas female foreheads are rounder and have a less prominent glabellar ridge that smoothly transitions into the nasal dorsum without increased projection over the nasofrontal area [11]. Parts of the zygoma, parietal bone, nasal bones, and maxilla also provide important landmarks for surgeons during many browlift approaches. Suture lines such as the nasofrontal, fronto-zygomatic, lambdoid, and coronal, are important landmarks to identify during the endoscopic forehead and browlift technique because they can represent limits of subperiosteal dissection and act as reference points for navigating the surgical equipment during the procedure [6]. Important anatomic structures can also be identified and protected once the suture lines are encountered, such as the sentinel vein, or the medial zygomaticotemporal vein, and frontal branch of the facial nerve which run just posterior and inferior to the fronto-zygomatico suture line (**Figure 3**).

The nasofrontal suture is an important bony landmark as endoscopic subperiosteal dissection only needs to proceed a few millimeters past this suture line onto the nasal bones for adequate release. If nasal tip rotation is indicated or if the nasofrontal angle needs to be slightly modified, the dissection can proceed further caudally along the nasal bones. The paired procerus muscle is also located near the nasofrontal suture and may be transected if necessary.

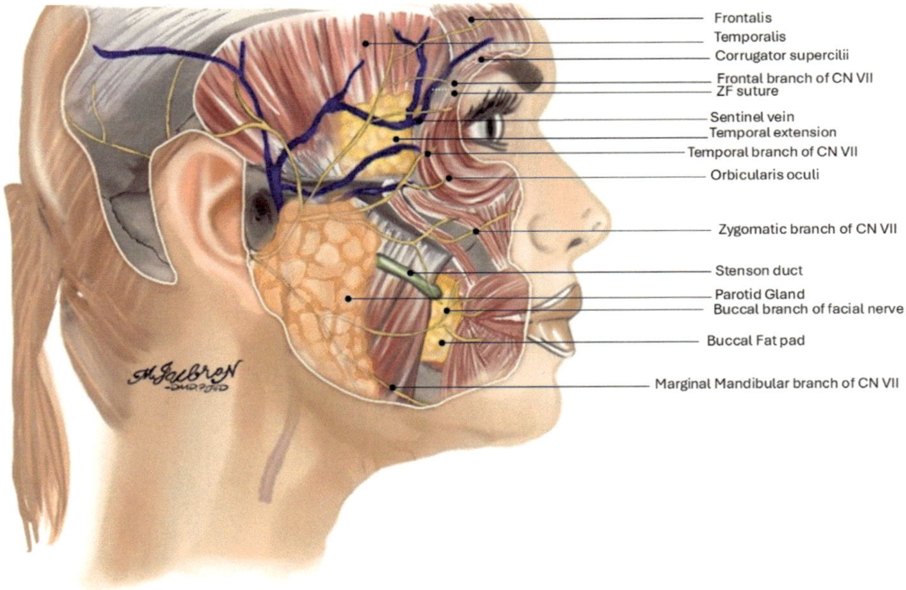

Figure 3.
Anatomy of the frontal branch of the facial nerve (CN VII) and its proximity to the sentinel vein, also called the medial zygomaticotemporal vein. As illustrated by the white dotted line, the sentinel vein is approximately 1–2 cm lateral to the zygomaticofrontal (ZF) suture. Damage to this vein may result in unwanted bruising and swelling in this area. It may also be difficult to achieve hemostasis. One should be aware of the frontal branch of the facial nerve nearby, which may be damaged while attempting to achieve hemostasis.

The superior orbital rim and its associated arcus marginalis represent the inferior limit of dissection over the orbit. These landmarks must be well-visualized endoscopically and freed of periosteal attachments in order to lift the brow and its associated fat pads for long-lasting results [6]. Along the superior orbital rim lies the supraorbital foramen or notch, which may be found within 1 mm of a line drawn in a sagittal plane tangential to the medial limbus [6, 12]. This landmark may be marked on the skin to give the surgeon a reference point that reveals the bony exit point of the supraorbital nerve. A deep division of the supraorbital nerve may be present in 10% of patients and may exit from another foramen which may be up to 1.5 cm above the orbital rim. This has led some surgeons to advocate the use of the endoscope once dissection has reached 2 cm from the superior orbital rim in order to reduce the risk of injury to the supraorbital nerve [6].

The temporal ridge is another important landmark that must be identified during dissection. Along this ridge lies a zone of fixation: a dense collection of fasciae approximately 1 cm wide that extends the length of the superior temporal line and ends inferiorly just above the fronto-zygomatico suture line at the fascial attachment known as the orbital ligament (**Figure 4**) [6]. Lateral to the orbital ligament lies the orbicularis-temporal ligament, which is where fibers from the orbicularis oculi, temporalis fascia and temporoparietal fascia fuse.

Bone thickness is another important anatomic factor to consider when using fixation methods that require drilling into the skull. Although bone thickness increases posteriorly near the occiput, fixation in this region is relatively difficult and not required. The safest site for bone tunnel or fixation screw placement for brow elevation is the frontal bone along a parasagittal line extended from the lateral limbus or

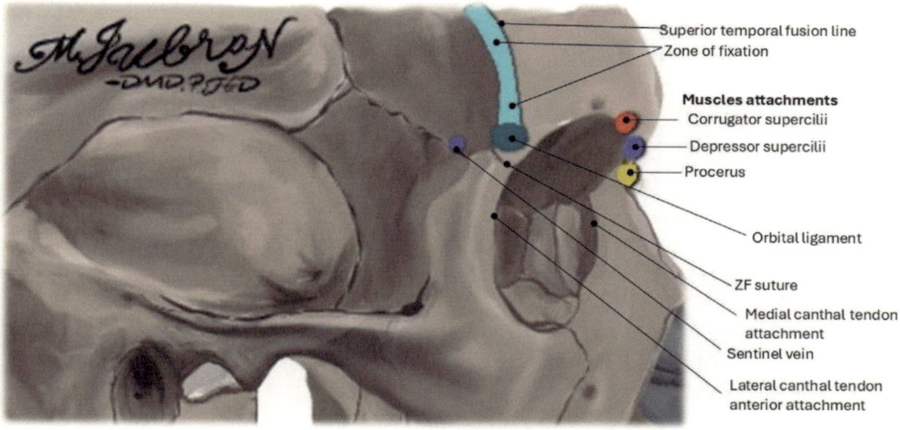

Figure 4.
The zone of fixation spans the length of the temporal ridge and ends just above the zygomaticofrontal (ZF) suture.

mid-pupil and anterior to the coronal suture [6]. Bone screw or tunnel fixation should not be near midline due to the presence of the sagittal sinus and a higher density of venous lakes on the inner surface of the skull near the sagittal suture. Also, caution must be taken to avoid bone penetration near the temporalis muscle laterally where potential injury to the middle meningeal artery, a branch of the internal maxillary artery, may occur.

The anatomy of the forehead is similar to the rest of the scalp, with some minor exceptions. Indeed, the acronym SCALP can be applied to forehead anatomy: *s*kin, sub*c*utaneous tissue, galea *a*poneurotica, *l*oose areolar tissue, and *p*eriosteum. In the forehead region, the galea aponeurotica, which is also continuous with the temporoparietal fascia in the temporal region, is fused into the frontalis muscle.

The muscles of the forehead and brow region are paired and include the frontalis, corrugator supercilii, procerus, depressor supercilii, orbicularis oculi, and temporalis muscles. The frontalis muscle is unique in that it is the only true elevator of the forehead and brows. The remaining aforementioned paired muscles act as forehead and brow depressors. The frontalis muscle originates from the galea aponeurotica and inserts into the orbital portion of the orbicularis oculi muscle. Its lateral extension fuses into the zone of adherence along the superior temporal line [6]. Laterally, the frontalis muscle's absence over the tail of the brow results in more unopposed action of the depressor muscles, causing the lateral tail of the brow to descend to a greater degree than its medial counterpart as one ages [13].

The procerus and corrugator supercilii muscles are the two most recognized depressors as they are often the target of many providers offering neuromodulator treatment for dynamic rhytids in the glabella region. The procerus muscles are paired superiorly and fuse into a single muscle belly inferiorly (**Figure 5**). They originate from the nasal bones and cartilages and insert into the medial frontalis muscle and overlying dermis. The procerus is responsible for brow depression at the midline, between the brows and eyes, that often create a horizontal crease across the upper art of the nose.

The corrugator supercilii muscles originate from the frontal bone near the midline, just above the nasal bones, and insert into the dermis of the medial brow. The two heads to the corrugator muscles, the oblique and transverse, act synchronously in

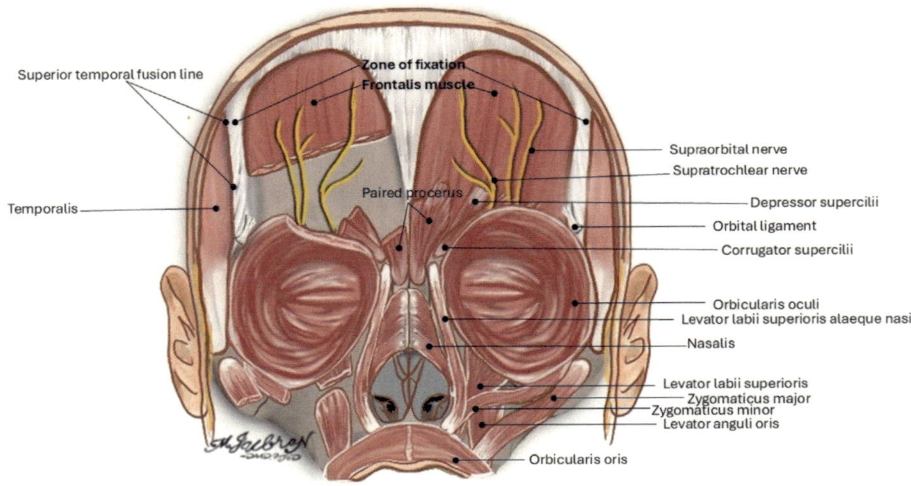

Figure 5.
Muscular anatomy of the forehead. The procerus and corrugator supercilii muscles are responsible for vertical rhytid formation ("11 s") in the glabellar region and are commonly targeted areas during browlift surgery and neuromodulator treatment.

order to pull the medial brow down and towards midline. The muscles act obliquely across the glabella and produce vertical lines or "11 s" while making certain facial expressions such as squinting and frowning and contribute to an "angry" or "grieving" appearance. The corrugator supercilii and procerus muscles are often transected during an endoscopic forehead or brow lift procedure to achieve a smooth, long-lasting result, akin to a "permanent Botox" effect.

The depressor supercilii muscle originates from the frontal process of the maxilla, just inferior and superficial to the origin of the corrugator supercilii. It inserts into the medial frontalis muscle and dermis just above the medial brow [6]. While performing an endoscopic forehead and browlift, this muscle may be transected via aggressive dissection through the corrugator muscle. This maneuver often leads to over-elevation of the medial brow to a position above the superior orbital rim, which may result in a post-operative "surprised" look [6, 14]. A similar outcome may occur if the depressor supercilii is inadvertently treated with neuromodulators: elevation of the medial brow.

More superficial to the depressor supercilii lies the orbital portion of the orbicularis oculi muscle which originates, in part, from the medial canthal tendon and inserts into parts of adjacent depressor muscles, the frontalis, and the dermis [6].

The temporalis muscles are located in the temporal fossa, from where they originate, and insert onto the coronoid process of the mandible. Its overlying fascia is useful and important to identify during upper facial cosmetic surgery because it aids in delineating surgical planes and may be used in fixation. The dense, shiny white temporalis fascia adheres to the underlying temporalis muscle and separates into superficial and deep layers in the lower half of the temporal fossa. Superficial to the temporalis fascia lies the temporoparietal fascia which is continuous with the superficial musculoaponeurotic system (SMAS) inferiorly and houses the frontal branch of the facial nerve under its deep surface (**Figure 6**).

Arterial blood supply to the forehead region is derived from branches of both the internal and external carotid arteries (**Figure 7**). The facial artery, a branch

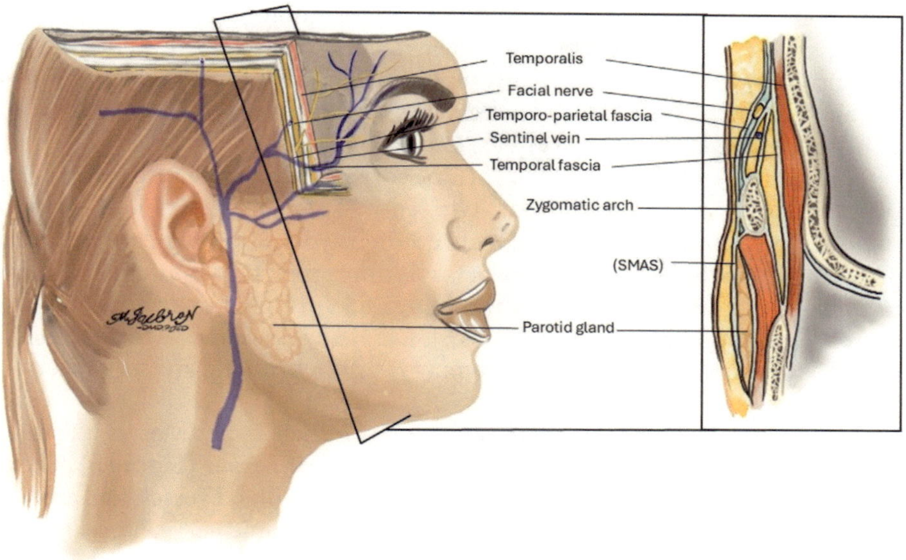

Figure 6.
Cross sectional anatomy of the frontal branch of the facial nerve and its proximity to the sentinel vein, also called the medial zygomaticotemporal vein. Damage to this vein may result in unwanted bruising and swelling in this area. It may also be difficult to achieve hemostasis. One should be aware of the frontal branch of the facial nerve nearby, which may be damaged while attempting to achieve hemostasis.

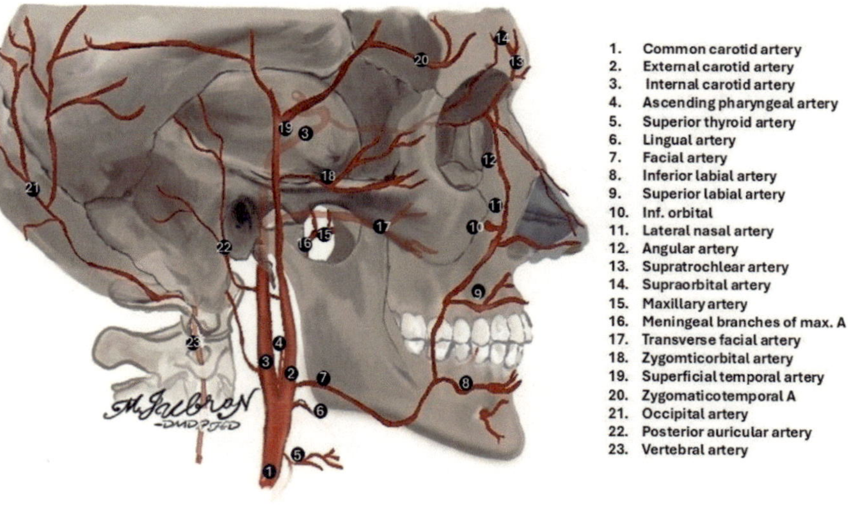

Figure 7.
Arterial blood supply to the face is derived from external carotid and internal carotid artery systems.

of the external carotid artery, gives rise to the angular artery, which supplies the medial canthal region. The superficial temporal artery, one of the terminal branches of the external carotid artery, gives rise to a frontal or anterior branch, which supplies the lateral canthal region. The maxillary artery, the other terminal branch of the external carotid artery, gives rise to the middle meningeal artery which supplies part of periosteum along the inner surface of cranial bones and the dura mater. Perforating branches of the middle meningeal artery also reach the diploe and may even at times reach the external surface of the skull [15]. The ophthalmic artery, a branch of the internal carotid artery, gives rise to the supra-orbital and supratrochlear arteries which exit their respective foramina to supply much of the forehead and mid-scalp regions [6].

Venous drainage of the upper facial third corresponds to the respective arterial supply, but may have some variations. The sentinel vein or the medial zygomaticotemporal vein remains relatively consistent in its course among patients. It runs perpendicularly through the temporalis fascia approximately 1–2 cm lateral or posterior to the fronto-zygomatico suture line and within 2 mm of the temporal branch of the facial nerve (**Figure 6**) [6, 8]. Careless dissection in this region may lead to injury to the sentinel vein which may result in bruising and a reduced field of visualization.

Nerve supply to the upper face also parallels its arterial supply. Most of the forehead is innervated by the supraorbital and supratrochlear nerves (**Figure 8**). These nerves exit the same foramina or notch as their respective blood vessels and are both divisions of the trigeminal nerve's first branch: the ophthalmic nerve. Once it exits its foramen, the supraorbital nerve gives off two divisions. The deep or lateral division supplies the lateral and posterior part of the forehead and scalp whereas the superficial or medial division pierces the frontalis muscle early in its course and travels superficially to the muscle supplying sensation to the lower and mid-forehead along the mid-pupillary line [6]. The deep branch is larger than the superficial branch and is located closer to the periosteum [12].

The supratrochlear nerve exits near the superior orbital rim, approximately 9 mm medial to the supraorbital foramen or notch, and supplies sensation to the mid-forehead region, with its territory overlapping somewhat with that of the supraorbital nerve. The infratrochlear nerve, which also originates from the ophthalmic nerve, exits just below the supratrochlear nerve around the medial orbital rim to supply sensation to the upper nose and medial orbit. The lateral orbit and temporal regions of the face receive sensory input from branches of the maxillary nerve, the second division of the trigeminal nerve: the zygomatico-frontal and zygomatico-temporal nerves.

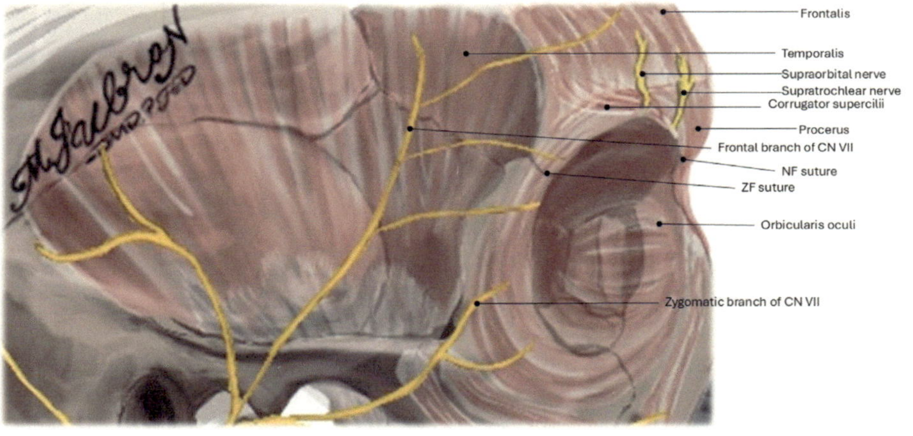

Figure 8.
Innervation of the upper facial third.

Part of the temporal region is also supplied by a branch of the mandibular nerve, the third division of the trigeminal nerve. The auriculotemporal nerve, supplies sensation to the front of the ear, the temporal skin above the zygomatic arch, and to the skin that is superficial to the superficial temporal artery [6]. It runs within 1 cm anterior to the tragus and parallel to the superficial temporal artery. Knowing its anatomic location will help prevent the surgeon from confusing it with the frontal branch of the facial nerve, which runs roughly 2 cm anterior to the tragus when it crosses the zygomatic arch at a more oblique angle and just deep to the SMAS and temporoparietal fascia above the arch.

Branches of the facial nerve, namely the frontal (or temporal) and zygomatic branches, are responsible for supplying motor innervation to the forehead and glabella. The temporal branch innervates the frontalis muscle, the superior portion of the orbicularis oculi muscle, the superior portion of the procerus muscle, and the transverse head of the corrugator supercilii muscle [6]. The nerve leaves the parotid gland deep to the SMAS and crosses the middle third of the zygomatic arch between the SMAS and periosteum. Once superior to the zygomatic arch, the temporal branch of the facial nerve travels within the temporoparietal fascia until it inserts into the deep site of the musculature [8]. The temporal branch has typically divided into two rami at the level of the zygomatic arch and into at least four branches at the level of the eyebrow. The zygomatic branch of the facial nerve supplies the medial orbicularis oculi muscle, the inferior portion of the procerus muscle, and the depressor supercilii muscle.

During an endoscopic forehead and browlift, the surgeon must identify key anatomic landmarks and create enough space in order to insert the endoscopic equipment. Once in the subperiosteal plane, the zone of fixation along the superior temporal crest becomes an important consideration during the dissection. While the less tenacious zone of adherence along the entire temporal crest may be elevated with blunt finger dissection, as the surgeon approaches the superior-lateral orbital rim and the inferior edge of the temporal crest, endoscopic guidance is used to achieve optimal release [6]. The attachments at the lateral orbital rim consist of an intermix of fibers from the periosteum, galea, temporalis, and temporoparietal fascia. During dissection, it is crucial to stay in the subperiosteal plane, against the bone, and in the sub-temporoparietal fascial plane, against the temporalis fascia, to avoid injury to the frontal branch of the facial nerve and the sentinel vein [6].

3. Pre-operative evaluation

As with all cosmetic surgical procedures, an accurate diagnosis and treatment plan is crucial to optimizing the final outcome and ensuring a high level of patient satisfaction. Knowing and understanding the patient's desires and expectations, while ensuring the patient understands the risks, benefits, and alternative treatments will help all parties develop trust among one another and the best outcome possible. After a forehead and browlift, new dynamic rhytids may appear as a result of the newly positioned tissue and, while some of the pre-existing rhytids may be improved, these lines will not be completely treated by browlifting, alone. Patients should be made to understand that other treatment modalities, such as neuromodulator injection, may be necessary to address these particular lines.

Patients should also be aware that forehead and browlifting, alone, will not change any intrinsic skin damage that has occurred due to sun exposure, age, and smoking. Topical medications and skin care along with skin resurfacing may be considered to address these changes. Chemical peels or laser resurfacing may be performed simultaneously with an endoscopic forehead and browlift, in which dissection is carried out in a subperiosteal and subgaleal plane. Patients who desire aggressive, high-fluence simultaneous ablative laser resurfacing require a deeper plane of dissection than a subcutaneous plane because the laser may place the thin lipocutaneous at risk of vascular after an aggressive laser [5].

Traditionally, the "ideal" female brow position is arched above the superior orbital rim, with it peaking between the middle and lateral third of the brow, which corresponds with the level of the lateral limbus of the iris [11]. This is known as a Westmore-shaped eyebrow and its point is typically 5–10 mm above the orbital rim [6, 14]. In reality, an ideal brow morphology is more dependent on one's facial shape: the Westmore eyebrow is not well-suited to long or square faces since it can negatively accentuate the angularity of these faces. Conversely, a laterally peaked Westmore eyebrow may add necessary angularity to a round face [14].

The male brow, on the other hand, is lower, usually at the level of the superior orbital rim, thicker, and tends to have a flatter, more horizontal contour [5, 11, 16]. Males undergoing browlift surgery typically require a more "straight-up" elevation of the entire brow to avoid feminization of their upper facial third, which may occur if the lateral brow was over-elevated. To achieve this, the parasagittal incisions may be placed in the scalp directly above the midline of the iris [17]. Relative contraindications for an endoscopic forehead and browlift include females with high hairlines, males with male pattern baldness, patients with thick adherent skin, and patients with extensive bone attachments [8].

Those who have brow ptosis or dermatochalasis may lead to subconscious frontalis muscle activity to lift the excess tissue and improve their visual field. Over time, this gives rise to deep forehead wrinkles (**Figure 9**).

Any bony irregularities that are noted upon examination may be further evaluated through use of a cephalometric radiograph or a computed tomography (CT) scan. Limited bony contouring may be performed via an endoscopic approach, however, major reduction for significant bony hypertrophy, such as frontal bossing, is best achieved by an open (coronal) approach [6]. Bone reduction may be limited by pneumatization of the frontal sinus, which may be evaluated pre-operatively with a CT scan. While CT scans are not necessary to treatment plan the location of bone tunnels for fixation, a cephalometric radiograph may be useful in determining the thickness of corticocancellous bone and provide reassurance to the surgeon [6].

Patients should be instructed to avoid medications that could increase the risk of intra-operative and post-operative bleeding such as aspirin and other nonsteroidal anti-inflammatory drugs, vitamin E, and several over-the-counter herbal medications, such as gingko, *Echinacea*, and St. John's wort, for at least 2 weeks pre-operatively [18]. Patients should also be instructed to wash their hair the night before and morning of surgery with antibacterial soap, such as Hibiclens®, or an antiseptic type of shampoo. Hairspray and other hair products are to be avoided immediately before surgery. Smokers and smokeless tobacco users should be instructed to discontinue nicotine products at least 3 weeks before and after their procedure.

Pre-operatively, five standard photographs of the patient are taken, along with close-up views of the eyes in closed and open gazes, lateral gaze, and upward gaze [8]. The patient is marked while sitting or standing in an upright position. The patient is then brought to the operating room and situated on the operating room table in a supine position. General anesthesia is induced by laryngeal masked airway or endotracheal intubation. The bed is rotated away from the anesthesia provider so that the

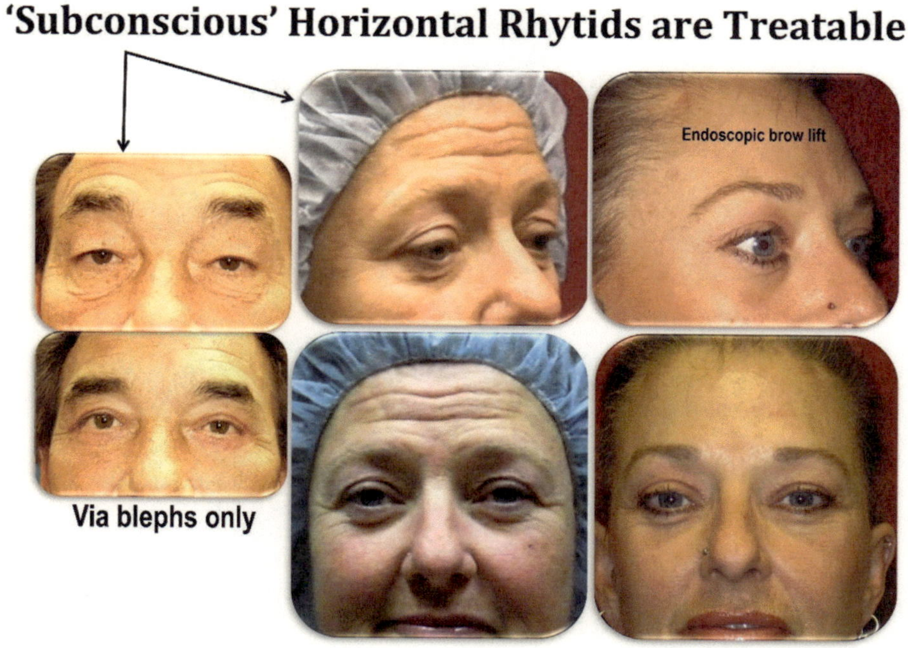

Figure 9.
The two patients in the image presented with deep forehead rhytids due to subconscious overactive frontalis activity. The patient on the left was treated with blepharoplasty only and the patient on the right was treated with an endoscopic forehead and brow lift. The removal of laxity over the eyes allowed for both patients to stop raising the eyebrows subconsciously, which improved the forehead wrinkles. The patient who underwent the brow lift procedure had a more dramatic improvement in subconscious forehead lines.

endoscopic tower or screen may be placed near the foot of the bed while the surgeon stands unobstructed at the head of the bed. The bed may be tilted in 5–10 degrees of reverse Trendelenberg position to facilitate insertion and maneuvering of the endoscopic equipment. Once the appropriate level of anesthesia has been achieved, the patient is prepped and local and tumescent anesthesia are administered. Lidocaine 1% with 1:100,000 epinephrine is injected along the superior orbital rim, glabella and lateral orbital rim. Tumescent anesthesia (250 mL normal saline with 1 mL 1:1000 epinephrine and 20 mL 2% lidocaine) is then injected into the forehead, temporal region, and posterior scalp. Alternatively, 20 mL (266 mg) of liposomal bupivacaine may be injected across the brow, the temple bilaterally, and circumferentially across the scalp, thus blocking supraorbital, supratrochlear, zygomaticofrontal, and zygomaticotemporal nerves regionally [19]. Shaving or cutting of the hair is usually not necessary, although it may be performed if the surgeon desires.

4. Surgical technique

Once the patient is prepped and draped, the author prefers to place five separate 2.5 cm incisions about 1 cm posterior to the hairline (**Figure 10**). The first incision is placed in the midline of the sagittal plane. Two more incisions are placed on either side of the first incision, in a line tangential to the lateral third of the brow. The final two incisions are placed in the temporal region in a line that is roughly parallel to the path of the temporal branch of the facial nerve.

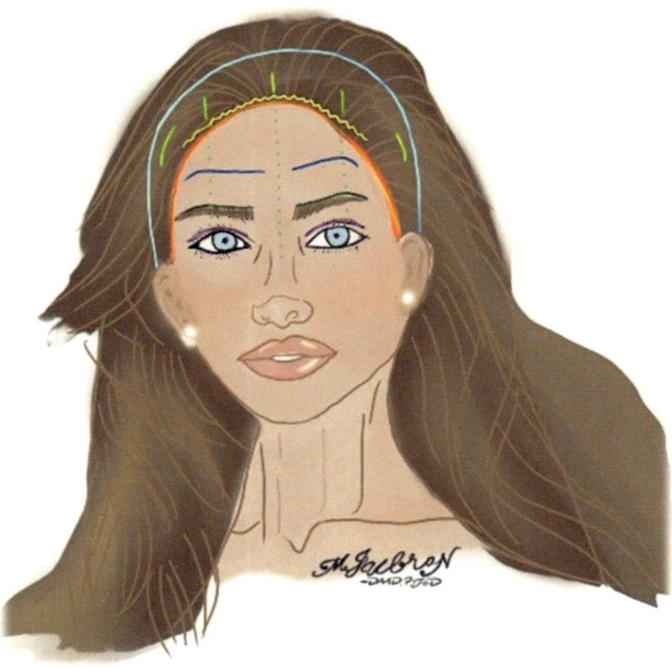

Figure 10.
Incisions of various browlift approaches. The endoscopic forehead and browlift incisions (green) are placed about 1 cm posterior to the hairline in the midline, parasagittal and temporal areas.

The location of these incisions is not arbitrarily decided upon. The midline incision, along with the two parasagittal incisions are parallel to each other and aligned vertically to avoid transection of branches of the supraorbital nerves originating inferiorly. The two parasagittal incisions are placed in line with the lateral third of the brow, where maximum lift is typically desired in female patients. For male patients, these parasagittal incisions may be placed slightly more medial in order to attain a more even brow elevation.

The decision to place the parasagittal incision in the described location is multifactorial. They are placed medial to the temporal crest to gain access to the skull, rather than the temporalis fascia, where bone tunnels will be placed and fixation will occur. Bony fixation may be safely performed in this area since it is one of the thickest regions of the frontal bone and it has a relatively low density of venous lakes to help prevent inadvertent intracranial injury. Another reason for placing the parasagittal incisions medial to the temporal crest is to easily gain access to the subperiosteal plane. If the incisions were further lateral, over the zone of fixation or the temporalis muscle, there would likely be increased bleeding and difficulty creating a subperiosteal pocket, making endoscopic visualization more obstructed.

In patients with receding hairlines, the incisions may become more noticeable. Instead of employing the aforementioned parasagittal incisions, 1-cm horizontal incisions may be placed at the upper forehead, at the level of the temporal limbus of the iris, within apparent horizontal forehead rhytids [20]. The midline and temporal incisions may be placed in the same locations as in those with non-receding hairlines.

The two temporal incisions are placed on either side of the head to allow for direct access to the thick deep temporal fascia. They are made perpendicularly to the desired vector of elevation from the lateral canthal region [6]. They are also designed to avoid injury to nerves and vessels: they are parallel to and 2–3 cm superior to the temporal branch of the facial nerve and also parallel the superficial temporal artery and vein.

Sharp dissection is performed through the aforementioned incisions down to pericranium medial to the temporal crest and down to the deep temporalis fascia lateral to the crest. With blunt finger dissection and with long, curved endoscopic periosteal elevators, the tissues are elevated to a point 2 cm above the orbital rims and the zygomatic arch [6]. Blunt dissection is used to release and elevate the temporal tissues to a few centimeters posterior to the ear, where the temporal fossa becomes self-limiting. At least 10 cm of posterior scalp elevation is required to achieve adequate undermining, but it can extend as far posterior as the lambdoid suture if needed. Blunt dissection is subsequently carried out to connect all incisions in the subpericranial and sub-temporoparietal fascial planes. It is recommended that blunt dissection occurs from the temporal incision towards the parasagittal incisions to avoid inadvertently releasing the deep temporal fascia from the temporal crest and creating a false tunnel, which would be easier to do if dissection were to proceed from medial to lateral. It is critical to stay firmly against the periosteum and deep temporal fascia in order to avoid facial nerve injury.

The endoscope is then carefully inserted through one of the three medial incisions (**Figure 11**). If it feels too tight, remove the endoscope and ensure that the scalp and forehead have been adequately elevated. The surgeon must be mindful to not apply excessive retracting forces on the undermined scalp and forehead to avoid skin perforation. Endoscopic dissection proceeds medially over the nasofrontal suture and the orbital rims with a curved, smooth, and rounded elevator. Once the entire rolled edge of the superior orbital rim is visualized, needle tip electrocautery is used to precisely incise the periosteum. A laser on a low power setting may also be used for this maneuver. The supraorbital nerves and vessels can be located near the orbital rim at a level tangential to the medial limbus. Periosteal release in this area should be avoided to prevent injury to these vital

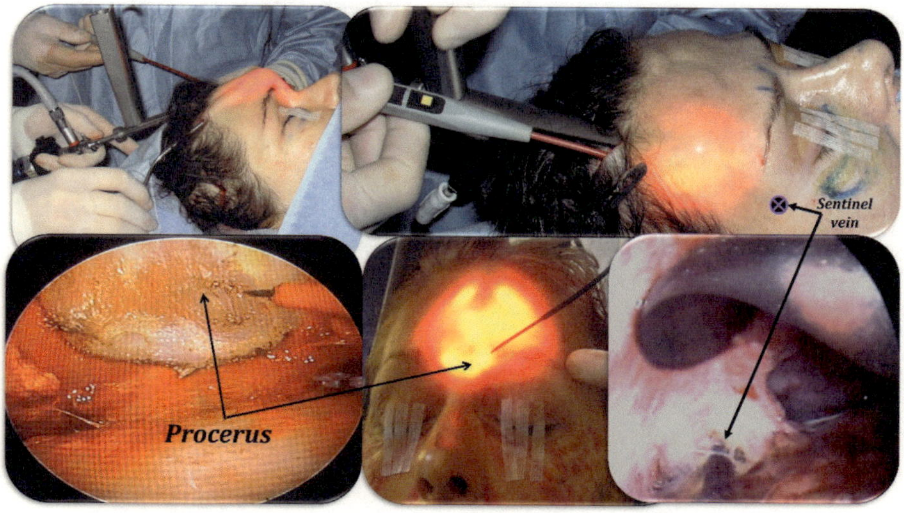

Figure 11.
The endoscope is inserted through the right parasagittal incision. Once the periosteum is released, the musculature of the forehead is visualized and may be transected if indicated.

structures. To maintain a clear visual field during electrocautery or laser use, the temporal incisions may be used as suction ports so that a suctioning tool, such as a Yankauer suction tip, can be inserted without interfering with the endoscope and other instruments utilizing the three medial incisions. With hemostatic control and an unobstructed visual field, the corrugator supercilii and procerus muscles are transected from their deep surfaces. Any bleeding that occurs that cannot be controlled easily may be managed by applying pressure over the external surface over the rim until visualization improves and pinpoint, accurate cauterization may be used to achieve hemostasis without nerve injury.

Transection of the corrugator supercilii and procerus muscles will improve vertical and horizontal glabellar rhytids, respectively (**Figure 12**). This leads to a more natural appearance in the upper facial third whereas more aggressive muscle removal and surgical avulsion of these muscles, as advocated by some surgeons, may lead to post-operative irregularities and abnormal facial expression unless otherwise corrected with adjunctive procedures such as fat grafting [6]. However, in a retrospective study that evaluated 31 post-operative endoscopic forehead and browlift patients, Jones et al. found that depressor muscle resection in conjunction with a brow lift reduces glabellar lines on short- and long-term follow-up [14].

Once the periosteum has been completely released across the orbital rims and muscle transection has occurred, periosteal elevators are used to separate the cut periosteal edges by at least 1 cm to facilitate release at the arcus marginalis [6]. This separation is crucial to achieving long-lasting results (**Figures 13** and **14**). Then, the orbital ligament and zone of fixation laterally must be released in order to expose the lateral orbital rim in the subperiosteal plane. One should stay close to periosteum and deep temporal fascia to prevent damage to the temporal nerve and for better hemostatic control. Aggressive retraction in this area may lead to nerve injury. Subperiosteal dissection should proceed in a clean plane inferiorly along the lateral

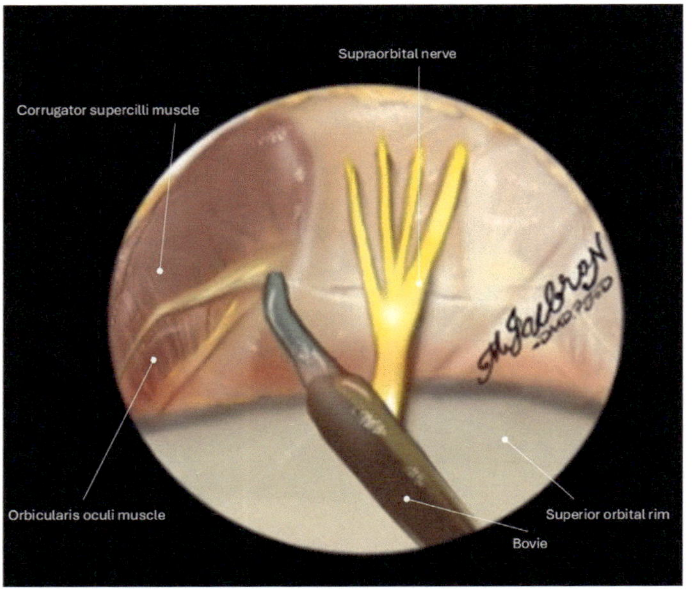

Figure 12.
Illustration of an endoscopic view of release of periosteum at the level of the superior orbital rim while protecting the supraorbital nerve.

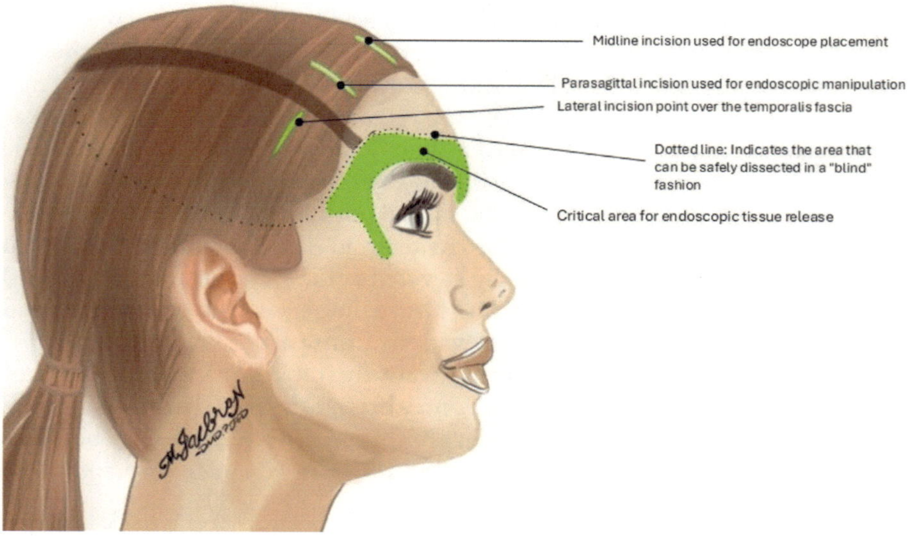

Figure 13.
The green highlighted area illustrates the area of subperiosteal release anteriorly, which extends along the lateral orbital rim into the malar region. The endoscope may be inserted through any of the three middle incisions for visualization.

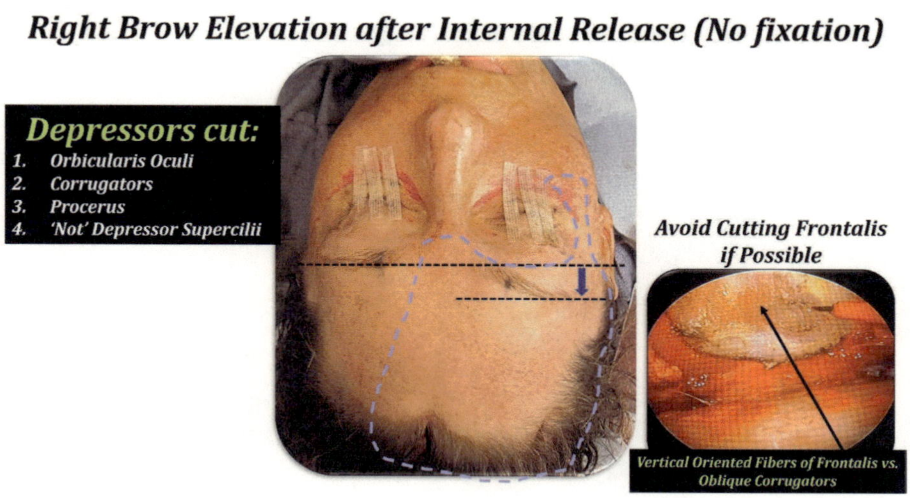

Figure 14.
The right brow has been sufficiently released and the depressor muscles have been transected. The frontalis muscle, the sole brow elevator, should be preserved. One can distinguish between the brow elevators and depressors by the muscle fiber orientation.

orbital rim, past the zygomaticofrontal suture, to about 1 cm from the level of the zygomatic arch.

Once adequate dissection has been completed, forehead and brow elevation with fixation is performed. There are several types of fixation techniques that the surgeon may choose such as tissue suture only, bone screws and plates, resorbable screws, bone tunnels, tissue glue, temporalis muscle exposure for added scarification, and others. Regardless of the method chosen, adequate lower forehead release remains the most important element in achieving adequate long-term fixation. Failure to sufficiently release the forehead tissues will inevitably lead to brow ptosis relapse.

The surgeon must now decide on the vector of lift to achieve the most esthetically pleasing result. For females, the lateral third of the brow is elevated most. This may be up to 1 cm above the superior orbital rim. The vector of pull is straight up and fixation may occur at or just posterior to the hairline. The galeal tissue may be secured to bone at this point while the lateral brow is held at its desired height or even a couple of millimeters above the desired level. The medial portion of the brow, however, should only be slightly elevated above the rim to avoid a more surprised or shocked appearance. The glabellar area is typically elevated without the need for fixation. One way of avoiding medial brow elevation is the leave the periosteum partially attached in this region so that there is little to no elevation of this part of the brow. During the recovery period, brow position remains relatively stable despite the presence of post-operative edema. Periosteal adhesions may begin to develop within the first few days post-operatively, adding to the stability of this procedure's long-term outcomes. Relapse of brow position is rare with proper technique and may only average 1–2 mm after 2 weeks of recovery [6].

It is the authors' preference to fixate the galea and periosteum just slightly posterior to the hairline to a bone tunnel created in the outer cortex of the calvarium in line with the parasagittal incisions. The bone tunnels should be placed in the frontal bone are created using a carbide fissure bur on a surgical drill or rotating osteotome [21]. The bur is held tangentially to the scalp to avoid inadvertent intracranial injury (**Figure 15**). The tissue is secured to the bone tunnel with a heavy suture, such as 0 Vicryl®. An alternative to creating a bone tunnel could be the use of a MicroAire forehead-specific endotine [3]. The lateral tail of the brow may be fixated through the

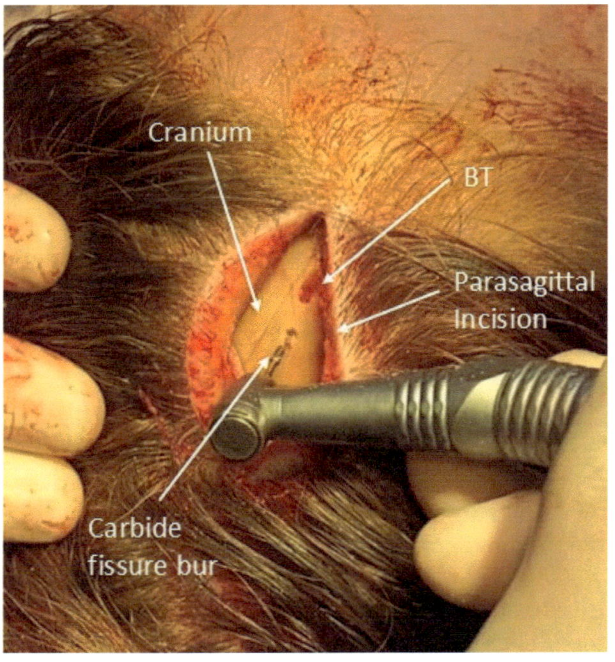

Figure 15.
A bone tunnel (BT) is created through a parasagittal incision using a carbide bur on a surgical handpiece held tangentially to the cranium. The bone tunnel should be in line with the point of desired maximal brow elevation.

temporal incisions, where a heavy suture is used to plicate the temporoparietal fascia to the deeper temporal fascia in a posterosuperior vector, following an imaginary line drawn from the outer nasal ala passing just lateral to the lateral canthus [6]. A small area of temporalis muscle may be exposed to facilitate scar formation and fixation. At the end of fixation, it is necessary to stop for a few minutes to evaluate the position of both sides of the eyebrows. This is an ideal time to assess the results and achieve the best possible outcome and symmetry.

Closure of the five incisions may be performed with skin staples alone. As there is no skin excised during the procedure and there is no tension on the incisions upon closure, patients have excellent scar formation. Although forehead and brow elevation does create some redundant and excess tissue in the scalp, it is easily redistributed over the previously elevated posterior scalp without any obvious signs of bunching [6]. The patient should be made aware pre-operatively that, because of the scalp elevation, the hairline may be slightly elevated post-operatively. No post-operative drains are typically placed for an isolated endoscopic forehead and browlift.

One main advantage of the endoscopic forehead and browlift is the ease with which it may be combined with other cosmetic surgery procedures. The temporal incisions may be connected with the preauricular incisions of a lower face and neck lift. Also, if performing a subperiosteal mid-facelift, the intraoral subperiosteal dissection can be connected to the subperiosteal plane from the endoscopic browlift near the lateral orbital rim.

A disadvantage of the endoscopic forehead and browlift is widening of the interbrow distance. In a retrospective cohort study, Hollabaugh et al. found that about 1.5 mm of widening does occur between the brows, even without corrugator muscle resection, but without an adverse effect on postoperative esthetics [3].

5. Post-operative instructions and care

Once the procedure is finished, the patient's head is wrapped in a compression bandage to limit edema, help prevent small hematoma formation, and possibly improve fixation. While resting during the first 3 days post-operatively, the head should be elevated at least 30–45 degrees. Cold compresses over the forehead, brows and eyelids are encouraged and the patient is instructed to limit physical activity. There should be no strenuous activity nor heavy lifting for at least 2 weeks post-operatively [6, 8]. Similarly, applying any hair products or chemicals should be avoided for at least 2 weeks to avoid unwanted hair loss.

On the first post-operative day, the patient may remove the compression bandage and replace it with a less compressive head wrap. This also gives the patient or his or her caretaker to inspect the surgical site for any issues. The patient is allowed to shower and gently shampoo their hair after 24 hours after surgery, but they are instructed to avoid the shower water from directly hitting the incision sites. The incision sites are cleaned daily with dilute hydrogen peroxide and a thin layer of antibiotic ointment for the first 7 days. The patient is also instructed to avoid bending over during the first few weeks post-operatively to avoid increased pressure on the face.

Due to the extensive release of scalp and deep facial tissues during the endoscopic forehead and browlift, post-operative pain control typically requires a short course of narcotic medication. Indeed, the browlift operation may be the most painful of the common facial cosmetic procedures [19]. Patients are also advised to take ibuprofen and acetaminophen, if there are no contraindications, to provide multi-modal post-operative pain control. To decrease the need for narcotic pain medication, patients may also elect to receive bupivacaine liposome injectable solution, which is typically administered intra-operatively and can provide up to 72 hours of post-operative pain relief [19].

Surgical staples are removed at the one-week mark. Patients are informed that areas of the scalp may be anesthetic for months after surgery and that the use of hot curling irons or similar devices should be used with extreme caution to prevent accidental self-inflicted burns or hair loss.

6. Complications

In order to decrease the likelihood of complications, the surgeon must be thorough in his or her patient selection process, preoperative planning, surgical technique, and postoperative care instructions. However, minor complications may be inevitable despite a surgeon's best efforts. Extensive edema and ecchymosis are typically not complications but may require the surgeon to provide comfort and reassurance to the concerned patient.

Complications after browlift surgery include poor scar formation, wound dehiscence, hematoma, skin sloughs or perforations, asymmetry, sensory disturbance, facial paralysis, eyelid ptosis, corneal abrasion, dry eye syndrome, alopecia, infection, relapse, contour irregularities, and irregular facial expressions [6, 9]. Expert knowledge of clinical anatomy and meticulous surgical technique are crucial in avoiding complications. While direct injury to the temporal branch of the facial nerve is rare, temporary post-operative neuropraxia is more common [9]. Hematomas must be diagnosed early and treated promptly: smaller collections may be aspirated, but larger ones may require surgical drainage. When bleeding occurs, the source is typically from either the superficial temporal and/or the zygomaticotemporal vessels [8]. Avoiding improper retraction, aggressive electrocautery, and excessive thinning of the flaps when transecting forehead muscles are ways to prevent complications from occurring during and after browlift surgery.

Alopecia and sensory disturbances can be troubling to the patient, but may not be permanent. With proper technique, an endoscopic forehead and browlift has a high rate of full sensory nerve recovery, but it may take several months for this to occur. The most crucial factor in preventing permanent sensory disturbances is careful and meticulous dissection around the supraorbital nerve. Alopecia is also usually temporary, but it is a matter of significant concern to many patients. Its risk is less with the endoscopic technique than with the coronal approach [8]. Local alopecia may resolve after a 4–8 month period of dormancy in the hair follicle. *Telogen affluvium* is a condition in which up to 70% of hair may fall out due to stress or a "shock" to the body [6]. This condition may take up to 6–8 months to resolve and is typically self-limiting. Permanent hair loss, on the other hand, is typically the result of excessive tension on the flaps, rough handling of wound margins, or excessive use of electrocautery near hair follicles.

Corneal abrasions are often painful and can be avoided with proper surgical technique. Eye lubricant should always be used and the eye should be additionally protected with corneal shields, placement of temporary sterile bandages, or a tarsorrhaphy suture so that the likelihood of inadvertent corneal scratches will be minimized. Severe pain requires prompt evaluation to rule out vision-threatening conditions such as a retrobulbar hematoma. Suspected corneal abrasions should be

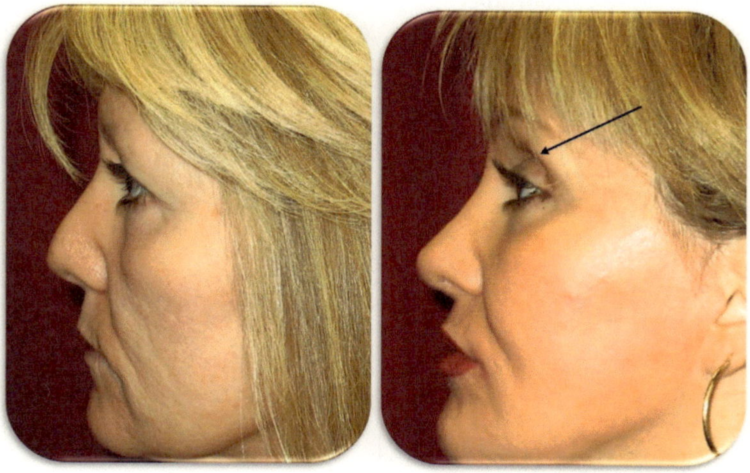

Figure 16.
Potential issues with aggressive brow lifting hollowing above and below the eyebrow may become evident and require fat grafting or filler at a later date.

treated with appropriate ophthalmic drops or bandage contact lenses for pain and with patching of the affected eye for 12–24 hours. Blurry vision for the first 12 hours post-operatively due to chemosis and the use of ophthalmic ointment is not unusual and the patient should have been made aware of this possibility pre-operatively.

Lagophthalmos is also a risk of browlift surgery. Once the arcus marginalis is released and the brow is elevated, upper eyelid elevation will also occur. Those at highest risk are patients who have had a previous upper blepharoplasty. One way to limit the risk of lagophthalmos is to perform the brow lift prior to the upper blepharoplasty [8]. An overly aggressive browlift, especially in conjunction with an upper blepharoplasty, may result in excessive hollowing under the eyebrow. This may be corrected at a later date with fat grafting or filler (**Figure 16**).

7. Conclusion

Complete facial rejuvenation begs the cosmetic surgeon to address the upper facial third. The widespread use of the endoscope and neuromodulators in this region have made treatment of the upper facial third increasingly popular. As with any cosmetic procedure, patient selection and proper diagnosis are key factors in obtaining great outcomes. Any brow lift procedure should stabilize the brow at an esthetically pleasing height, shape and orientation, provide long-lasting results, have concealed scars, preserve forehead sensation, and avoid an unfavorable hairline position (**Figure 17**) [8].

While the endoscopic forehead and browlift provides well-hidden scars, some surgeons argue that its significant learning curve, extensive armamentarium, effect on forehead length, and "unpredictable" longevity make other approaches, such as the subcutaneous browlift, more favorable [5]. A subcutaneous browlift offers certain advantages such as no specialized instrumentation needed, minimal concern for frontal nerve injury, lesser degree of a learning curve, and no need for osseous fixation [5].

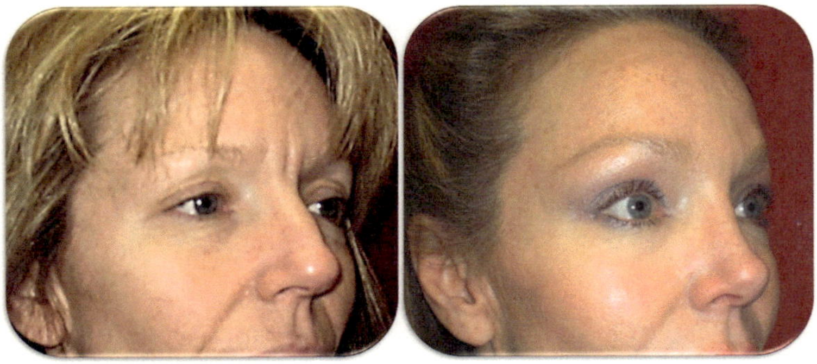

Figure 17.
Endoscopic browlift longevity. The patient is shown before and 5 years following an endoscopic forehead and browlift, fat grafting and laser resurfacing.

While foreheads, brows, and skin problems may vary widely among patients, no one can escape the effects of gravity. Brow ptosis and wrinkles will inevitably occur, but the degree to which it happens and when it happens is variable. While patients above the age of 40 years old may be candidates for facelift surgery, patients in their 20s and 30s may be candidates for brow lifting. It behooves the cosmetic surgeon to be well versed in various browlift, blepharoplasty and injectable techniques to address patients' upper facial thirds.

The aging population wants to feel and look more youthful while today's younger population wants to remain looking youthful. Patients are becoming more educated and well-versed in cosmetic surgery thanks, in part, to social media. It is the surgeon's duty and responsibility to provide the patient with the best and safest techniques available to achieve their realistic, desired outcomes.

Author details

Anthony Congiusta[1*], Angelo Cuzalina[2] and Maria Jubran-Khoury[3]

1 Connecticut Surgical Arts, Norwich, Connecticut, USA

2 Tulsa Surgical Arts, Tulsa, Oklahoma, USA

3 Independent Researcher, Tel Aviv, Israel

*Address all correspondence to: anthony.congiusta.90@gmail.com

References

[1] Darwin C. The Project Gutenberg eBook of the Expression of Emotion in Man and Animals. 1998. Available from: https://www.gutenberg.org/files/1227/1227-h/1227-h.htm#link2HCH0007

[2] Knize DM. Anatomic concepts for brow lift procedures. Plastic and Reconstructive Surgery. 2009;**124**(6):2118-2126. DOI: 10.1097/PRS.0b013e3181bd0726

[3] Hollabaugh B, Perenack J, Christensen B. Endoscopic brow lift without muscle resection: Objective and subjective changes in intereyebrow width. The American Journal of Cosmetic Surgery. 2020;**37**(2):97-103. DOI: 10.1177/0748806819884424

[4] Sundaram H, Signorini M, Liew S, et al. Global aesthetics consensus: Botulinum toxin type A--Evidence-based review, emerging concepts, and consensus recommendations for aesthetic use, including updates on complications. Plastic and Reconstructive Surgery. 2016;**137**(3):518e-529e. DOI: 10.1097/01.prs.0000475758.63709.23

[5] Niamtu J. The subcutaneous brow- and forehead-lift: A face-lift for the forehead and brow. Dermatologic Surgery. 2008;**34**(10):1350-1361; discussion 1362. DOI: 10.1111/j.1524-4725.2008.34288.x

[6] Cuzalina A, Sohn A. Forehead and eyebrow lift techniques. In: Ferneini EM, Goupil MT, MA MN, Niekrash CE, editors. Applied Head and Neck Anatomy for the Facial Cosmetic Surgeon. Cham, Switzerland: Springer; 2021. pp. 149-166. Chap 18

[7] Cuzalina A, Bedi M. Forehead and brow lift. In: Fonseca RJ, editor. Oral and Maxillofacial Surgery. 3rd ed. St. Louis, Missouri: Elsevier; 2014. pp. 395-428. Chapter 22. Orthognathic Surgery Esthetic Surgery Cleft and Craniofacial Surgery

[8] Terella AM, Wang TD. Technical considerations in endoscopic brow lift. Clinics in Plastic Surgery. 2013;**40**(1):105-115. DOI: 10.1016/j.cps.2012.06.004

[9] Guthrie A, Kadakia S, Cranford J, Sawhney R, Ducic Y. A review of complications and their treatments in facial aesthetic surgery. The American Journal of Cosmetic Surgery. 2017;**34**(2):73-80. DOI: 10.1177/0748806816689619

[10] Dhaliwal H. Analysis and diagnosis of upper facial region. Atlas of the Oral and Maxillofacial Surgery Clinics of North America. 2016;**24**(2):87-93. DOI: 10.1016/j.cxom.2016.05.002

[11] Ramly EP, Katave C, Ranganathan K. Facial feminization: Upper third of the face. Oral and Maxillofacial Surgery Clinics of North America. 2024;**36**(2):183-194. DOI: 10.1016/j.coms.2024.01.002

[12] Cuzalina AL, Holmes JD. A simple and reliable landmark for identification of the supraorbital nerve in surgery of the forehead: An in vivo anatomical study. Journal of Oral and Maxillofacial Surgery. 2005;**63**(1):25-27. DOI: 10.1016/j.joms.2004.04.026

[13] Punthakee X, Mashkevich G, Keller GS. Endoscopic forehead and brow-lift. Facial Plastic Surgery. 2010;**26**(3):239-251. DOI: 10.1055/s-0030-1254335

[14] Jones BM, Lo SJ. The impact of endoscopic brow lift on eyebrow

morphology, aesthetics, and longevity: Objective and subjective measurements over a 5-year period. Plastic and Reconstructive Surgery. 2013;**132**(2):226e-238e. DOI: 10.1097/PRS.0b013e3182958b9f

[15] Chmielewski P, Skrzat J, Walocha J. Clinical importance of the middle meningeal artery. Folia Medica Cracoviensia. 2013;**53**(1):41-46

[16] Fisher O, Zamboni WA. Endoscopic brow-lift in the male patient. Archives of Facial Plastic Surgery. 2010;**12**(1):56-59. DOI: 10.1001/archfacial.2009.109

[17] Geroulis A, Kemker B. Endoscopic forehead and brow-lift surgery for male patients. The American Journal of Cosmetic Surgery. 1996;**13**(4):315-319. DOI: 10.1177/074880689601300404

[18] Cuzalina A, Bedi M. Management of complications associated with upper facial rejuvenation. Atlas of the Oral and Maxillofacial Surgery Clinics of North America. 2016;**24**(2):175-180. DOI: 10.1016/j.cxom.2016.05.001

[19] Richards BG, Schleicher WF, Zins JE. Putting it all together: Recommendations for improving pain management in plastic surgical procedures-surgical facial rejuvenation. Plastic and Reconstructive Surgery. 2014;**134**(4 Suppl 2):108S-112S. DOI: 10.1097/PRS.0000000000000673

[20] Rammos CK, Mardini S. Endoscopic browlift in the receding hairline patient. The Journal of Craniofacial Surgery. 2016;**27**(1):156-158. DOI: 10.1097/SCS.0000000000002266

[21] Jugan M, Sellers V, Waite P. Endoscopic forehead rejuvenation: Using bone channels for soft-tissue suspension. The American Journal of Cosmetic Surgery. 2002;**19**(2):77-85. DOI: 10.1177/074880680201900202

Chapter 3

The Lip Lift, Pearls about the Procedure, How to Avoid Complications and How to Obtain Patient's Satisfaction

Alicia Sigler

Abstract

In this study, the author shares her experience from performing 488 lip lift procedures. The procedure technique is shared with all the details of the preop and postop instructions in order to avoid complications. The success of the procedure was based on the assessment of scar appearance, length of the upper lip, and patients' satisfaction with their upper lip length.

Keywords: lip lift procedure, lip lift technique, lip lifting, patient satisfaction, complication prevention

1. Introduction

It has been described that a youthful and beautiful upper lip should allow the upper teeth to show when the person is talking and to be fully seen when the person poses a big smile [1–4]. There is a standard distance between the base of the nose and the white roll of the upper lip for an attractive upper lip height such as 10–12 mm for women and 15 mm for men [5, 6].

Height shortening of the upper lip or lip lift procedure has been challenging for some surgeons since the resulting scar may be visible or unpleasant, that's why the bull-horn pattern was designed to hide the scar in the area where the shadow of the nasal base covers it [7]. If the plastic surgeon considers the characteristics of the patient and follows the correct surgical steps to obtain normal wound healing and good scar tissue, the results will be beautiful and will bring a youthful appearance to the aging lip.

2. Methods

The patients that participated in this study agreed to getting a bullhorn lip lift by the author, and patients were excluded when they could not be located after the procedure or when they declined to be part of it.

Assessment of the results in scar appearance, length of the upper lip, and patients' satisfaction with their upper lip length were performed by the author 3 and 6 months

IntechOpen

after the lip lift procedure. Ideally, the surgeon should have the patient's input on how much tissue should be excised. The author suggests having the patient face a mirror and pull with the index fingers the upper lip to provide the resulting shape and height of her/his ideal upper lip, that way the surgeon will be able to calculate the amount in millimeters of tissue to be removed (**Figures 1–4**). A Bullhorn pattern was designed before the skin removal and was based on measurements to obtain the total ideal length of the upper lip without including the vermilion part: ideally 10-12 mm for female patients and 15 mm for male patients (**Figure 5**) etc. After locally injecting with lidocaine 2% and epinephrine, the first incision was made on the marking located superiorly (on the base of the nose) and only included skin. The dissection was performed only under the skin that had the area to be removed. After performing a test where traction was done on the inferior limit of the marked area to observe if the result would be as planned and requested by the patient, the amount of skin that is contained inside those markings

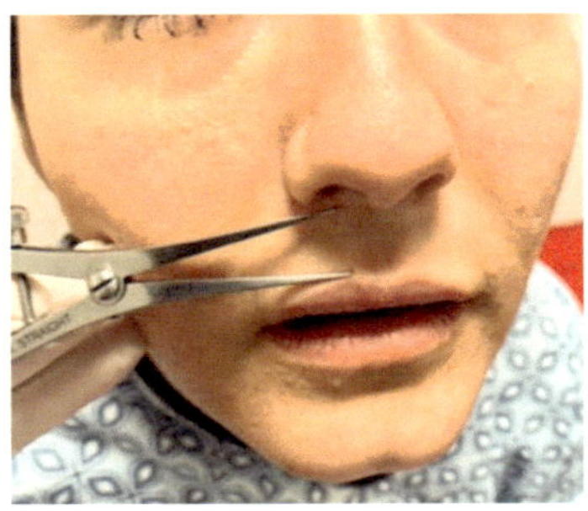

Figure 1.
Measurement of the upper lip at rest from the base of the nose to the white roll of the lip.

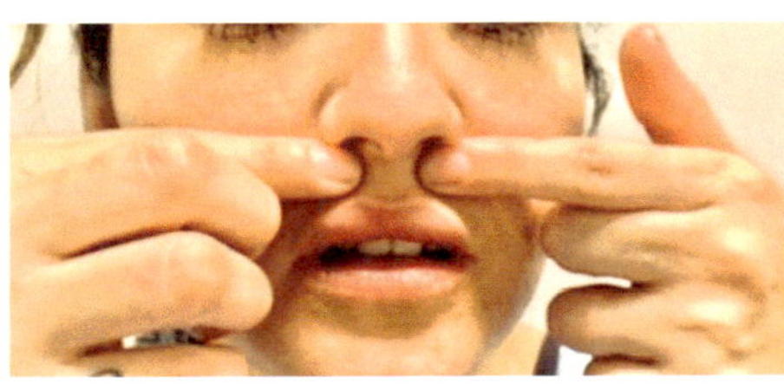

Figure 2.
The patient is asked in front of a mirror to pull with index fingers the appearance and height she/he would like her/his upper lip to get.

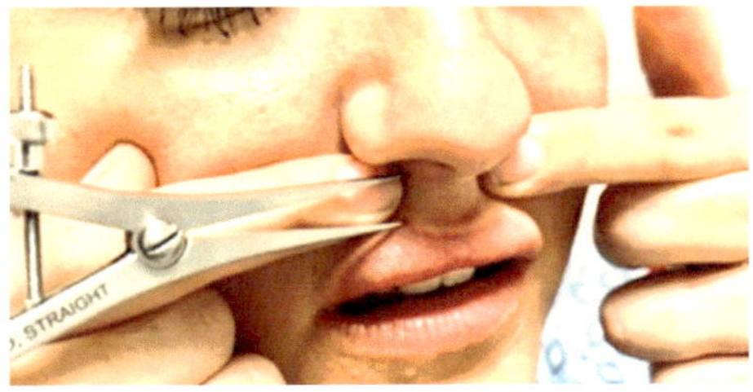

Figure 3.
The desired height of the upper lip is measured from the base of the nose to the white roll.

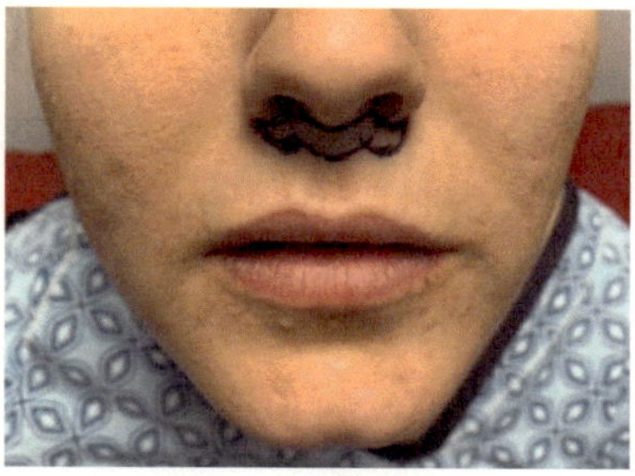

Figure 4.
The desired height measurement is subtracted from the total height of the upper lip at rest and the resulting measurement is equal to the measurement in millimeters that will need to be excised.

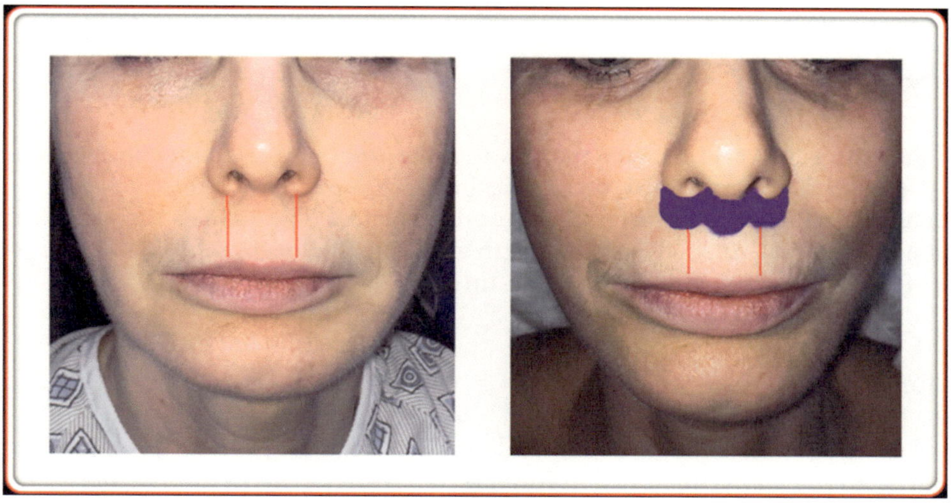

Figure 5.
Measurements method suggested by the author.

was removed. The edge of the lower incision was released from tension trimming under the skin about one or two millimeters more. No dissection nor management was performed on the SMAS nor on the orbicularis oris muscle of the upper lip. The wound was closed with 5-0 nylon stitches for the deep dermis layer and 6-0 nylon stitches for the superficial skin layer (**Figure 6**). The superficial stitches were removed after 2 weeks of the procedure. Very detailed instructions were given to the patients before the surgery such as avoiding smoking and vaping, NSAIDs, herbal medications, and vitamin E 1 month before the surgery. After the lip lift, the patients were instructed to cleanse the wound with peroxide and apply triple antibiotic ointment three times a day for 1 week, avoid sunlight, and heat to the lip area, and all anti-edema measures after a facial surgical procedure for 2 weeks, such as sleeping at a 45-degree angle, avoid heavy lifting, exercising, bending over, etc. One week after the stitch removal, the patients massaged the wound in the process to become a scar with scar treatment gel and moderate pressure for 5 minutes, 3 times a day, until the scar felt soft, and its color was resembling the color of the patient's skin. It was also recommended to cover the scar with sunscreen with a 50 SPF (sun protection factor).

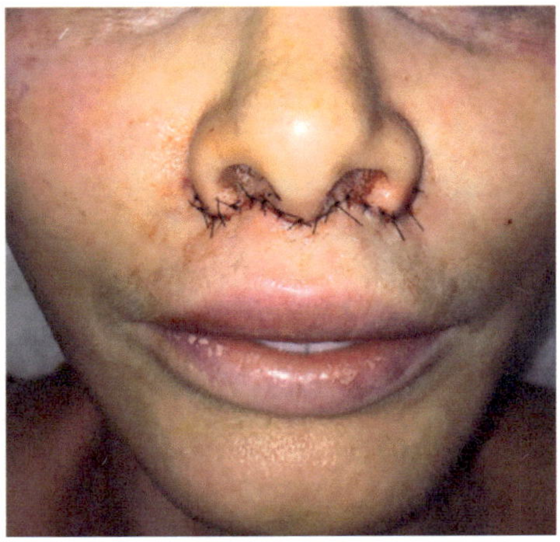

Figure 6.
Lip lift sutures.

Patients were seen 1, 3, and 6 months after the procedure for follow-up, and at 3 and 6 months follow-up visits, the total length of the upper lip without including the vermilion and the scar characteristics were documented. The patients answered to the questions: are you satisfied with the length of your upper lip after the lip lift? Are you satisfied with the scar resulting from the lip lift?

3. Results

During a period of 10 years, the author has performed 488 lip lifts on patients with ages ranging between 18 and 76 years old. Ninety eight percent of the patients were female including 5 trans women (**Figures** 7 and **8**), and 2% were male patients (**Figures 9** and **10**). From the total: 88% were Caucasian, 10% were Hispanic, 1% were Asian, and 1% were Afro-American. The amount of skin removed from 98% of the patients was 6–8 mm to obtain the length of 10–12 mm in women and 15 mm in men. From all the patients, 98% of the patients were satisfied with the result in length of the upper lip as well as the scar (**Figures 11–16**). Long-term results will be the subject for another study. Only 2% of the patients in

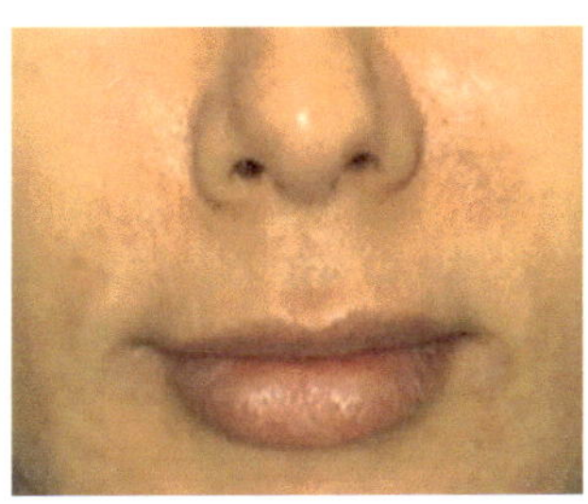

Figure 7.
Lip lift preop female patient.

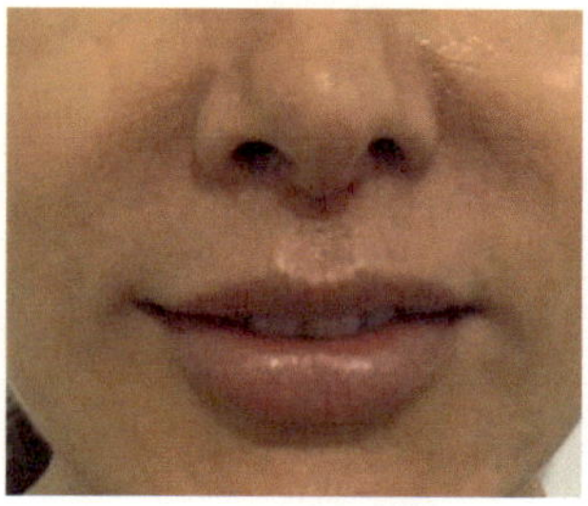

Figure 8.
Lip lift postop female patient.

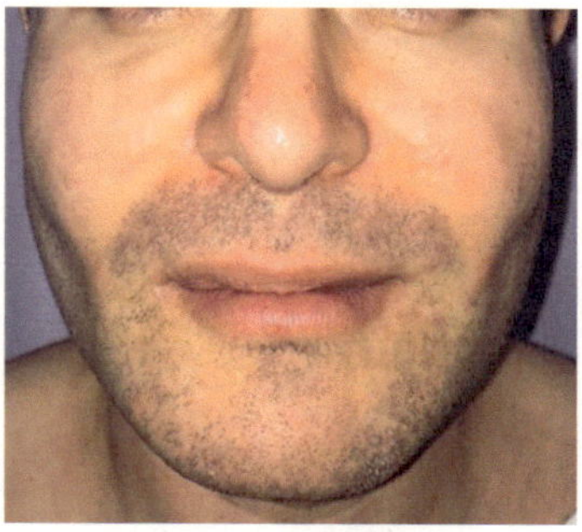

Figure 9.
Lip lift preop male patient.

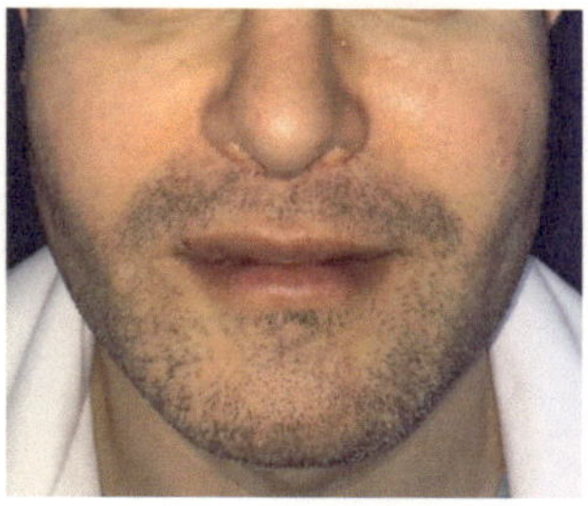

Figure 10.
Lip lift postop male patient.

this study required surgical revisions to reduce even more the length of the upper lip. Three patients, all Hispanic, two females and one male, developed hypertrophic scars, they requested treatment for them due to their appearance that was difficult to hide. These three patients were the ones not satisfied with their scars even when they were satisfied with the length obtained with the procedure. The hypertrophic scars improved with the intralesional triamcinolone injections to the point of patients' satisfaction, and they stated the scars were not noticeable anymore. The hypertrophic scars were diagnosed due to their characteristics: they were pink in color, painless, felt hard to touch and they raised less than 1 mm from the skin surface. The scars did not extend beyond the initial site of the wound (**Figure 17**) [8].

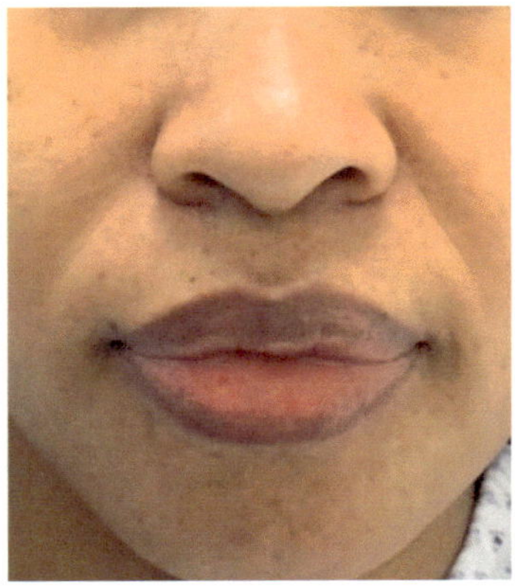

Figure 11.
Preoperative appearance of upper lip.

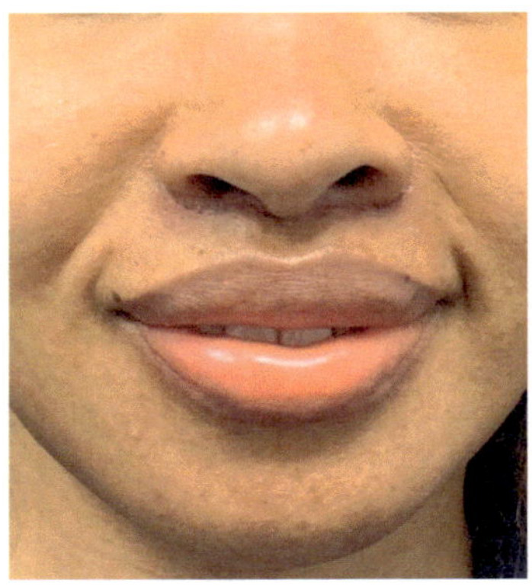

Figure 12.
Lip lift postoperative result.

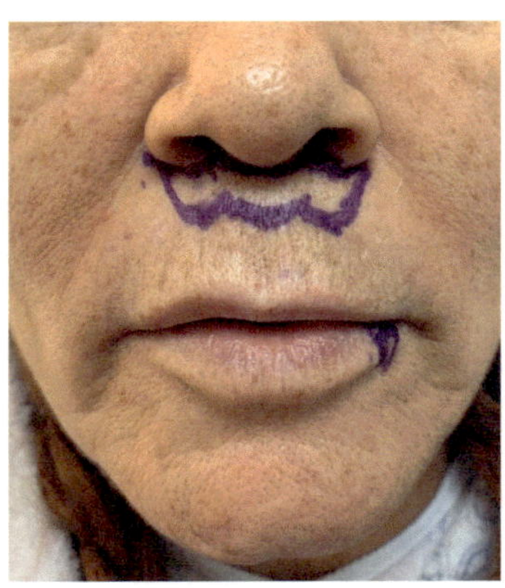

Figure 13.
Asymmetrical preoperative markings for a lip lift in a female patient's lip with asymmetrical length. She also was having a lower lip lesion removed.

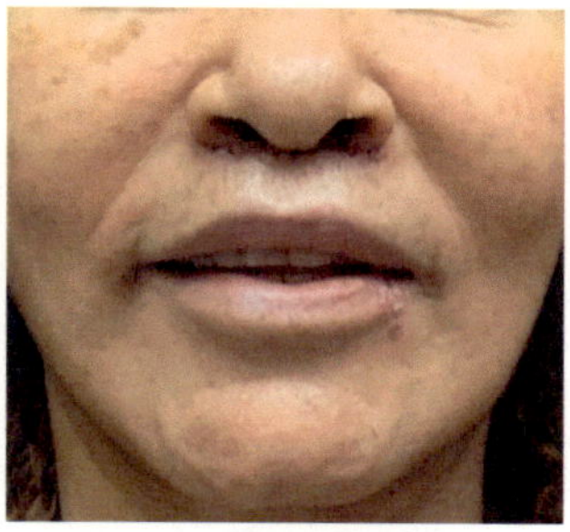

Figure 14.
The postoperative result of a lip lift procedure with asymmetrical markings, to obtain height symmetry of the upper lip.

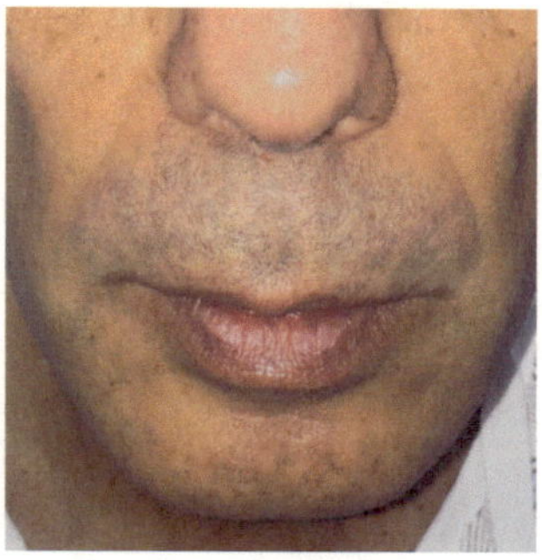

Figure 15.
Preoperative appearance of a long upper lip in a male patient.

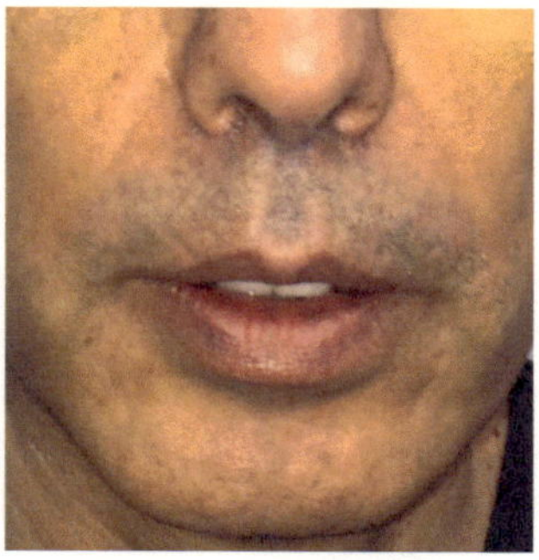

Figure 16.
Postoperative result of the lip lift in a male patient.

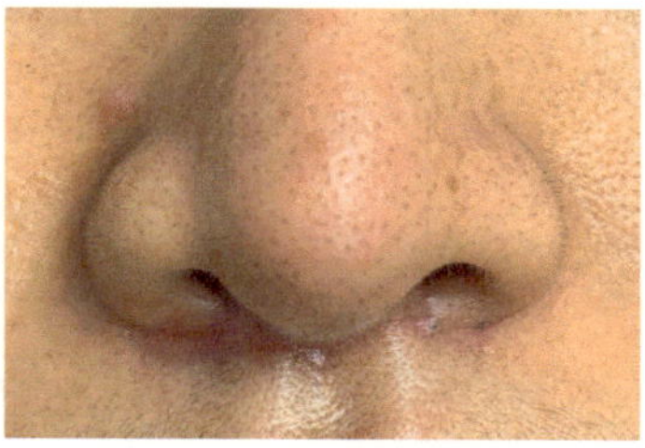

Figure 17.
Hypertrophic scar from a lip lift procedure.

4. Discussion

There have been multiple authors providing information about their experience related to the pattern they prefer for the lip lift skin resection and how they determine the measures of that pattern. They also share and describe the surgical technique of their preference [9–12]. Zhang et al. added a T-shaped resection of the orbicularis oris to the lip lift procedure [13]. Talei and Pearlman propose suturing the SMAS of the upper lip to the piriform ligament before suturing the skin which allows the wound edges to approximate without tension [14]. In this series of patients treated by the author, there was no need to treat the SMAS nor the orbicularis oris muscle. The three patients that developed hypertrophic scars had more than 10 mm of lip length removed, and there is a possibility that this caused tension on the wound edges and predisposed them to develop this type of scar. The author recommends removing less than 10 mm of lip height to avoid this kind of scar tissue. It is important for the surgeons who will be more involved with this procedure to create their own protocol based on what has been described to avoid complications and to provide their patients with the best results. The strategies used in this protocol to obtain good scar formation are the creation of a moisture-rich environment for faster epithelialization by the prophylactic local antibiotics and the avoidance of tension on the suture line. It is also of great importance to prevent wound infection by the topical application of the triple antibiotic ointment, and to massage the scar for the degradation of excessive and nonpliable collagen. The use of sunscreen reduces the scar hyperpigmentation when exposed to the ultraviolet light stimulation [15]. Patients should adhere to all the preoperative and postoperative instructions for their prompt recovery and an unnoticeable scar.

5. Conclusion

The lip lift has become a popular procedure since the upper lip is considered a feature to project beauty and youth. To obtain the optimal results and avoid complications, the surgeon must consider the patient's expectations, plan very carefully the design of the pattern to be used and the amount of skin to be removed, and perform the procedure following all the principles to avoid suture tension, wound infection, and excessive use of the electrocautery to prevent increased edema. Most of the patients undergoing this approach are satisfied with the length obtained on their upper lips.

Compliance with ethical standards

Conflict of interest statement

The author declares that she has no conflict of interests to disclose.

Statement of human or animal rights, or ethical approval

This article does not contain any studies with human participants or animals performed by the author.

Informed consent

For this type of study informed consent is not required.

Author details

Alicia Sigler
Hospital Ángeles, Tijuana, Mexico

*Address all correspondence to: aliciasiglerplasticsurgeon@gmail.com

References

[1] Rozner L, Isaacs GW. Lip lifting. British Journal of Plastic Surgery. 1981;**34**(4):481-484

[2] Fanous N. Correction of thin lips: "Lip Lift". Plastic and Reconstructive Surgery. 1984;**74**(1):33-41

[3] Austin HW. The lip lift. Plastic and Reconstructive Surgery. 1986;**77**(6):990-994

[4] Raschke GF, Rieger UM, Bader RD, et al. Perioral aging and athropometric appraisal. Journal of Cranio-Maxillo-Facial Surgery. 2014;**42**(5):a312-a317

[5] Farkas LG, Katic MJ, Hreczko TA, Deutsch C, Munro IR. Anthropometric proportions in the upper lip-lower lip-chin area of the lower face in young white adults. American Journal of Orthodontics and Dentofacial Orthopedics. 1984;**86**(1):52-60

[6] Popenko NA, Tripathi PB, Devcic Z, et al. A quantitative approach to determining the ideal female lip aesthetic and its effect on facial atractiveness. JAMA Facial Plastic Surgery. 2017;**19**(4):261-267

[7] Ramirez OM et al. The upper Lip Lift using the "Bull's Horn" approach. Journal of Drugs in Dermatology. 2003;**2**(3):303-306

[8] Gauglitz GG et al. Hypertrophic scarring and keloids: Pathomechanisms and current and emerging treatment strategies. Molecular Medicine. 2011;**17**(1-2):113-125

[9] Weston GW, Byron DP, Sigal RK, Austin HW. Lifting lips: 28 years of experience using the direct excision approach to rejuvenating the aging mouth. Aesthetic Surgery Journal. 2009;**29**(2):83-86

[10] Waldman SR. The subnasal lift. Facial Plastic Surgery Clinics of North America. 2007;**15**(4):513-516

[11] Winslow C. Surgical and nonsurgical perioral/lip rejuvenation. Beyond volume restoration. Clinics in Plastic Surgery. 2018;**45**(4):601-609

[12] Tonnard PL, Verpaele AM, Ramaut LE, Blondeel PN. Aging of the upper lip: Part II. Evidence-based rejuvenation of the upper lip. A review of 500 consecutive cases. PRS. 2019;**143**(5):1333-1342

[13] Zhang GL et al. T-shaped excision of the orbicularis oris muscle: An innovative technique for upper lip lift procedures. Aesthetic Surgery Journal. 2015;**35**(4):456-461

[14] Talei B, Pearlman SJ. CUPID lip lift: advanced lip design using the deep-plane upper lip lift and simplified corner lift. Aesthetic Surgery Journal. 2022;**42**(12):1357-1373

[15] Commander SJ et al. Update on postsurgical scar management. Seminars in Plastic Surgery. 2016;**30**(3):122-128

Chapter 4

Upper and Lower Face Lifting Surgery

Artem Krutyansky and Angelo Cuzalina

Abstract

The face is often the first area to exhibit signs of aging. Over the past two decades, the popularity of rejuvenating the aging face has grown significantly. Historically, traditional incisional face-lifting was the primary technique for facial rejuvenation. However, in the past 10 years, cosmetic surgery has evolved to include a variety of procedures such as alloplastic facial implants, chemodenervation, injectable fillers, and skin resurfacing through laser or chemical exfoliation. Despite the availability of these diverse methods for addressing facial aging, the "modern" face-lift remains the benchmark for treating generalized facial cutis laxa (rhytidosis), jowling, excess skin in the cervicomental region, and platysmal banding. This chapter will examine upper and lower facelifting with the experience of Dr. Cuzalina in 30 years of clinical practice.

Keywords: facelift, submentoplasty, jowling, neck laxity, jaw-line

1. Introduction

The main factors contributing to facial aging are genetics, age, and smoking. The primary concerns addressed by current face-lifting techniques include loose skin in the jowls and neck area, pronounced nasolabial folds, and platysmal banding. Typically, patients seek lower face-lifting and neck-lifting treatments between the ages of 45 and 65, though this range can vary widely. Esthetic concerns related to the forehead and brow areas affect individuals across various age groups. Unlike the traditional lower face and neck rhytidectomy, which is typically sought by patients over the age of 45, cosmetic issues in the upper third of the face can become noticeable in patients as young as their twenties and thirties, often due to genetic factors. The second subsection of this chapter will concentrate on upper face lifting.

1.1 Lower face lifting

1.1.1 Body

1.1.1.1 History

The early descriptions of face-lifts in the literature focused solely on skin excision. Despite the temporary benefits and often unnatural appearance, some surgeons still employ this method for patients with unique anatomy or for revision procedures. Nowadays, face-lifting techniques are diverse, with most involving the manipulation of the superficial musculoaponeurotic system (SMAS). This approach was first introduced by Mitz and Peyronie in their landmark 1976 article [1].

Historical details regarding face-lifting are documented in various publications. During that period, both surgeons and patients were hesitant to publicly acknowledge their interest in cosmetic surgery [2]. Consequently, technical advancements were slow to emerge and spread. Despite extensive undermining of skin flaps in face-lifts performed decades ago, the outcomes were only partially effective and did not address issues related to the neck and platysma. A significant advancement in understanding facial anatomy was made by Skoog in 1974, whose techniques in manipulating facial tissue paved the way for future improvements in face-lifting surgery [3]. Subsequently, Webster and colleagues highlighted that extensive subcutaneous dissection exposed larger raw areas, increasing the risk of complications [4]. Richard Webster was among the first to advocate for a "short flap" with basic SMAS plication, suggesting that the skin would adequately advance from its attachment to the elevated deep tissue.

Experienced surgeons now have a deeper understanding of achieving long-lasting, significant results. Cosmetic surgery has always focused on contouring and sculpting. Since 1999, we have been advancing rhytidectomy, beginning with Dr. Cuzalina's pioneering partial resection of the submandibular glands (**Figures 1** and **2**).

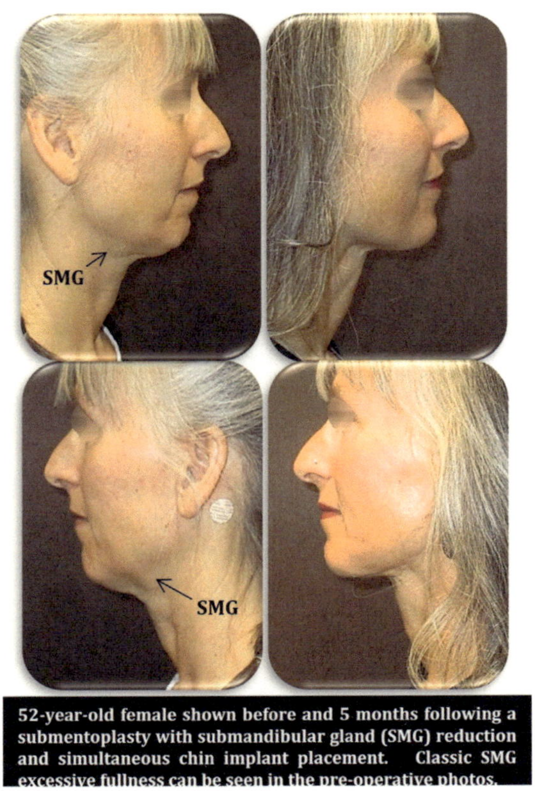

Figure 1.
52-year-old female shown before and 5 months following a submentoplasty with submandibular gland (SMG) reduction and simultaneous chin implant placement. Classic SMG excessive fullness can be seen in the pre-operative photos.

DOI: http://dx.doi.org/10.5772/intechopen.1008262

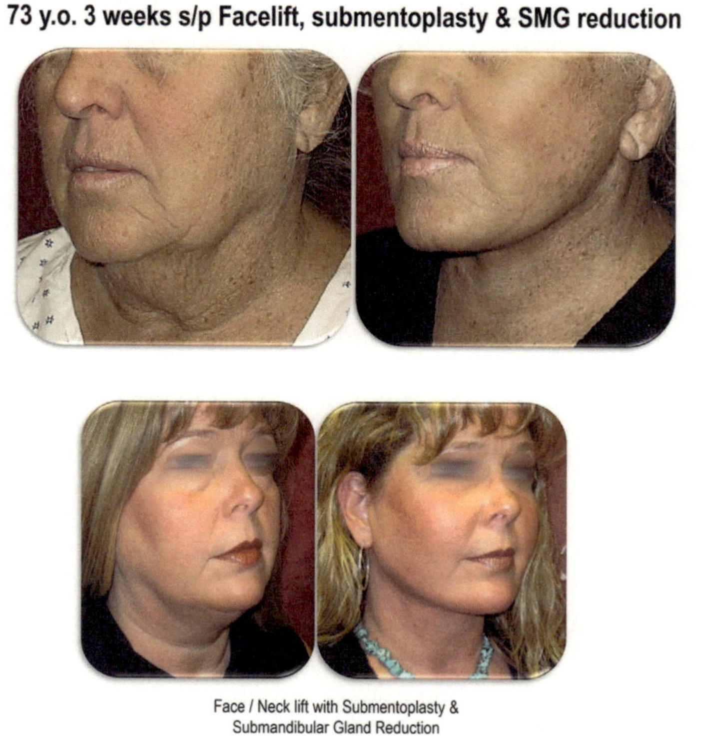

Figure 2.
73 y.o. 3 weeks s/p Facelift, submentoplasty & SMG reduction. Face/Neck lift with Submentoplasty & Submandibular Gland Reduction.

This procedure resulted in sharper jawlines and prevented bulging in the submandibular area. Additionally, Dr. Cuzalina performed superficial parotidectomies on patients with excess masseter hypertrophy to soften the face. These techniques are now being adopted by experienced cosmetic surgeons to create more defined, enduring results.

1.1.2 Anatomy

A surgeon must be vigilant of three primary danger zones: the mid-zygomatic temporal region, the malar eminence region, and the area along the inferior border of the mandible near the angle. The mid-zygomatic arch area houses the temporal or frontal branch of the facial nerve, which crosses over the arch approximately 2 cm from the external auditory meatus [5]. This nerve is particularly vulnerable in the area over the bony prominence, where there is minimal soft tissue coverage.

The second zone is located at the zygomatic/malar eminence. This area contains a network of vessels connecting the transverse facial artery and the facial artery proper, along with the zygomatic branch of the facial nerve, which crosses upward near the outer corner of the eye. This region is referred to as the "MacGregor patch" due to the strong fibrous attachments between the zygomatic bone and the skin.

The third zone is at the lower border of the mandible, slightly in front of the mandibular angle. The marginal mandibular branch of the facial nerve runs just below the mandible's lower border approximately 20–50% of the time, but it can be found up to 1.5 cm below this border [6]. Initial dissection over the platysma muscle helps avoid damaging the marginal mandibular nerve, while further dissection below the platysma must be performed with greater caution to preserve the nerve's integrity.

Several sensory nerves may be injured during a rhytidectomy, with the most notable being the greater auricular nerve. It is essential for patients undergoing any cosmetic procedure to have reasonable expectations. Undermining the skin or any fascial plane typically results in some degree of numbness. However, if this potential outcome is communicated to the patient preoperatively, it transforms the "complication" into a nonissue for the patient.

Anatomically, it is crucial to understand that during a deep plane facelift, the deep plane becomes subcutaneous beyond the masseter muscle or in the region of McGregor's patch (**Figure 3**). Otherwise, there is a risk of facial nerve injury, a detail often not elaborated upon in the literature. In the biplane technique, a short deep plane SMAS flap is utilized. Despite this, the results can be comparable due to the equivalent extent of dissection performed.

1.1.3 Procedure

As with any surgical procedure, obtaining informed consent and proper documentation is essential before moving forward. Ideally, the consent form should be reviewed by the patient well before the surgery date.

Depending on the patient's medical history, specific laboratory tests might be necessary. For patients over 40 years old, a 12-lead electrocardiogram, urinalysis, and hematocrit are recommended. The need for additional advanced tests, such as electrolytes, prothrombin time, partial thromboplastin time, or chest radiography, will be determined based on a thorough history and physical examination.

Patients should be advised to avoid aspirin and non-steroidal anti-inflammatory drugs, and to stop taking Vitamin E 2 weeks prior to surgery to reduce platelet dysfunction and the risk of bleeding.

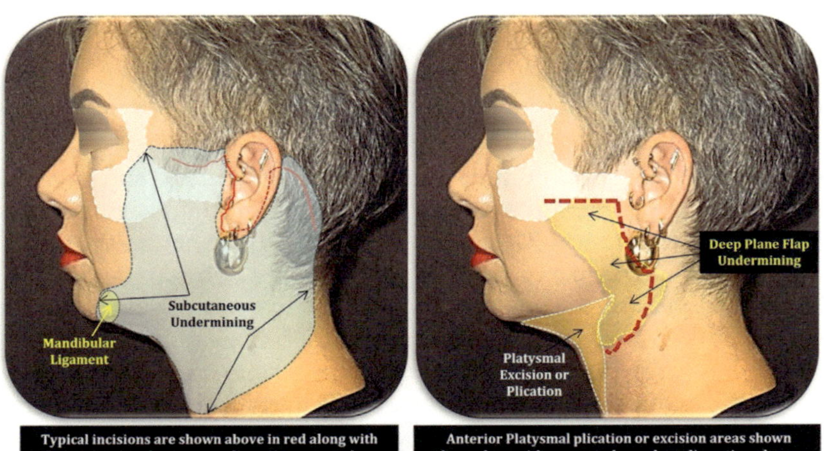

Figure 3.
Typical incisions are shown above in red along with the maximum subcutaneous dissection extent along with mandibular ligament release. Anterior Platysmal plication or excision areas shown above along with common deep-plane dissection planes.

Many patients may not realize that the instruction to fast does not mean they should skip their regular morning blood pressure medications; they can take these with a small sip of water. For patients with borderline preoperative blood pressure but no history of hypertension, preoperative clonidine may be beneficial. A small dose of clonidine before surgery can help stabilize blood pressure during the procedure [7].

Other preoperative procedures involve having the patient thoroughly wash their hair and face with germicidal soap on the morning of the surgery. Some patients may benefit from mild benzodiazepine sedation administered the night before and on the morning of the procedure.

Before transporting the patient to the operating room, the incision site should be marked, and the hair should be taped, shaved, or braided. Following sedation or general anesthesia, wrap paper tape around the patient's hair and head just posterior to the incision sites in the temporal and mastoid regions. Hair in front of the temporal incision site can be twisted and secured with a rubber band or paper tape. If incisions are planned entirely within the hairline, shaving is not required. Wrapping the patient's hair with paper tape helps prevent loose hair from interfering with suturing. During surgery, K-Y jelly or Polysporin ointment can be useful if hair encroaches on the wound.

A light preparation with alcohol or povidone-iodine (Betadine) is recommended prior to the infiltration of local anesthetic. Additionally, during skin preparation, administer 1 g of cefazolin and 8 mg of dexamethasone (Decadron) intravenously. Since it takes about 15 minutes to achieve maximal local vasoconstriction, this step should ideally be completed before the surgeon scrubs and drapes.

We believe that submentoplasty is essential for most candidates undergoing rhytidectomy. With 30 years of experience in performing facelifts, it's evident that the primary concern often lies in neck laxity and rhytids. Referring to it simply as a facelift may be somewhat misleading; a more accurate term would be a lower face and neck lift.

Face-lift scissors are employed to carefully undermine the skin while maintaining an even layer of subdermal fat. The dissection extends inferiorly to the lower border of the thyroid cartilage and laterally to the posterior border of the mandible. Extensive skin undermining is essential to facilitate proper skin redraping once the deep tissues have been treated. Insufficient skin undermining can result in bunching after midline plication of the platysma. If skin elasticity is assessed as inadequate during the preoperative evaluation, a combination of face-lift and submentoplasty is generally required.

A flat spatulated cannula can then be utilized for liposuction of the fat overlying the platysma under direct visualization. A lighted Aufricht retractor enhances visibility through the small submental incision. Any excess submental fat is subsequently excised. A Kelly clamp or large hemostat is positioned in the midline to hold the platysma and fat, while a needle-tipped cautery or scissors is used for resection. At this stage, the anterior jugular veins may be encountered.

Achieving proper hemostasis is crucial for the successful completion of the operation and to minimize the risk of postoperative hematoma. After resecting the midline fat, the anterior borders of the platysma and the hyoid bone should be identified. The platysma is then backcut starting at the level of the hyoid bone. This backcut extends approximately 5 to 7 cm, remaining parallel to the inferior border of the mandible and well below the inferior extent of the submandibular gland (**Figure 4**). Caution is required to avoid damaging the facial vessels or nerve during this incision. The platysma is then undermined superior to the backcut area. In cases of submandibular

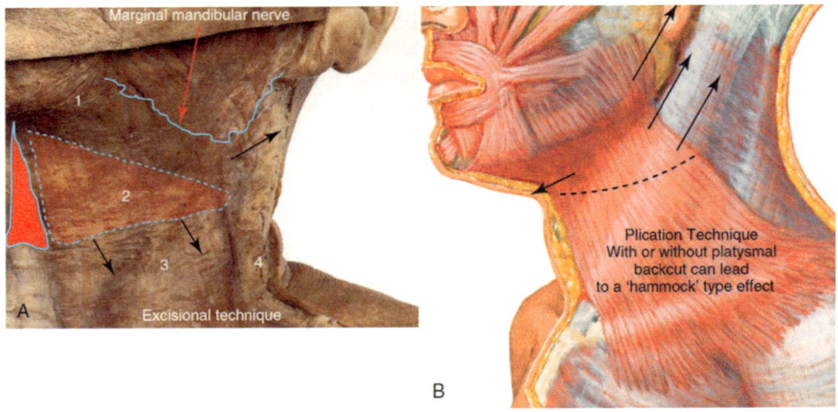

Figure 4.
Dueling face-lift and anterior platysmal plication may compete, but some surgeons believe that it may also create a positive "hammock" effect on the neck.

gland ptosis or enlargement, resection of the gland's superficial portion with a needle-tipped cautery may be necessary; however, this procedure is complex and not recommended for novice surgeons. Bleeding may be challenging to control due to the small incision and limited access.

Following bilateral mobilization of the platysma, a corset platysmaplasty is performed using a running 2–0 Vicryl suture. The inferior edges of the platysma are plicated at the midline to the fascia over the hyoid bone. If a chin implant is required to improve a poorly defined cervicomental angle caused by a low hyoid position, it should be inserted at this stage (**Figure 5**).

The temporal incision may extend directly upward from the preauricular sulcus incision, or it might curve around the front edge of the temporal hair tuft. The latter approach is especially useful if the temporal tuft is high, such as in patients who have had previous face-lifts. The superior portion of the incision curves slightly forward but remains well concealed within the dense temporal hair. It extends upward into the hair as needed (typically 3 to 4 cm) to facilitate lifting of the mid-face region. The incision in the hair should follow the direction of the hair follicles, or the upper edge should be beveled to ensure that hair growth covers the scar.

A standard face-lift incision is generally divided into three main sections: temporal, periauricular, and mastoid. For men, the incision is placed in the preauricular sulcus, just in front of the tragus, to prevent hair growth over the tragus after surgery. Women may also use this incision, but many surgeons place it at the posterior edge of the tragus to better camouflage the scar.

Retroauricular or mastoid incisions can be made in the hair-bearing scalp or just in front of the hairline. These incisions start at the upper end of the retroauricular sulcus incision, level with the external auditory canal, or where the post-auricular hair meets the ear helix. The skin incision should be about 90 degrees to avoid necrosis. Incisions in front of the mastoid hairline are straightforward and prevent postoperative changes to the hairline or hair loss but might leave a noticeable, widened scar if there's excessive tension during closure. Fortunately, even short hairstyles will eventually cover this incision. When incisions extend directly into the hair, the scar is well hidden, but this may lead to hair loss and complications in aligning the hairline properly.

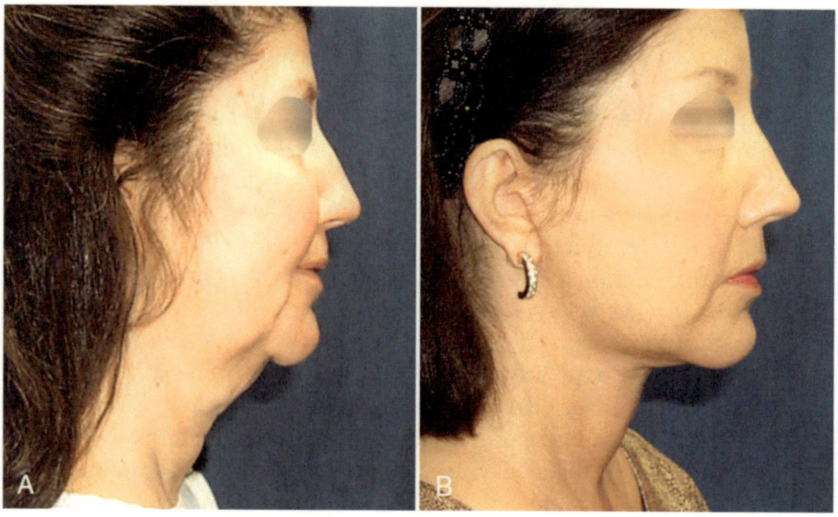

Figure 5.
A: A 52-year-old patient before undergoing a facelift and submentoplasty, which involved the removal of deep fat, a minor reduction of the digastric muscle, platysmal back cuts with undermining, and anterior plication. B: Six months after surgery.

Using double-pronged hooks to lift and separate the skin edges allows for dissection with minimal trauma to the skin. It is crucial to maintain a well-controlled subcutaneous plane with a healthy fat layer during the development of a long subcutaneous flap.

To avoid damaging the branches of the superficial temporal artery or vein, stay superficial to these structures, just beneath the temporal tuft hairline incision. Care must be taken to ensure an adequate superficial flap thickness of approximately 6–8 mm, while staying above the deep fascia. The thickness of the flap can vary across different facial areas and from patient to patient. The region over the sternocleidomastoid and the greater auricular nerve is often the thinnest and most fibrotic. Direct blade or cautery over this cervical area helps avoid external jugular vein injury compared with other nondirect or blind elevation techniques.

In the mastoid and occipital regions, the dissection plane should be positioned well beneath the hair follicles to prevent alopecia. Initially, flap elevation posterior to the ear is performed immediately above the occipital fascia and the investing fascia of the sternocleidomastoid muscle using needle-tip electrocautery. The flap is thickest in the occipital scalp and gradually thins as it extends distally over the cervical fascia. The scalp is also elevated superiorly from the occipital region by 1 to 2 cm to facilitate more precise closure and alignment with the posterior hairline. The dissection continues inferiorly and anteriorly to connect with the subcutaneous flap created during the anterior submentoplasty, which is performed prior to lateral dissection from the ears.

We utilize the deep posterior biplane dissection technique. This method is referred to as an opportunistic technique because the extent of deep plane dissection is guided not by anatomical landmarks but by what is necessary to achieve the desired elevation for the patient. The biplane and opportunistic aspects of this facelift are performed through the submental incision and the posterior dissection.

The initial incision starts along or just below the zygomatic arch and extends forward by 2 to 3 cm from a point approximately 1 cm in front of the helix. The horizontal superior incision continues downward in front of the ear and curves back anteriorly across the posterior platysmal border, approximately 2 cm below the mandibular border.

The flap is initially elevated using electrocautery and is further lifted with facelift scissors. The inferior dissection of the musculofascial flap often connects with the anterior platysmal myotomy below the mandibular border.

The depth of dissection is easily determined when there is a sufficient SMAS layer, staying just above the parotideomasseteric fascia and below the cervical platysma. The upper limit of dissection is near the zygomatic arch, and care must be taken to maintain adequate tissue coverage over the frontal nerve branches.

As the dissection proceeds anteriorly, it approaches the anterior margin of the parotid gland, potentially exposing the underlying masseter fascia. The buccal branch of the facial nerve and Stensen's duct should be carefully avoided.

At the inferior border of the mandible, it is crucial to avoid damaging the marginal mandibular nerve by carefully observing the underside of the platysma and ensuring the fascial coverage over the nerve remains intact. Once the flap is sufficiently elevated and hemostasis is achieved, it can be secured in place. The approach to releasing the deep flap depends on the quality of the tissue, the retention of ligaments, and the surgeon's comfort with the anatomy.

If tissues are insufficient for deep elevation, a basic plication may be used. Typically, the elevation is directed posterior-superiorly, but the vectors are adjusted slightly in front of and behind the ear to achieve the most natural and esthetically pleasing result. In front of the ear, the deep plane is elevated more superiorly, while the skin is angled slightly more obliquely anteriorly. Conversely, behind the ear, the direction is reversed.

Key anchoring sutures include one from the temporal region, running superiorly along the cut edge, down to the cervical platysma, which is elevated and plicated to the mastoid fascia. Due to the release of deep tissue, the tension on the tissue suture anchorage is minimal, allowing for the use of resorbable sutures.

After folding, the skin is readjusted around the ear. Any slight skin dimples or folds should be smoothed out before continuing. Sometimes, additional loosening of the skin is required. The excess skin is then gradually removed to ensure the wound can be closed without undue tension. Starting the skin removal process from the earlobe is recommended, with careful attention to avoid pulling the earlobe downward (**Figure 6**).

If the hairline was crossed by the initial incisions, it should be realigned at this stage. Using isolated staples at key points during skin excision helps prevent overtrimming and the formation of dog-ears. Subcutaneous sutures are then placed, ensuring enough space is left in the postauricular sulcus to insert a closed suction drain behind each ear and potentially extending down into the neck, if desired. Staples are applied to the hair-bearing incisions, and the preauricular incisions are closed with 6–0 nylon or plain gut sutures, starting at the earlobe and progressing towards the temple (**Figure** 7).

After sutures are placed, Polysporin ointment is applied to the incisions. If dressings are used, they should be applied with gentle pressure to avoid disrupting the blood flow to the skin flaps.

A dressing made of 3 M Reston foam 1563 L (3 M Medical-Surgical, St. Paul, Minn) and a Nexcare Coban (3 M Medical-Surgical) head wrap is then placed over the submental area and worn for 24 hours. The following day, after the patient returns, the wrap is removed and replaced with a compression garment, such as a face-lift

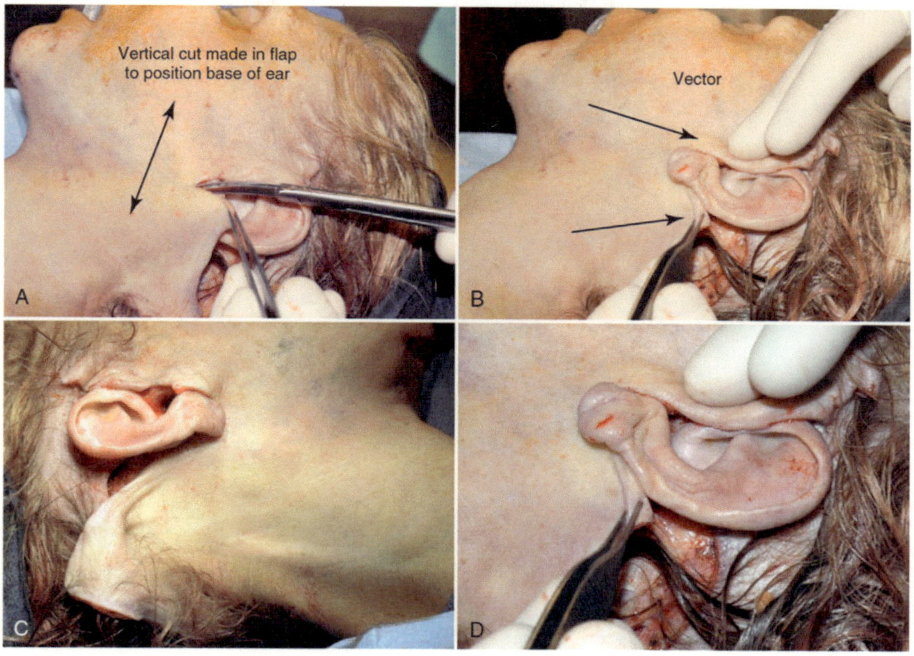

Figure 6.
Positioning the base of the ear is crucial once the primary work is finished. The angle of lift should be guided by what appears most esthetically pleasing and natural. Proper placement of the ear's base in relation to the flap is essential for normal skin redraping and proper alignment of the posterior hairline. Cutting too far in either direction can lead to significant challenges during closure.

bra, which should be worn as much as possible, both day and night, for the first week. After 1 week, the garment should be worn only at night for an additional 2 weeks.

Based on extensive experience, we have found that pressure dressings are generally unnecessary. Although patients might expect them, you can use this as a marketing advantage by highlighting that they are not needed with your facelifts. The key to success is ensuring complete hemostasis and maintaining consistency in the sequence of the facelift to enhance efficiency and smoothness.

Sutures in the preauricular area are taken out 5 days post-surgery, while final staple removal happens between 8 to 10 days later. The next follow-up appointment is typically set for 1 month after the procedure, provided there are no complications. Patients are advised against driving due to the risk of sudden neck movements. Smoking is prohibited for at least 2 weeks following the surgery.

1.2 Conclusion

There is ongoing debate about the most effective facelift technique due to the numerous variables involved, which prevent a purely scientific comparison. Proponents of the deep plane technique believe it yields superior and longer-lasting results, though this has not been scientifically validated and remains contested by many surgeons.

The senior author has employed the biplane facelift technique for over 25 years, performing nearly 1500 procedures with excellent outcomes. Our experience shows that the biplane facelift enhances esthetics and durability while minimizing complications. This technique, when executed correctly, effectively elevates the submalar,

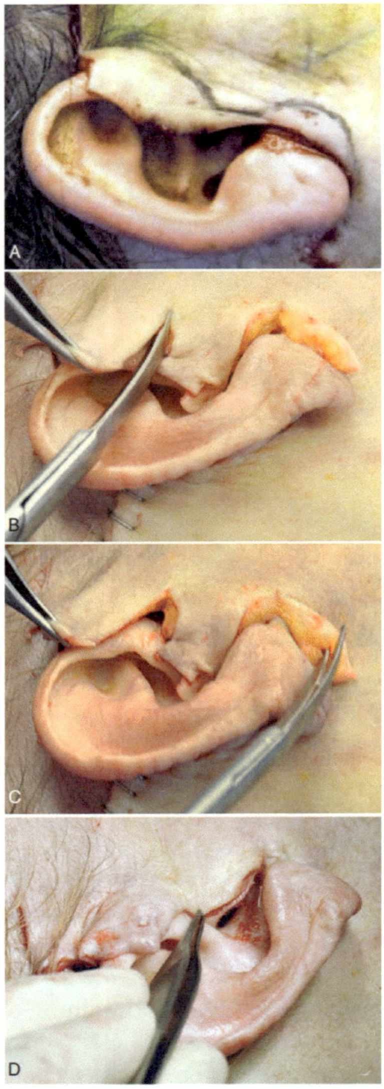

Figure 7.
Trimming the skin around the tragus is essential. It's best to work from the bottom up. Making horizontal pre-cuts on both sides of the tragus simplifies the process of removing excess skin and helps prevent skin tension.

jowl, and neck areas (**Figure 8**). The pronounced effects of facial aging are primarily due to changes in the deeper musculofascial plane, which the biplane facelift addresses by allowing precise elevation of this layer. The sharply dissected, long subcutaneous flap minimizes damage to the underlying fat and vascular networks, and the flexibility of the deep flap elevation is based on the patient's needs rather than anatomical landmarks.

The biplane facelift offers several advantages and some drawbacks. Benefits include a smoother deep musculofascial flap, which may provide fewer irregularities and more lasting results compared to basic plication or short flap techniques. The release of zygomatic and mandibular ligaments, along with thorough platysma

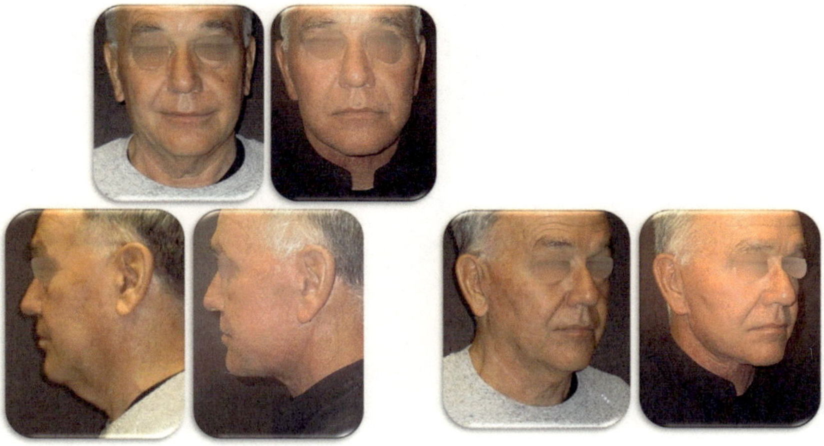

Figure 8.
Male patient status post rhytidectomy including superficial parotidectomy. Angle of the jaw is more defined with this maneuver.

treatment, can significantly improve challenging cases. Additionally, the biplane approach in the anterior neck can achieve a more acute chin-neck angle than many other facelift methods that restrict anterior and subplatysmal manipulation. However, the procedure is more labor-intensive in the anterior neck and technically challenging in the posterior facial region.

It is important to recognize that not every patient requires a full biplane dissection. Treatment plans should be tailored to each patient's specific needs and anatomical constraints (**Figure 9**). Due to the extensive dissection involved, this technique is not recommended for novice surgeons.

1.3 Upper face lifting

1.3.1 Body

1.3.1.1 History

Elevation and rejuvenation of the forehead, brow, and upper eyelids have been achieved by reducing the forces responsible for dynamic forehead wrinkles and restoring the involved structures to their natural anatomical positions. Endoscopic brow lifting, first introduced by Keller in 1991 [8], has been part of our practice since 1996. Over time, our patients have generally favored the endoscopic method over more traditional open approaches. However, open techniques may still be preferred in patients with a high hairline or deep forehead rhytids. In this chapter we will focus on the endoscopic approach as it has become a staple for long term results in the primary authors' practice. The endoscopic forehead and eyebrow lift has gained significant popularity due to its minimally invasive nature compared to traditional coronal and trichophytic procedures. This technique allows cosmetic surgeons to effectively address signs of aging in the forehead, eyebrows, and glabella while reducing the risks of hypoesthesia and hair loss [9].

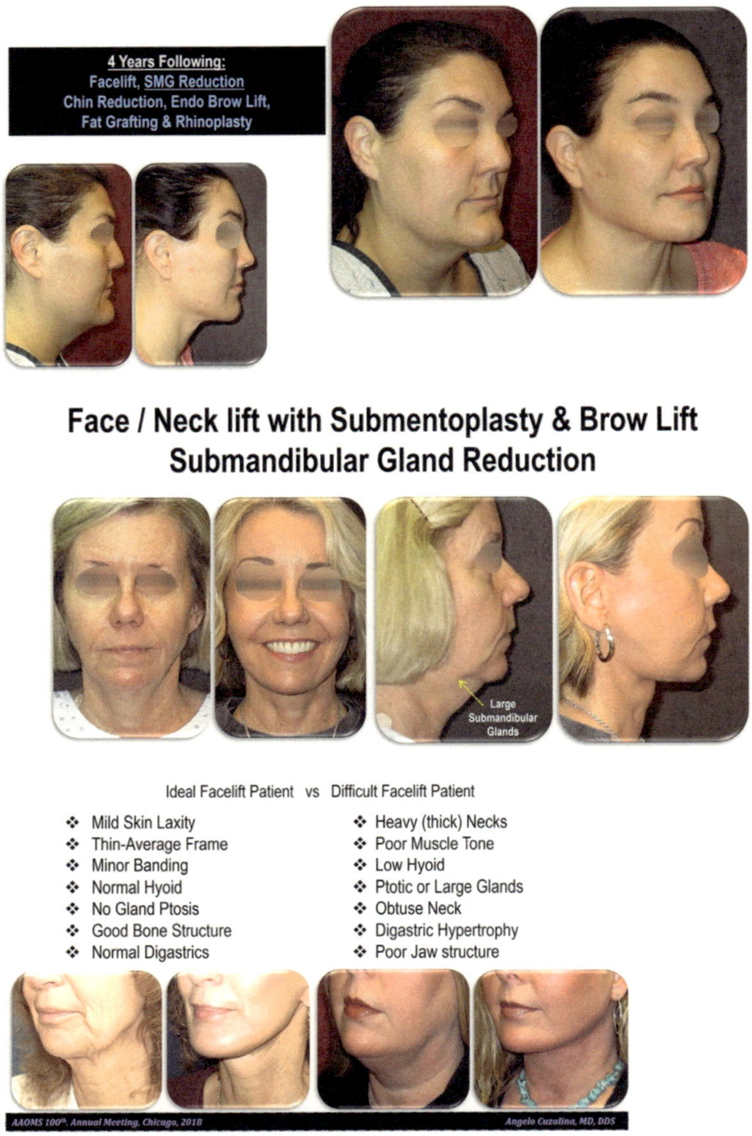

Figure 9.
Face/neck lift with submentoplasty & brow lift submandibular gland reduction.

2. Anatomy

The frontalis muscle is the primary elevator of the brow, while several other depressor muscles significantly contribute to facial expression and the appearance of aging. These depressor muscles include the corrugator supercilii, procerus, depressor supercilii, and orbicularis oculi (**Figure 10**). The procerus muscle is an extension of the frontalis muscle. It originates from the nasal bones and inserts upward into the frontalis muscle fibers before attaching to the dermis. When this pyramid-shaped muscle contracts, it forms horizontal wrinkles (bunny lines) over the nasal radix [10]. Typically, this muscle is transected during an endoscopic brow lift procedure. Some of the primary authors colleague believe that transection is not necessary as the

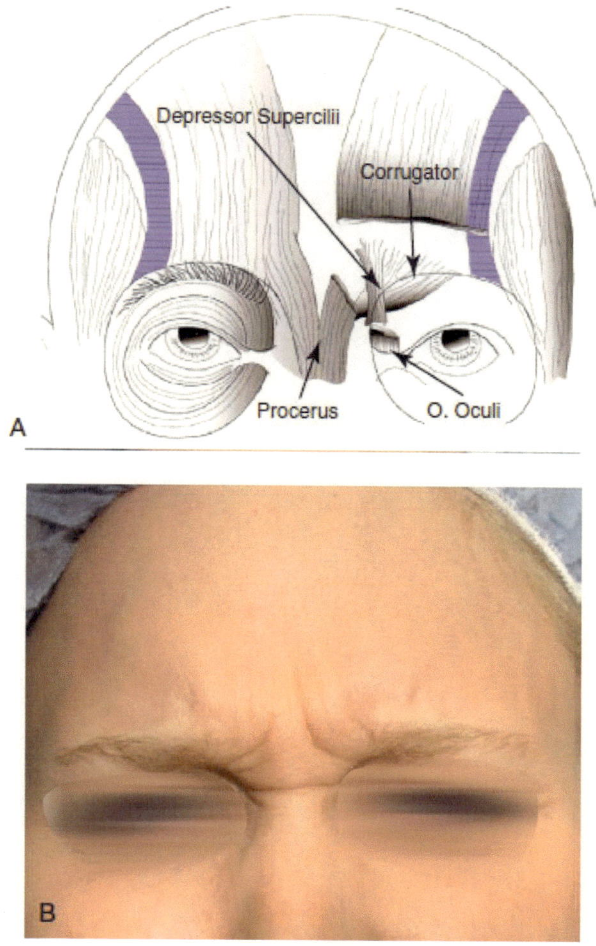

Figure 10.
A. The primary muscle responsible for elevating the eyebrow and forehead is the frontalis. Several depressor muscles are visible beneath the cut frontalis, including the corrugator supercilii, procerus, depressor supercilii, and orbicularis oculi. B. The patient exhibits typical wrinkles caused by two major depressor muscles. The horizontal wrinkle (commonly known as bunny lines) at the nasal radix is produced by the procerus, while the vertical wrinkles in the glabella are formed by the corrugator muscles.

muscle heals, these fibers reattach. Over resection of the depressor muscles can lead to an overlifted medial brow (**Figure 11**). However, Transection of the lateral orbital portion of the orbicularis oculi muscle is typically required to achieve a satisfactory upper third facelift procedure.

In the lateral temporal region, the frontalis muscle merges with a dense fascial layer referred to as the zone of adherence. This zone establishes a connection between the galea of the upper face and the superficial fascial system of the lower face. A thorough understanding of the fascial layers in this area is essential, as their release is necessary to achieve the desired long-term lifting effect during an endoscopic brow lift [11, 12].

The temporoparietal fascia, which is spongy in texture, is continuous with the galea aponeurotica. This layer houses the superficial temporal artery and the frontal branch of the facial nerve. The deep temporal fascia exhibits a thicker structure and a white, glistening appearance. Beneath the zygomatic arch, this fascia divides into

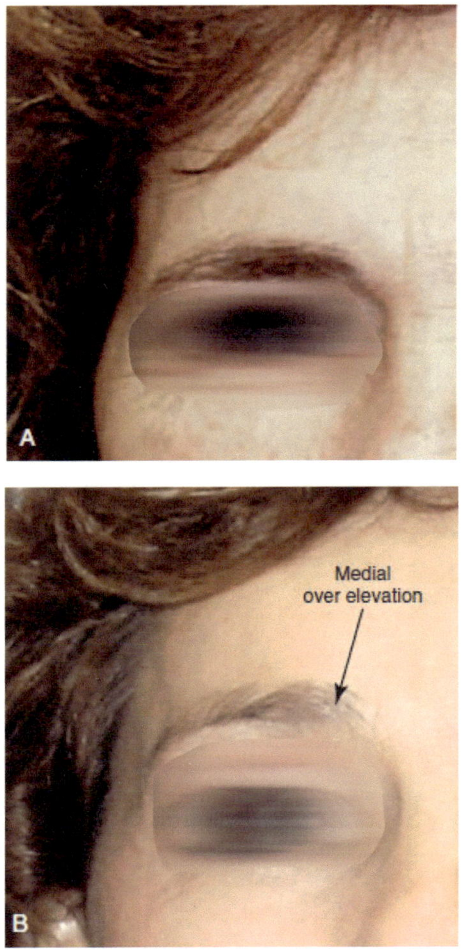

Figure 11.
Excessive dissection of the depressor supercilii muscle may result in an unnaturally elevated brow. If the medial eyebrow is raised higher than the lateral eyebrow, it can create a "surprised" expression, which is generally considered esthetically undesirable.

two layers known as the intermediate temporal fascia and the deep temporal fascia. The temporoparietal fascia is continuous with the superficial musculoaponeurotic system (SMAS) below the zygomatic arch and the galea aponeurotica, which is also connected to the frontalis muscle [13].

For the endoscopic browlift blunt dissection is done up to 2 cm away from the orbital rim. The final 2 cm should be dissected under endoscopic visual guidance. It is recommended by the authors to perform the dissection above the superficial temporal fascia through the lateral incisions, allowing access to the central subperiosteal plane, referred to as the "safe zone" (**Figure 12**).

Maintaining depth to the periosteum is crucial for preventing injury to the deep divisions and branches of the supraorbital nerve, which are located within the subgaleal plane near the fixation zone. Dissection towards the occiput is conducted subperiosteally, or occasionally in the subgaleal plane, to facilitate scalp elevation and to enhance the maneuverability of the endoscope [14].

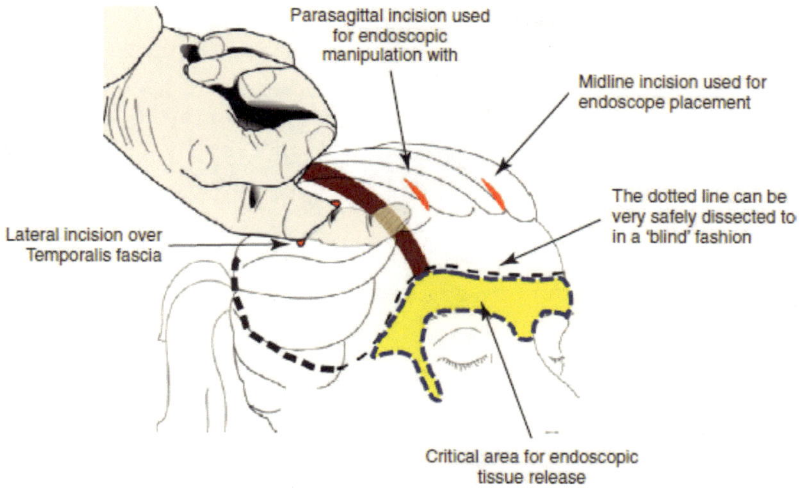

Figure 12.
Access to the subperiosteal plane is achieved through finger dissection following the elevation of the medial portion of the scalp with instruments. Blunt and blind dissection can be safely conducted up to 1.5 cm above the orbital rims. Additional dissection in the yellow-shaded area should be carried out under direct visualization.

The initial focus is on the lateral aspect of the elevated forehead flap, where the fixation zone begins at the lateral corner of the superior orbital rim. This location represents the convergence point of all fascial layers. Lateral dissection in this area aims to expose the lateral orbicularis oculi while carefully releasing the zone of fascial convergence. It is important to proceed with precision, as the temporal branch of the facial nerve curves medially in this region on its ascent towards the forehead, necessitating caution to avoid injury. Additionally, the surgeon should be aware of the sentinel vein, located approximately 1 cm lateral to the zygomaticofrontal suture line, which traverses the temporoparietal fascia at a perpendicular angle. While the sentinel vein can be sacrificed, it is critical to avoid cauterizing the area where the vein can retract and continue to bleed [15, 16].

The central dissection plane advances to the level of the superior orbital rim, ensuring that the entire superior rim is adequately visualized. The endoscope should provide a clear view of the periosteum raised in a relatively bloodless plane. Dissection through the periosteum will expose the subgaleal fat, except at the location of the supraorbital nerve. The nerve, along with its accompanying artery and branches, can be observed as they penetrate the fascial layers towards the frontalis and subcutaneous tissue, originating from the supraorbital notch and aligning with the medial limbus. As the surgeon continues superficial dissection towards the muscles of the glabella and medial eyebrow, it is essential to remain aware of the position of the supraorbital nerve and artery. The supraorbital nerve runs in alignment with the medial limbus of the eyebrow, and medial to this nerve bundle, the corrugator supercilii is identifiable with its two heads. Upon transecting the oblique head of the corrugator, the supratrochlear nerve and depressor supercilii muscle will be encountered, which should be preserved unless transection of the depressor supercilii is warranted due to over-elevation (**Figure 13**).

2.1 Procedure

The procedure commences with the creation of five distinct incisions in the scalp. Each incision measures approximately 3 cm in length, beginning 1 cm posterior to the

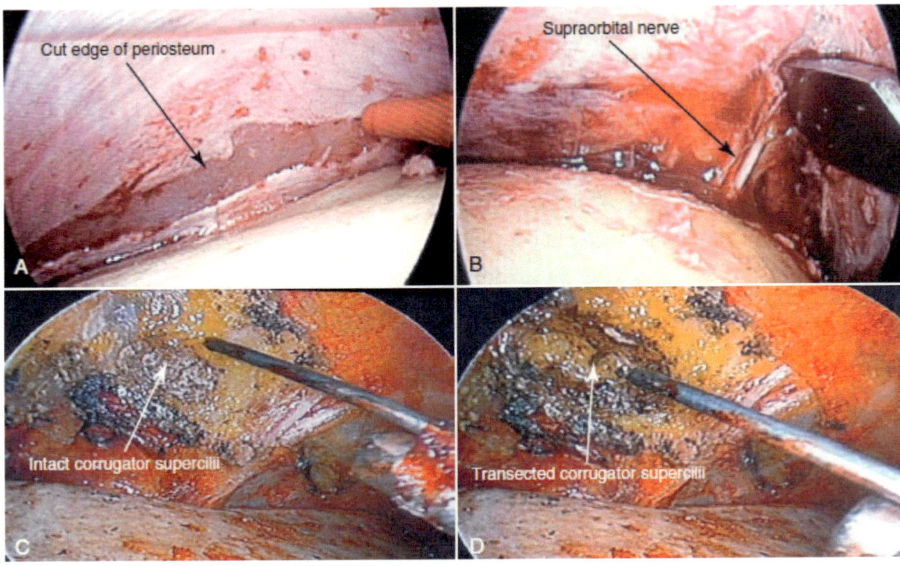

Figure 13.
The left corrugator muscle is in close proximity to the supraorbital nerve, with the muscle belly positioned superficially to the nerve on both the medial and lateral sides.

hairline and extending backward. The first incision is positioned along the midline in a sagittal plane, followed by two paramedian incisions made in a parasagittal plane, approximately 3 to 4 cm apart and parallel to the midline incision. This vertical arrangement of incisions helps prevent the transection of sensory nerves to the scalp, facilitating access to the entire anterior forehead and eyebrow regions. Care must be taken to ensure that the parasagittal incisions are not placed too laterally over the zone of fixation. These incisions should be located over the thick region of the frontal bone, preparing for the creation of bone tunnels or the placement of bone screws, while also being positioned as far as possible from the venous lakes of the skull.

The final two lateral incisions are made obliquely over the temple, running parallel to the temporal branch of the facial nerve and the temporal artery and vein, thereby reducing the risk of damage to sensory and vascular supply to the scalp. The position of the supraorbital nerve is marked by tracing a line from the medial limbus of the iris to the eyebrow. Dissection begins in the central area of the subperiosteal plane, remaining medial to the temporal lines. The posterior elevation is carried out to approximately 10 cm behind the incisions, while anteriorly, the subperiosteum is elevated to a horizontal line 2 cm above the superior orbital rims and the zygomatic arch (**Figure 14**). Blunt finger dissection can facilitate complete elevation of the forehead and scalp within the specified limits.

Upon completion of this step, a connection is established from the lateral incisions to the subperiosteal plane through the upper portion of the zone of fixation, utilizing blunt finger dissection. Dissection below this level, where the branches of the facial nerve are located, should be avoided. The direction of finger placement should move from the lateral incisions towards the central subperiosteal space, rather than the reverse, to prevent inadvertent tunneling within the spongy temporoparietal fascia, which contains the superficial temporal artery and the frontal branch of the facial nerve. It is crucial to maintain close contact with the periosteum and temporalis fascia during the initial elevations.

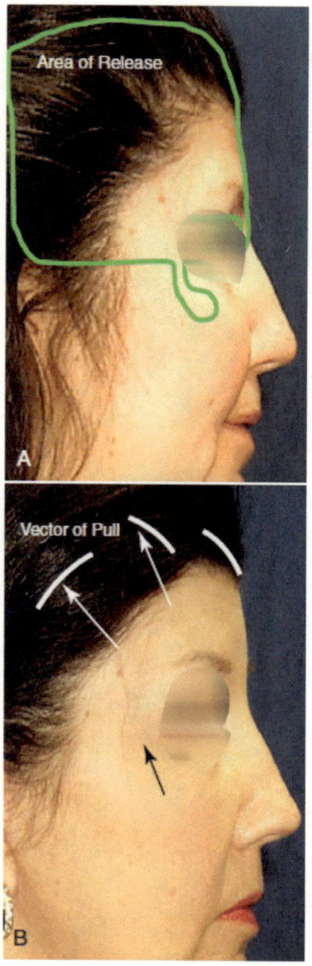

Figure 14.
This is a previous patient from the lower facelifting subsection. This image shows a before and after. Take notice on the vector of pull. The green area shows subperiosteal dissection.

Direct visualization is essential for continuing the dissection down to the superior orbital rims and the nasofrontal junction. The endoscope is carefully inserted through one of the three median incisions, taking particular care in the area of the elevated flap. Excessive retraction may lead to skin perforation or significant postoperative neurapraxia. A smooth, curved periosteal elevator is utilized to release the periosteum over the superior orbital rims bilaterally and in the nasofrontal region. The dissection should be performed bimanually, with the non-dominant hand positioned over the patient's face to control the tip of the elevator. The assistant should hold the endoscope and suction cannula. The dissection should progress laterally over the lateral orbital rim and the zygomatic bone (**Figure 15**).

The periosteum is incised using either a needle-tipped electrocautery device or a laser set to low power. It is essential for the surgeon to be aware of the trajectory of the supraorbital vessels towards the frontalis muscle and forehead at the level of the medial limbus on both sides. The use of three ports facilitates the maneuverability of the endoscope, cautery or laser, and suction cannula. Temporal incisions can serve

A.

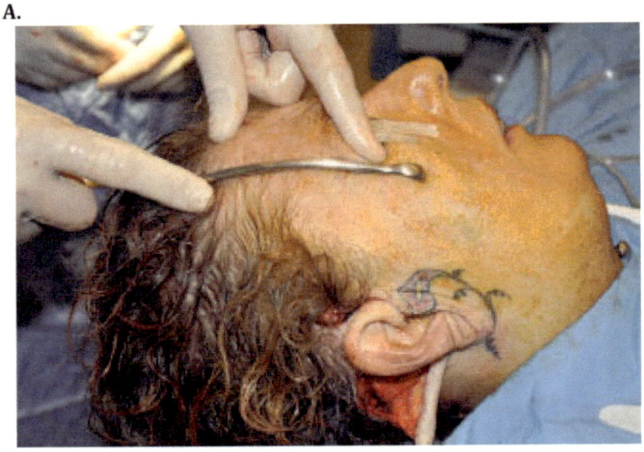

B.

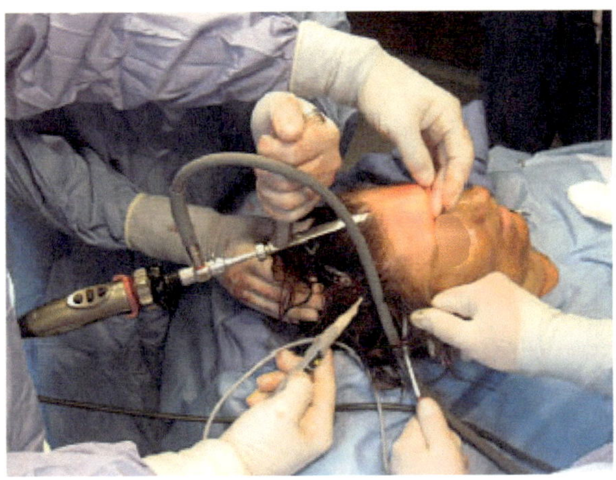

Figure 15.
A. An intraoperative image illustrating the subperiosteal dissection, which is tunneled over the lateral orbital rim into the malar prominence. The elevator is utilized through a parasagittal incision located just behind the hairline. The globe is consistently protected throughout the procedure. B. The typical configuration of the surgeon and assistants during an endoscopic brow lift procedure involves the surgeon managing the cautery with one hand while applying counterpressure to the skin with the opposite hand to maintain control and prevent perforation. The first assistant is responsible for holding the endoscope, while the second assistant, if present, operates the suction device and ensures the correct positioning of the patient's head.

as effective suction ports if the medial ports are congested with the endoscope and cautery device. Bimanual cauterization is recommended due to the relatively short distance the cautery must traverse to penetrate the skin, particularly in the glabellar region and nasofrontal junction.

Following the exposure of the corrugator supercilii and procerus muscles, careful transection is performed with precise cauterization to minimize bleeding. If bleeding occurs at the muscle edges, gentle cauterization may be applied after exerting external pressure to enhance visualization. Hypertrophy of the depressor muscles can be addressed through muscle avulsion. The authors have observed that muscle debulking poses a significant risk of nerve damage and postoperative irregularities in the glabellar region. It is advisable to gently separate the muscle edges using a periosteal elevator by at least 1 cm to facilitate the release of the arcus marginalis, which may lead to a notably prolonged brow elevation effect.

Subsequently, dissection is conducted along the anterior and inferior aspects of the temporal crest, extending down to the zygomaticofrontal suture line. It is crucial to be aware of the proximity of the sentinel vein (zygomaticotemporal vein), which lies laterally to the dissection pathway and may need to be sacrificed to achieve adequate exposure for surgical intervention (**Figure 16**). The lateral dissection and elevation are essential for determining the degree of eyebrow elevation and fixation upon the completion of the endoscopic brow lift procedure (**Figure 17**).

This dissection area demonstrates significant compatibility with various facelift procedures when utilizing an endoscopic approach. In cases where an extended mid-face lift is planned, the tissue over the zygomatic arch can be elevated between the superficial and deep temporal fascia layers. Alternatively, abbreviated mid-face lifts can be performed by remaining in the subperiosteal plane along the lateral orbital rim. Another option includes a mid-face lift using intraoral dissection, which allows for a connection between the subperiosteal forehead plane and the intraoral zygomatic periosteal plane laterally.

Once periosteal dissection and muscle transection are completed, flap elevation and fixation are the next steps. Several techniques have been described for securing the forehead flap to the underlying bone in its new retracted position, such as suture fixation, bone screws and plates, resorbable screws, bone tunnels, local skin excision, tissue adhesive, tight head wraps, and temporalis muscle unroofing to enhance scarring. While many of these options are effective, it is crucial to highlight that an inadequately released tissue flap may revert to its original position, regardless of the

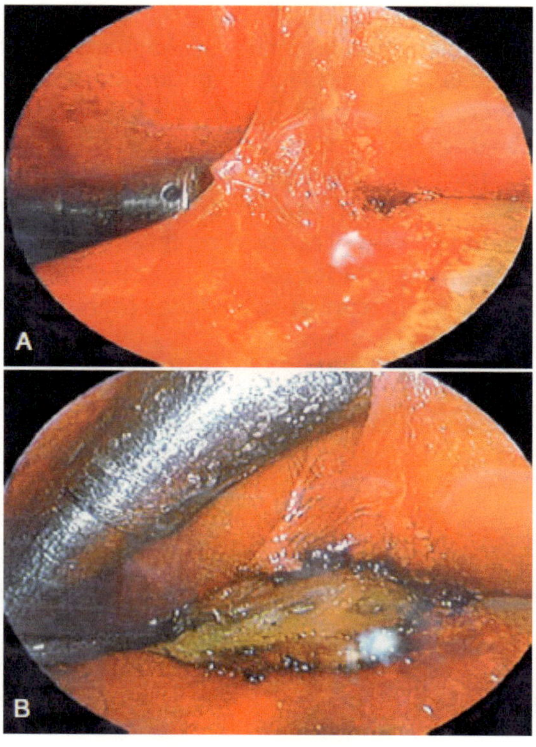

Figure 16.
The left lateral orbital ligament (A) prior to release and at the moment of initial release (B). This ligament is observed during the release process over the lateral orbital rim.

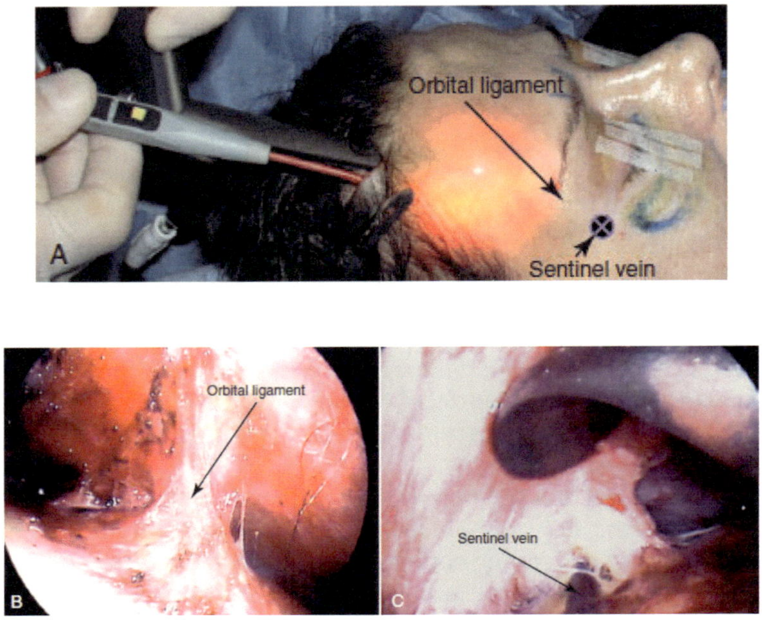

Figure 17.
The release of the orbital ligaments is essential for achieving sufficient stability in brow lift procedures. The image illustrates the endoscopic release of the orbital ligaments, which allows access to the lateral orbicularis oculi. The sentinel vein, located at the inferior border of the ligament, can be cauterized, ligated, or preserved during this process.

fixation method employed. Fixation is achieved through parasagittal incisions by elevating the lateral third of the brow to its maximum height and securing the periosteum to the cranial structure (**Figure 18**). The medial brow and glabella will naturally elevate with the maximal stretching of the lateral eyebrow, ensuring that the medial brow remains lower than the lateral side and preventing overcorrection, which could lead to patient dissatisfaction due to a long-term surprised appearance. For enhanced effect, fixation of the lateral brow tail can be accomplished through imbrication of the temporoparietal fascia in a posterior and superior direction via the lateral incisions. This vector can be visually represented by a line connecting the outer nasal ala to a point just behind the lateral canthus.

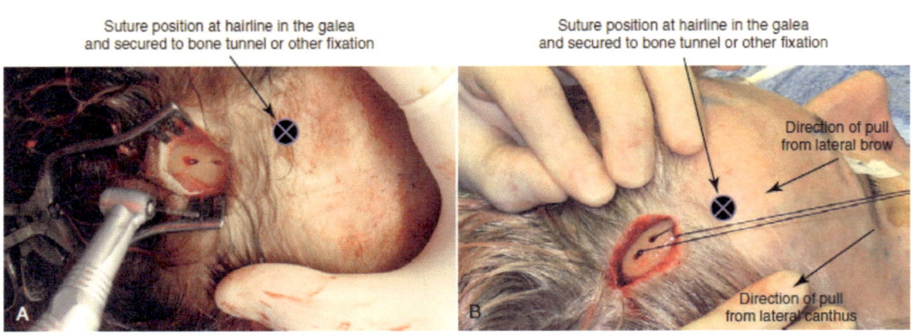

Figure 18.
Bone tunnels are one method of fixation. The image depicts a right parasagittal bone tunnel located near the coronal suture. A secure galeal suture is sutured from the hairline below to the bone tunnel above. The parasagittal bone of the skull is quite thick, enabling the safe placement of a shallow tunnel.

Minimal relapse is anticipated in the early postoperative phase, with a typical 1- to 2-mm descent expected within the first 2 weeks. Various estimates exist regarding the time required for the periosteum to adhere to its new position, with recent findings indicating that sufficient fusion occurs within 7 to 9 days, contrary to earlier suggestions of 12 weeks. This is evidenced by the efficacy of transcutaneous bone screws, which are usually removed after 1 week and exhibit excellent long-term retention. The incision is closed using skin staples, resulting in anticipated excellent healing outcomes. Redundancy of the forehead flap is resolved through redistribution over the posterior 10 to 20 cm of occipital periosteal elevation, accounting for the acceptable minimal elevation of the hairline.

2.2 Conclusion

Upper facial rejuvenation has reached a pivotal turning point. The successful implementation of minimally invasive brow lifting and chemodenervation (Botox) has established the endoscopic forehead and brow lift as the gold standard for addressing brow ptosis. This subsection focused on endoscopic brow lifting and its ability to address the upper face. A thorough understanding of anatomical structures

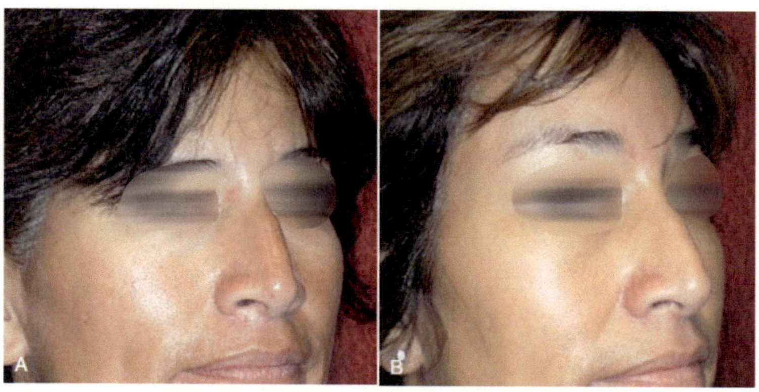

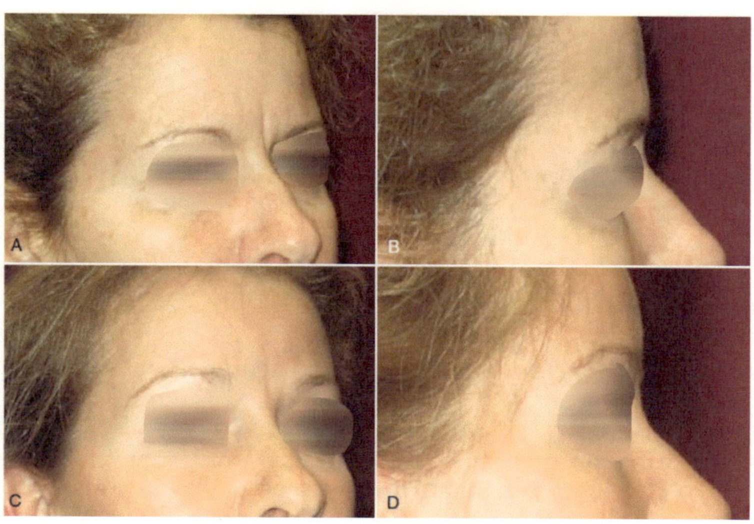

Figure 19.
Primary authors dramatic before and after changes with isolated endoscopic upper face lift.

and the locations of critical nerves has enhanced the safety of cosmetic procedures on the upper face, yielding excellent long-term outcomes (**Figure 19**).

Rejuvenating the upper face requires proficiency in multiple techniques by the cosmetic surgeon. The current demand for minimal downtime, reduced invasiveness, and exceptional results has propelled endoscopic forehead and brow lifting to the forefront of upper facial rejuvenation. This chapter emphasizes the importance of ensuring a safe surgical procedure through comprehensive knowledge of relevant anatomy and the meticulous application of endoscopic techniques. Ultimately, the procedure has demonstrated safety, consistency, and favorable long-term results for patients with aged, ptotic eyebrows (**Figure 19**).

Author details

Artem Krutyansky[1*] and Angelo Cuzalina[2]

1 Columbia University, New York, USA

2 Tulsa Surgical Arts, Oklahoma, USA

*Address all correspondence to: ak5329@cumc.columbia.edu

References

[1] Mitz V, Peyronie M. The superficial musculo-aponeurotic system (SMAS) in the parotid and cheek area. Plastic and Reconstructive Surgery. 1976;**58**:80-88

[2] Larrabee W, Ridenour B. Rhytidectomy: Technique and complications. American Journal of Otolaryngology. 1992;**13**:1-15

[3] Skoog T. Plastic Surgery: New Methods and Refinements. Vol. 6. Philadelphia: WB Saunders; 1974. pp. 300-330

[4] Webster RC, Davidson TM, White MF, et al. Conservative face-lift surgery. Archives of Otolaryngology. 1976;**102**:657-662

[5] Ellis E, Zide MF. Surgical Approaches to the Facial Skeleton. Baltimore: Williams & Wilkins; 1995

[6] Baker PC, Conley J. Avoiding facial nerve injuries in rhytidectomy: Anatomical variations and pitfalls. Plastic and Reconstructive Surgery. 1979;**64**:78-795

[7] Man D. Premedication with oral clonidine for facial rhytidectomy. Plastic and Reconstructive Surgery. 1994;**94**:214-215

[8] Bernstein G. Surface landmarks for the identification of key anatomic structures of the face and neck. The Journal of Dermatologic Surgery and Oncology. 1986;**12**:722-726

[9] Grant JCB, editor. Grant's Atlas of Anatomy. 6th ed. Baltimore: Williams & Wilkins; 1972

[10] Knobloch K, Gohritz A, Reuss E, et al. Nicotine in plastic surgery: A review. Chirurgie. 2008;**79**:956-962

[11] Baker TJ, Gordon HL, Mesienko P. Rhytidectomy. Plastic and Reconstructive Surgery. 1977;**59**:24-30

[12] Goldwyn RM. Late bleeding after rhytidectomy from injury to the superficial temporal vessels. Plastic and Reconstructive Surgery. 1991;**88**:443-445

[13] Alexander RW. Cosmetic alterations of the aging neck: Rhytidectomy. Oral and Maxillofacial Surgery Clinics of North America. 1990;**2**:247-257

[14] Huntley JE. The Divine Proportion. New York: Dover; 1970

[15] Rickets RM. Divine proportion of facial aesthetics. Clinics in Plastic Surgery. 1982;**9**:401-422

[16] Tolhurst DE, Carstens MH, Greco RJ, et al. The surgical anatomy of the scalp. Plastic and Reconstructive Surgery. 1991;**87**:603-612, discussion 613-614

Chapter 5

Perspective Chapter: Facial Implants – Enhancing Aesthetics and Reconstructive Outcomes

Mohammad K.H.B. Abdulaziz and Mohammad Kamal

Abstract

The choice of aesthetic operations is much influenced by facial looks; a disparity between perceived and actual age could cause discontent and affect self-esteem. Beautiful faces influence social and professional contacts by often being connected with success and ability. As such, good facial aesthetic treatments can improve social contact and self-awareness. Wrinkles, poor skin texture, and uneven, soft tissue define facial aging, which alters youthful, symmetrical features and consequently affects attractiveness and self-esteem. These developments can also influence personality and emotional perception, therefore causing misunderstandings of emotions. Treatments that restore a young, balanced look can help with these problems, boosting self-confidence and social contacts. Rising desire for facial beauty has resulted in the creation of several cosmetic operations targeted on volume restoration and facial augmentation, including less invasive techniques like lifting procedures, injectable fillers, fat transfer, and facial implants. Research shows that people view faces as a whole rather than by individual characteristics; hence, a comprehensive approach including several modalities is utilized increasingly to evaluate the full face. Available in metals, polymers, and ceramics, facial implants give long-lasting support and may be less expensive than regular injections. Modern techniques and materials are made possible by historical developments in cosmetic surgery, therefore greatly improving facial repair and augmentation. Improvements in materials and surgical techniques, as well as a greater knowledge of facial aging, keep improving the effectiveness and results of facial implant operations. The present chapter aims to cover the fundamental aspects of facial implantology and explore future advancements.

Keywords: facial skeletal, alloplastic, aesthetic, craniofacial, infections, implant

1. Introduction

Facial appearance plays a key role in selecting aesthetic procedures, as a mismatch between perceived and actual age can lead to dissatisfaction and affect self-esteem. Attractive faces are often viewed as more competent and successful, influencing social and professional interactions. Thus, effective facial aesthetic treatments can improve self-image and social relationships [1–3]. Facial aging signs, such as wrinkles, poor skin texture, and uneven, soft tissue, disrupt youthful, symmetrical features, impacting attractiveness and self-esteem. These changes can alter how others perceive one's emotions and personality, often leading to miscommunication of feelings. Addressing these issues with treatments that restore a youthful, balanced appearance can enhance self-image and improve social interactions [4, 5]. The rising demand for facial beauty has led to the development of various cosmetic procedures focused on volume replacement and facial augmentation. Advances in aesthetic medicine now include less invasive techniques such as lifting procedures, injectable fillers, fat transfer, and facial implants. A holistic approach, assessing the entire face with diverse modalities, is increasingly used as research shows that people perceive faces as a whole rather than by individual features [6, 7].

Restoring facial form and function after trauma, tumors, infection, or congenital deficiencies is essential in facial plastic surgery. Aging often causes volume loss in the maxilla and mandible, leading to the use of facial implants for augmenting areas like the malar eminences, chin, and mandibular angle. Implants, available in metals, polymers (silicone, porous polyethylene, Gore-Tex, MMA), and ceramics (hydroxyapatite), provide lasting support and may be more cost-effective compared to repeated injections [8–11]. Overall, facial aging involves epidermal thinning, soft tissue volume loss, and skeletal resorption, transforming the face from a youthful to a more rectangular shape. While injectable fillers are popular for their minimal invasiveness, skeletal implants offer durable results by providing lasting support and reducing the need for frequent treatments [12, 13].

1.1 A historical perspective

The history of aesthetic surgery began in 1845 when Johann Friedrich Dieffenbach first described reducing large noses through external incisions [14]. Although he did not illustrate it, Julius von Szymanowski later detailed the procedure in his handbook [15, 16]. In 1881, Edward T. Ely performed one of the first purely aesthetic surgeries for correcting prominent ears [17]. Around the same time, John Orlando Roe demonstrated bulbous nose reduction and hump removal under local anesthesia [18, 19]. Robert Weir introduced the "Weir operation" for alar base excision [20]. Meanwhile, in Berlin, Jacques Joseph refined otoplasty and rhinoplasty techniques, which remain largely unchanged today [21].

In the late 19th and early 20th centuries, the rising focus on personal appearance led to a surge in charlatans and "beauty doctors" operating commercially in salons. These practitioners, advertised in newspapers and magazines, promised quick, simple cosmetic enhancements at high costs, claiming that improved appearance could boost job prospects and social relationships. Charles C. Miller (1880–1950), considered by some a charlatan and by others the "father of modern cosmetic surgery," published "The Correction of Featural Imperfections" in 1907. His work included illustrations of facial procedures and promoted paraffin injections for improving facial features and wrinkles [22].

2. Types of facial implants

Facial implants are utilized for post-traumatic reconstruction, congenital abnormality correction, and aesthetic enhancement. Traditionally, facial skeletal augmentation used autogenous bone grafts, but advancements now favor alloplastic materials. These implants offer benefits such as greater availability and avoidance of donor-site issues like scarring and resorption. Additionally, they simplify graft shaping, reducing surgical time and complexity [23, 24]. The following section provides an overview of autogenous and alloplastic implants in further detail.

2.1 Autogenous implants

Autogenous options (e.g., bone, cartilage, fat, dermis, fascia) have long been viewed as the gold standard for facial profile modifications, embodying the principle of "replacing self with self" for both the facial skeleton and soft tissues. It is a process that uses the patient's body tissues to rebuild or improve facial structures while reducing the possibility of rejection and fostering good tissue integration [25].

2.1.1 Bone grafts

Bone grafts from the calvarium or iliac crest often face stability issues due to resorption. Calvarial grafts are more stable than iliac crest grafts, but alloplastic materials are preferred for their predictability and avoidance of donor-site complications [26, 27].

2.1.2 Cartilage grafts

Autogenous and lyophilized allogeneic cartilage are used for facial augmentation. Lyophilized cartilage integrates well with tissue and has low infection rates, but can resorb up to 20%. Fresh frozen allogeneic cartilage is effective in rhinoplasty with low complication rates [28, 29].

2.1.3 Autologous fat transfer

Used for facial balancing, autologous fat transfer cannot replace skeletal augmentation. Fat retention ranges from 50 to 80%, and it provides only temporary contour improvements [30, 31].

Autograft use in cosmetic augmentation is limited by unpredictable bony resorption. According to Wolff's Law, bone remodels in response to stress, so insufficient stimulation at implant sites leads to decreased density and increased resorption [23, 32]. Although once considered the gold standard in facial implantology, autologous options have drawbacks, including donor-site morbidity, longer surgery times, and less stable outcomes due to predictable attrition [27].

2.2 Alloplastic implants

The synthetic materials used in facial reconstruction and augmentation are grouped into alloplastic implants. These implants provide customizable shape and volume, enhance symmetry, avoid donor-site issues, and offer lower complication risks with shorter operative times. They are also potentially reversible. Standard alloplastic facial implants are listed below and detailed in the succeeding section.

2.2.1 Titanium mesh

Rigid, non-resorbable, and inert. Used for recontouring deficient mandibular angles, with fenestrations for tissue growth and stability.

2.2.2 High-density porous polyethylene (HDPE)

Rigid and noncompressible, with pore sizes ranging from 80 to 400 microns, influencing tissue ingrowth (bone or fibrous). Implants with 100–250 micron pore size allow bony ingrowth but require fixation to prevent disruption of neovascularization. Can be recontoured by heating to 180°F.

2.2.3 Silicone

Nonporous, available as solid silicone or dimethylsiloxane subunits. Requires fixation to prevent encapsulation, migration, and bony resorption, reducing tissue ingrowth and seroma formation [33].

3. Common materials used in facial implants and their ideal properties

Facial implants are categorized based on their location, such as chin, paranasal, malar, submalar, and more. They can be prefabricated, anatomical, or custom-made and come in various shapes and sizes. These implants are made from different materials, each with its own advantages and disadvantages. Therefore, surgeons must be well-acquainted with these materials [34].

3.1 Metal used in facial implants

3.1.1 Stainless steel (Fe-Cr-Ni alloys)

The biocompatibility of metals is largely determined by their resistance to corrosion and the tissue reactions, both local and systemic, to the products of corrosion [35]. A stainless-steel implant is a biomedical device crafted from iron-chromium-nickel alloys, which have been in use since the 1920s. These implants are utilized extensively in plastic surgery, particularly for craniofacial and hand surgeries. They are also employed in hemoclips, cranial plates, artificial joints, and dental implants. Despite their widespread use, stainless-steel implants are susceptible to corrosion over time, which can lead to implant failure [36–38].

3.1.2 Titanium

Titanium is the preferred material for craniofacial plating systems due to its high mechanical strength, corrosion resistance, biocompatibility, and non-ferromagnetic properties. It is suitable for MRI imaging and has low artifacts on CT scans. Its stability and rigidity make it ideal for craniofacial fracture fixation, but it is less suitable for aesthetic augmentation due to its high elastic modulus. This rigidity can cause a "stress shielding effect," weakening adjacent bone and potentially loosening the implant. Titanium plates used in mandibular reconstruction have a high complication rate, including infection and plate removal. Despite its benefits, titanium can be visible under thin skin, particularly in the periorbital region, and can cause thermal sensitivity and discomfort, often necessitating removal [35, 39, 40].

3.1.3 Vitallium (CoCrMo alloys)

Vitallium, a base metal alloy (CoCrMo), has been used in dentistry and medicine since 1929. It is widely used in orthopedic and maxillofacial surgery and is well tolerated. Single case reports from the 1990s documented its use in midface bone defect reconstruction without significant morbidity or complications [41]. Initially, Vitallium was particularly recommended for orbital fracture cases to maintain normal eye appearance and function. In large follow-ups, no postoperative orbital infections or implant removals were necessary. However, Vitallium is not recommended without rigid fixation. Studies in animal models found it to be less biocompatible than titanium, showing decreased biomechanical fixation and increased metal ion accumulation around the implant. Additionally, Vitallium presents challenges in shaping and causes radiographic scatter. Despite these issues, the choice between titanium alloy and CoCrMo should be based on a comprehensive review of factors influencing clinical implant survival [42].

3.1.4 Tantalum

Tantalum is gaining significant attention as a biomaterial due to its exceptional biocompatibility. It boasts an outstanding ability to form bone-like apatite, does not release cytotoxic ions, and resists dissolution in local, systemic, and remote organs, contributing to excellent osseointegration. Renowned for its strength and anti-corrosion properties, tantalum stands out as a promising material for bioperformance applications [43]. Since the 1940s, it has been utilized in the medical field, with Burke pioneering its use in skin applications, subcutaneous and tendon sutures, and various plates. Tantalum's ability to form a compact, passive, and extremely thin yet robust and tenacious oxide layer that adheres strongly to its surface is noteworthy. This oxide layer supports bone ingrowth in vivo by developing bone-like apatite, promoting adhesion of both hard and soft tissues [44].

3.2 Polymer

Polymers are large organic macromolecules composed of numerous equivalent sub-molecules. While metallic implants are commonly used for skeletal fixation and bone augmentation, polymers are preferred for soft tissue augmentation and contouring. The use of polymers in these applications has increased significantly over the past decade. Naturally occurring polymers like collagen (tropocollagen polymer) have been utilized, but facial implantology primarily employs synthetic polymers such as medical-grade polysiloxane (silicone) and polyethylene. These materials are chosen for their effectiveness in enhancing soft tissue contours and their biocompatibility [45].

3.2.1 Polyethylene

Polyethylene, a polymer made from ethylene monomers, has several forms used in facial implants, including HDPE and ultra-high-molecular-weight polyethylene. HDPE, used in products like Medpor, is firm and porous, allowing for tissue ingrowth, which helps stabilize implants but complicates their removal. Though their removal is more difficult, porous polyethylene implants offer better integration with

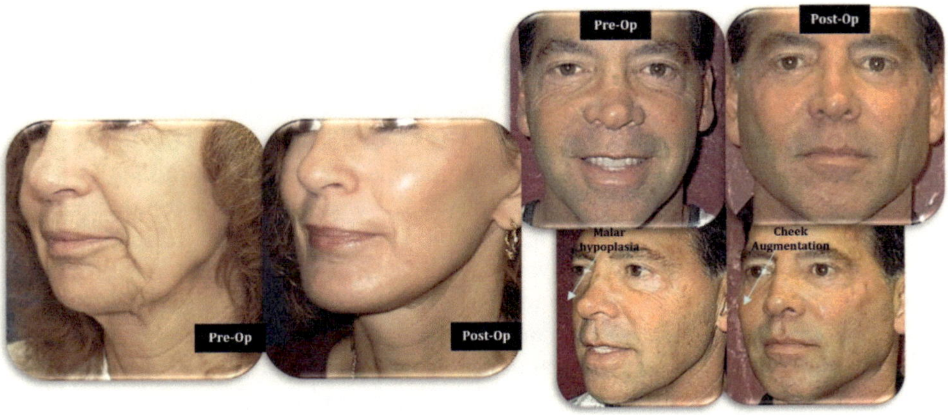

Figure 1.
Female and male patients of Dr. Cuzalina, after placement of prefabricated silicone mandibular angle implants, a chin implant, as well as cheek implants for each patient, with good aesthetic outcomes.

tissue and are less prone than silicone implants to migrate. Commonly used in facial reconstruction, polyethylene implants provide several consistencies and mechanical characteristics fit for different uses [46].

3.2.2 Silicone (Polysiloxane)

Made in solid, gel, or liquid forms, silicone implants, known for their biocompatibility and adaptability, have fibrous tissue capture them; it makes removal easier but may cause problems like seroma development and migration. Silicone implants may promote bone resorption and are more prone to displacement, even with a low infection rate and good aesthetic results, as shown in **Figure 1**. Their simplicity of molding and sterilizing makes them extensively applied in facial implantology [34, 47, 48].

3.3 Hydroxyapatite (bioceramic)

Highly osteo-conductive and inductive, hydroxyapatite (HaP), a ceramic made of calcium and phosphate, shines in bone tissue engineering. It is less likely to need removal since it encourages better cellular adhesion and integration than other implants. Usually used without screw fixation in face augmentation, HaP is volume stable and available in block and granular forms. With recent research demonstrating that HaP granules are replaced by neo-bone and well-encased by host collagen, they progressively blend into host bone. HaP is sometimes used with polylactic acid to increase mechanical strength and thereby enhance its brittleness [49, 50].

4. Indications and common areas for implantation

4.1 Aesthetic augmentation, improving aesthetics

Facial reconstruction and augmentation in plastic surgery address trauma, tumors, infections, and congenital defects. Aesthetic concerns, such as age-related volume loss and reduced projection, often reflect predictable changes in the facial skeleton. Facial balance is a critically important concept for aesthetic and reconstructive treatment planning of the facial skeleton [50]. Procedures for volume replacement and facial augmentation include lifting techniques, injectable fillers, autologous fat transfer, and facial implants [51–55]. Facial implants are often ideal due to their permanence, diverse shapes and sizes, ease of placement, minimal recovery time, and low complication rate. In particular, alloplastic implants provide a durable solution for skeletal augmentation, facial irregularity correction, and rejuvenation [34, 56].

4.2 Reconstructive needs (post-traumatic post-oncologic reconstruction)

Besides enhancing aesthetics, facial implants are used to reconstruct post-traumatic defects and address developmental and congenital abnormalities [47]. Craniofacial deformities affecting vision, breathing, and chewing typically require skeletal osteotomies for treatment. For less severe midface and mandibular hypoplasia, where occlusion is normal or has been corrected with orthodontics, extensive surgery may not be necessary. Instead, facial implants can effectively simulate the results of osteotomies, offering a less invasive and more appealing alternative. Patients with craniofacial syndromes or corrected deficiencies can benefit from implant augmentation with proven results in Treacher-Collins syndrome and Stickler syndrome [27, 57, 58]. Alloplastic implants can be effective for reconstructing post-traumatic and post-ablative craniofacial deformities. However, they are best suited for non-load-bearing areas, as implants in load-bearing sites risk micromotion, bone erosion, and extrusion. Chronic exposure to the sinuses can lead to bacterial contamination and infection. Reliable applications of alloplastic implants include parts of the cranial vault and internal orbit [27]. A flowchart presentation of facial deformity classifications and recommended treatment options is provided in **Figure 1** [59].

4.3 Mandible, malar region, chin, and nasal areas

Facial implants are frequently used to enhance the chin, zygomas, and mandibular angles. According to a 2020 American Society of Plastic Surgeons survey, malar implants are the most common facial implant procedure and the third most popular cosmetic surgery, with a 938% increase in popularity since 2000. Chin implants have risen by 63% over the same period. Implants are less commonly used on other bony areas, such as the nose, glabella, and temple [33]. Facial implants are classified by their placement sites (e.g., malar, submalar, paranasal, chin) and can be prefabricated, anatomical, or custom-made. They come in various shapes and sizes. Submalar implants restore lost volume in the midface due to aging, whereas malar implants augment and alter the patient's appearance. Smaller implants typically restore a previous look, while larger ones change the facial profile. The submalar area, experiencing significant atrophy, is often treated with smaller implants for women and medium ones for men. Larger implants are used for both volume restoration and enhancing unsatisfactory appearances. Chin augmentation addresses microgenia effectively with alloplastic implants, which are safe and straightforward to place. Mild to moderate chin deficiencies are well treated with these implants, while severe cases may require additional soft tissue filling and tension restoration for optimal results [34]. **Figure 2** illustrates the effectiveness of chin implants in improving the patient's jaw appearance.

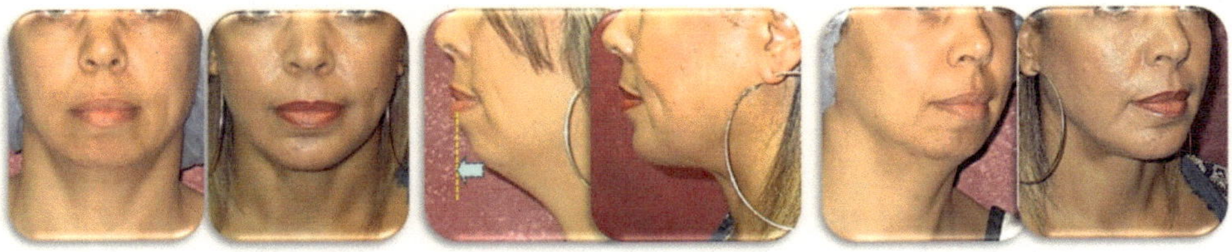

Figure 2.
Two years s/b submentoplasty, chin implant, and submandibular gland reduction by Dr. Cuzalina. The patient was also a candidate for a jaw crease, but she preferred an implant. Her lip apposition pre-op was relatively normal, so that a chin implant could be used and not deepen her labiomental crease beyond normal. The chin implant greatly improved the results from neck surgery by increasing chin projection and neck length.

5. Surgical techniques and considerations

5.1 Preoperative planning procedure choice and implant shaping

Effective patient selection is crucial for facial reconstruction with implants. Avoid high-risk candidates, such as diabetics or smokers [60]. Assess whether malar, submalar, or combined implants are needed for midface reconstruction, and note that chin implants mask rather than correct issues like micrognathia. Evaluate occlusion and facial proportions, and present all options, including implants, orthognathic surgery, and genioplasty if implants alone are unsuitable [61]. Proper shaping of implants, both preoperatively and intraoperatively, is essential to prevent complications. Yang et al.'s modified Gore-Tex carving technique involves V-grooves for improved curvature and fit, minimizing visible edges and gaps [62]. Wong's technique for silicone forehead implants includes corrugated edges and central perforations for better contour and fixation, reducing capsule contraction [63].

5.1.1 Preoperative antibiotic loading and implant infection control

Intraoperative antibiotics are standard in head and neck surgeries, including facial reconstruction with implants, to prevent infections. Ridwan-Pramana et al. noted a 7.2% infection rate in Medpor implants with pre- and/or intraoperative antibiotics but without antibiotic-soaked implants or reported postoperative oral antibiotics [64]. Some experts recommend short courses of intravenous (IV) and oral corticosteroids to mitigate inflammatory responses.

Antibiotic preloading of alloplastic implants has been explored with methods such as dipping, immersing, and using negative pressure. A 2009 study by Keefe and Keefe found negative pressure most effective in reducing Staphylococcus growth on Gore-Tex and Medpor implants [65]. However, there is limited evidence on the effectiveness of these methods in preventing infections. Niechajev's study, using suction to impregnate Medpor implants with cloxacillin, achieved a 2.8% infection rate in nasal reconstructions. Despite some advocacy for preoperative antibiotic impregnation, controlled trials are lacking [46]. Godin and collaborators (2003) found no significant difference in infection rates with preoperative antibiotic soaking for Gore-Tex chin implants and did not address perioperative or postoperative antibiotic use [66].

5.2 Surgical procedure and techniques

5.2.1 Nasal alloplastic implants

Made from either silicone, ePTFE, or porous polyethylene, nasal alloplastic implants are used for nasal augmentation. While less prone to infection than ePTFE, which has a greater infection rate but can be readily removed, silicone implants need anchoring to stop movement. Porous polyethylene implants might induce tissue ingrowth, which would complicate removal. Autologous cartilage is often preferred to avoid complications [8, 67, 68].

5.2.2 Premaxillary augmentation

Often used in rhinoplasty, particularly for enhancing nasal projection and midface contour. Implants are placed via an intranasal incision after elevating the periosteum of the premaxilla. Options include prefabricated silicone or ePTFE implants.

5.2.3 Midface augmentation

Aims to address volume loss and aging signs. Implants restore midface volume, improving projection and reducing nasolabial folds. These implants can be used alone or with rhytidectomy for enhanced results.

5.2.4 Mandibular augmentation

5.2.4.1 Anterior mandibular implants

Provide 6–9 mm of projection in men and 4–7 mm in women. Severe cases may require 10–12 mm. Access is through intraoral or submental approaches.

5.2.4.2 Mandibular angle implants

Inserted via a mucosal incision along the retromolar trigone, with subperiosteal dissection and secured with a titanium screw. **Figure 3** illustrates a CT-guided custom mandibular angle implant.

5.2.4.3 Total mandibular implants

Address comprehensive micrognathia, using both submental and retromolar approaches, and can be customized with computer-aided design [8, 59].

5.2.5 Lip augmentation

Traditionally done with fillers, but ePTFE implants like Advanta offer a longer-lasting solution. Implants are inserted through small incisions near the oral commissure, requiring proper dermal placement to prevent visibility and extrusion. Fillers and surgical lifts are alternative options [8, 68, 69]. An overview of essential principles for intraoperative techniques in facial implants is depicted in **Figure 2** [68].

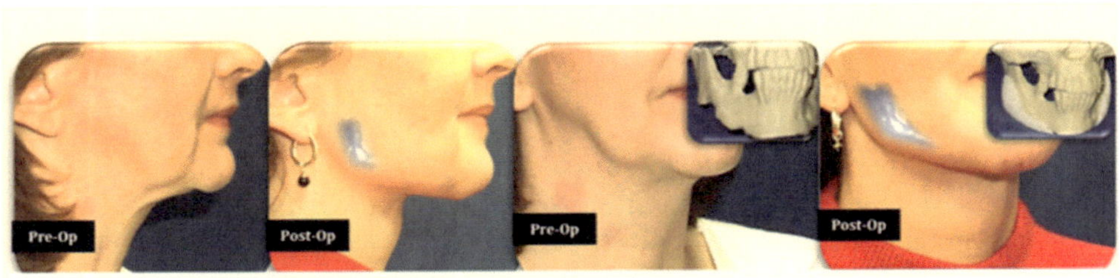

Figure 3.
Female patient of Dr. Cuzalina following placement of 3D CT-guided custom mandibular angle implants with prejowl implant fill and submentoplasty (no facelift).

5.3 Postoperative care and monitoring

Opinions on postoperative antibiotic use vary. Some advocate a short 5–7-day prophylactic course, while others argue it has no impact on infection rates. Villarreal et al. [70] found no significant difference in infection rates among patients who received amoxicillin-clavulanate, clindamycin, or no postoperative antibiotics after orbital floor reconstruction with Medpor implants ($p = 0.958$) [70]. All patients had received pre- or intraoperative IV antibiotics, and the infection rate was 12.5%. In contrast, Shadfar and colleagues reported a 2.9% infection rate in nasal reconstructions with Medpor implants, using a 7-day postoperative antibiotic course but no preoperative antibiotic soak [60].

6. Complications and risk management

Postoperative implant complications are usually minor and temporary. Prevention through proper patient selection, planning, and protocol is essential. Early issues can often be treated with anti-inflammatories and pain relievers. Numbness may occur, but it typically resolves within a week. A follow-up visit at 1–2 weeks is recommended to check for complications [71, 72]. A summary of the common complications associated with different sites of reconstruction is mentioned in **Figure 3** [68].

6.1 Short-term outcomes

6.1.1 Infection, extrusion, and inflammation

In the immediate postoperative period, patients may experience a range of short-term complications, primarily due to the surgical procedure itself and the initial response by the body triggered due to the implant. In facial reconstruction, *infection* remains a significant concern, particularly with alloplastic materials such as titanium, porous polyethylene (Medpor), and polyetherketone (PEEK) [46]. These materials, while advantageous for reducing donor site morbidity and enhancing surgical efficiency, are not immune to infection risks and can harbor bacteria [64, 73]. Biofilm formation is a key factor in these infections. Biofilms are dense clusters of microorganisms encased in a protective matrix, making them highly resistant to antibiotics and immune responses. Contamination of implants before surgery can lead to the development of biofilms, which are difficult to manage and may require implant removal for treatment [74, 75]. Malaisrie and coworkers demonstrated the development of biofilms in guinea pig models within one week after contamination with *Staphylococcus aureus*. Their study showed anatomical evidence of biofilm formation on various facial bioimplants, including titanium, silicone, ion-bombarded silicone, expanded polytetrafluoroethylene (e-PTFE; GORE-TEX), and porous high-density polyethylene (PHDPE; Porex Surgical Inc.). This highlights the rapid onset and complexity of biofilm-related infections in facial implants [76]. The incidence of infections, though, varies between different implant materials. Rojas and colleagues, following a literature search, revealed significant differences in infection rates between Medpor and silicone implants. Specifically, the infection rate for silicone implants stands at 2.2%, whereas Medpor implants have a considerably lower infection rate of 0.7% [9].

Implant *extrusion* is rare but often linked to underlying infection, which weakens the overlying tissues. It occurs when the implant breaches the skin or incision site, such as through the intraoral approach for cheek implants or into the maxillary sinuses. Factors like poor vascularization, previous surgeries, and excessively large implants increase the risk [71, 77]. Implant extrusion rates are higher in mobile soft tissue regions, like the columella or ala, due to muscle contracture. The orbicularis oris muscle's role in facial movement, swallowing, and respiration increases the risk of infection and extrusion [8]. Immediate intervention, including repositioning or removal of the implant, may be necessary to prevent further complications.

Inflammation is another common issue, and even a well-tolerated alloplastic implant acts as a foreign body, triggering a host response. Host proteins adhere to the implant, denature, and cause inflammation, leading to collagen deposition on and around the implant [78]. Uncontrolled inflammation can increase morbidity at implant sites. A meta-analysis conducted by Oliver and colleagues reported that the methyl methacrylate (2.50%) and Lactosorb (8%) implants had higher inflammation rates, with frontal implants also having poor cosmetic outcomes (5.20%). Orbital implants had an 8% inflammation rate [56]. Choi and colleagues describe how a silicone implant was moved into the frontal sinus following a nose job, emphasizing the dangers of inflammation and other difficulties that come with artificial implants as opposed to autologous tissues [30]. Proper surgical technique, with meticulous hemostasis and gentle tissue handling, is crucial to minimize risks. Postoperative care includes anti-inflammatory medications, fluid drainage, and close monitoring. Complications of facial implants have also included edema, postoperative asymmetry, lipid dysfunction, neuropraxia, seroma, and hematoma [34, 79].

6.2 Long-term complications and safety profiles

6.2.1 Chronic infections, migration, and resorption

Chronic infections may manifest long after the initial surgery, often presenting subtle signs such as chronic pain or low-grade fever. Chronic inflammation, on the other hand, may also lead to the formation of a fibrous capsule around the implant [68, 71]. Migration of the implant is another long-term issue, typically resulting from mechanical factors such as poor fixation or the absence of adequate tissue encapsulation. Migration can cause noticeable asymmetry, discomfort, and dissatisfaction with the aesthetic outcome. Surgical revision may involve re-securing the implant or using a different material to better match the patient's anatomy [34]. Recently, two cases of eyelid implant migration cases, with facial palsy have been discussed in implant migration. In both cases reported, the decision was made to remove the implant without reimplantation [80].

Bone resorption is a common and high-risk issue with alloplastic chin implants, particularly beneath the implant's surface in contact with the mandible [81, 82]. Resorption of the underlying bone can occur due to the pressure exerted by the implant, particularly if the implant is too large or improperly positioned. The first failures of alloplastic implants were reported by Robinson in 1972, where 12 of 14 patients with acrylic and silicone implants experienced up to 5 mm of bone resorption. This was attributed to implant shape, position, pressure from large implants, subperiosteal placement, and implant hardness [83, 84]. In a case series, the authors discussed four patients with alloplastic chin implants, where three exhibit varying degrees of bone erosion beneath the prostheses, while one has a normal bony contour [82]. In another recent report, the authors present two clinical cases of anterior chin cortex bone resorption associated with silicone implants [85].

6.2.2 Stability and integration of implants

The long-term stability of facial implants depends on the material and surgical technique used. Porous implants, such as porous polyethylene material (Medpor), foster fibrovascular ingrowth for better stabilization but are difficult to remove if complications occur. Smooth implants like silicone are less integrated with surrounding tissues, making them prone to movement but easier to remove if needed. Bone resorption, especially with oversized implants, can alter facial contours and affect both aesthetics and function, making radiographic monitoring crucial for early detection [34, 71].

6.3 Management of complications

Historically, implant infections were treated with antibiotics, incision, and removal. Recent methods in cardiothoracic, vascular, and orthopedic surgery now use debridement and systemic and local antibiotics to salvage implants. Orthopedics employs two-stage revisions with antibiotic-loaded spacers, and trauma surgery uses gentamicin beads and collagen sheets. These techniques are now being explored for facial implants, with mixed results [86–88].

Studies on Medpor grafts have identified higher failure risks in certain sites (nose, maxilla, ear) and patient conditions (syndromic patients) [89]. Porous polyethylene implants, especially when placed transorally or without proper coverage, have shown increased infection and exposure risks [90, 91]. Biofilms on implants, such as those found in a GORE-TEX dorsal nasal implant case, complicate treatment, requiring prolonged antibiotic use and often implant removal [92].

Bacterial infections vary, with common skin flora and atypical bacteria like mycobacteria requiring different treatments. Mycobacterial infections often evade routine cultures and need specialized testing and extended antibiotics [93]. Exposed implants usually require surgery, with techniques like tissue flaps and antibiotic irrigation showing partial success but still facing high complication rates [94]. Future treatments might include non-antibiotic methods to disrupt biofilms, such as laser waves and ultrasound. Preventing infections through thorough preoperative evaluation, sterility, debris minimization, and careful site selection is crucial [88, 95].

Summarizing this, effective management of chronic complications often requires long-term antibiotics and surgical removal of infected implants. For migration, resorption, or capsular contracture, surgical intervention, such as repositioning or replacing the implant, is typically necessary.

7. Case studies and clinical outcomes

7.1 Review of significant studies

The overview of some of the studies on facial implants, the success rates, patient satisfaction, and functional outcomes is presented in **Table 1**.

Implant material	Uses	Patients	Results	Reference
Polyethylene (Medpor)	Midface contouring in cleft patients	51	Reliable, long-term stable materials for effectively enhancing paranasal, subnasal, and malar areas, as well as a solid nasal dorsum in cleft patients, Medpor implants have few problems.	Schwaiger et al. [96]
	Skeletal augmentation	44	For face skeletal augmentation, high-density porous polyethylene is a dependable substitute for autogenous grafts; with enough soft tissue covering, it produces good long-term results with few complications.	Deshpande & Munoli [97]
	Single oral and maxillofacial surgeon	61	Results showed a 2.5% complication rate over a three-year follow-up, demonstrating that this midfacial correction technique is successful in both the short and long term.	French et al. [98]
	Correction of secondary unilateral cleft lip nasal deformity	32	One patient experienced delayed incision healing, with no other complications, resulting in a 96.9% satisfaction rate.	Zhuwei et al. [99]
Silicone	Mentoplasty	17	There were no permanent complications, with 15 patients (88.2%) extremely pleased with the procedure. Additionally, 16 patients (94.12%) showed significant improvement after solid silicone augmentation mentoplasty, and no revisions were needed.	Altintas et al. [100]
	Mandibular angle augmentation	58	Patients received 116 bilateral silicone implants at the mandibular angle, with 96 intact and no complications.	Al-Jandan & Marei [101]
	Chin alloplastic augmentation	10	Silastic alloplastic chin implants effectively augment moderate chin retrusion, with all patients showing significant profile improvement and high satisfaction according to the Genioplasty Outcome Evaluation.	Abdelmabood et al. [102]
	Chin augmentation	28	There were no complications with the implants, and all patients reported satisfaction with facial symmetry and cosmetic results, benefiting from the absence of visible scars.	Alasseri et al. [103]

Implant material	Uses	Patients	Results	Reference
Hydroxyapatite	Malarplasty	430	Hydroxyapatite/collagen composite used in malarplasty yields successful outcomes, though it has a longer learning curve compared to more commonly used implantable biomaterials.	D'Agostino et al. [104]
	Facial Skeleton	17	The study confirmed that only the placement of hydroxyapatite granules leads to initial collagen formation, followed by bone conversion, integrating the implant with the host bone for long-term stability.	Huggins & Mendelson [105]
	Neck rejuvenation	15	93.3% of patients showed at least a 1-grade improvement on the 5-point scale, with no serious adverse events reported, most being mild and transient.	de Sanctis Pecora [106]
Titanium	Aesthetics, deformity, and malformation surgery	12	3D printing accuracy of 0.1 mm facilitates precise jaw angle implant planning, with patients valuing preoperative renderings, while infections can be managed through careful selection and technical recommendations.	Mommaerts [107]
	Maxillofacial bones	16	Patient-specific titanium implants yielded satisfactory outcomes for various oral and maxillofacial defects.	Lim et al. [108]
	Maxillofacial surgery	32	Significant improvement and total recovery were observed in 32 cases, concluding that building anatomical models based on CT studies is financially viable for repairing orbital floor fractures.	Yusupov [109]

Table 1.
Here is an overview of some studies on facial implant success rate, patient satisfaction, and functional results:

7.2 An insight into case studies

Used for both cosmetic and reconstructive objectives, facial implants have shown great success rates over several anatomical areas. These implants give those with facial abnormalities resulting from disease, trauma, or congenital problems structural support and enhance their appearance. Often concentrating on certain areas such as the orbital, nasal, and auricular areas, several studies have assessed the effectiveness and longevity of various implants.

The success and survival rates of extraoral implants in the orbital, nasal, and auricular areas were evaluated in a 2017 Heitor Batista dos Reis et al. With no appreciable variation depending on anatomical area or past radiation exposure, this study indicated that the success rates were 95.9% for orbital implants, 92.9% for nasal implants, and 92% for auricular implants [110]. With a 79.5% total implant survival rate, Subramaniam et al. [111] also published long-term results showing temporal implants had the highest success rate (97.0%) compared to nasal (87.5%) and orbital implants (63.3%) [111].

Yoshino et al. [112] investigated the value of connective tissue grafting combined with instantaneous implant implantation. With an overall implant success rate of

100% at the one-year mark [112], their study found that connective tissue grafts helped preserve the facial gingival level. Moreover, a 2011 study by Kan and colleagues verified that although constant monitoring of facial gingival tissue was essential due to possible recession, favorable implant success rates and peri-implant tissue responses could be obtained with immediate placement and provisionalization [113].

Generally speaking, facial implants show good success rates, especially in non-irradiated areas and under appropriate surgical methods. Outcomes are significantly influenced by the implant material and anatomical placement; auricular and nasal implants usually show better success rates than orbital implants. Constant developments in surgical methods and materials will probably help to raise these success rates and lower complications.

8. Future perspective

Facial implants are expertly positioned as a permanent medical device inside the face to shape and fashion a patient's characteristics. For individuals interested in these surgeries, there are plenty of choices ranging from cheek to jaw implants; now, there is another choice utilizing your own tissue. Facial implants have bright futures with continuous technological and medical innovation opening the path for more efficient, safer, and aesthetically acceptable solutions. Highly tailored implants that better fit patients' anatomical needs are resulting from technological advancements, including 3D printing and the creation of biocompatible materials (especially polyetheretherketone and titanium alloy plates), therefore lowering problems and increasing satisfaction [114–116]. Furthermore, regenerative medicine and tissue engineering's stem cell integration and bioengineered implants created from a patient's own cells are providing amazing opportunities for natural tissue regeneration and lowering the danger of rejection. Minimally invasive techniques are also becoming more popular since they shorten recovery times and cause little scarring, therefore reducing the risk of operations [117, 118].

Furthermore, the merging of robotics and artificial intelligence is revolutionizing the planning and execution of facial implant procedures, therefore enabling perfect design and customized treatment plans [119, 120]. While highlighting aesthetic and functional improvements, future implants will most likely solve hereditary defects, injuries, or diseases affecting facial features. More tailored treatment plans will result from genetic testing and improved imaging as personalized medicine advances. Along with technology advancements, ethical and legal concerns will shift to ensure patient safety and management of costs. As these technologies become more readily available, offering more opportunities and more acceptance among a bigger audience, the market for facial implants is expected to develop. Using computer-designed patient-specific implants nowadays helps to more precisely reconstruct maxillofacial abnormalities. Higher patient satisfaction results from this method, which also removes the typical difficulties connected with previous implants. The great expense is the main disadvantage, though [121]. Advancement of implant technology depends on the improvement of biocompatibility, durability, and infection control. Crucially, there are innovations in individualized implants, minimally invasive approaches, and neural interfaces. Furthermore, greatly improving health outcomes and quality of life will involve addressing cost, accessibility, ethical issues, and patient-centered results.

9. Conclusion

Facial implants play a critical role in both aesthetic and reconstructive facial surgeries. They address the complex needs arising from trauma, congenital abnormalities, and age-related volume loss. The evolution of materials from metals and polymers to bioceramics has significantly enhanced the durability, safety, and integration of implants. Historical progress in aesthetic surgery has laid the foundation for modern techniques that ensure better patient outcomes. Despite the high success rates of facial implants, ongoing research and technological advancements promise even greater improvements in biocompatibility, customization, and minimally invasive procedures. The future of facial implants looks promising, with potential innovations in regenerative medicine and personalized treatment plans offering new possibilities for enhancing facial aesthetics and function.

Additional materials

This video provides a step-by-step breakdown of the cheek implant surgery process. Download the video here: https://bit.ly/4dTp5qV.

Author details

Mohammad K.H.B. Abdulaziz[1*] and Mohammad Kamal[2]

1 Plastic Surgery Department, University Hospitals Birmingham, NHS Trust, Warwickshire, United Kingdom

2 Kuwait University Faculty of Dentistry, Kuwait

*Address all correspondence to: drbaqer1988@gmail.com

References

[1] Ehlinger-Martin A, Cohen-Letessier A, Taïeb M, Azoulay E, du Crest D. Women's attitudes to beauty, aging, and the place of cosmetic procedures: Insights from the QUEST observatory. Journal of Cosmetic Dermatology. 2016;**15**(1):89-94

[2] Sezgin B, Findikcioglu K, Kaya B, Sibar S, Yavuzer R. Mirror on the wall: A study of women's perception of facial features as they age. Aesthetic Surgery Journal. 2012;**32**(4):421-425

[3] Zebrowitz LA, Montepare JM. Social psychological face perception: Why appearance matters. Social and Personality Psychology Compass. 2008;**2**(3):1497-1517

[4] Reilly MJ, Tomsic JA, Fernandez SJ, Davison SP. Effect of facial rejuvenation surgery on perceived attractiveness, femininity, and personality. JAMA Facial Plastic Surgery. 2015;**17**(3):202-207

[5] Swift A, Liew S, Weinkle S, Garcia JK, Silberberg MB. The facial aging process from the "inside out". Aesthetic Surgery Journal. 2021;**41**(10):1107-1119

[6] Maurer D, Le Grand R, Mondloch CJ. The many faces of configural processing. Trends in Cognitive Sciences. 2002;**6**(6):255-260

[7] Taubert J, Apthorp D, Aagten-Murphy D, Alais D. The role of holistic processing in face perception: Evidence from the face inversion effect. Vision Research. 2011;**51**(11):1273-1278

[8] Hsieh T-y, Dhir K, Binder WJ, Hilger PA. Alloplastic facial implants. Facial Plastic Surgery. 2021;**37**(06):741-750

[9] Rojas YA, Sinnott C, Colasante C, Samas J, Reish RG. Facial implants: Controversies and criticism. A comprehensive review of the current literature. Plastic and Reconstructive Surgery. 2018;**142**(4)

[10] Rubin PJ, Yaremchuk MJ. Complications and toxicities of implantable biomaterials used in facial reconstructive and aesthetic surgery: A comprehensive review of the literature. Plastic and Reconstructive Surgery. 1997;**100**(5)

[11] Wong C-H, Mendelson B. Newer understanding of specific anatomic targets in the aging face as applied to Injectables: Aging changes in the craniofacial skeleton and facial ligaments. Plastic and Reconstructive Surgery. 2015;**136**(5S)

[12] Dhir K, Binder W. Solid midfacial implants: When fillers are not enough. Facial Plastic Surgery. 2016;**32**(05):480-487

[13] Shaw RB Jr, Katzel EB, Koltz PF, Yaremchuk MJ, Girotto JA, Kahn DM, et al. Aging of the facial skeleton: Aesthetic implications and rejuvenation strategies. Plastic and Reconstructive Surgery. 2011;**127**(1)

[14] Dieffenbach J. Die Operative Chirurgie. In: Leipzig FA, editor. Brockhaus. Vol. 1. 1845. pp. 744-746

[15] Rogers BO. Julius von Szymanowski (1829-1868): His life and contributions to plastic surgery. Plastic and Reconstructive Surgery. 1979;**64**(4):465-478

[16] Marck K, Marck R. On the origin of our specialty: The conceptual thinking

in plastic reconstructive surgery. European Journal of Plastic Surgery. 2022;**45**(3):495-501

[17] Ely ET. An operation for prominence of the auricles. Plastic and Reconstructive Surgery. 1968;**42**(6):582-583

[18] Roe JO. The deformity termed 'Pug nose' and its correction by a simple operation. Archives of Otolaryngology–Head & Neck Surgery. 1989;**115**(2):156-157

[19] Roe JO. The deformity termed "pug nose" and its correction, by a simple operation. Plastic and Reconstructive Surgery. 1970;**45**(1):78-81

[20] Weir RF. On restoring sunken noses without scarring the face. Plastic and Reconstructive Surgery. 1970;**45**(4):382-390

[21] Joseph J. Über die operative Verkleinerung einer nase (rhinomiosis). Berlin Klin Wochenschr. 1898;**40**:822

[22] Miller CC. The Correction of Featural Imperfections: The Author; 1907

[23] Frodel JL, Lee S. The use of high-density polyethylene implants in facial deformities. Archives of Otolaryngology–Head & Neck Surgery. 1998;**124**(11):1219-1223

[24] Gear AJ, Lokeh A, Aldridge JH, Migliori MR, Benjamin CI, Schubert W. Safety of titanium mesh for orbital reconstruction. Annals of Plastic Surgery. 2002;**48**(1):1-9

[25] Goldsmith D, Horowitz A, Orentlicher G. Facial skeletal augmentation using custom facial implants. Atlas of the Oral and Maxillofacial Surgery Clinics of North America. 2012;**20**(1):119-134

[26] Chen NT, Glowacki J, Bucky LP, Hong H-z, Kim W-K, Yaremchuk MJ. The roles of revascularization and resorption on endurance of craniofacial onlay bone grafts in the rabbit. Plastic and Reconstructive Surgery. 1994;**93**(4):714-722

[27] Yaremchuk MJ. Atlas of Facial Implants E-Book. Elsevier Health Sciences; 2019

[28] Sailer H, Marentette L, Makek M. Lyophilized cartilage in nasal reconstruction. The American Journal of Cosmetic Surgery. 1987;**4**(1):21-25

[29] Sailer HF. Experiences with the use of lyophilized bank cartilage for facial contour correction. Journal of Maxillofacial Surgery. 1976;**4**:149-157

[30] Choi JY, Ko E, Lee CR, Choi J, Moon S-H, Oh DY, et al. Frontal sinus displacement of silicone implant after previous rhinoplasty. Journal of Craniofacial Surgery. 2024;**10**(1097)

[31] Kaufman MR, Miller TA, Huang C, Roostaien J, Wasson KL, Ashley RK, et al. Autologous fat transfer for facial recontouring: Is there science behind the art? Plastic and Reconstructive Surgery. 2007;**119**(7):2287-2296

[32] Rowe P, Koller A, Sharma S. Physiology, Bone Remodeling. StatPearls. Treasure Island (FL) ineligible companies. Disclosure: Adam Koller declares no relevant financial relationships with ineligible companies. Disclosure: Sandeep Sharma Declares no Relevant Financial Relationships with Ineligible Companies.: StatPearls Publishing, Copyright © 2024, StatPearls Publishing LLC.; 2024

[33] Sharma EM, Smith KD. Facial Implants. StatPearls [Internet]: StatPearls Publishing; 2024

[34] Sarkarat F, Bohluli B, Kahali R. Facial augmentation with implants. In: A Textbook of Advanced Oral and Maxillofacial Surgery. Vol. 2. London, UK: IntechOpen; 2015

[35] Thakur A, Kumar A. Recent advancements in the surface treatments for enhanced biocompatibility and corrosion resistance of titanium-based biomedical implants. Applied Chemical Engineering. 2024;**7**(1)

[36] Panje WR, Hetherington HE. Use of stainless steel implants in facial bone reconstruction. Otolaryngologic Clinics of North America. 1995;**28**(2):341-349

[37] Saini M, Singh Y, Arora P, Arora V, Jain K. Implant biomaterials: A comprehensive review. World Journal of Clinical Cases: WJCC. 2015;**3**(1):52

[38] Hasirci V, Hasirci N. Fundamentals of Biomaterials. Springer; 2018

[39] Pan Z, Patil P. Titanium osteosynthesis hardware in maxillofacial trauma surgery: To remove or remain? A retrospective study. European Journal of Trauma and Emergency Surgery. 2014;**40**:587-591

[40] Kreppel M, Kauke M, Grandoch A, Safi A-F, Nickenig H-J, Zöller J. Evaluation of fronto-orbital advancement using titanium-based internal fixation for corrective pediatric craniofacial surgery. Journal of Craniofacial Surgery. 2018;**29**(6):1542-1545

[41] Sargent LA, Fulks KD. Reconstruction of internal orbital fractures with vitallium mesh. Plastic and Reconstructive Surgery. 1991;**88**(1):31-38

[42] Pacifici L, de Angelis F, Orefici A, Cielo A. Metals used in maxillofacial surgery. ORAL & implantology. 2016;**9**(Suppl 1/2016 to N 4/2016):107

[43] Huo W, Zhao L, Yu S, Yu Z, Zhang P, Zhang Y. Significantly enhanced osteoblast response to nano-grained pure tantalum. Scientific Reports. 2017;**7**(1):40868

[44] Bakri MM, Lee SH, Lee JH. Improvement of biohistological response of facial implant materials by tantalum surface treatment. Maxillofacial Plastic and Reconstructive Surgery. 2019;**41**:1-8

[45] Mohutsiwa R, van der Walt J, van den Heever H. Polymeric materials and processes to produce facial reconstruction implants: A review. In: MATEC Web of Conferences. EDP Sciences; 2022

[46] Niechajev I. Facial reconstruction using porous high-density polyethylene (medpor): Long-term results. Aesthetic Plastic Surgery. 2012;**36**:917-927

[47] Ahmed MG, AlHammad ZA, Al-Jandan B, Almohammadi T, Alam MK, Bagde H. Silicone facial implants, to fixate or not to fixate: A narrative review. Cureus. 2023;**15**(2)

[48] Quatela VC, Chow J. Synthetic facial implants. Facial Plastic Surgery Clinics of North America. 2008;**16**(1):1-10

[49] Bogala MR. Three-dimensional (3D) printing of hydroxyapatite-based scaffolds: A review. Bioprinting. 2022;**28**:e00244

[50] Kauke-Navarro M, Knoedler L, Knoedler S, Deniz C, Stucki L, Safi A-F. Balancing beauty and science: A review of facial implant materials in craniofacial surgery. Frontiers in Surgery. 2024;**11**:1348140

[51] Funt DK. Nonsurgical facial enhancement and rejuvenation—Fillers, neurotoxins, and fat transfers. Tips and tricks in plastic. Surgery. 2022:85-110

[52] Kang K. Sequential autologous fat injection techniques for volumetric face lifting in young Korean females. Journal of Cosmetic Medicine. 2020;**4**(2):57-63

[53] Narciso R, Basile E, Bottini DJ, Cervelli V. PEEK implants: An innovative solution for facial aesthetic surgery. Case Reports in Surgery. 2021;**2021**(1):5518433

[54] Schultz KP, Raghuram A, Davis MJ, Abu-Ghname A, Chamata E, Rohrich RJ. Fat grafting for facial rejuvenation. In: Seminars in plastic surgery. Thieme Medical Publishers; 2020

[55] Toplu G, Altınel D. Facial contouring and rejuvenation with the use of fat injection. Düzce Üniversitesi Sağlık Bilimleri Enstitüsü Dergisi. 2021;**11**(1):61-66

[56] Oliver JD, Eells AC, Saba ES, Boczar D, Restrepo DJ, Huayllani MT, et al. Alloplastic facial implants: A systematic review and meta-analysis on outcomes and uses in aesthetic and reconstructive plastic surgery. Aesthetic Plastic Surgery. 2019;**43**:625-636

[57] Cabanillas-Aquino AG, Rojas-Yauri MC, Atoche-Socola KJ, Arriola-Guillén LE. Assessment of craniofacial and dental characteristics in individuals with treacher collins syndrome. A review. Journal of Stomatology, Oral and Maxillofacial Surgery. 2021;**122**(5):511-515

[58] Snead M, Martin H, Bale P, Shenker N, Baguley D, Alexander P, et al. Therapeutic and diagnostic advances in stickler syndrome. Therapeutic Advances in Rare Disease. 2020;**1**:2633004020978661

[59] Binder WJ, Dhir K. Internet access to advanced 3-dimensional software for the prototyping and design of complex and precise custom mandibular implants. The American Journal of Cosmetic Surgery. 2016;**33**(2):83-90

[60] Shadfar S, Farag A, Jarchow AM, Shockley WW. Safety and efficacy of expanded polytetrafluoroethylene implants in the surgical management of traumatic nasal deformity. JAMA Otolaryngology–Head & Neck Surgery. 2015;**141**(8):710-715

[61] Brandt MG, Moore CC. Implants in facial skeletal augmentation. Current Opinion in Otolaryngology & Head and Neck Surgery. 2013;**21**(4):396-399

[62] Yang P, Yang Q, Liu T, Zeng J, Bi B, Zhou Y, et al. A modified technique for expanded polytetrafluoroethylene shaping in chin augmentation: Parallel groove carving technique. Journal of Craniofacial Surgery. 2015;**26**(2):e146-e1e8

[63] Wong JK. Forehead augmentation with alloplastic implants. Facial Plastic Surgery Clinics. 2010;**18**(1):71-77

[64] Ridwan-Pramana A, Wolff J, Raziei A, Ashton-James CE, Forouzanfar T. Porous polyethylene implants in facial reconstruction: Outcome and complications. Journal of Cranio-Maxillofacial Surgery. 2015;**43**(8):1330-1334

[65] Keefe MS, Keefe MA. An evaluation of the effectiveness of different techniques for intraoperative infiltration of antibiotics into alloplastic implants for use in facial reconstruction. Archives of Facial Plastic Surgery. 2009;**11**(4):246-251

[66] Godin M, Costa L, Romo T, Truswell W, Wang T, Williams E.

Gore-Tex chin implants. Archives of Facial Plastic Surgery. 2003

[67] Dresner HS, Hilger PA. An overview of nasal dorsal augmentation. In: Seminars in Plastic Surgery. © Thieme Medical Publishers; 2008

[68] Patel K, Brandstetter K. Solid implants in facial plastic surgery: Potential complications and how to prevent them. Facial Plastic Surgery. 2016;**32**(05):520-531

[69] Yaremchuk MJ. Facial skeletal reconstruction using porous polyethylene implants. Plastic and Reconstructive Surgery. 2003;**111**(6):1818-1827

[70] Villarreal PM, Monje F, Morillo AJ, Junquera LM, González C, Barbón JJ. Porous polyethylene implants in orbital floor reconstruction. Plastic and Reconstructive Surgery. 2002;**109**(3):877-885

[71] Ferneini EM, Di Pasquale L, Mommaerts M. Facial Implants. In: Complications in Maxillofacial Cosmetic Surgery: Strategies for Prevention and Management. 2018. pp. 237-249

[72] Rayess HM, Svider P, Hanba C, Patel VS, Carron M, Zuliani G. Adverse events in facial implant surgery and associated malpractice litigation. JAMA Facial Plastic Surgery. 2018;**20**(3):244-248

[73] Yaremchuk MJ. Secondary malar implant surgery. Plastic and Reconstructive Surgery. 2008;**121**(2):620-628

[74] Ussia M, Urso M, Kment S, Fialova T, Klima K, Dolezelikova K, et al. Light-propelled nanorobots for facial titanium implants biofilms removal. Small. 2022;**18**(22):2200708

[75] Walker TJ, Toriumi DM. Analysis of facial implants for bacterial biofilm formation using scanning electron microscopy. JAMA. Facial Plastic Surgery. 2016

[76] Malaisrie SC, Malekzadeh S, Biedlingmaier JF. In vivo analysis of bacterial biofilm formation on facial plastic bioimplants. The Laryngoscope. 1998;**108**(11):1733-1738

[77] Schatz C, Ginat D. Imaging of cosmetic facial implants and grafts. American Journal of Neuroradiology. 2013;**34**(9):1674-1681

[78] Sclafani AP, Romo T III. Biology and chemistry of facial implants. Facial Plastic Surgery. 2000;**16**(01):003-006

[79] Lutz J-C, Vitale LSA, Graillon N, Foletti J-M, Schouman T. Standard and customized alloplastic facial implants refining orthognathic surgery: Outcome evaluation. Journal of Oral and Maxillofacial Surgery. 2020;**78**(10):1832. e1-. e12

[80] Krajewska-Węglewicz L. Migration and extrusion of eyelid implant in patients with facial palsy–two case reports. Klinika Oczna/Acta Ophthalmologica Polonica. 2023;**125**(1)

[81] Matarasso A, Elias AC, Elias RL. Labial incompetence: A marker for progressive bone resorption in silastic chin augmentation. Plastic and Reconstructive Surgery. 1996;**98**(6):1007-1014

[82] Polo M. Bone resorption under chin implants: The orthodontist's role in its diagnosis and management. American Journal of Orthodontics and Dentofacial Orthopedics. 2017;**151**(1):201-208

[83] Cuzalina LA, Hlavacek MR. Complications of facial implants. Oral

and Maxillofacial Surgery Clinics of North America. 2009;**21**(1):91-104

[84] Robinson M. Bone resorption under plastic chin implants: Follow-up of a preliminary report. Archives of Otolaryngology. 1972;**95**(1):30-32

[85] Ramalho GC, Miranda SLD, Moreno R, Silva HCLE, Miranda MVDF. Bone reabsorption associated with silicone implants in mentoplasty: A clinical case report. Revista Brasileira de Cirurgia Plástica. 2023;**32**:291-294

[86] Diefenbeck M, Mückley T, Hofmann GO. Prophylaxis and treatment of implant-related infections by local application of antibiotics. Injury. 2006;**37**(2):S95-S104

[87] Lapid O. Use of gentamicin collagen sponges for the treatment of periprosthetic breast implant infection. Journal of Plastic, Reconstructive & Aesthetic Surgery. 2011;**64**(12):e313-e3e6

[88] Mohan K, Cox JA, Dickey RM, Gravina P, Echo A, Izaddoost SA, et al. Treatment of infected facial implants. In: Seminars in Plastic Surgery. Thieme Medical Publishers; 2016

[89] Cenzi R, Farina A, Zuccarino L, Carinci F. Clinical outcome of 285 Medpor grafts used for craniofacial reconstruction. Journal of Craniofacial Surgery. 2005;**16**(4):526-530

[90] Fialkov JA, Holy C, Forrest CR, Phillips JH, Antonyshyn M. Postoperative infections in craniofacial reconstructive procedures. Journal of Craniofacial Surgery. 2001;**12**(4):362-368

[91] Menderes A, Baytekin C, Topcu A, Yilmaz M, Barutcu A. Craniofacial reconstruction with high-density porous polyethylene implants. Journal of Craniofacial Surgery. 2004;**15**(5):719-724

[92] Desai SC, Moradzadeh A, Branham G. Anatomical evidence of microbial biofilms in an alloplastic nasal implant. Aesthetic Plastic Surgery. 2013;**37**:468-471

[93] Rhie JW, Jeong YJ, Kim SW. Nontuberculous mycobacterial infection related to nasal implant. Journal of Craniofacial Surgery. 2013;**24**(4):1257-1259

[94] Lu L, Shi W, Luo M, Sun Y, Fan X. Repair of exposed hydroxyapatite orbital implants by subconjunctival tissue flaps. Journal of Craniofacial Surgery. 2011;**22**(4):1452-1456

[95] Hasson O, Levi G, Conley R. Late infections associated with alloplastic facial implants. Journal of Oral and Maxillofacial Surgery. 2007;**65**(2):321-323

[96] Schwaiger M, Echlin K, Atherton D, Haers P. The use of Medpor implants for midface contouring in cleft patients. International Journal of Oral and Maxillofacial Surgery. 2019;**48**(9):1177-1184

[97] Deshpande S, Munoli A. Long-term results of high-density porous polyethylene implants in facial skeletal augmentation: An Indian perspective. Indian Journal of Plastic Surgery. 2010;**43**(01):034-039

[98] French K, Gormley M, Kana A, Deacon S, Revington P. Outcomes and complications associated with malar onlays: Literature review and case series of 119 implants. British Journal of Oral and Maxillofacial Surgery. 2020;**58**(9):1110-1115

[99] Zhuwei W, Jie L, Ligang X. Application of porous high-density polyethylene in the correction of secondary unilateral cleft lip

nasal deformity. Journal of Tissue Engineering and Reconstructive Surgery. 2024;**20**(2):212

[100] Altintaş A, YegIn Y, ÇelIk M, Kayabaşoğlu G. Our Outcomes of Augmentation Mentoplasty with Solid Silicone. 2018

[101] Al-Jandan B, Marei HF. Mandibular angle augmentation using solid silicone implants. Dental and Medical Problems. 2018;**55**(4):367-370

[102] Abdelmabood A, Abdullah W, Amer M. Clinical evaluation of Genioplasty with either Silastic (solid silicone) and Medpor (porous polyethylene) as chin alloplastic augmentation. Egyptian Dental Journal. 2022;**68**(4):3161-3169

[103] Alasseri N, Khubrani AM, Al-Moraissi E. Minimally invasive approach for chin augmentation using a silicone implant. European Journal of Plastic Surgery. 2023;**46**(4):525-532

[104] D'Agostino A, Trevisiol L, Favero V, Gunson MJ, Pedica F, Nocini PF, et al. Hydroxyapatite/collagen composite is a reliable material for malar augmentation. Journal of Oral and Maxillofacial Surgery. 2016;**74**(6):1238. e1-. e15

[105] Huggins RJ, Mendelson BC. Biologic behavior of hydroxyapatite used in facial augmentation. Aesthetic Plastic Surgery. 2017;**41**:179-184

[106] de Sanctis PC. The gold protocol: A combined treatment approach for neck rejuvenation with calcium hydroxyapatite, botulinum toxin, and hyaluronic acid in the same session. Journal of Cosmetic Dermatology. 2024

[107] Mommaerts MY. Guidelines for patient-specific jawline definition with titanium implants in esthetic, deformity, and malformation surgery. Annals of Maxillofacial Surgery. 2016;**6**(2):287-291

[108] Lim H-K, Choi Y-J, Choi W-C, Song I-S, Lee U-L. Reconstruction of maxillofacial bone defects using patient-specific long-lasting titanium implants. Scientific Reports. 2022;**12**(1):7538

[109] Yusupov S. Clinical application of 3D pre-bent titanium implants for fractures of inferior wall of the orbit. International Journal of Medical Science and Public Health Research. 2023;**4**(11):81-88

[110] Dos, Reis HB, de Oliveira JAP, Pecorari VA, Raoufi S, Abrahão M, Dib LL. Extraoral implants for anchoring facial prostheses: Evaluation of success and survival rates in three anatomical regions. International Journal of Oral & Maxillofacial Implants. 2017;**32**(2)

[111] Subramaniam S, Breik O, Cadd B, Peart G, Wiesenfeld D, Heggie A, et al. Long-term outcomes of craniofacial implants for the restoration of facial defects. International Journal of Oral and Maxillofacial Surgery. 2018;**47**(6):773-782

[112] Yoshino S, Kan JY, Rungcharassaeng K, Roe P, Lozada JL. Effects of connective tissue grafting on the facial gingival level following single immediate implant placement and provisionalization in the esthetic zone: A 1-year randomized controlled prospective study. International Journal of Oral & Maxillofacial Implants. 2014;**29**(2)

[113] Kan JY, Rungcharassaeng K, Lozada JL, Zimmerman G. Facial gingival tissue stability following immediate placement and provisionalization of maxillary anterior single implants: A 2- to 8-year follow-up. The International

Journal of Oral & Maxillofacial Implants. 2011;**26**(1):179-187

[114] Jindal S, Manzoor F, Haslam N, Mancuso E. 3D printed composite materials for craniofacial implants: Current concepts, challenges and future directions. The International Journal of Advanced Manufacturing Technology. 2021;**112**(3):635-653

[115] Davis R, Singh A, Jackson MJ, Coelho RT, Prakash D, Charalambous CP, et al. A comprehensive review on metallic implant biomaterials and their subtractive manufacturing. The International Journal of Advanced Manufacturing Technology. 2022;**120**(3):1473-1530

[116] Anghelina F, Mitroi AA, Ciuca E, Tumbar LT, Boicea AR, Anghelina L, et al. Biomaterials used in the prosthetics of facial fractures. 2024;**61**(1):11

[117] Charbe NB, Tambuwala M, Palakurthi SS, Warokar A, Hromić-Jahjefendić A, Bakshi H, et al. Biomedical applications of three-dimensional bioprinted craniofacial tissue engineering. Bioengineering & Translational Medicine. 2023;**8**(1):e10333

[118] Meghe S, Ramapure R, Jaiswal S, Jawade S, Singh S. A comprehensive review of minimally invasive dermatosurgical procedures. Cureus. 2024;**16**(3)

[119] Memon AR, Li J, Egger J, Chen X. A review on patient-specific facial and cranial implant design using artificial intelligence (AI) techniques. Expert Review of Medical Devices. 2021;**18**(10):985-994

[120] Miragall MF, Knoedler S, Kauke-Navarro M, Saadoun R, Grabenhorst A, Grill FD, et al. Face the future—Artificial intelligence in oral and maxillofacial surgery. Journal of Clinical Medicine. 2023;**12**(21):6843

[121] Alasseri N, Alasraj A. Patient-specific implants for maxillofacial defects: Challenges and solutions. Maxillofacial Plastic and Reconstructive Surgery. 2020;**42**:1-8

Chapter 6

Injection Techniques for Perioral Enhancement

Riekie Smit

Abstract

This chapter will focus on the injection techniques for perioral rejuvenation using botulinum toxin and dermal filler injections. The perioral region is a very mobile region that shows aging changes at various levels. The most common concerns of patients include perioral wrinkling, mouth corners turning down, lip inversion and volume loss. The correct use of botulinum toxin A could minimize perioral wrinkles, give slight eversion ("lip flip") and help to reduce mouth corner drooping. Fillers can be utilized to treat perioral volume loss and to manage the fine wrinkles around the lips. These procedures require in-depth knowledge of the perioral anatomy and the layers of structures, good knowledge of the products and their respective pharmacokinetics and rheology, and lastly, good injection skills. This will ensure minimizing side effects or complications.

Keywords: botulinum toxin A, lip wrinkles, perioral lines, lip fillers, perioral aging, lip flip, mouth corners

1. Introduction

The aging changes in the perioral region have a significant impact on appearance, attractiveness and revealing one's age.

There are numerous factors contributing to the aging changes that are visible in the perioral region, ranging from skin aging due to chronological, intrinsic and extrinsic aging; soft tissue, fat and muscular changes; and also dental factors and bony resorption [1, 2]. Another important factor affecting the perioral and, specifically, lip aging process is the hormonal decline in females, especially after menopause [3].

The need for esthetic enhancement in the perioral region is high due to the impact that this region has on the perception of age and attractiveness [4–6].

There are numerous types of treatments and protocols for perioral rejuvenation. It is very important that the physician understand the aging pathology in the perioral region, know how to evaluate the perioral region and choose the correct individualized treatment plan to ensure patient satisfaction.

2. Perioral evaluation

The perioral region should be evaluated in relation to the whole face. Ideal proportions of the perioral region should be considered according to the ethnicity of the patient and care should be taken not to measure all patients according to the generally defined Caucasian proportions.

The relation of the perioral region to the whole face is often described by the artistic proportions dividing the face into thirds (**Figure 1**) [7–9].

The upper third of the face extends from the hairline to the nasion. The middle third of the face then extends from the nasion to the subnasale, and the lower third then to the menton. The inferior third is then further divided into the height of the upper lip compared to the height of the lower lip and chin.

On a lateral view, Rickett's e-line is used to evaluate the lip prominence and relation to nose and chin [7–9].

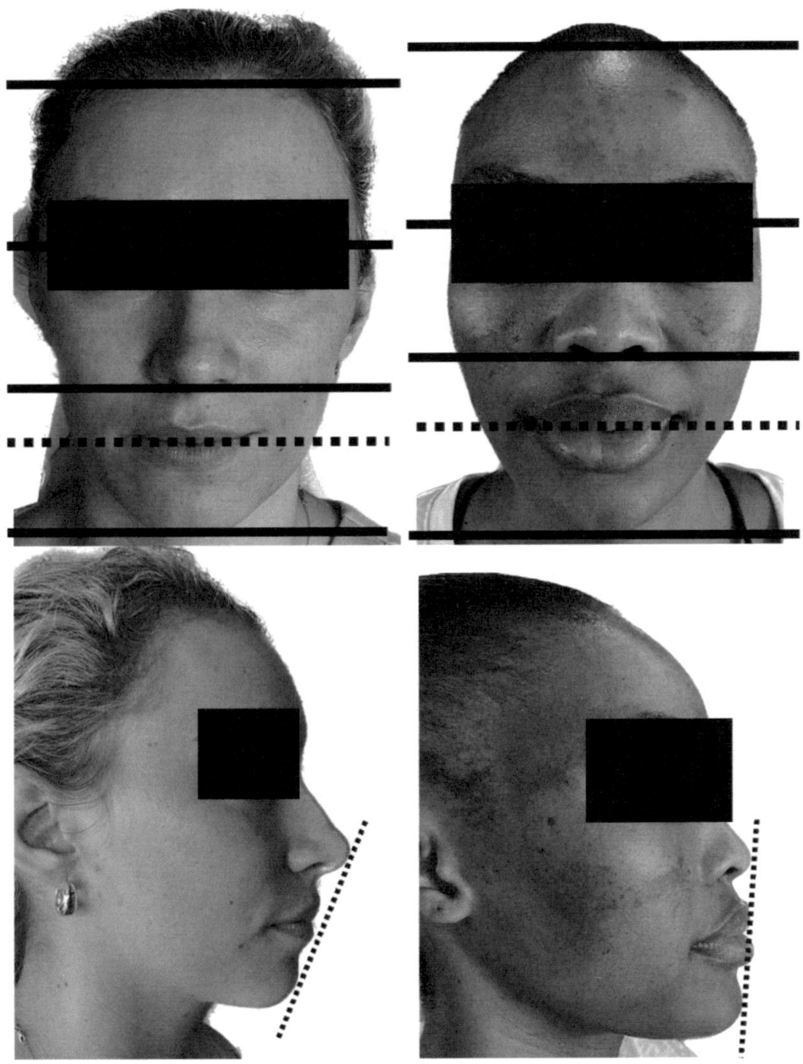

Figure 1.
The proportions of the facial thirds on frontal view and the lateral view proportions using Rickett's e-line. Image by Dr. Smit with permission from patients.

The major differences in the perioral region between different races are noticeable in the lateral view. There are numerous different proportional lines, reference planes and angles that can be used for the evaluation of lip prominence and its relation to the nose and chin. The Rickett's line is an easy line to use during evaluation and during treatment. This line is described as the line from the tip of the nose to the pogonion. In Caucasian patients the upper lip should be 3–4 mm behind this line and the lower lip 2 mm behind this line [9–12]. This is not the same for ideal proportions in other ethnicities [9]. In the Asian and African populations, the lips will often cross this line and still remain esthetically pleasing and attractive [9–12].

It remains important to take into consideration that skeletal and dental factors also influence the lower face proportions. This may necessitate a referral to a dentist or maxillofacial surgeon in some cases.

3. Perioral aging

The perioral region is one of the first regions in the face to show signs of facial aging due to intrinsic factors and is often aggravated by extrinsic factors, especially smoking and excess sun exposure [1, 2].

The aging signs in the peri-oral region may include the following visible changes:

- Loss of lip volume
- Vermillion border and Cupid's bow loss
- Inversion of upper lip
- Vertical lines extending from upper and lower lip (often referred to as barcode wrinkles or smoker's lines)
- Down-turned mouth corners and marionette folds
- Worsening of nasolabial and melo-labial folds
- Pre-jowl sulcus
- Chin dimpling (**Figure 2**).

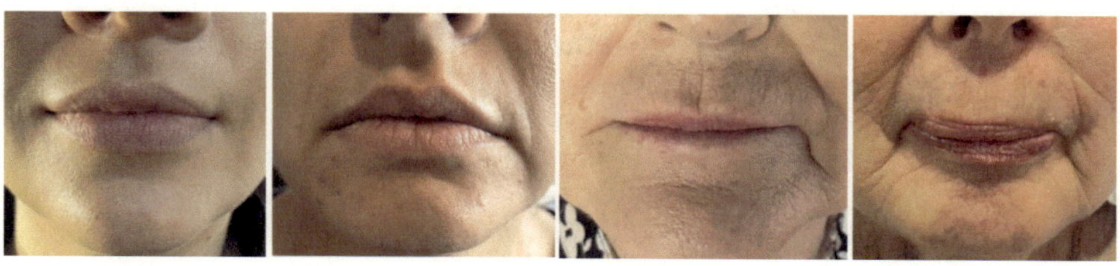

Figure 2.
Aging changes that occur perioral, starting from younger to older perioral region. Images by Dr. Smit with permission from patients.

4. Perioral rejuvenation

The perioral enhancement techniques are focused on managing the aging pathology in this region. Often, a combination of techniques may be required to address the various pathological aspects of skin aging, volume loss, or muscular hyperactivity.

Treatments for perioral rejuvenation are not exclusively injection techniques, as chemical peels and energy-based devices are other successful treatments for perioral rejuvenation, particularly for skin aging changes.

The injection techniques for perioral rejuvenation include:

1. Skin rejuvenation injections

2. Botulinum toxin injections

3. Filler injections

Non-invasive esthetic procedures for rejuvenation of the perioral region have advanced significantly, offering satisfactory outcomes in a minimally invasive and uncomplicated way. The three mentioned treatments are often used in combination, and their success in combination has been published [13, 14].

Skin rejuvenation injections, often referred to as esthetic or anti-aging mesotherapy injections, involve the use of dermal injection techniques of revitalizing, nourishing and hydrating solutions to improve skin quality, firmness and superficial wrinkles [13–16].

Botulinum toxin injections are used to reduce hyperactive mimetic muscles that lead to wrinkles of expression or depression of facial features, such as the depressor anguli oris muscle depressing the mouth commissure.

Subdermal filler injections are used to address wrinkles and fold with medium-density products or volume restoration using high-density products for injection.

4.1 Skin rejuvenation injections in the perioral region

The purpose of skin rejuvenation techniques is to reverse cutaneous aging signs including wrinkles. Ablative and exfoliative treatments are commonly used for skin rejuvenation, such as peelings, lasers and microdermabrasion. In contrast to exfoliation or ablation, revitalizing or rejuvenation injections focus on replenishment and nourishment to improve skin aging signs. This concept, unique to the technique of skin rejuvenation mesotherapy or revitalization, focuses on the replacement and nourishment of the vital components of the skin with mostly poly-vitamin solutions and especially non-cross-linked hyaluronic acid [17].

The injectable products used for skin rejuvenation should be sterile, registered for injection within the dermis and suitable for intradermal injections. The ideal product to use should contain ingredients that will replenish the extracellular matrix, reduce oxidation, nourish the fibroblasts and stimulate neocollagenesis. Polycomponent preparations for mesotherapy or intradermal injections are developed to supply the necessary substrates to aging skin that are needed for optimal functioning of the fibroblast [14, 15]. This will typically include free hyaluronic acid, vitamins, minerals, antioxidants, coenzymes and new types of ingredients with scientific evidence of fibroblast stimulation or collagen-boosting properties [14–17]. There are many new products entering the market for improving skin quality including innovative substances such as peptides, enzymes and exosomes.

Various injection techniques have been recommended, used, or studied to deliver these substances to the dermal fibroblasts and the surrounding extracellular matrix.

Different techniques for delivering skin-replenishing or revitalizing substances include:

- Classic mesotherapy injection techniques—epidermal, dermo-epidermal and dermal techniques
- Intradermal injections with a needle (such as 32G × 4 mm needles)
- Intradermal injections with needle devices (such as Nanosoft™)
- Skin needling rollers (dermal rollers)
- Electronic skin needling devices (Demapen®, Mesopen®)
- No-needle injection devices (**Figure 3**).

To achieve successful results without complications, there are some important rules to follow, which include but are not limited to the following:

- Use a good quality product with scientific evidence of efficacy.
- Use good-quality injection needles or devices.
- Good skills in injection techniques.
- Thorough cleansing and disinfection before injections.
- Do not mix solutions.
- Use only new, unopened vials for injections.
- Check the expiry date of products.
- Be careful of topical anesthesia that may cause skin reactions.

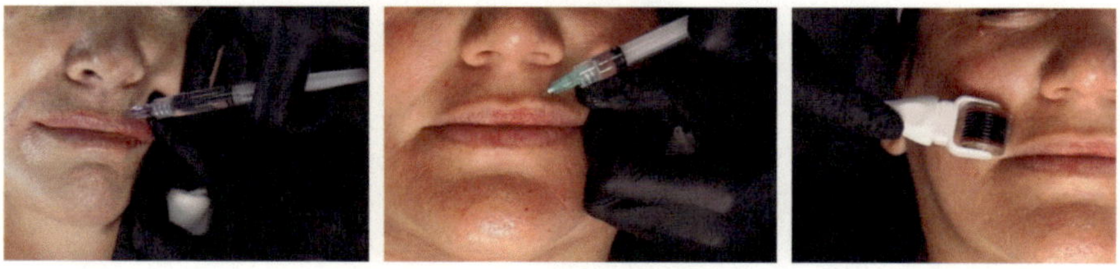

Figure 3.
Skin rejuvenation techniques. This method of replenishment of the skin and reverse aging signs are often combined with either fillers, botulinum toxin or both [13, 17]. Image by Dr. Smit with permission from patients.

- There are many reports in literature of contact dermatitis to topical anesthesia [18]. These reactions may be further aggravated with multiple needle punctures to the skin barrier as performed by these techniques.

4.2 Botulinum toxin injections in the perioral region

Botulinum toxin injections have been used for various esthetic indications, particularly for the upper face, but also for the middle and lower face and the neck [19].

Several consensus recommendations for the use of botulinum toxin in the lower face have been developed despite this region being off-label indications.

The use of botulinum toxin in the perioral region includes:

- Treatment of perioral wrinkles with small doses in the superficial orbicularis oris muscle.

- Reduction of gummy smile (excessive gingival exposure on smiling) by reducing the activity of the relevant lip elevators.

- Reducing the activity of the depressor anguli oris muscle will give an elevation of the mouth corner.

- Reducing the chin dimpling effect and melomental crease with the relaxation of the mentalis muscle.

The use of botulinum toxin injections in the perioral region requires an in-depth knowledge of the location of the muscles, their depths, their relation to surrounding muscles and their vectors of movement (**Figure 4**).

When treating perioral wrinkles with botulinum toxin injection, the depth of injection should be superficial and close to the vermillion border of the lip [19–21].

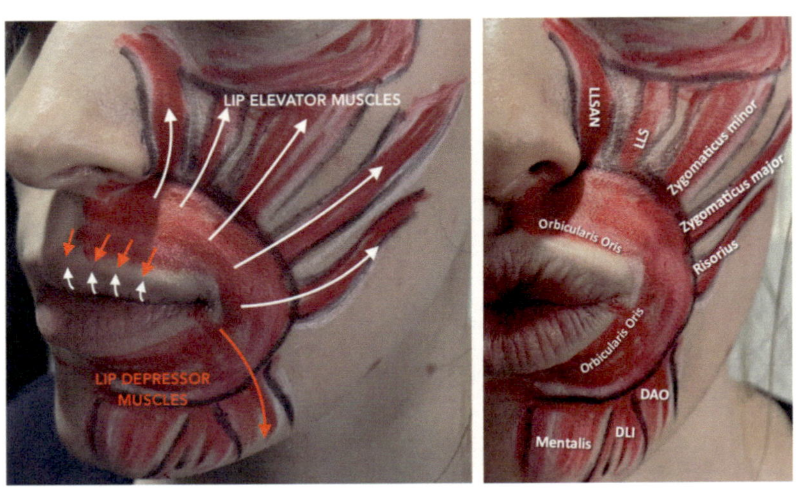

Figure 4.
Perioral muscles. DAO: depressor anguli oris muscle; DLI: depressor labii inferioris muscle; LLSAN: levator labii superioris alaeque nasi muscle; LLS: levator labii superioris muscle. Image and illustration by Dr. Smit with permission from patient.

This will ensure that the deep fibers of the orbicularis oris muscle are not injected, ensuring effective reduction of the perioral wrinkles and mild eversion of the upper lip (**Figures** 5 and **6**).

4.3 Filler injections in the perioral region

The use of fillers for lip rejuvenation and lip enhancement remains a very popular esthetic medical procedure [21]. The most widely used filler material remains hyaluronic acid fillers due to their natural properties, numerous scientific studies and safety aspects, especially since they can be reversed with the enzyme hyaluronidase. Hyaluronic acid fillers are widely used in esthetic medicine for facial rejuvenation and volume enhancement in different body regions and their popular use includes the lips [21, 22].

A frequently misunderstood aspect of beauty is the notion that beautiful lips are synonymous with full lips. While full lips are commonly associated with attractiveness compared to thinner lips, the reality is more complex. Attractive lips encompass more than just their fullness, encompassing factors beyond the absence of perioral wrinkles and the presence of a well-defined Cupid's bow [23].

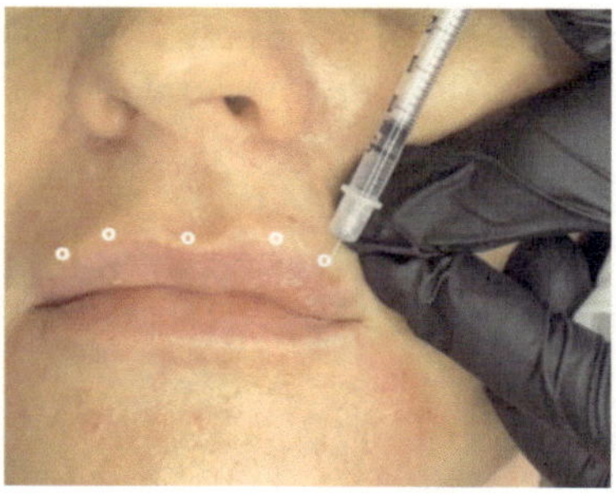

Figure 5.
Perioral wrinkle treatment with botulinum toxin. The recommended dosage for this indication is 2 Units of Abobotulinum toxin A or 1 unit of Onabotulinum toxin A per point of injection superficially [19, 20]. Image by Dr. Smit with permission from patient.

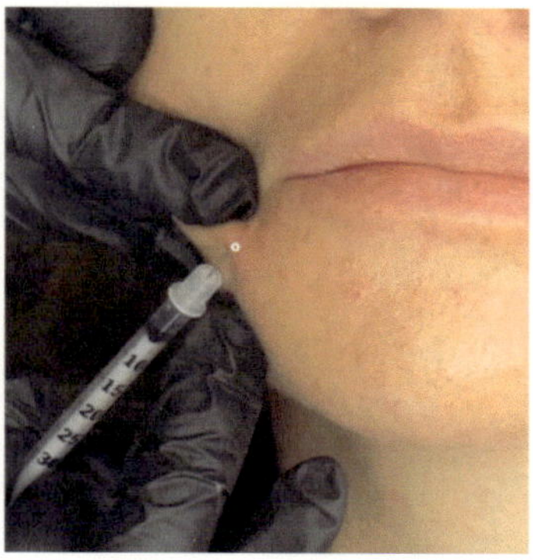

Figure 6.
Mouth corner lifting treatment with botulinum toxin. The recommended dosage for this indication is 4–6 units of abobotulinum toxin A or 2–4 units of onabotulinum toxin A per point of injection very superficially to avoid spread to the depressor labii inferioris muscle. The location of injection of the depressor anguli oris can also be determined by drawing a line from the mouth corner 1 cm lateral and then 1 cm inferior [19, 20]. Image by Dr. Smit with permission from patient.

In many cases of perioral rejuvenation, augmenting fullness can certainly address and improve specific concerns in the perioral area. However, it may not constitute a comprehensive or suitable treatment strategy for the patient's unique indications or concerns. Unfortunately, a common issue that arises is not just an excess of fullness but, more frequently, the improper placement of that fullness within the patient's lips.

The most important step in achieving successful results with lip enhancement is a good proportional evaluation of the lips and the perioral region from a frontal and lateral view, as discussed earlier. The lips themselves also need to be evaluated according to their subunits as known by artists and originating from the embryological development of the lips (**Figure 7**).

These lip subunits need to be evaluated according to loss of volume or excess volume and this will help guide the treatment plan for lip enhancement.

Further to this, the perioral region needs to be evaluated. Only enhancing the lips and leaving perioral concerns untreated will not result in a satisfactory result (**Figure 8**).

Perioral lines or wrinkles may reduce the attractiveness of the lips. This may include perioral (barcode or smoker's lines) (A), nasolabial folds (B) or marionette folds (C) or even an unaesthetic chin profile.

Following the evaluation of the lip subunits and the perioral region, the treatment can be planned according to the aims of treatments for the lips, which may be volumization, contouring, restoration or purely perioral rejuvenation (**Figure 9**).

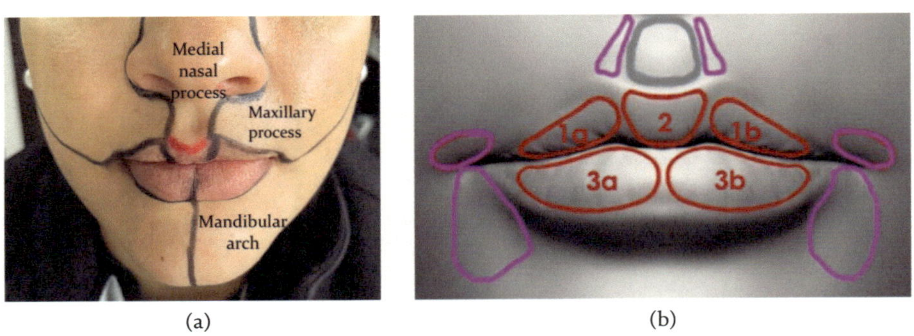

Figure 7.
Lip subunits. a: the lip subunits, according to embryological development. The lip subunits can be evaluated according to the following subunits: superolateral subunits (1a and 1b), the superomedial subunit (2) and the inferolateral subunits (3a and 3b) [23]. Images and illustrations done by Dr. Smit and with permission from patient.

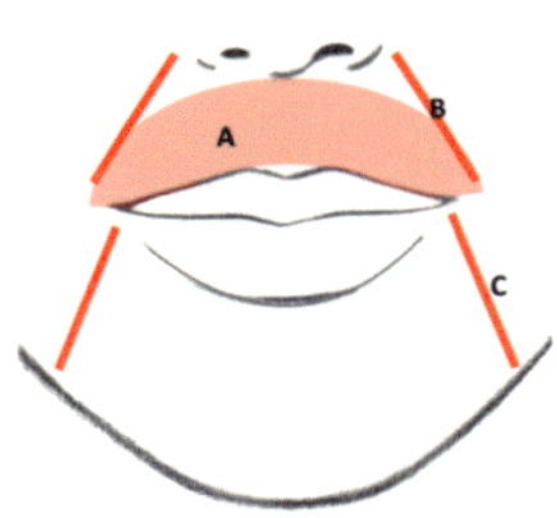

Figure 8.
The evaluation of the perioral region when planning lip enhancement. Illustration by Dr. Smit with permission.

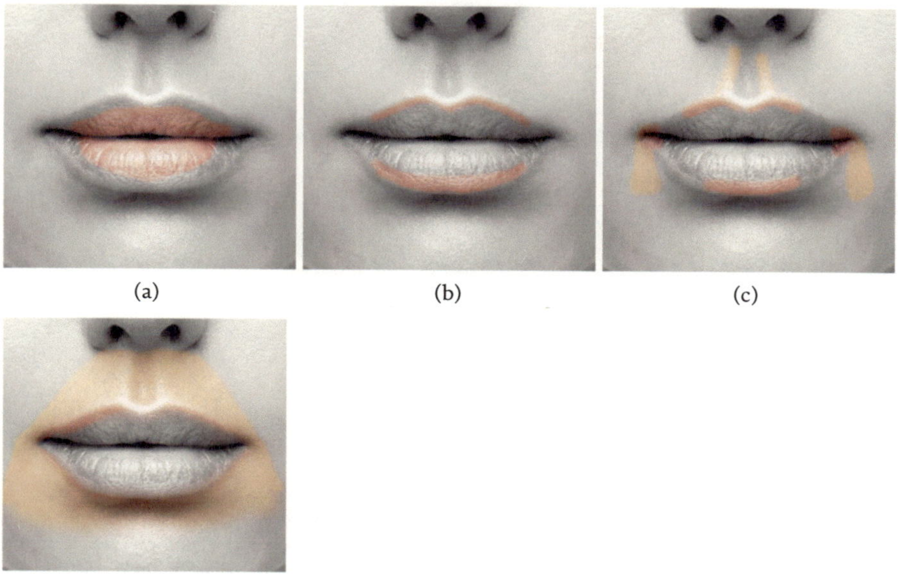

(a) (b) (c) (d)

Figure 9.
Different aims of treatments with lip filler injection techniques. a: lip volumization; b: lip contouring; c: perioral restoration; d: perioral rejuvenation. Illustrations by Dr. Smit with permission.

Techniques of injection of fillers will depend on the product rheology and the aim of treatments. The lip region remains a highly vascularized and highly dangerous zone for the risk of intravascular injection. The vascular supply of the lips derives from the superior and inferior labial arteries branching from the facial artery [21]. Safe and successful procedures in the perioral region depend on a thorough, comprehensive knowledge of facial anatomy, in particular vascular anatomy. Insufficient familiarity with this aspect can result in significant complications [25].

The use of cannula of 25G or thicker (22 or 23G) reduces the risk of intravascular injection but does not completely eliminate the risk. When using needles, smaller needles and the use of smaller amounts per injection with continuous monitoring of capillary refill are recommended to reduce the risk for intravascular complications [21–25]. Other complications with fillers in the perioral region could arise due to lack of sterility, incorrect choice of product for the depth, existing localized infection, recent viral infections and other side effects, which are often classified into technique-related or product-related adverse events. All professionals performing these procedures should be familiar with the risks of adverse events, how to avoid or reduce the risks, as well as knowledge of managing such events.

Further to injection techniques, one needs to understand the rheology of the hyaluronic acid (HA) fillers to ensure that the correct product is used for the specific indication. The various factors influencing the viscosity and elasticity such as the length of HA chains, the amount of cross-linking, the molecular weight, G-prime and other factors should be taken into consideration when choosing the product for the indication, the depth of injection and the region of injection (**Figures 10–12**) [24].

When treating the perioral region, it may also be necessary to balance the profile of the nose, lip and chin region. The evaluation of the frontal and lateral profile measurements is vital to ensure the profile remains balanced and esthetically pleasing (**Figure 13**).

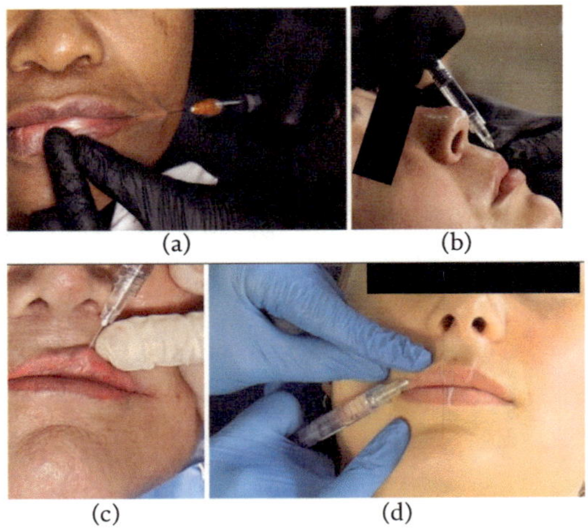

Figure 10.
Techniques of injections for lip enhancement. a: using a blunt cannula remaining in the superficial plane of the lips; b: superficial retro-tracing technique with a needle for eversion of the upper lip; c: superficial retro-tracing technique with a needle for eversion of the upper lip; d: superficial needle technique for contouring the lip vermillion border. Images by Dr. Smit with permission from patients.

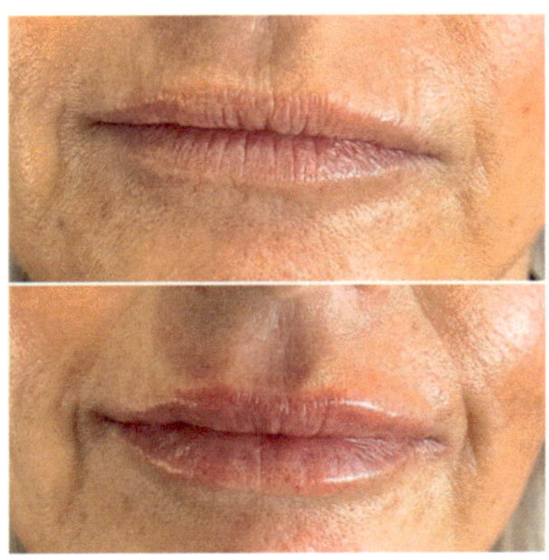

Figure 11.
Results before and after with hyaluronic acid fillers for lip enhancement. 1 ml of a medium cross-linked HA filler was used.

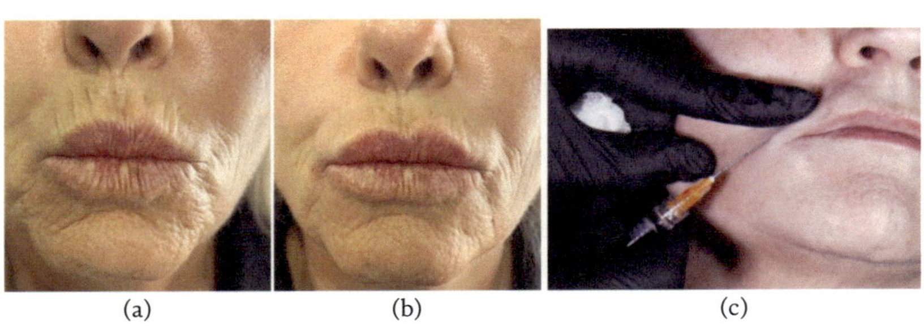

Figure 12.
Results of injection of the perioral region with a low cross-linked HA filler using a cannula in a fanning pattern on the upper and lower white lip perioral region. a: before treatment; b: after treatment; c: technique of injection with a cannula in the perioral region. Images by Dr. Smit with permission from patients.

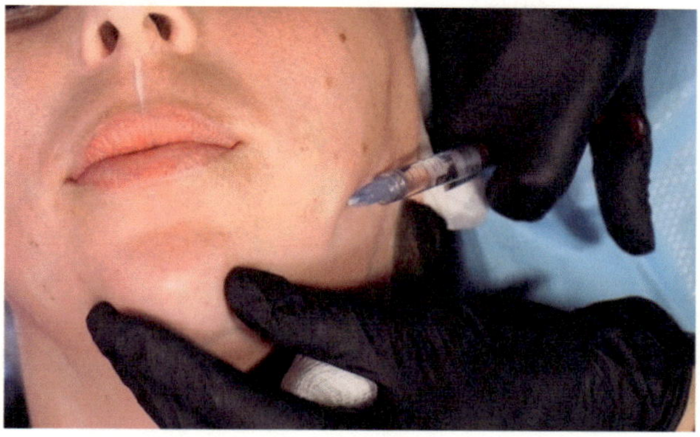

Figure 13.
Balancing of the perioral region with fillers. Image by Dr. Smit with permission from patient.

5. Conclusion

Injection techniques for perioral enhancement remain an important tool to enhance patient self-esteem and satisfaction with their appearance [2].

There are various tools available for rejuvenating and restoring perioral concerns and there are numerous developments in this field of medicine to ensure higher satisfaction and safety. The treatment options for the perioral region does not only include injectable treatments with botulinum toxin A, dermal fillers and skin revitalizers; but also, energy-based devices for skin rejuvenation and tightening [2, 21].

The duty of the practitioner is to remain updated on the knowledge of the existing and new products that can be used, the techniques of use, the anatomical knowledge, safety precautions and management of adverse events with techniques in the perioral region [24].

Artistic insight and an understanding of profilometry, facial measurements and the differences between races and genders are other important factors that ensure success with perioral procedures.

The perioral region requires insight from an injector into the holistic facial proportions in relation to the lips, as well as the understanding of the lip subunits and how these should be respected to maintain natural proportions during enhancement procedures [23]. Respecting these natural proportions while also considering the inter-ethnic and gender variations will ensure natural results that will enhance the attractiveness of the patient. Furthermore, it remains vital to understand the different types of techniques of injection for specific indications combined with the knowledge of the specific rheology of fillers needed for the indication, especially when treating the lips.

It is also important that only qualified and experienced professionals perform such procedures to minimize the risk of complications.

Lastly, the importance of combination treatments should be understood for success with perioral rejuvenation, especially with progressing age. The multifactorial aging of the perioral region occurs in various layers from bone to skin [2]. Therefore, the need of a multilayered and combination approach will be necessary to ensure patient satisfaction. Practitioners treating the perioral region should thus have knowledge and be skilled to use these different methods to treat the perioral region.

Conflict of interest

The author declares no conflict of interest.

Author details

Riekie Smit
Dr. Riekie Smit Practice, Pretoria, South Africa

*Address all correspondence to: riekiesmit@icloud.com

References

[1] Tonnard PL, Verpaele AM, Ramaut LE, Blondeel PN. Aging of the upper lip. Plastic and Reconstructive Surgery. 2019;**143**:1333-1342

[2] Wollina U. Perioral rejuvenation: Restoration of attractiveness in aging females by minimally invasive procedures. Clinical Interventions in Aging. 2013;**8**:1149-1155

[3] Gubanova E, Gubanova Y. Functional condition of the lip skin: Effect of the age and hormone replacementtherapy. Vestnik dermatologii i venerologii. 2010;**86**:94-99. DOI: 10.25208/vdv874

[4] Nicksic PJ, Karczewski AM, Zhao Q, Garcia NA, Michelotti BF, Mahajan AY, et al. The contribution of the lower third of the face to perceived age: Do masks make you appear younger? Aesthetic Surgery Journal Open Forum. 2021;**3**(3):ojab017. DOI: 10.1093/asjof/ojab017

[5] Beer K, Beer J. Overview of facial aging. Facial Plastic Surgery. 2009;**25**(5):281-284

[6] Forte AJ, Andrew TW, Colasante C, Persing JA. Perception of age, attractiveness, and tiredness after isolated and combined facial subunit aging. Aesthetic Plastic Surgery. 2015;**39**:856-869

[7] Perkins S, Sandel H. Anatomic considerations, analysis, and the aging process of the perioral region. Facial Plastic Surgery Clinics of North America. 2007;**15**:403, 7. DOI: 10.1016/j.fsc.2007.08.006

[8] Prendergast P. Facial Proportions. 2012. DOI: 10.1007/978-3-642-17838-2_2

[9] Fang F, Clapham PJ, Chung KC. A systematic review of inter-ethnic variability in facial dimensions. Plastic and Reconstructive Surgery. 2011;**127**(2):874-881

[10] Popenko NA, Tripathi PB, Devcic Z, Karimi K, Osann K, Wong BJF. A quantitative approach to determining the ideal female lip aesthetic and its effect on facial attractiveness. JAMA Facial Plastic Surgery. 2017;**19**(4):261-267. DOI: 10.1001/jamafacial.2016.2049

[11] Pradhan R, Rajbhandari A, Bajracharya M, Manandhar P, Maharjan S. Lip prominence using different reference planes. Orthodontic Journal of Nepal. 2019;**9**:50-53. DOI: 10.3126/ojn.v9i1.25691

[12] Ricketts RM. Planning treatment on the basis of the facial pattern and an estimate of its growth. The Angle Orthodontist. 1957;**27**:14-37

[13] Braccini F, Dohan Ehrenfest DM. Intérêt des thérapies combinées en médecine esthétique pour le traitement du vieillissement du visage: Toxine botulique, fillers et mésothérapie (advantages of combined therapies in cosmetic medicine for the treatment of face aging: Botulinum toxin, fillers and mesotherapy). Revue de Laryngologie—Otologie—Rhinologie. 2010;**131**(2):89-95

[14] Grand-Vincent A, Boisnic S, Salomon C, Prinderre P, Piccerelle P. Clinical assessment of a mesotherapy formulation for skin rejuvenation in healthy volunteers. Journal of Cosmetics, Dermatological Sciences and Applications. 2017;**7**:291-305

[15] Robin S, Fanian F, Courderot-Masuyer C, Tordjman M, Braccini F, Boisnic S, et al. Efficacy of a biorevitalizing-filler solution on all skin

aspects: 10 years approach through in vitro studies and clinical trials. Journal of Cosmetics, Dermatological Sciences and Applications. 2021;**11**:18-37

[16] Prikhnenko S. Polycomponent mesotherapy formulations for the treatment of skin aging and improvement of skin quality. Clinical, Cosmetic and Investigational Dermatology. 2015;**8**:151-157. DOI: 10.2147/CCID.S76721

[17] Smit R. Bio-skin-gineering: A novel method to focus cutaneous aging treatment on each individual layer of the skin specifically and precisely. Aesthetic Medicine. 2019;**5**:1

[18] Cox B, Durieux ME, Marcus MA. Toxicity of local anaesthetics. Best Practice and Research. Clinical Anaesthesiology. 2003;**17**:111-136

[19] Galadari H, Galadari I, Smit R, Prygova I, Redaelli A. Use of abobotulinumtoxin A for cosmetic treatments in the neck, and middle and lower areas of the face: A systematic review. Toxins. 2021;**13**:169

[20] Hong SO. Cosmetic treatment using botulinum toxin in the oral and maxillofacial area: A narrative review of esthetic techniques. Toxins. 2023;**15**:82. DOI: 10.3390/toxins15020082

[21] Wollina U, Goldman A. Lip enhancement and mouth corner lift with fillers and botulinum toxin A. Dermatologic Therapy. 2020;**33**:e14231

[22] Zanella R, Padoin A, Valente D. Lips enhancement using hyaluronic acid. Journal of Investigative Cosmetology. 2023;**37**:44. DOI: 10.15406/jdc.2023.07.00232

[23] Smit R. Improving Lip Enhancement. Apr 2020;**10**(2). Available from: https://www.prime-journal.com/improving-lip-enhancement/

[24] Wick E, Ostby E, Grunebaum L. Lip rejuvenation and filler complications in the perioral region. Plastic and Aesthetic Research. 2022;**9**:1-7. DOI: 10.20517/2347-9264.2021.58

[25] Florin L, Catalina-Petruta I, Mihaly E, Cosmin P, Florin-Mihail F, Ioan B, et al. The assessment of the anatomical risk in the perioral region. MAEDICA—A Journal of Clinical Medicine. 2022;**17**:820-825. DOI: 10.26574/maedica.2022.17.4.820

Section 2

Breast and Body Cosmetic Surgery

Chapter 7

Simultaneous Breast Augmentation with Mastopexy

Chase Nelson, Angelo Cuzalina and Sebastian Gutierrez De Pineres

Abstract

Breast lift and augmentation are often desired by the female patient to address ptotic breasts. Historically, this was performed with a staged mastopexy followed by augmentation at a later date. More recently, the two procedures have been found to be safely and effectively performed as a single stage procedure. This affords the patient a more cost effective (only one operation and one anesthesia fee) and timely strategy for reaching their esthetic goals. Furthermore, prior literature describes fairly stringent restrictions on implant size. We present our technique of using a superomedial-central pedicle with total submuscular implant placement to achieve appropriate breast position with preserved nipple-areola-complex vascularization whilst having the freedom to place a proportionately sized implant, even relatively large implants if so desired by the patient. The described technique has proven to have extremely durable results leaving the patient with a youthful appearing breast with a propensity to withstand future ptosis and/or waterfall deformity.

Keywords: breast augmentation, mastopexy, breast lift, breast augmentation with mastopexy, wise pattern, total submuscular breast augmentation, superomeidal central pedicle

1. Introduction

Deflated, ptotic breasts are commonplace complaints in cosmetic surgery practice. Loss of breast fullness and descent of the nipple-areola-complex (NAC) below the inframammary fold (IMF) can occur as a result of pregnancy, lactation, weight loss, and congenital deformity. The desired outcome of affected patients is generally "larger, perkier" breasts. Simultaneous breast augmentation and mastopexy offers a single stage solution. This procedure is among the most challenging cosmetic surgical procedures as the surgeon strives for symmetric manipulation of the breast skin envelope, parenchyma, NAC, IMF, and chest wall anatomy whilst maintaining adequate vascularization. While it is a challenging procedure to perform, it is extremely rewarding for both patient and surgeon when performed in an expert manner. Complications, revisions, and litigation are higher than many other cosmetic surgeries. This Chapter is aimed at providing detailed clarity on the anatomy, clinical evaluation and decision making process, surgical marking,

 IntechOpen

surgical technique, and potential complications of simultaneous breast augmentation and mastopexy with the goal of helping surgeons appropriately plan and execute this enjoyable procedure.

2. Anatomy of the breast

2.1 Surface anatomy

The female breast assumes a conical form with rounding at the inferior pole. The gland extends from the 2nd to the 6th rib along the midclavicular line in the vertical plane and from the sternocostal junction across to the midaxillary line in the horizontal plane [1]. Superolaterally, the mammary gland extends toward the axilla to form the tail of Spence [2]. The breast overlies the pectoralis major, external oblique, serratus anterior and upper rectus muscles (**Figure 1**) [1, 2].

2.2 Nipple-areola complex

The NAC is composed of stratified squamous epithelium. The lactiferous ducts converge and open into mammary pits that elevate and form the nipple. Failed formation of this lactiferous duct convergence and elevation results in an inverted nipple which affects 2–4% of females [2]. The NAC measures 2–4 cm in diameter and is ideally located in the center of the breast mound [2]. Ideally the NAC should be approximately 1/3rd of the overall breast diameter and the nipple itself should be 1/3rd of the areolar diameter [2, 4]. The NAC is ideally positioned slightly above the IMF [5]. A 21 cm sternal notch-to-nipple distance is often considered ideal with a nipple-to-IMF distance of 7–10 cm (**Figure 2**) [2, 7]. However, these distances do vary based on certain factors discussed in the "preoperative marking" section of this chapter.

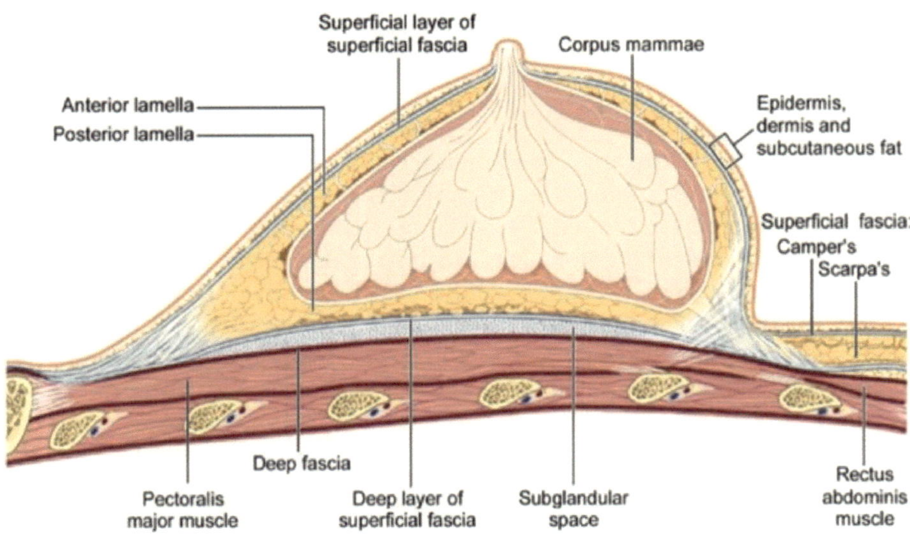

Figure 1.
Surface anatomy of the breast including underlying pectoralis major and rectus upper rectus abdominis muscle [3].

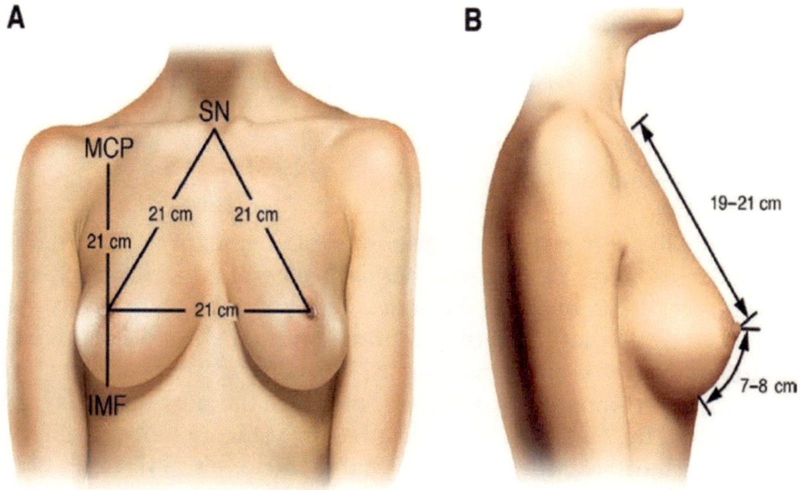

Figure 2.
A. MCP - midclavicular point, IMF - inframammary fold, SN - sternal notch. Ideally, the sternal notch-to-nipple distance and nipple-to-nipple distance are ideally equidistant. B. The superior measurement shows the ideal sternal notch-to-nipple distance of 19–21 cm and a nipple-to-IMF distance of 7–8 cm [6].

2.3 Glandular anatomy

The glandular tissue is composed of 15–25 lobes, the functional unit of the breast, which extend toward the NAC as lactiferous ducts and open at the nipple (**Figure 3**). The breast gland has no discrete fascia, instead it has fibrous Cooper's ligaments that provide scaffolding support to the glandular breast. Additionally, the inframammary crease ligament contributes to a well defined inframammary crease and extends from the medial aspect of the 5th rib and laterally to the fascia of the 5th and 6th ribs [4]. The inframammary crease ligament that gives rise to the inframammary fold and acts a sling for the breast parenchyma. During augmentation mammaplasty, the release of the pectoralis muscle with preservation of the ligament to the bony framework

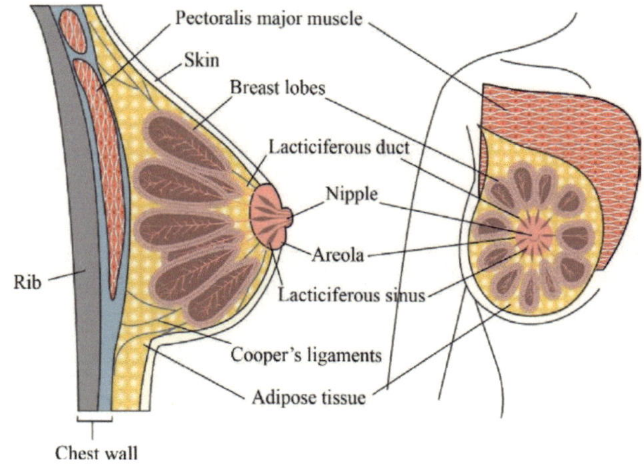

Figure 3.
Schematic view of the breast parenchyma anatomy [8].

will minimize risk of bottoming out [9]. Weight fluctuation, pregnancy and aging can attenuate Cooper's ligaments and lead to varying degrees of mammary ptosis (**Figure 4**, **Table 1**) which is based on the nipple position in relation to the inframammary fold [2, 4].

2.4 Neurovascular supply

Arterial supply to the breast is from perforating branches of the internal thoracic artery (internal mammary artery), branches of the lateral thoracic artery, and direct branches from the 2nd-5th intercostal arteries. The internal mammary artery is the primary blood supply to the NAC with perforators from the 2nd-5th intercostal spaces immediately lateral to the parasternal border (**Figure 5**).

Venous outflow is through an anastomotic plexus in the subcutaneous tissue beneath and around the NAC that drain peripherally via large subcutaneous veins that empty into the intercostal, axillary, and internal thoracic veins [4]. The most important and reliable venous routes are located in the superomedial and inferior pedicles and congestion of these routes can be a primary cause of NAC ischemia and necrosis in mastopexy procedures [4, 11].

Nerve supply of the NAC includes the 3rd- 5th anterior/medial intercostal cutaneous branches, and most prominently the lateral cutaneous branch of the 4th intercostal nerve and its deep branch which tends to run along the fascia of the pectoralis major before emerging to innervate the nipple from its posterior surface (**Figures 6** and 7) [4]. Additionally, the cervical plexus contributes to sensory innervation of the superior aspect of the breast [12].

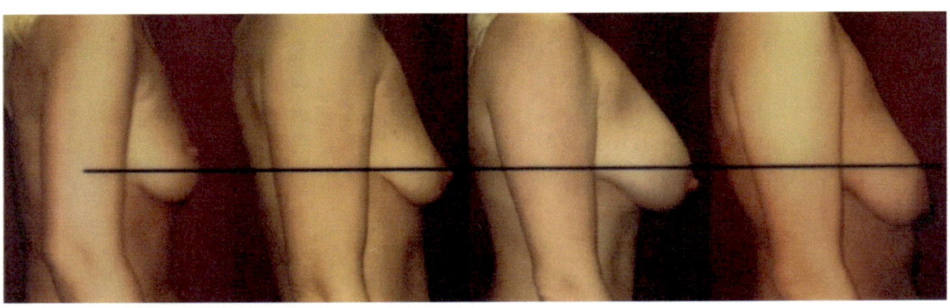

Figure 4.
Ptosis grading. Dark like indicates the IMF which is used as the reference point for ptosis grade.

Regnault's classification of ptosis	
Minor ptosis (1st degree)	Nipple at the IMF or 1 cm inferior to IMF
Moderate ptosis (2nd degree)	Nipple inferior to IMF & superior to lower breast contour
Severe ptosis (3rd degree)	Nipple inferior to IMF & at lower breast contour
Glandular ptosis	Nipple superior to IMF & breast tissue inferior to the breast fold
Pseudoptosis	Nipple superior to IMF; breast is hypoplastic & inferior to the breast fold

Table 1.
Ptosis as described by regnault.

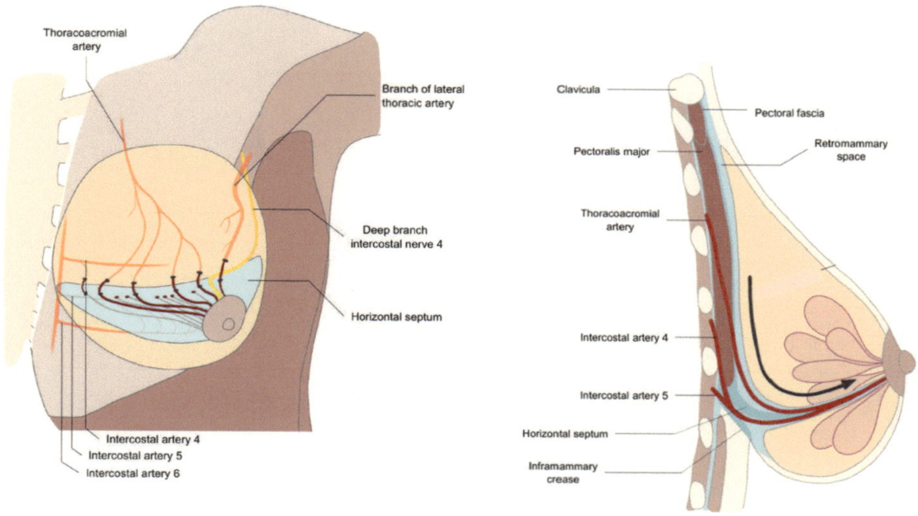

Figure 5.
Left: Anterior view schematic of the breast's arterial supply. Right: Lateral view schematic of the breast's arterial supply [10].

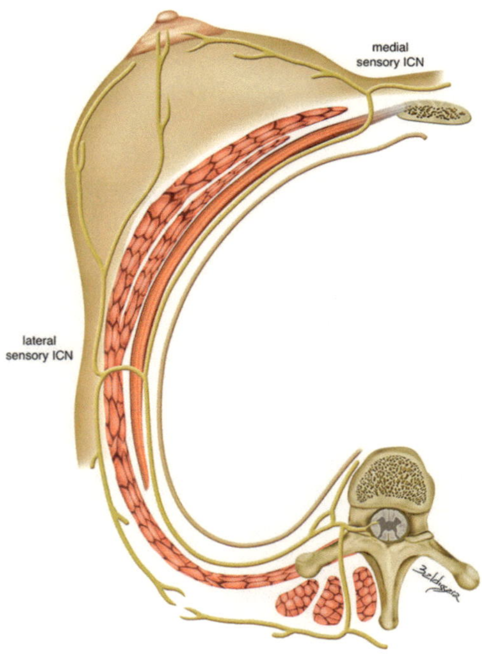

Figure 6.
Axial view schematic showing the cutaneous nerve supply of the breast [12].

2.5 Lymphatics

The primary lymphatic drainage of the breast flows into the axilla through the external mammary nodal group, however, additional drainage occurs through the medial, transpectoral and postpectoral routes as well [4].

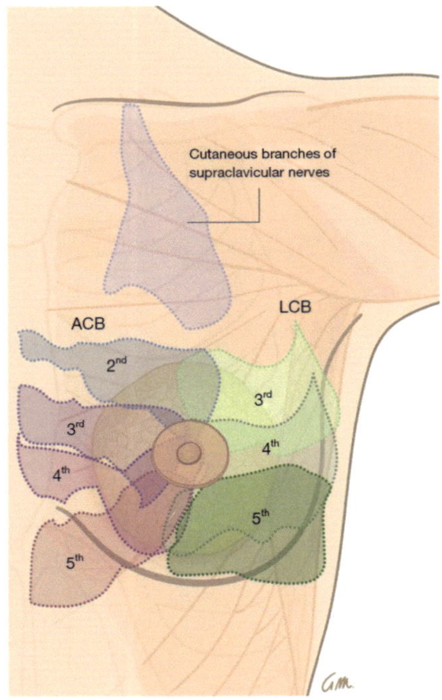

Figure 7.
Schematic representation of the nerve supply of the anterior chest wall, indicating the individual contributions of the 2nd–5th anterior, and 3rd–5th lateral cutaneous branches of the intercostal nerves. ACB, anterior cutaneous branch; LCB, lateral cutaneous branch [13].

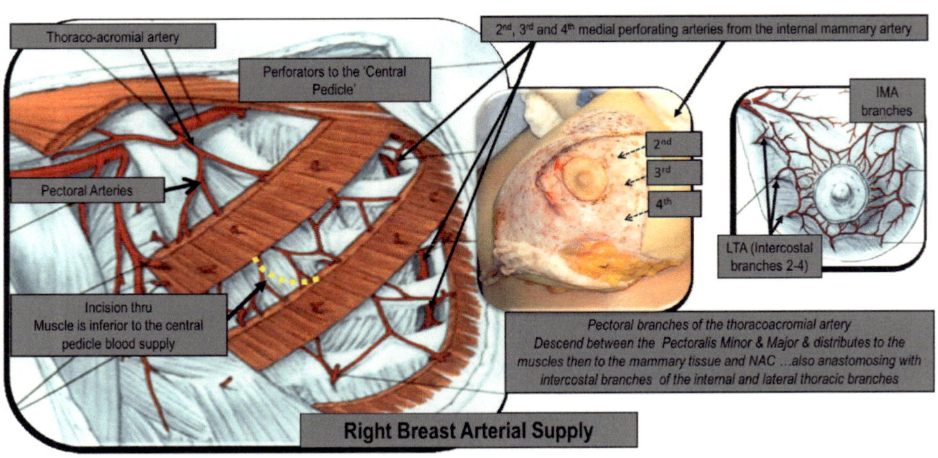

Figure 8.
The figure demonstrates the two major sources of blood supply to the superomedial-central (SMC) pedicle. The medial source from branches of the internal mammary artery and central component from the pectoral perforators. The 2nd medial perforator supplies the most superomedial area of the SMC pedicle. Maintaining all these sources during dissection produces a robustly vascularized pedicle.

2.6 Chest musculature

The chest wall musculature includes the Pectoralis Major, Pectoralis Minor, Serratus Anterior, External Oblique, Rectus Abdominis, and Intercostal muscles.

When performing total submuscular placement of a breast implant, the implant is below the pectoralis major muscle, preserving the perforating pectoral branch vessels of the pectoral branch of the thoracoacromial artery [4, 9]. Of key importance, the 2nd-4th medial perforating arteries from the internal mammary artery along with pectoral arterial branches from the thoracoacromial artery supply the NAC in the majority of our combined mastopexy with or without augmentation cases; which utilize a superomedial central pedicle (SMC) (**Figure 8**).

3. Clinical evaluation

3.1 Patient interview

A thorough preoperative evaluation permits an understanding of the most appropriate options available to achieve the desired result, and allows the surgeon to obtain medical and social history, perform a physical exam, and partner with the patient to set achievable expectations based on anatomical limitations that may exist. The patient's desired breast size is ascertained. In addition, this is an opportunity to explain the postoperative process, as well as the risks and benefits of alternative options.

When performing clinical evaluation we focus on obtaining a thorough medical history and social history including use of nicotine products, i.e. vaping, chewing tobacco, and cigarettes, as these can impact the healing process. History of breast-feeding and number of pregnancies is discussed in order to appreciate the associated changes in breast volume and position. For patients over the age of 40 or patients who are at high risk of breast cancer, i.e. strong family history, breast masses, +BRCA test should undergo mammography prior to surgery [14].

3.2 Physical exam

Physical examination of the patient begins with inspection of the breasts and evaluating the skin envelope with regard to laxity and quality, breast volume, position

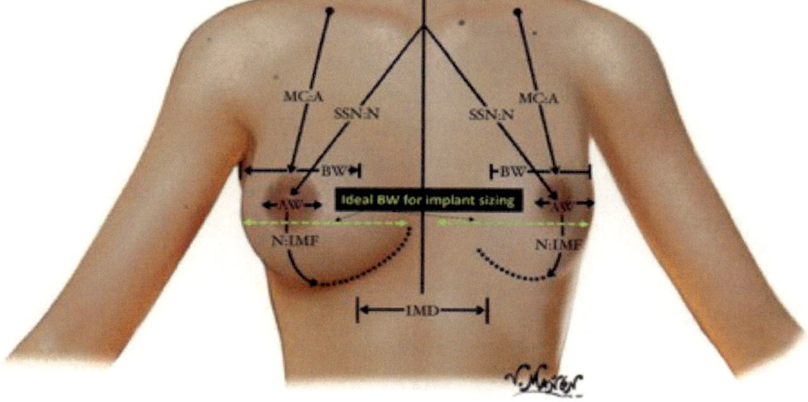

Figure 9.
Schematic showing the markings that are obtained during initial patient evaluation. SSN:N - suprasternal notch-to-nipple distance, N:IMF - nipple-to-IMF distance, BW - base width or breast width, IMD - Inframammary distance, MC:A - midclavicular axis, AW - areola width.

of the NAC, areolar size, asymmetries including deformities of the chest or spine that can contribute to such asymmetries [9]. The degree of ptosis is assessed which is defined as the position of the nipple in relation to the inframammary fold and skin envelope.

Topographical measurements from fixed points on the torso on the breast itself are used to analyze the breast (**Figure 9**) [9].

Sternal Notch-to-Nipple: Determines the location of the NAC complex on the chest wall. The nipple is most often situated 19–25 cm from suprasternal notch [9].

Nipple to IMF: The appropriate distance from the nipple to the IMF is approximately 7 cm [9]. This is critical to establish an esthetic lower fullness and overall breast shape. The upper pole slope is linear or slightly concave, and the lower pole is convex.

Breast Width/Base Width: Typically different from the actual breast width of the native breast tissue, and can be measured as the distance from the Anterior Axillary line to within 1 cm from chest midline. This measurement dictates the appropriate implant width.

Intermammary Distance: Distance from nipple to nipple; usually 21 cm [9].

4. Treatment planning

4.1 Pedicle design

The operative plan depends largely on physical exam and evaluation of topographic measurements of both breasts in conjunction with noting the location of the breast mound and its location on the chest wall. A Sternal Notch-to-Nipple distance >25 cm and/or Nipple-IMF distance >10 CM usually signifies that the patient will require a mastopexy alone or in conjunction with augmentation [2]. Indications for augmentation with simultaneous mastopexy include any patient that requires correction of ptosis and desires increased breast volume [2]. Generally, pedicle design is based on sternal notch to nipple distance (**Table 2**, **Figure 10**). We have found the following measurements (**Table 2**) and their respective pedicle designs to yield reliable vascular supply to the NAC while permitting good areola rotation without significant kinking of the pedicle.

The SMC pedicle provides the most robust blood supply in combined mastopexy augmentation procedures when the the sternal notch-to-nipple distance is </= 30 cm as the majority of the blood supply to this pedicle originates from the Internal mammary artery iva intercostal perforators and a central component with trans-pectoral perforators from the pectoral branch of the thoracoacromial artery. Of note, the central vascularization can only be maintained well when placing implants in a subpectoral plane. Placing implants in the subglandular plane sacrifices the central pedicle (**Figure 11**) [4].

Sternal notch to nipple distance	Pedicle choice
<30 cm	Superomedial Central (SMC)
30–36 cm	Medial Central (MC)
> 36 cm	Inferior pedicle or No pedicle w/ Free nipple grafting

Table 2.
Pedicle design choice based on the sternal notch-to-nipple distance.

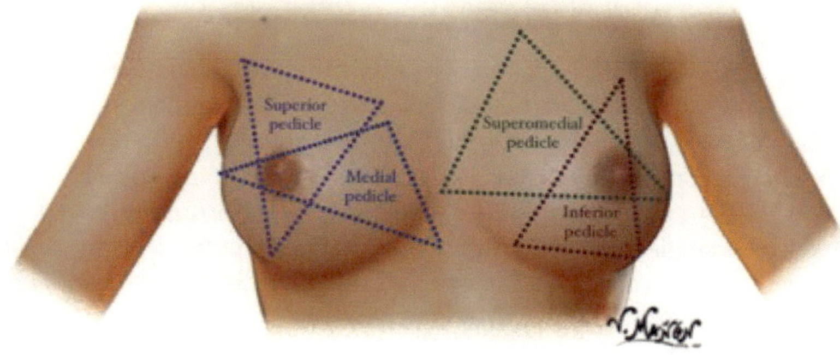

Figure 10.
Schematic showing the different axes associated with different pedicle choices.

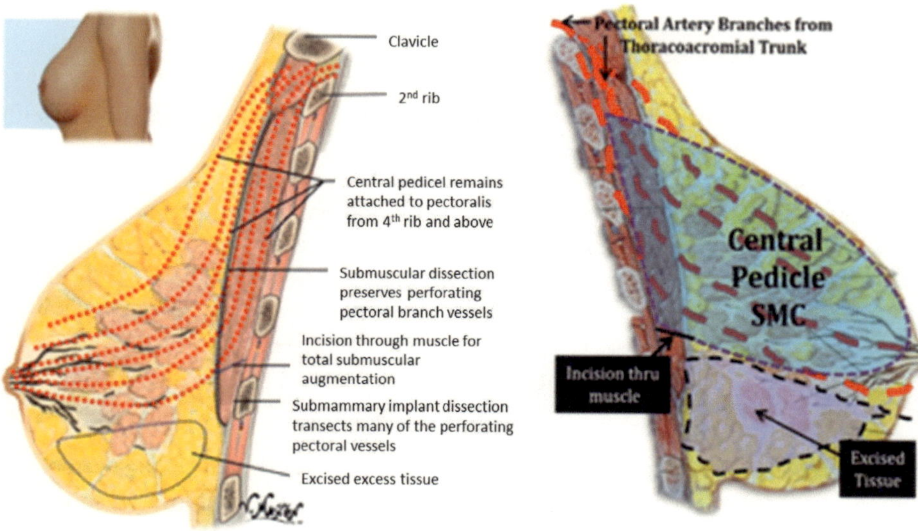

Figure 11.
Schematic lateral view of the breast showing the central component of the SMC and MC pedicles which is only maintained with a subpectoral dissection.

The MC Pedicle provides a good alternative when the sternal notch-to-nipple distance is >30 CM but <36 cm. This option maintains the medial mammary and pectoral perforator arterial branches while allowing a better arc of rotation of the pedicle into its final position without excessive kinking or tension to the pedicle [4].

The Inferior Pedicle is used in very long sternal notch-to-nipple distance whilst also having a comparatively short nipple-IMF distance of <5 cm. Since the inferior pedicle bottoms out more than other pedicles, the vertical limbs should be reduced close to 5 cm compared to the usual 7 cm length of the SMC and MC pedicles that exhibit very limited stretching [4].

A free nipple graft, obviating the use of a pedicle, is considered for a sternal-notch-to-nipple distance of >36 cm, in a breast that has had previous surgeries to have likely violated the blood supply relied upon in a SMC or MC pedicle, or in any other situation in which vascular supply is deemed compromised.

4.2 Implant size

Determining appropriate implant size can prove difficult. The patient's desired breast size must be balanced with what can be safely accommodated. Implant size will be limited to a degree based on the patient's anatomy, tissue quality, and breast skin laxity. Undoubtedly, the appropriate implant size that is used in simultaneous mastopexy with augmentation varies among surgeons. The plastic surgery literature suggests that most implants used in this single stage procedure are less than 400 cubic centimeters [15–17]. However, in select patient's larger implants can and have been safely placed. An acceptable upper limit of implant size has not been defined as breast characteristics will dictate what size can be safely accommodated. Intraoperative sizers, as discussed below, are informative as to the tension that will be placed on the breast for a given implant size. Caution must be exercised regarding implant size as to avoid overaggressive sizing resulting in excess breast tension, compromised blood supply, and wound breakdown. Conservative implant sizing is the rule in order to minimize complications.

4.3 Preoperative markings

There are few if any cosmetic surgical markings that are as nuanced and difficult to correctly perform as the mastopexy. The Wise pattern mastopexy is the most widely used method to address moderate to severe breast ptosis and is appropriate for a nipple to IMF distance >10 cm. A vertical or "lollipop" lift is appropriate in most cases in which the nipple-IMF distance is <10 cm, minimal lifting is needed, and a large amount of breast tissue excision is not indicated or desired. There are markings common to all mastopexy procedures as they are used for reference regardless of the incision pattern chosen.

4.4 Reference markings

The patient is in the standing position with arms relaxed at the sides. The midline sternal notch is marked. A vertical line extending from the sternal notch is drawn down the midline of the sternum between the breasts. The mid clavicular line is marked. The breast meridian is marked by extending a straight line from the mid clavicular point down the breast through the NAC and down through the inframammary fold. The inframammary fold position is transposed and marked on the anterior surface of the breast (**Figure 12**). The medial aspect of the planned breast implant pocket is marked at 1 cm lateral to the midline. This marking is carried superiorly and laterally with a gentle arc to define the superomedial limits of the breast implant position. NAC position is then determined. Several factors are considered in marking its position. (1) The NAC should sit at or slightly above the inframammary fold. (2) Appropriate nipple position has been described as being level with the midpoint of the humerus (3) sternal notch to nipple distances usually ranges from 19 to 21 cm, (4) finally the planned NAC position is looked at subjectively to ensure it lies in an esthetic position. Based on these factors, the top of the new areola position is marked. Once the new areola position is determined, the reference markings are concluded and incision marking takes place.

4.5 Wise pattern mastopexy

A template is then used to make the "Wise pattern" incision markings. First the incision for the new areola position is marked in semicircular fashion. Vertical

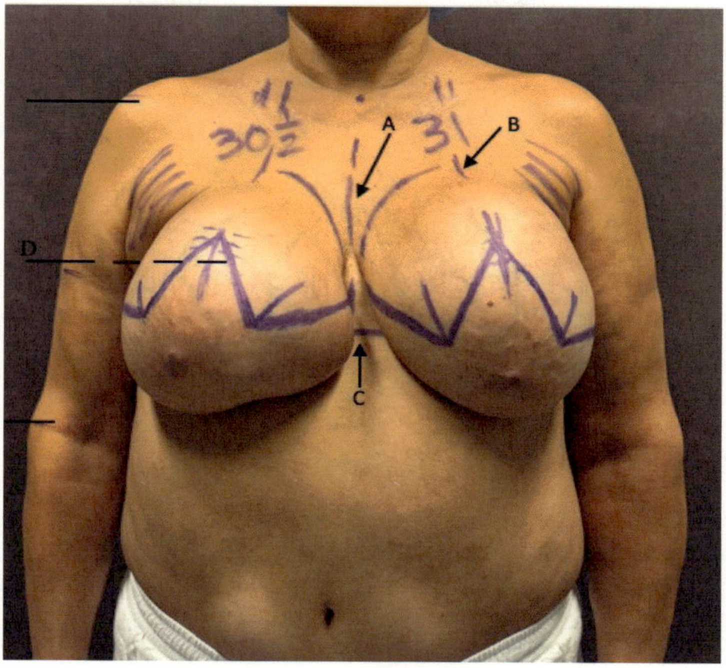

Figure 12.
(A) vertical line extending from the sternal notch is drawn down the midline of the sternum between the breasts. (B) The breast meridian is marked by extending a straight line from the mid clavicular point down the breast through the NAC and down through the inframammary fold. (C) The inframammary fold position is transposed and marked. (D) The NAC should sit at or slightly above the inframammary fold.

limbs are then drawn. The vertical limbs define the new nipple to fold distance and should be 7 cm in length. Great care is taken to ensure both limbs are the same length. A judgment must be made as to what angle the vertical limb incisions diverge from the areola marking. Clearance of the native areola will in part dictate this angle. A more obtuse angle equals more parenchymal excision while a more acute angle will yield less parenchymal excision. Hence, for the wider breast a more obtuse vertical incision is marked and for a more narrow breast, a more acute vertical incision is marked. The IMF incision is then marked approximately 1 cm superior to the actual fold. The length of the IMF incision changes based on the preoperative breast size and extent of lifting required. Larger, more ptotic breasts require a longer fold incision while those that require less lifting but are not candidates for a vertical mastopexy are best addressed with a rather short fold incision. The vertical limb markings are then connected via a horizontal limb to the medial and lateral ends of the IMF incision marking (**Figure 13**). One must keep in mind that with a short IMF incision there will be minimal excision of lateral and medial breast tissue at the breasts inferior pole. In a patient with large breasts, particularly a wide inferior pole, too little medial and lateral breast parenchyma excision at the inferior pole of the breast will result in a wide, boxy, even square shaped breast. Conversely, an IMF incision that is excessively long will not necessarily result in a displeasing inferior pole shape, but produces an unnecessarily long scar. Finally, areas planned for liposuction are made. As with all cosmetic surgery, an eye of esthetic judgment must be maintained whilst following a dogmatic approach to surgical marking.

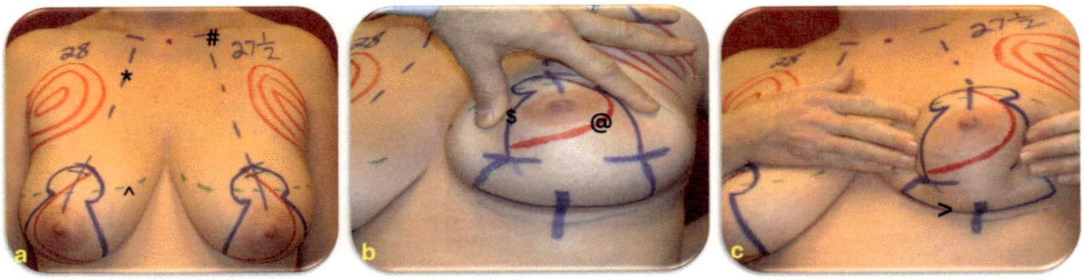

Figure 13.
*Reference markings and incision marking for wise pattern mastopexy. Dashed lines represent reference markings. Solid blue lines are incision markings. Red concentric circles are areas of planned liposuction. a. # midclavicular point, * midclavicular line extending through breast meridian, ^ transposed IMF. b. $ 7 cm medial vertical limb incision, @ SMC pedicle design. c. > IMF.*

4.6 Vertical mastopexy

When the nipple-IMF distance is normal or near normal, i.e. <10 cm, omitting the horizontal incisions of the Wise pattern mastopexy may be appropriate. One situation in which vertical mastopexy would not be appropriate with a near normal nipple-IMF distance is in a wide breast with a voluminous inferior pole necessitating a large amount of inferior pole breast tissue excision. In such a case, the only way to eliminate skin redundancy after an abundant inferior pole parenchymal excision is to excise the skin which is accomplished via the Wise pattern.

A template is used to mark the new areola position and vertical incisions. The vertical incisions again need to clear the edges of the areola and are then tapered medially to come to a point above the inframammary fold. There are times when the gentle tapering of the vertical incisions comes to a point below the IMF. In this situation, the vertical incision markings are gently curved laterally to avoid the incision crossing the IMF (**Figure 14**).

4.7 Anesthesia

It is extremely difficult and technically challenging to achieve adequate local anesthesia of the chest wall musculature which will be heavily manipulated during

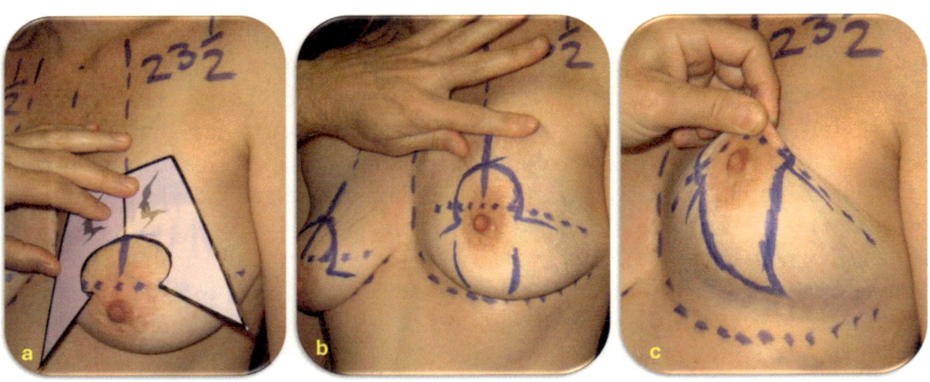

Figure 14.
Vertical mastopexy markings. Dashed lines are reference markings indicating the IMF and transposed IMF onto the breast skin. a. Template being used to mark the new areola position. b. Vertical limbs are drawn. c. vertical limb is completed by bringing the tapered end laterally to avoid the incision crossing the IMF; the nipple-to-IMF distance is approximately 7 cm.

submuscular implant pocket creation, therefore, the procedure is best performed under general anesthesia. To aid in limiting the amount of analgesia administered systemically, local tumescent anesthesia is used. With anesthesia induction complete, modified Klein Solution made up of 1 L Normal Saline, 30 mL 1% lidocaine, and 1 mL of 1:1000 epinephrine is infiltrated into the planned incisions, the area to be de-epithelialized, and into the subpectoral space with care not to violate the chest wall and inadvertently causing a pneumothorax.

5. Operative technique

5.1 Liposuction

Liposuction is a wonderful adjunct to breast surgery and offers improved definition of the breast resulting in a more refined, rounded shape. Unaddressed fullness adjacent to the breast diminishes its contour and underwhelms the expected result. Prior to surgery, the decision is made as to whether liposuction of the perimammary fat is indicated. The areas to be liposuctioned are marked preoperatively. Liposuction is performed in the patient with excess subcutaneous fat causing abnormal fullness overlying the anterior aspect of the superolateral pectoralis major, within the axilla and lateral thorax, and/or the upper abdomen. .

5.2 Areola diameter and marking

Areola diameter is marked with an areola marker with a 38–42 mm diameter while the breast is compressed circumferentially to stretch or expand the areola. Care is taken to ensure stretching is symmetric in order to avoid overstretching or understretching a portion of the areola thus resulting in an oblong segment of areola following incision.

5.3 Skin incisions and de-epithelialization

Initial skin incisions are made 360° around the areolar only down to the dermis. Remaining incisions based on preoperative markings are made. The areolar inset incision and vertical limb incisions are made down to the dermis. The horizontal limbs and IMF incisions are made full thickness down through the dermis.

De-epithelization is performed in a superior to inferior direction. One must remain aware of the areola position so that it is not inadvertently undermined. De-epithelization is continued inferiorly to just beyond the level of the horizontal limb incisions where the skin is left attached and removed en bloc with the breast parenchyma to be excised later.

5.4 Pedicle design—Superomedial central and medial central pedicle

Pedicle design is based on sternal notch-to-nipple distance as described previously. The SMC pedicle is marked with a curvilinear incision beginning superiorly at 12 o'clock with respect to the de-epithelialized skin and extending in an inferolateral direction around the NAC and then medially to end at the corner of the vertical and horizontal limb of the medial pillar.

For a medial pedicle, the incision is made beginning at 2 o'clock for the right breast, 10 o'clock for the left breast with respect to the areola inset incision. Again the incision is brought laterally and curved around the NAC, then medially to the corner of the vertical and horizontal limb of the medial pillar. This slight positional change compared to the SMC pedicle allows for rotation of the more ptotic NAC into its new position without undue tension and kinking of the pedicle (**Figure 15**).

5.5 Parenchymal excision

At this point, full thickness horizontal limb incisions and IMF incisions have been made. The medial extent of parenchymal excision is defined by the border of the pedicle. At this point, there will be a small area of dermis that has not yet been incised just lateral to the pedicle. This dermis is incised following the already made skin incisions (**Figure 15c**).

Initial parenchymal dissection is begun inferiorly at the inframammary fold. The parenchyma is incised and dissection is carried deeply with a bevel headed in the superior direction at an angle of approximately 30° until the pectoralis fascia is encountered. The pectoralis fascia is followed superiorly to the level of the inferior limits of the pedicle. Any undermining beyond the inferior edge of the pedicle will violate the pectoral perforator vascular supply of the central component of the pedicle. The horizontal limb incisions are carried through the parenchyma at 90° respective to the skin down to the pectoralis fascia. The lateral vertical limb incision is likewise carried at 90° down through the parenchyma to the pectoralis fascia. The pedicle defining incision (at the pedicle's lateral edge) is then carried deeply through the parenchyma down to the pectoralis fascia. The parenchymal dissection around the pedicle is performed with a bevel away from the NAC, thus forming a pyramid of parenchyma beneath the NAC (**Figure 16**). The parenchyma defined by these incisions down to the pectoral fascia is then divided off of the pectoral fascia and removed.

5.6 Pectoralis major entry and total submuscular pocket creation

The entry point for a total submuscular pocket is through the pectoralis major at the point which underlies the new NAC position (**Figure 17**). The pectoralis muscle

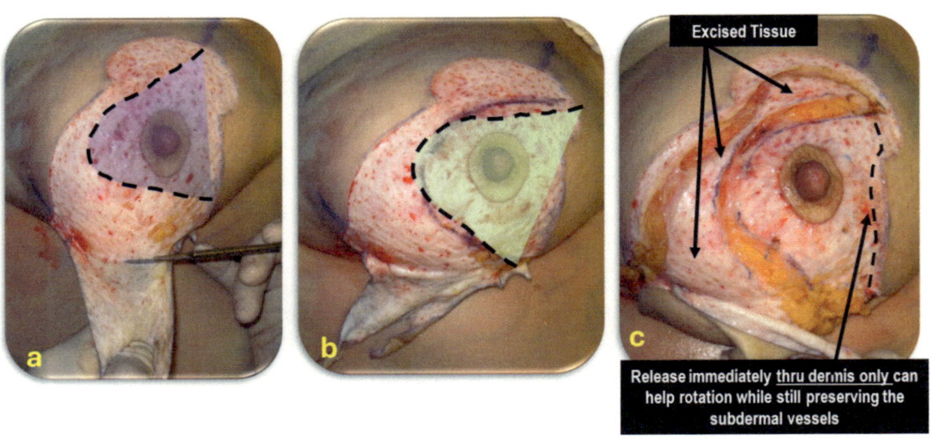

Figure 15.
Right breast. Pedicle design and parenchymal incision. a. Superomeial-central pedicle design for a sternal notch-to-nipple distance <30 cm. b. Medial central pedicle design for sternal notch-to-nipple distance of >30 cm and < 36 cm. c. A medial pedicle has been delineated and incisions through the dermis have been made. These incisions define the area of parenchyma that will be excised.

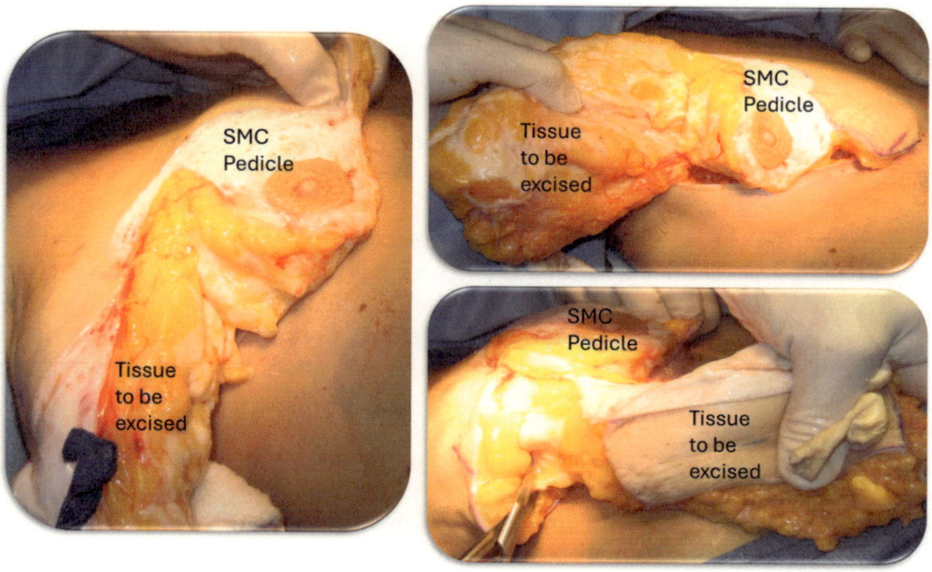

Figure 16.
*Right breast. A superomedial central pedicle has been defined. Parenchymal incision takes place down to the pectoralis fascia and parenchyma is excised lateral and inferior to the pedicle. ** The pedicle is not undermined. The parenchyma underlying the pedicle is full thickness down to the pectoralis fascia.*

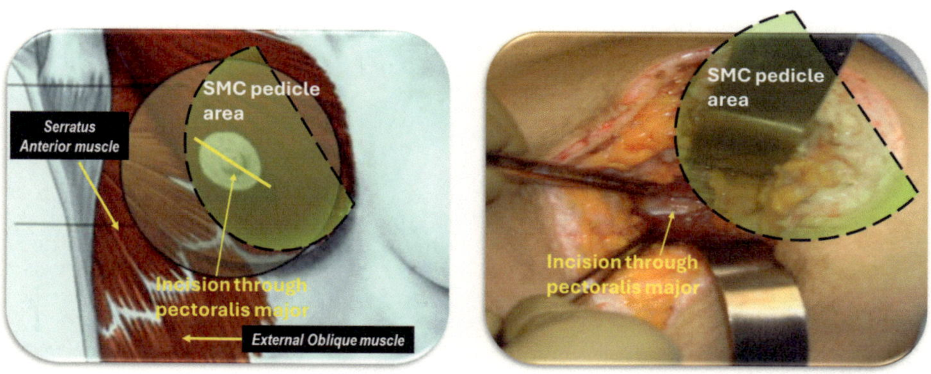

Figure 17.
Right breast. The pectoralis entry point directly underlies the new areola position.

is incised parallel to the muscle fibers. The incision should be 3–4 cm in length and initially quite superficial. A safe entry is aided with an alice clamp at each side of the incision lifting the pectoralis major off of the chest wall. The incision is then carried through the pectoralis major muscle to the subpectoral fibrofatty tissue.

At this point a finger is inserted into the submuscular space and directed superiorly along the chest wall. As with any breast implant surgery, care is taken not to violate the limits of the anterior axillary line laterally and the medial implant placement marking. Finger sweeping is first performed from superior to medial to inferior, then from superior to lateral, ensuring not to breach the anterior axillary line. To achieve total submuscular coverage, an effort is made laterally to finger dissect beneath a portion of the serratus anterior and external oblique. Finally, blunt finger dissection is carried out inferiorly. At the inferior portion of the pocket, the muscular attachments can be quite adherent and must be elevated off of the chest wall with care not to perforate the overlying tissue. The inferior dissection is taken down to the inframammary fold (**Figure 18**). In instances where the inferior dissection seems likely to perforate or where a perforation has already been made, monopolar diathermy can be used to complete the dissection without causing additional perforations or extension of already present perforations. When dissecting the inferior portion of the pocket, care must be taken to avoid going beneath the rectus abdominis fascia which is palpated as a thick, tight, horizontal band of fascia approximating the inframammary fold. The defining factor in total submuscular implant placement is the incorporation of the chest wall musculature lateral and inferolateral to the pectoralis major, namely the serratus anterior and occasionally the external oblique.

5.7 Freeing the pedicle to permit rotation

Using monopolar diathermy on cut function and Adson forceps to lift the dermis, the dermis is incised along the medial aspect of the pedicle (**Figure 15c**). This is performed slowly, with great precision in a "layer by layer" fashion until the full thickness of the dermis has been incised. Subdermal vessels are visualized and kept intact.

Next, the parenchyma at the inferomedial aspect of the pedicle, immediately adjacent to the medial pillar is minimally incised with the monopolar diathermy to a depth of approximately 1 cm. This step is necessary to permit rotation of the NAC into position without distorting the medial pillar and avoid undue tension on the pedicle.

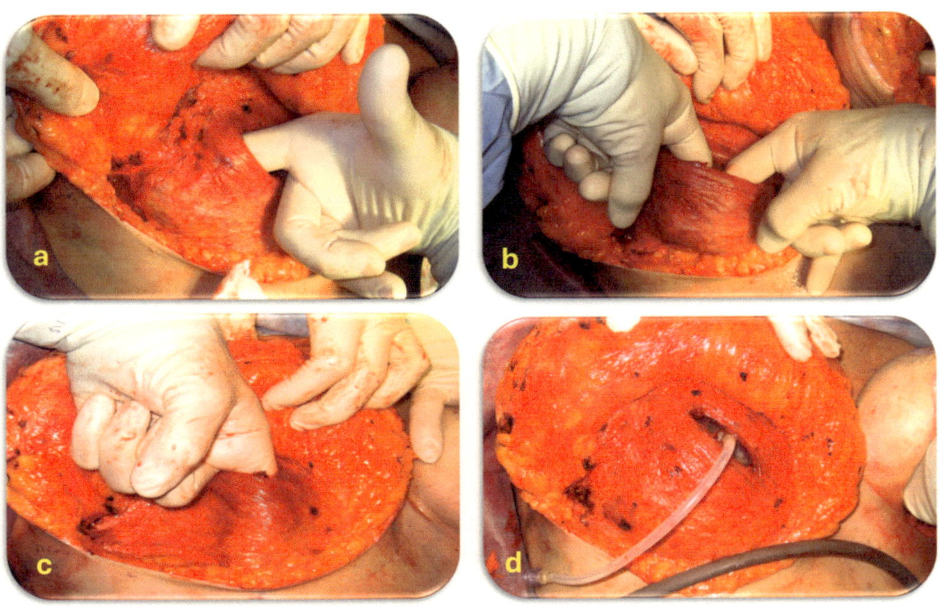

Figure 18.
Right breast. a. Blunt finger dissection is performed superiorly initially. b. The pocket is further developed with finger dissection more inferiorly. c. Finger dissection is performed down to the level of the IMF. d. A sizer has been placed showing total coverage within the total submuscular pocket.

5.8 Initial sutures

A 2-0 polyglactin (Vicryl) suture is used to approximate the superior portion of the vertical limbs by placing two sutures in the deep dermis. The NAC is then rotated into its new position and secured in place with a buried, deep dermal 2-0 polyglactin suture at 12, 3, 6, and 9 o'clock positions. Four 4-0 poliglecaprone (Monocryl) sutures are then placed in the dermis between the polyglactin sutures in buried fashion. This initial closure permits evaluation of the breast size, shape and tension when the sizer is introduced into the pocket.

5.9 Sizers and implant size selection

A temporary sizer is inserted and filled to the volume estimated pre-operatively. Once inflated, the overlying breast tissue tension is assessed. The breast at this point is not fully closed, therefore some manual manipulation of the breast tissue, particularly the pillars is performed to estimate breast tissue tension if the breast were to be closed at the current sizer volume. The sizer volume is adjusted accordingly to balance the patient's desired breast size with minimal breast tissue tension. If obvious areas of restriction inhibit proper positioning of the sizer, blunt finger dissection and stretching of the pocket can be performed to relieve these restrictions.

5.10 Hemostasis

The sizer is removed. Hydrogen peroxide soaked lap sponges, usually 3–4 of them, are placed into the implant pocket and left in place for 2–3 minutes. The sponges are then removed and the pocket is visually assessed for any bleeding. Meticulous hemostasis is achieved using monopolar diathermy.

5.11 Implant delivery

The implant pocket is irrigated with betadine and antibiotic solution containing 1 g cefazolin and 80 mg gentamicin in 500 ml of saline. The implant is soaked in the same solution and is then delivered into the pocket using a Keller Funnel. Valve position is confirmed. Again, blunt finger dissection and/or stretching of the pocket is performed as needed to accommodate proper implant position. The patient is sat up at this point and implant height is assessed and the pocket is adjusted as needed to achieve symmetry.

5.12 Closure

Closure of the pectoralis entry point is often unnecessary, but can be closed if desired. A strong suture such as a 0 polyglactin suture is used in "three-way" fashion to place a parenchymal suture that approximates the inferior aspect of the pillars and then approximates the pillars to scarpa's fascia at the inframammary fold. Deep dermal sutures are then placed in buried interrupted fashion to reapproximate the remaining portion of vertical incision and the inframammary fold incision. The authors prefer to use a 2-0 polyglactin suture for this. These sutures should bear the majority of any tension placed on the breast. The skin of the inverted-T incision and the areola are then closed with a 3-0 barbed poliglecaprone (Mondoderm Quill) suture.

5.13 Dressings

Mastasol and Robbins tape is placed over all incisions. A supportive bra is then placed and often a superior strap is used.

6. Post-operative care

6.1 Breast support and incision care

A supportive post-surgical bra is worn for 1 week. If a superior strap is used to prevent superior displacement of the implant, it is generally worn for 1 week. After 1 week, a supportive sports bra is worn for 3 months. Robbins tape is left on for 1 week. At the 1 week post operative appointment, tape is replaced with brown paper tape which is left in place for 5 additional weeks. Silicone tape is then recommended to be worn whenever feasible for the following 3 months.

6.2 Activity/restrictions

- Week 1:
    - *No:* lifting >10 lbs., lifting the arms above 90°, exercise, submerging the incision in water, doing anything that engages the pectoralis muscle
    - *Yes*: daily showering using hibiclens soap, light walking
- Week 2:
    - *No:* lifting >10 lbs., exercise, submerging the incision in water, doing anything that engages the pectoralis muscle
    - *Yes*: daily showering using hibiclens soap, light walking, slowly progressing to raise the arms over the head
- Week 3–6:
    - *No:* resistance training that flexes the chest or shoulder, i.e. bench press, shoulder press, push ups, dips, tricep presses.
    - *Yes*: resume cardiovascular exercise as long as there is no bouncing, i.e. walking at incline, elliptical, stationary bike with plenty of bra support.

7. Complications

Complication rates of simple breast surgery are notable. Studies have consistently shown a 15–25% reoperation rate post primary augmentation, and clinical experience shows that this rate is consistent when augmentation is combined with mastopexy [18]. Interestingly, these studies have shown that combined surgery complication rates are not exponential nor additive compared to two stage approaches [19]. Significant complications like implant extrusion, infection and nipple necrosis are very uncommon. More prevalent complications include Implant displacement, Hematoma, and capsular contracture.

7.1 Infection

Meticulous sterile technique is paramount in any surgery, but even more so when dealing with an implant of any kind. Studies show that in addition to meticulous sterility, infection following breast implant surgery is mitigated by soaking the implant and irrigating the implant pocket prior to insertion with povidone-iodine (PI) with or without antibiotic solution [20]. Our preference is to soak the breast implant and irrigate the implant pocket in solution containing PI with 1 g Ancef and 80 mg gentamicin. A Keller funnel is used for implant placement. Keller funnel for placement of implant reduces the amount of skin contact and has been shown to decrease potential parenchyma contamination compared to digital insertion technique [21].

7.2 Capsular contracture

Capsular contracture is the most common reason for reoperation following breast implant surgery. The reported incidence of capsular contracture varies by source. A recent database search of MEDLINE shows an incidence of 10.6% [22]. Certain factors have been shown to decrease this incidence. Less than a decade ago, implant choice between textured, polyurethane coated implants and smooth implants was an option. Capsular contracture rates were noted to be less with micro-textured and polyurethane coated implants. In 2019, a link between breast implant associated-anaplastic large cell lymphoma was found and such implants were recalled. The remaining implant choices are between manufacturers and silicone vs. saline filled. New generation silicone implants, which dominate the current implant market, show acceptably low capsular contracture rates of approximately 4% [22].

Surgical technique used has also been shown to affect capsular contracture rates. It is well known that subglandular implant placement confers increased risk of capsular contracture. Submuscular implant placement was shown to have a 2.8% rate of capsular contracture vs. 8.6% for subglandular placement [23].

Management of capsular contracture depends on degree of contracture and implant integrity [9]. For Baker grades I and II, the patient may be instructed to perform daily massages to soften the breast capsule or take a leukotriene inhibitor (montelukast/zafirlukast) for several months to prevent worsening and reduce the degree of contracture. Leukotriene inhibitor therapy (Zafirlukast/Montelukast) has been shown to reduce capsular contracture grade and even decrease the risk of capsular contracture development [14]. For moderate to severe cases with Baker grades III or IV, surgical intervention is indicated with either capsulotomy, capsulectomy, implant pocket exchange, use of acellular dermal matrices, or soft tissue/muscle flaps (**Figures 19** and **20**) [9]. The success rate of resolution after reoperation and implant exchange is 79%. Unfortunately, the recurrence rate is ~54% [24]. However, a more recent systematic review performed by Wan and Rohrich, found that implant exchange is associated with 0–26% recurrence rate of capsular contracture compared with no implant exchange.

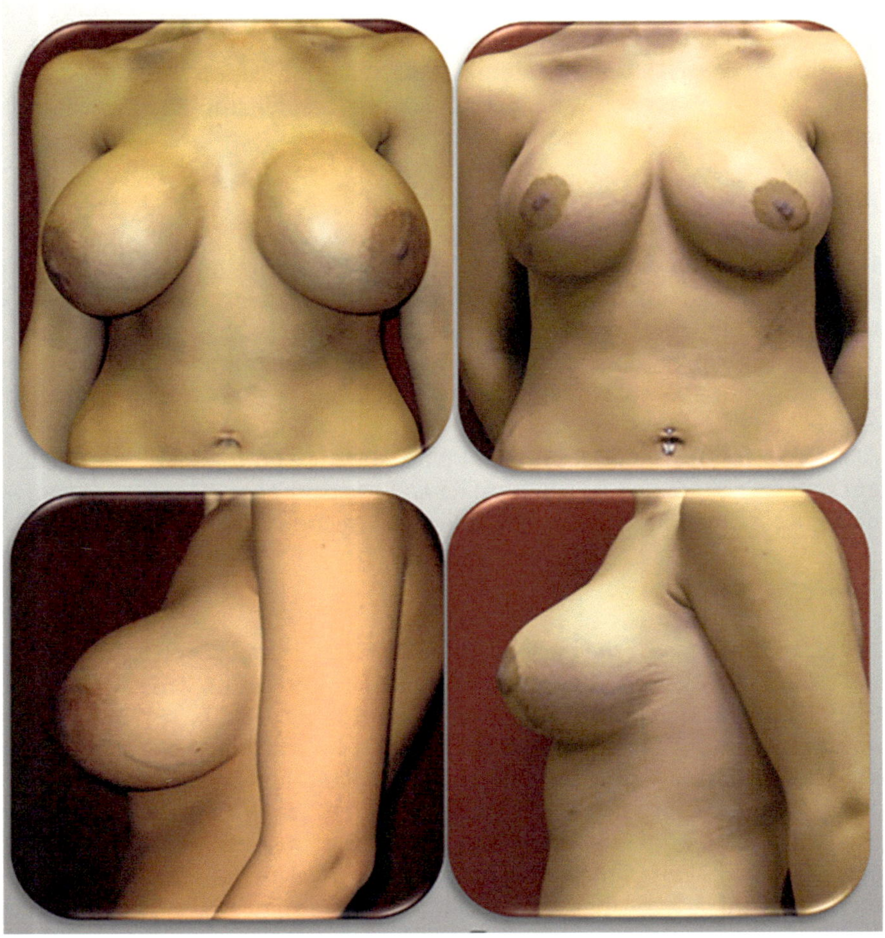

Figure 19.
Grade IV capsular contracture. Patient with Grade IV capsular contracture. Patients with capsular contraction who desire a breast lift with augmentation must be informed of the high revision rate and risk of complications.

7.3 Hematoma

Hematoma is among the more common postoperative complications related to breast implant surgery. The obvious remedy is avoidance with meticulous hemostasis. Untreated hematoma results in increased risk of capsular contracture, results in increased breast tissue tension and potentially reduced perfusion of at risk breast tissue. In the event of hematoma, the implant pocket should be explored and hematoma evacuated.

7.4 Implant displacement

Implant displacement is mitigated by submuscular placement of the implant. It is important to avoid inadequate release of the inferior aspect of the breast pocket to avoid superior displacement, however, care must also be taken not to dissect beyond the IMF as this too predisposes the implant to displacement but in the inferior direction. Similarly, avoid lateral or medial malposition by avoiding over dissection of the submuscular pocket. Clear post operative instructions are given that are conducive to adequate healing and breast support.

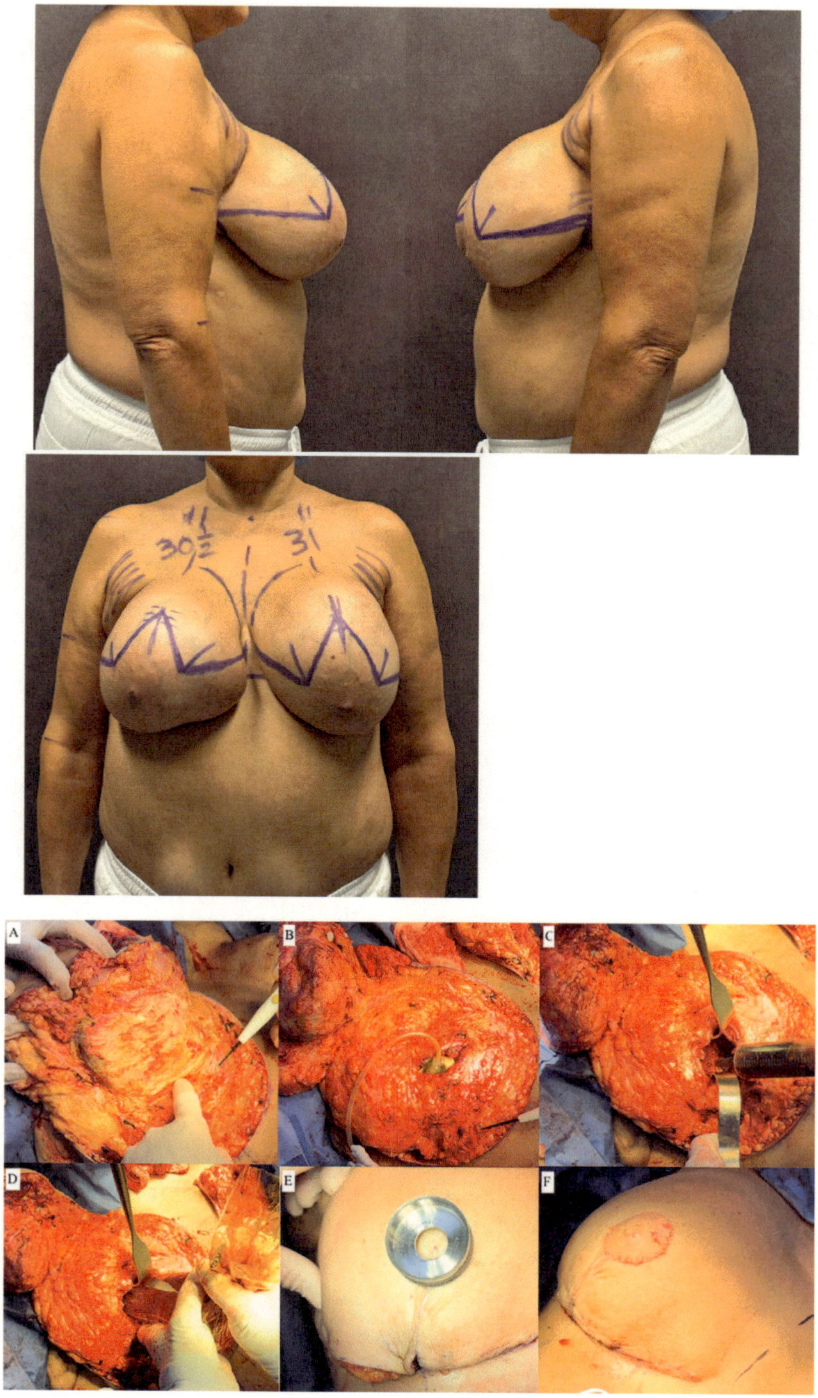

Figure 20.
Grade IV capsular contracture. 64 year old female with 30 year history of subpectoral 300 cc silicone implants desiring softer but equal or slightly larger size. Planned for removal and replacement of implant, total capsulotomy, augmentation with silicone implants, and free nipple graft. (A) Dissection of Capsulotomy (B) Utilizing Sizers to determine appropriate implant size (C) Implant pocket irrigated in solution containing PI with 1 g Ancef and 80 mg gentamicin (D) Keller funnel is used for placement of 450 cc SRF silicone implant (E) Areolar marker to outline position of new nipple and area to deepithelialize. (F) Free nipple graft positioned and sutured with 5-0 plain gut suture.

In the event of early malposition of the implant, manual force applied to the breast overlying the implant in the direction of needed movement is applied 3× daily for a constant 60 seconds until implant position is appropriate. Alteration to the patient's sports bra can be made such as placing a gauze padding inferiorly or laterally to apply a medially or superomedially directed force. In the event of impending medial displacement and symmastia, a thong bra should be worn.

7.5 NAC necrosis

Fortunately, NAC necrosis is rare. Its prevention is best assured by appropriate pre-operative planning i.e. proper patient selection, patient avoidance of nicotine-containing substances, and appropriate pedicle design.

If signs of mild NAC vascular compromise are noted intraoperatively, any periareolar hematoma should be evacuated and hemostasis assured. Nitropaste application is also helpful in relieving minor venous congestion. Further intervention to relieve vascular compromise includes removal of suture around the NAC and/or implant removal. These maneuvers decrease extrinsic vascular pressure leading to decreased venous congestion and increased tissue perfusion. Finally, hyperbaric oxygen has shown promise in avoiding NAC necrosis when vascular compromise is present or suspected.

7.6 Wound breakdown

The most common site of wound breakdown is at either point trifurcation. Surgical technique that leaves adequate subcutaneous tissue underlying the corners of the trifurcation is requisite for successful healing. Overzealous implant sizing resulting in increased tissue tension upon closure potentially compromises wound healing. Finally, tension bearing suture placement directly at the trifurcation should be avoided as this tends to be a source or inflammation leading to suture spitting and skin breakdown.

8. Summary

Simultaneous mastopexy with breast augmentation, while technically challenging, when performed with appropriate patient evaluation and selection and proper surgical planning provides the patient and surgeon a single stage, rewarding experience with a high probability of success. The SMC and MC pedicles with total submuscular implant placement provide ideal implant coverage with a robust NAC vascular supply. Combined mastopexy with augmentation should be part of the armamentarium of the cosmetic breast surgeon as it obviates a second stage procedure with its associated increased patient costs and delay in achieving the patient's ultimate desired result.

9. Case studies

9.1 Case 1

See **Figure 21**.

9.2 Case 2

See **Figure 22**.

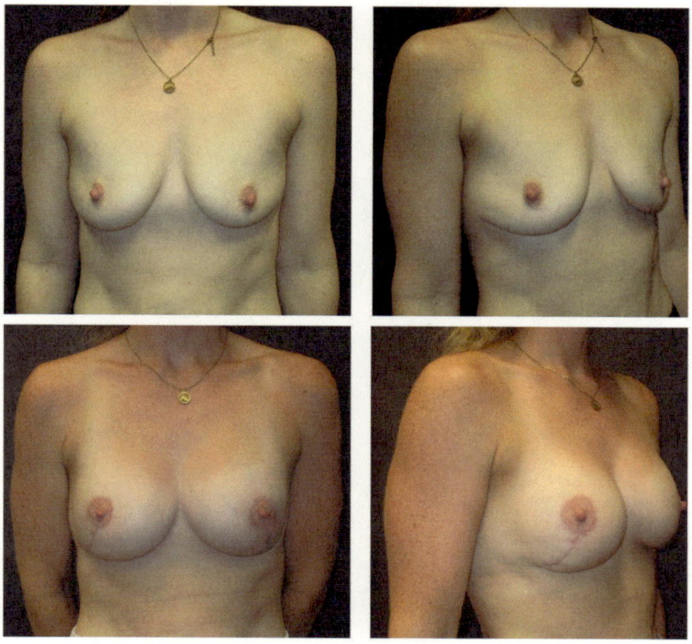

Figure 21.
33 year old woman with grade 2 ptosis and significant deflation. Sternal notch-to-nipple distance: right 23.5 cm, left 23 cm; nipple-IMF distance: right 7 cm, left 7.5 cm. 6 weeks after vertical mastopexy was performed using a SMC pedicle. 320 cc silicone implant. Total submuscular placement.

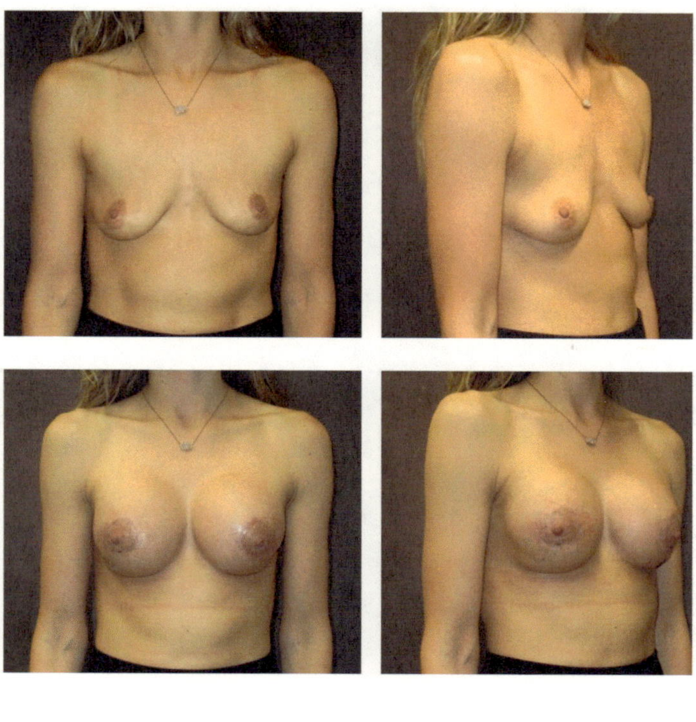

Figure 22.
32 year old female, grade 1 ptosis with significant deflation. Sternal notch-to-nipple distance: right 21 cm, left 19.5 cm; nipple-IMF distance: right 6 cm, left 4.5 cm. 6 weeks after vertical mastopexy was performed using a SMC pedicle. 345 cc silicone implant, total submuscular placement.

9.3 Case 3

See **Figure 23**.

9.4 Case 4

See **Figure 24**.

9.5 Case 5

See **Figure 25**.

9.6 Case 6

See **Figure 26**.

9.7 Case 7

See **Figure 27**.

9.8 Case 8

See **Figure 28**.

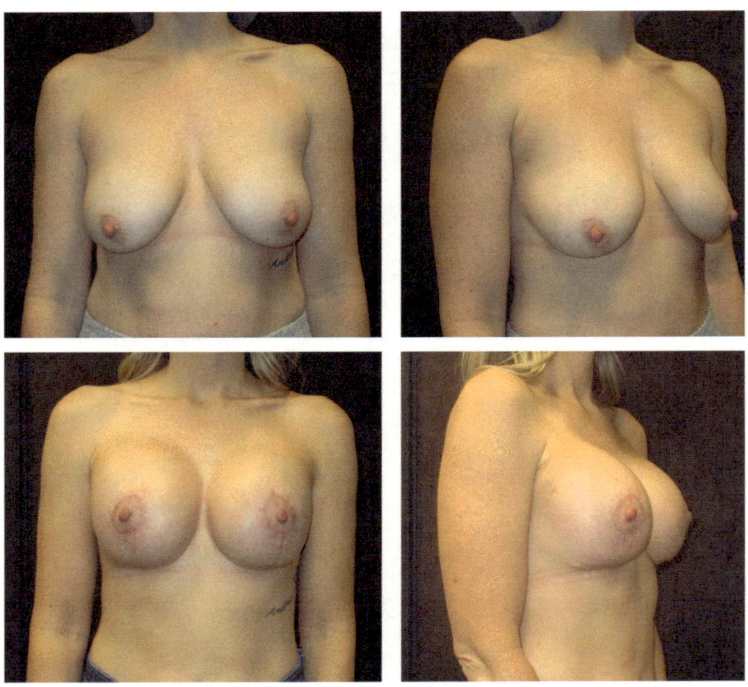

Figure 23.
34 year old female, grade 2 ptosis. Sternal notch-to-nipple distance: right 26 cm, left 25 cm; nipple-IMF distance: right 7 cm, left 8 cm. 6 weeks after Wise pattern mastopexy was performed using a SMC pedicle. 365 cc silicone implant, total submuscular placement.

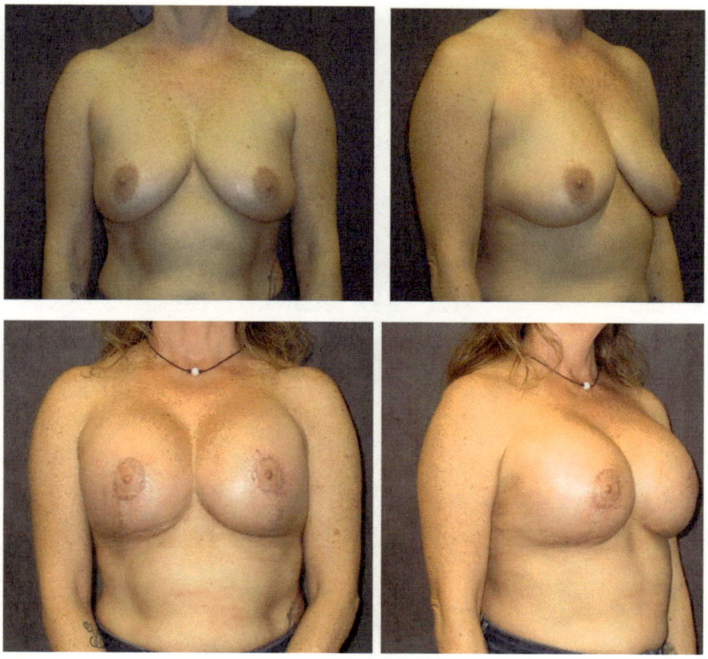

Figure 24.
54 year old female, grade 2 ptosis. Sternal notch-to-nipple distance: right 25 cm, left 25.5 cm; nipple-IMF distance: right 9 cm, left 9.5 cm. 6 weeks after Wise pattern mastopexy was performed using a SMC pedicle. 485 cc silicone implant, total submuscular placement.

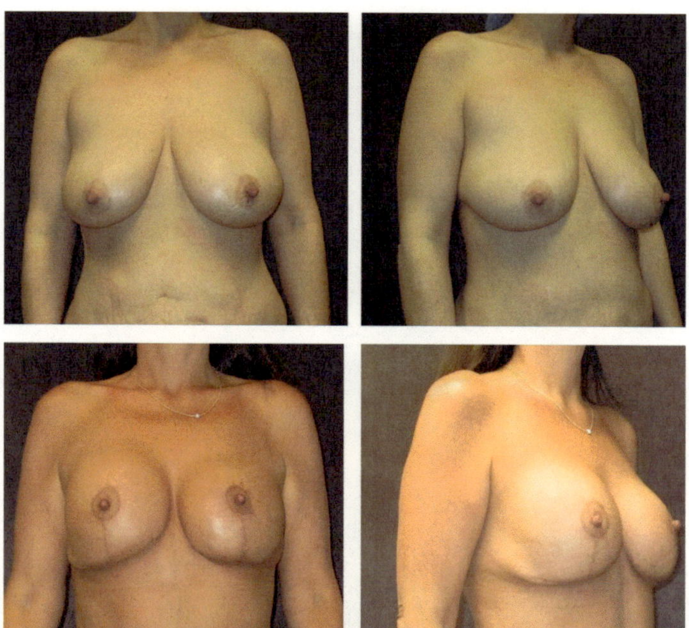

Figure 25.
44 year old female, grade 2 ptosis. Sternal notch-to-nipple distance: right 28 cm, left 29 cm; nipple-IMF distance: right 9 cm, left 10 cm. 6 weeks after Wise pattern mastopexy was performed using a SMC pedicle. 295 cc silicone implant, total submuscular placement.

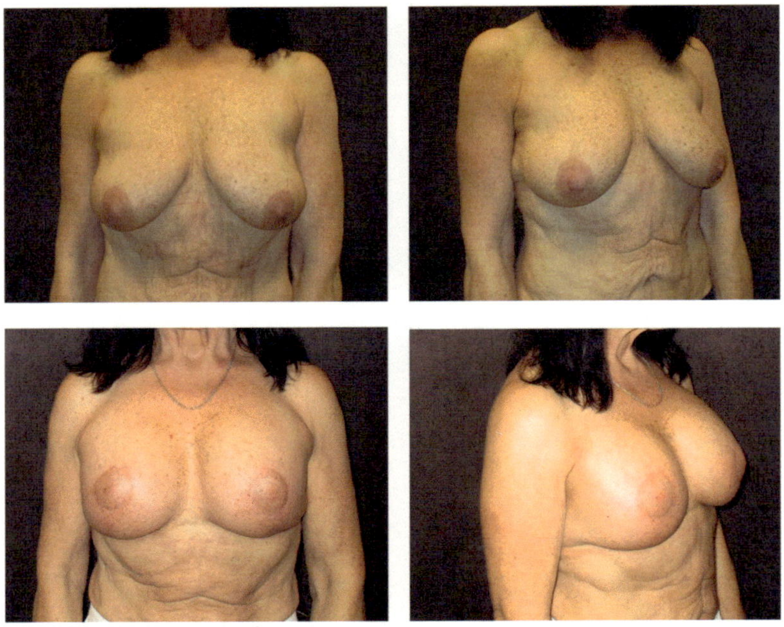

Figure 26.
68 year old female, grade 3 ptosis. Sternal notch-to-nipple distance: right 27.5 cm, left 27 cm; nipple-IMF distance: right 7 cm, left 8 cm. 6 weeks after Wise pattern mastopexy was performed using a SMC pedicle. 360 cc silicone implant, total submuscular placement.

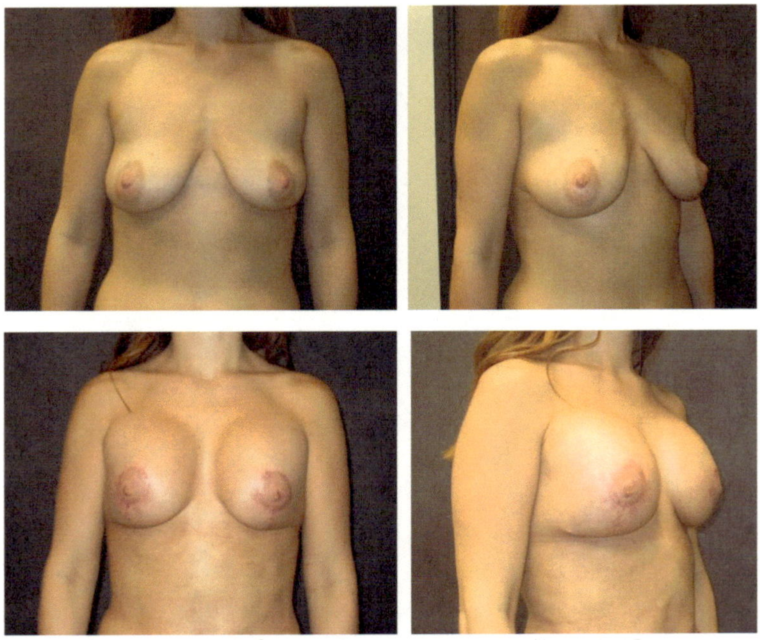

Figure 27.
32 year old female, grade 2 ptosis. Sternal notch-to-nipple distance: right 23 cm, left 22.5 cm; nipple-IMF distance: right 8 cm, left 7.5 cm. 6 weeks after Wise pattern mastopexy was performed using a SMC pedicle. 365 cc silicone implant, total submuscular placement.

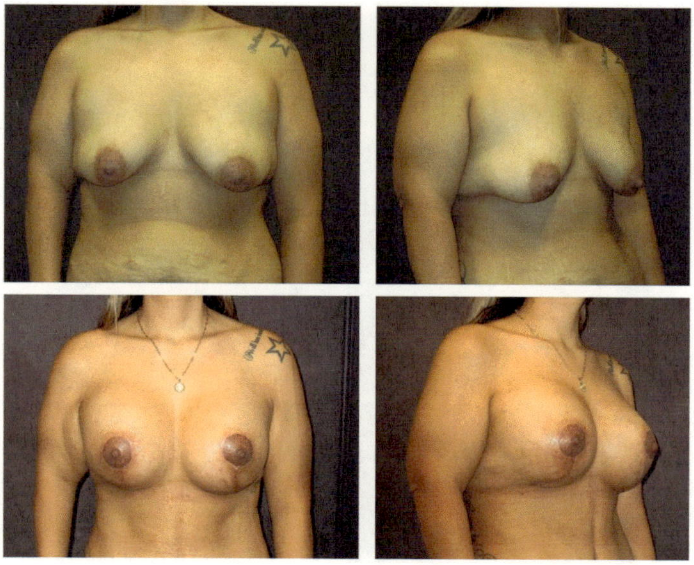

Figure 28.
36 year old female, grade 3 ptosis, tubular breasts. Sternal notch-to-nipple distance: right 26.5 cm, left 27.5 cm; nipple-IMF distance: right 8 cm, left 9 cm. 6 weeks after Wise pattern mastopexy was performed using a SMC pedicle. 520 cc silicone implant, total submuscular placement.

9.9 Case 9

See **Figure 29**.

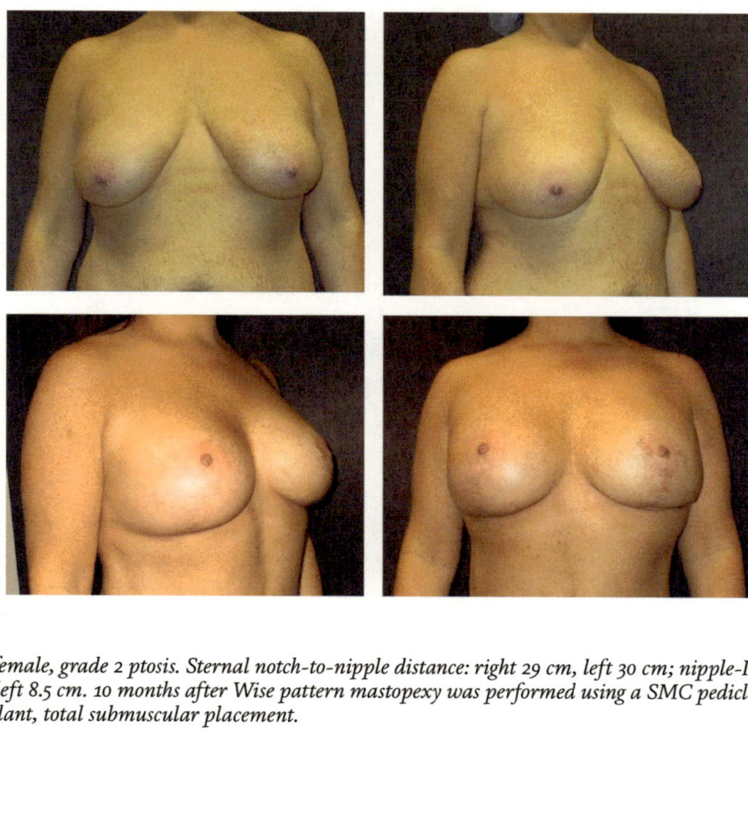

Figure 29.
39 year old female, grade 2 ptosis. Sternal notch-to-nipple distance: right 29 cm, left 30 cm; nipple-IMF distance: right 8 cm, left 8.5 cm. 10 months after Wise pattern mastopexy was performed using a SMC pedicle. 445 cc silicone implant, total submuscular placement.

9.10 Case 10

See **Figure 30**.

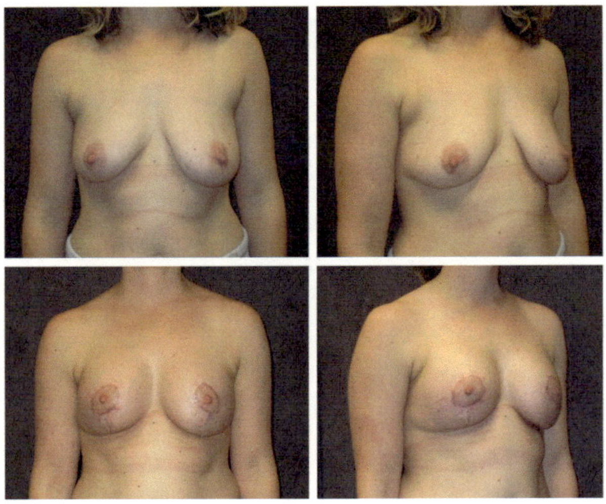

Figure 30.
39 year old female, grade 2 ptosis. Sternal notch-to-nipple distance: right 21.5 cm, left 22 cm; nipple-IMF distance: right 7 cm, left 9 cm. 6 weeks after Wise pattern mastopexy was performed using a SMC pedicle. 295 cc silicone implant, total submuscular placement.

9.11 Case 11

See **Figure 31**.

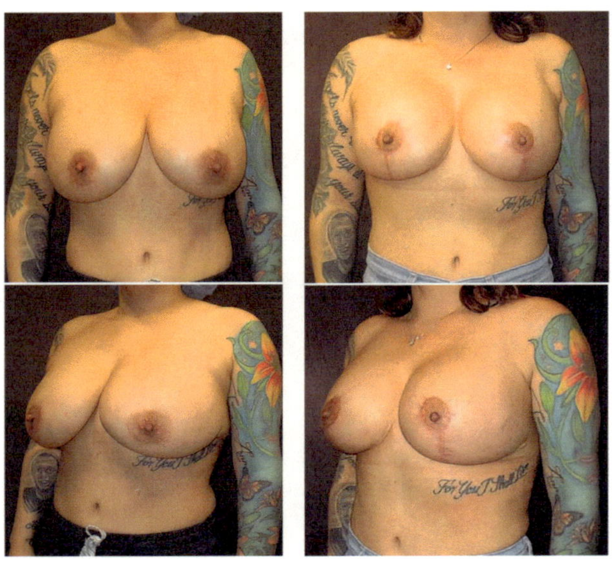

Figure 31.
35 year old female, grade 2 ptosis. Status post implant replacement and breast lift. Implant 575 cc silicone implants replaced with SRD 485 cc Silicone implants. Capsulotomy and capsulorrhaphy were performed. Left implant was found to be ruptured intraoperatively.

DOI: http://dx.doi.org/10.5772/intechopen.1008688

Author details

Chase Nelson*, Angelo Cuzalina and Sebastian Gutierrez De Pineres
Tulsa Surgical Arts, Tulsa, Oklahoma, USA

*Address all correspondence to: cnelson.do@gmail.com

References

[1] Schünke M, Ross LM, Lamperti ED, Schumacher U, Schulte E. Neurovascular Systems: Topographical Anatomy; Anterior Trunk Wall: Nerves, Blood Vessels, and Lymphatics in the Female Breast. New York, NY, USA: Thieme; 2010. pp. 180-181. Atlas of anatomy. general anatomy and musculoskeletal system. Thieme

[2] Nahai F, Nahai F. The Art of Aesthetic Surgery, Three Volume Set. 3rd ed. New York, NY, USA: Thieme; 2020

[3] Rehnke RD, Groening RM, Van Buskirk ER, Clarke JM. Anatomy of the superficial fascia system of the breast: A comprehensive theory of breast fascial anatomy. Plastic and Reconstructive Surgery. 2018;**142**(5):1135-1144. DOI: 10.1097/PRS.0000000000004948

[4] Cuzalina A, McLain L. Simultaneous mastopexy with augmentation. In: The Art of Body Contouring. London, UK: IntechOpen; 2019. DOI: 10.5772/intechopen.84967

[5] Shestak KC. Reoperative Plastic Surgery of the Breast. Philadelphia, PA, USA: Lippincott Williams & Wilkins; 2006

[6] Ramanadham SR, Rose JA. Breast lift with and without implant: A synopsis and primer for the plastic surgeon. Plastic and Reconstructive Surgery. Global Open. 2020;**8**(10):e3057. DOI: 10.1097/gox.0000000000003057

[7] Liu YJ, Thomson JG. Ideal anthropomorphic values of the female breast: Correlation of pluralistic aesthetic evaluations with objective measurements. Annals of Plastic Surgery. 2011;**67**(1):7-11. DOI: 10.1097/SAP.0b013e3181f77ab5

[8] Chen J, Sun Y, Liu Q, Yip J, Yick KL. Construction of multi-component finite element model to predict biomechanical behavior of breasts during running and quantification of the stiffness impact of internal structure. Biomechanics and Modeling in Mechanobiology. 2024;**23**:1679-1694. DOI: 10.1007/s10237-024-01862-2. Epub ahead of print

[9] Cuzalina AG, Tolomeo P, Mañón AV. Revisions for Complications of Aesthetic Breast Surgery. London, UK: IntechOpen; 2024. DOI: 10.5772/intechopen.112915

[10] Würinger E. Localization of central breast lymphatics and predefined separation of lobes along the horizontal septum. Plastic and Reconstructive Surgery. Global Open. 2023;**11**(12):e5446. DOI: 10.1097/GOX.0000000000005446

[11] Netter FH. Atlas of Human Anatomy. 2nd ed. Philadelphia, PA: Novartis; 1997. p. 525

[12] Coopey S, Keleher A, Daniele K, Peled AW, Gomez J, Julian T, et al. Careful where you cut: Strategies for successful nerve-preserving mastectomy. Plastic and Reconstructive Surgery. Global Open. 2024;**12**(5):e5817. DOI: 10.1097/GOX.0000000000005817. Erratum in: Plast Reconstr Surg Glob Open. 2024;12(5):e5943. doi: 10.1097/GOX.0000000000005943

[13] Bubberman JM, Van Rooij JAF, Van der Hulst RRWJ, Tuinder SMH. Sensory recovery and the role of innervated flaps in autologous breast reconstruction-a narrative review. Gland Surgery. 2023;**12**(8):1094-1109. DOI: 10.21037/gs-23-40. Epub 2023 Aug 11

[14] Shin K, Whitman GJ. Clinical indications for mammography in men and correlation with breast cancer. Current Problems in Diagnostic Radiology. 2021;**50**(6):792-798. DOI: 10.1067/j.cpradiol.2020.11.001. Epub 2020

[15] Payer J, Chalkidis N, Polackova P, Patzelt M. MAMAS (mastopexy–augmentation made applicable and safer): A standardized template of pre-operative marking and step-by-step surgical procedure. JPRAS Open. 2024;**40**:293-304. ISSN 2352-5878. DOI: 10.1016/j.jpra.2024.03.007

[16] Abdelkader R, Raafat S, Sakr W, Abdelaziz M, ElNoamany S. Augmentation mastopexy: A five-step standardized strategy approach. Plastic and Reconstructive Surgery. Global Open. 2022;**10**(6):e4349. DOI: 10.1097/GOX.0000000000004349

[17] Hubaide M, Ono MT, Karner BM, Martins LV, Pires JA. Safe augmentation mastopexy: Review of 500 consecutive cases using a vertical approach and muscular sling. Plastic and Reconstructive Surgery-Global Open. 2024;**12**(1):e5504. DOI: 10.1097/GOX.0000000000005504

[18] Gutowski KA, Mesna GT, Cunningham BL. Saline-filled breast implants: A plastic surgery educational foundation multicenter outcomes study. Plastic and Reconstructive Surgery. 1997;**100**:1019-1027

[19] Adams WP. Discussion: Simultaneous augmentation mastopexy a retrospective 5-year review of 332 consecutive cases. Plastic and Reconstructive Surgery. 2013;**131**(1):157-158

[20] Jewell ML, Bionda N, Moran AV, Bevels EJ, Jewell HL, Hariri S, et al. In vitro evaluation of common antimicrobial solutions used for breast implant soaking and breast pocket irrigation-part 2: Efficacy against biofilm-associated bacteria. Aesthetic Surgery Journal. 2021;**41**(11):1252-1262. DOI: 10.1093/asj/sjaa308

[21] Moyer HR, Ghazi B, Saunders N, Losken A. Contamination in smooth gel breast implant placement: Testing a funnel versus digital insertion technique in a cadaver model. Aesthetic Surgery Journal. 2012;**32**(2):194-199. DOI: 10.1177/1090820X11434505 Epub 2012 Jan 18

[22] Headon H, Kasem A, Mokbel K. Capsular contracture after breast augmentation: An update for clinical practice. Archives of Plastic Surgery. 2015;**42**(5):532-543. DOI: 10.5999/aps.2015.42.5.532. Epub 2015 Sep 15

[23] Namnoum JD, Largent J, Kaplan HM, et al. Primary breast augmentation clinical trial outcomes stratified by surgical incision, anatomical placement and implant device type. Journal of Plastic, Reconstructive and Aesthetic Surgery. 2013;**66**:1165-1172

[24] Lardi AM, Farhadi J. Physiopathology, prevention, and treatment of capsular contracture. In: Urban C et al., editors. Oncoplastic and Reconstructive Breast Surgery. New York: Springer; 2019. pp. 601-607

Chapter 8

Breast Reduction

Chandler Hinson, Victoria Bouillon, Hallie Masters, Polly Jasper and Ronald Brooks

Abstract

This chapter on breast reduction provides a comprehensive overview of the surgical and non-surgical procedures aimed at reducing the size and reshaping the breasts. It delves into the goals of breast reduction surgery, including alleviating physical discomfort, improving body proportions, and enhancing overall quality of life. This chapter discusses the surgical planning involved, considering factors such as desired breast size, nipple placement, and patient anatomy. Various breast reduction techniques are discussed, including the traditional wise pattern and vertical scar methods. The chapter also discusses the use of various pedicles versus free nipple grafting. Lastly, this chapter discusses the importance of monitoring and following patient outcomes post-surgery, assessing factors such as healing, scarring, and patient satisfaction. Through a comprehensive examination of these components, this chapter serves as a valuable resource for both patients considering breast reduction and healthcare professionals involved in their care.

Keywords: breast reduction surgery, mammaplasty, reduction mammoplasty, breast hypertrophy, pedicles, free nipple grafts, macromastia, gigantomastia, wise pattern reduction, vertical pattern reduction

1. Introduction

1.1 Definition

Breast hypertrophy, also known as macromastia, is a medical condition characterized by the excessive growth of adipose and fibrous tissue [1]. This overgrowth can lead to significant physical and psychological discomfort for affected individuals [2–4]. Extensive breast hypertrophy is known as gigantomastia, which is a rare medical condition characterized by the rapid and excessive growth of breast tissue to an exceptionally large size [5]. While there is no standardized definition of gigantomastia, it is arbitrarily defined as excessive breast growth of over 1.5 kilograms per breast [5]. This condition, along with macromastia, can cause significant chronic back, neck, and shoulder pain, skin infections under the breast from retained moisture, impaired posture, and psychological distress from body dysmorphia. The exact cause of macromastia and gigantomastia is not well understood, but both are believed to be linked to hormonal imbalances, the use of certain medications, and genetic factors [6]. Lifestyle modifications and weight loss is the first step in treatment. Definitive management involves a reduction mammoplasty to remove excess breast tissue.

1.2 Pathogenesis

The pathogenesis of breast hypertrophy results from the pathologic imbalance of hormones and growth factors. Estrogen and progesterone, which regulate normal breast development, are believed to play a significant role in the excessive growth seen in breast hypertrophy [7, 8]. During periods of hormonal change, such as puberty, pregnancy, and menopause, some women experience an exaggerated response to these hormones, leading to the rapid and excessive growth of breast tissue. Genetic factors may predispose individuals to breast hypertrophy, as evidenced by cases of familial macromastia [9]. Other contributing factors may include obesity because increased body fat can elevate estrogen levels. Certain medications that influence hormone levels, such as steroids, penicillamine, or bucillamine have also been linked to macromastia [10, 11].

1.3 Epidemiology

While breast hypertrophy can affect women of all ages, it is most common during periods of significant hormonal fluctuation, such as puberty and pregnancy. The prevalence of breast hypertrophy is not well-documented due to the variability in severity of the condition and its subjective nature [9, 12, 13]. Specifically for gigantomastia, studies have estimated incidences ranging from 1 in 28,000 to 1 in 100,000 [14]. It is important to note that breast hypertrophy can also occur in men and referred to as gynecomastia. Gynecomastia is often associated with hormonal imbalances or certain medical conditions that result in elevated estrogen levels. Nevertheless, the incidence of gynecomastia in men is far less that macromastia in women [15, 16].

1.4 Symptoms and physical findings

Women affected by excess breast hypertrophy frequently report back, neck, and shoulder pain due to the excessive weight of their breasts [17–19]. Shoulder grooving from the pressure of bra straps on the shoulders also results from the excess weight. Skin irritation and infections can occur under the breast crease where moisture accumulates [17–19]. The excess weight tends to shifts the individuals center of gravity and can lead to poor posture [19]. Physical findings in breast hypertrophy include enlarged and pendulous breasts, stretched skin with striae (known as 'stretch marks'), and downwardly displaced nipples and areolas [2, 20, 21]. In addition to physical symptoms, affected individuals may experience psychological distress, including self-consciousness and social embarrassment [9].

1.5 Breast ptosis

Breast ptosis, or breast sagging, is a condition usually associated with breast hypertrophy but can occur independently due to aging, rapid weight gain or loss, or pregnancy [22, 23]. Ptosis refers to the downward displacement of the breast tissue and nipple-areolar complex (NAC). There is a grading system based on the position of the nipple relative to the inframammary fold (IMF). **Figure 1** is a visual schematic of grades of breast ptosis [24].

1.5.1 Grades of breast ptosis

- *Grade I (mild ptosis)*: The nipple is at the level of the IMF but above the lowest point of the breast gland.

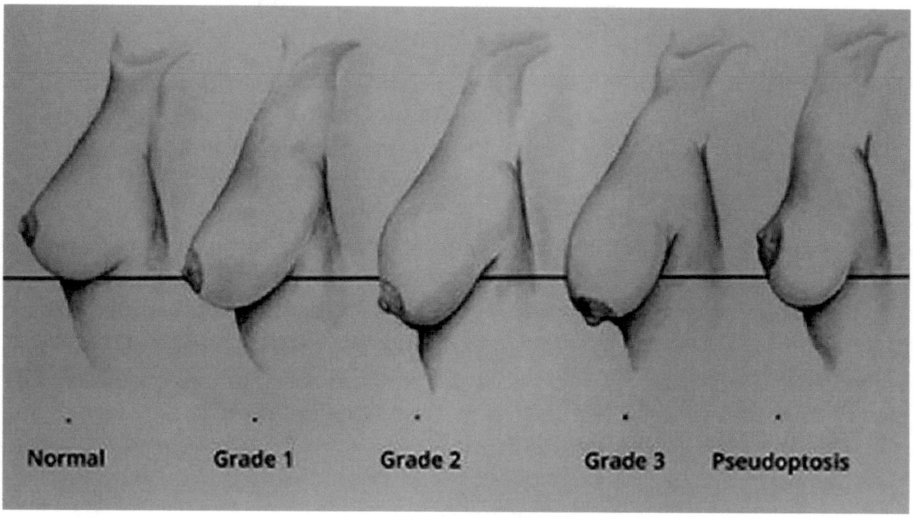

Figure 1.
A depiction of the breast ptosis grading system proposed by Regnault et al. Normal: Areola above the inframammary fold (IMF) and above the gland contour; Grade I: Areola at the IMF and above the gland contour; Grade II: Areola below the IMF and above the gland contour; Grade III: Areola below the IMF and below the gland contour; Pseudoptosis: Areola at the IMF with glandular ptosis.

- *Grade II (moderate ptosis)*: The nipple is below the level of the IMF but still above the lowest point of the breast gland.
- *Grade III (severe ptosis)*: The nipple is below the level of the IMF and at the lowest point of the breast gland, often pointing downward.
- *Pseudoptosis*: The nipple is at or above the level of the IMF, but the breast gland hangs below the fold.

Breast ptosis can significantly impact a woman's body image and self-esteem. The severity of ptosis influences the surgical approach in reduction mammaplasty and mastopexy procedures. Effective management involves a detailed assessment of the degree of ptosis and a tailored surgical plan to reposition the NAC and reshape the breast for a more youthful and esthetically pleasing contour.

2. Anatomy

The anatomy of the breast involves a complex arrangement of soft tissue, vasculature, nerves, and lymphatics. The breast is composed primarily of glandular tissue whose primary function is milk production and delivery of that milk via the lactiferous ducts to the NAC during times of childbearing. The adipose and connective tissue, known as Cooper's ligaments, give the breasts their fullness, maintain their shape and integrity, and generate the esthetic appearance of the female chest. The breast is situated on the chest wall and is anchored to the pectoralis major muscle by the pectoralis fascia. **Figure 2** illustrates the internal structure of the breast [25].

2.1 Breast borders and measurements

The anatomical borders of the breast are defined by specific landmarks on the chest. Superiorly, the breast extends to the second or third rib. Inferiorly, it terminates at the sixth rib. The medial border lies along the lateral edge of the sternum, and the lateral border extends to the mid-axillary line. The areola, the pigmented area surrounding the nipple, marks the central point of the breast. Many key measurements for surgical planning are in relation to the position of the nipple. These include the distance from the sternal notch to the nipple (SNN), the nipple-to-inframammary fold distance (NIMF), and the nipple-to-nipple distance (**Figure 3**) [26]. These measurements are crucial for ensuring symmetry during breast procedures.

2.2 Arterial and venous blood supply

The breast has a robust blood supply (**Figure 4**) [27]. The primary arterial supply comes from perforator branches of the internal mammary artery, also known as the internal thoracic artery, which is a branch of the subclavian artery. Additionally, the lateral thoracic artery, a branch of the axillary artery, supplies the lateral aspect of the breast. Smaller contributions come from the thoracoacromial artery and the intercostal arteries. The venous drainage of the breast mirrors the arterial supply and involves a network of veins that drain into the axillary vein, the internal thoracic vein, and the intercostal veins. This extensive vascular network is vital for maintaining the health of breast tissue and for healing post-surgery.

2.3 Nerve supply

The sensory innervation of the breast can be broken into three groups: intercostal nerves, lateral cutaneous nerves, and supraclavicular nerve branches (**Figure 5**) [28]. The fourth, fifth and sixth intercostal nerves provide sensation to the medial breast tissue. The lateral breast receives its sensory innervation from the third, fourth, fifth,

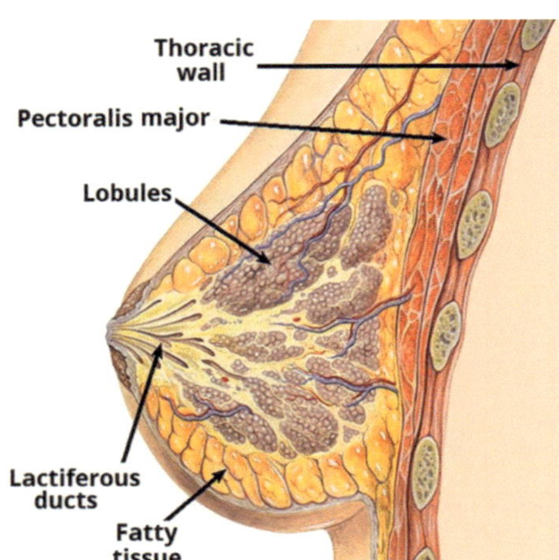

Figure 2.
The internal structure of the breast.

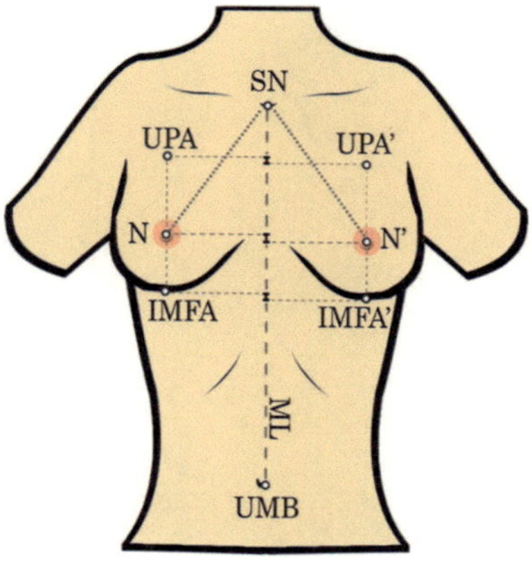

Figure 3.
Illustration of important landmarks and measurements of the breast. SN = sternal notch, UPA = upper pole apex, N = nipple, IMFA = inframammary fold apex, ML = medial line, UMB = umbilicus.

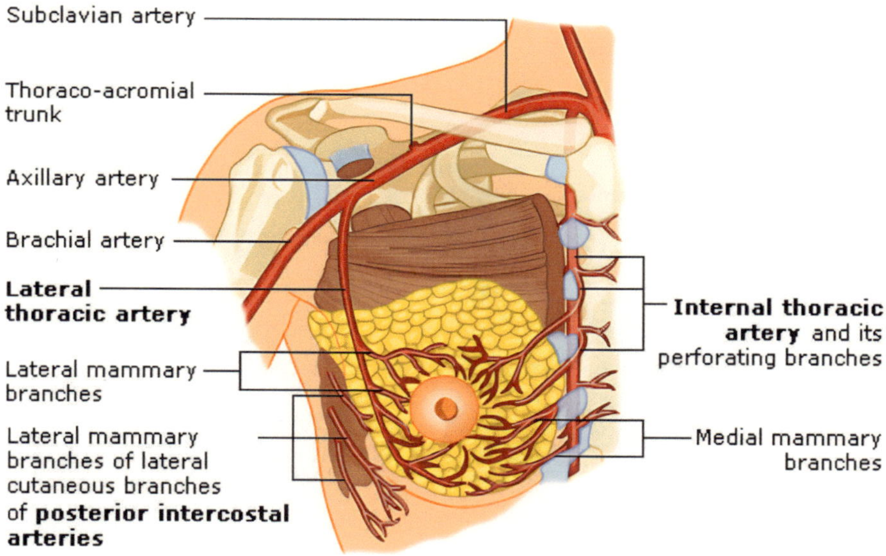

Figure 4.
Figure of the three main arterial systems within the breast.

and sixth branches These nerves are not only important for sensation of the breast and its overlying skin, they also play a key role in activation of the reflexes involved in lactation. The NAC is supplied by the fourth lateral cutaneous branch which travels medially in the deep fascia to the midclavicular line and then directs itself toward the deep surface of the nipple. The supraclavicular nerves, originating from the cervical plexus, contribute to the sensory innervation of the upper portion of the breast.

2.4 Lymphatic system

The lymphatic system of the breast is an essential component for maintaining fluid balance and facilitating immune responses. Lymph drainage flows via two main pathways: the axillary and internal mammary lymph channels (**Figure 6**) [29].

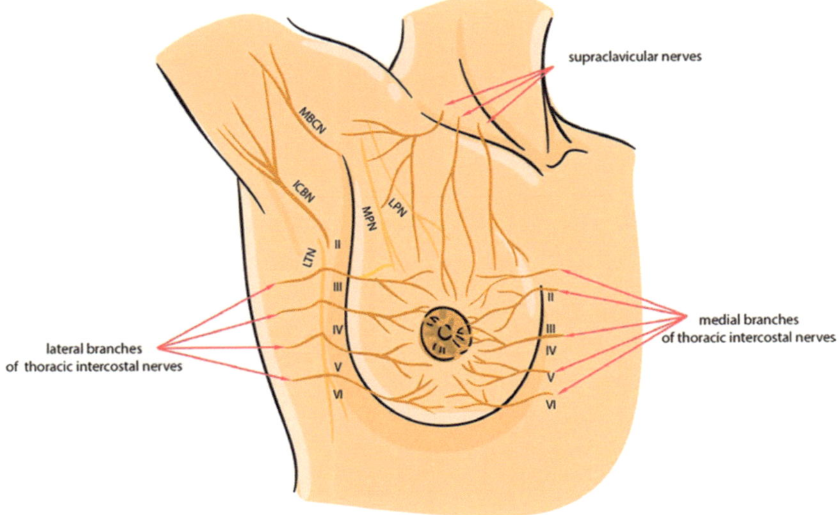

Figure 5.
Innervation of the axilla and breast. ICBN = intercostobrachial nerve; LTN = thoracic nerve; LPN = lateral pectoral nerve; MBCN = medial brachial cutaneous nerve; MPN = medial pectoral nerve. Figure created by Dr. Barbara Versyck.

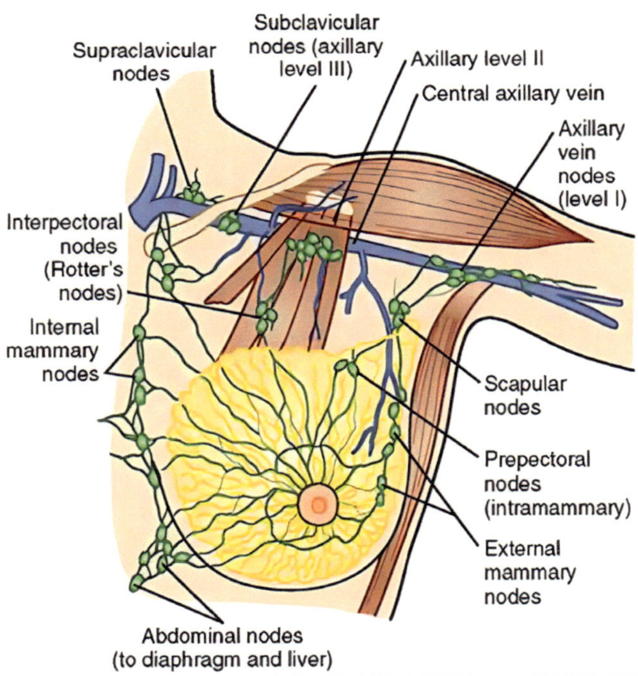

Figure 6.
Lymphatic drainage schematic created by Dr. Iram Dubin.

Approximately 75% of the breasts' lymphatic fluid drains to the axillary lymph channels. The superficial axillary nodes are divided by location: lateral, central, apical, and subscapular groups of nodes. The deep axillary lymph nodes are subdivided into three levels based on their anatomical position relative to the pectoralis minor muscle. The minor lymphatic drainage routes lymph toward the internal mammary nodes located along the internal thoracic vessels.

3. Surgical management

Breast reduction surgery, known as reduction mammaplasty, is a procedure designed to decrease breast size and alleviate discomfort associated with overly large breasts. This surgery consists of two main components: parenchymal excision and skin excision. Parenchymal excision is the removal of glandular tissue and fat from the breast to reduce its overall volume. Skin excision removes excess skin to reshape and lift the breast, thereby providing a more esthetically pleasing and proportionate appearance. Together, these components achieve the desired reduction in breast size and improve the overall contour of the breasts.

3.1 Parenchymal excision

Parenchymal excision is a critical component of breast reduction surgery. Excess glandular tissue and fat are removed to decrease breast volume.

Several excisional techniques exist including pedicle-based excisions and free nipple grafting. The technique utilized is determined by the planned volume of tissue resection. Other important considerations include desired final breast size, shape, preoperative degree of ptosis, and the preoperative position of NAC. A pedicle-based excision preserves the NAC on a tissue stalk, or pedicle, in order to maintain native blood and nerve supply to the nipple. This method is preferred because it maintains nipple sensation and function, and cosmetic outcomes are thought to be superior. In contrast, FNG involves the complete removal of the NAC and reattaching a portion of the areola as a skin graft, which may be necessary in some cases of macromastia or significant ptosis. The chosen technique is driven by the patient's specific anatomical needs and desired outcomes.

3.1.1 Inferior pedicle

The inferior pedicle technique preserves the NAC via a stalk that stems from the inferior pole breast tissue. Vascular supply of this pedicle includes the lateral thoracic artery and intercostal artery perforators. Preservation of the blood supply allows for the safe relocation of the NAC higher on the breast mound while reducing the overall breast volume.

Creating the inferior pedicle involves several critical steps (**Figure** 7) [30]. First, The pedicle is de-epithelialized. The pedicle is then incised and dissected free from the surrounding tissue that will later be excised. Excess breast tissue, fat, and skin are removed from the upper, lateral, and medial portions of the breast. It is crucial not to incise or violate the base of the pedicle in order to preserve the blood supply. The goal base width of the pedicle is approximately 8 cm with a length to width ratio of 3:1 as to reduce risk of pedicle ischemia [30, 31]. The resultant pedicle is about 2 cm in thickness and will resemble an inverted 'U' with a broad base. The de-epithelialized dermis and underlying parenchyma remains attached to the inframammary fold. Plication of the inferior portion of the pedicle is performed when necessary to achieve the appropriate pedicle length and IMF to NAC distance as depicted in **Figure 8** [32]. Once the desired volume is excised, the NAC is positioned cephalad. The incisions are

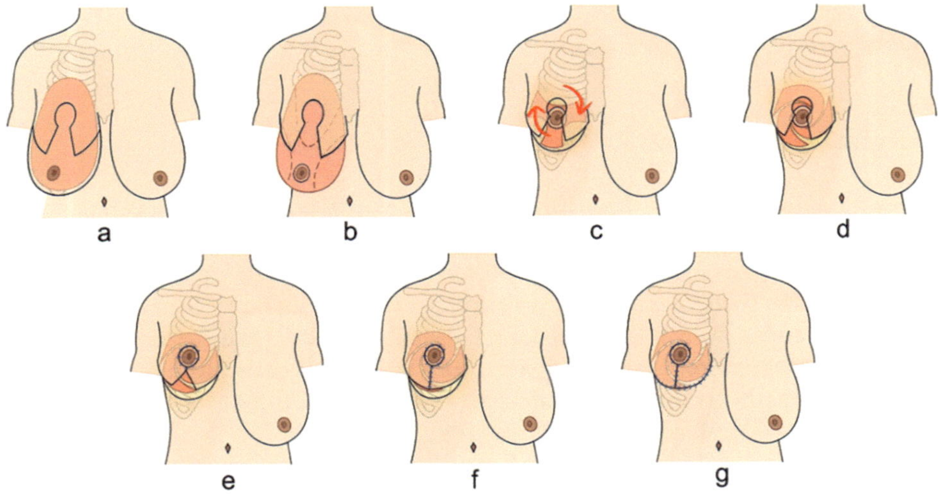

Figure 7.
Schematic drawing of the inferior pedicle mammoplasty operation steps with a wise pattern skin incision. (a) Flap design. (b) De-epithelialized skin and designed gland removal. (c) Shifted and rotated flap to reshape the breast. (d) Sutured and fixed breast gland. (e) Periareolar incision suturing. (f) Vertical incision suturing. (g) Breast IMF incision suturing.

closed in multiple layers to support the new position of the breast mound. While not recommended by the American Society of Plastic Surgeon, drains may be placed to prevent fluid accumulation [30].

The inferior pedicle technique is reliable for achieving large volume reductions while maintaining sensation to the NAC [33]. It also ensures a robust blood supply to the NAC, reducing the risk of ischemia and necrosis [30, 34]. This technique is highly versatile and can be adapted to various breast sizes and shapes [31]. It is particularly effective for patients with severe macromastia and significant breast ptosis because it allows the surgeon to substantially decrease the length between the IMF and the NAC which allows for repositioning the NAC and eliminating ptosis. The primary disadvantage of the inferior pedicle technique is the risk of "bottoming out," in which the lower pole of the breast becomes overly full and droops over time creating a phenomenon known as pseudoptosis [35, 36]. Pseudoptosis occurs because the bulk of the remaining breast tissue is below the NAC. Therefore, if the patient should experience glandular hypertrophy or the breast skin becomes more compliant, the most likely affected area will be the inferior pole of the breast causing pseudoptosis. While the technique can be used in various patients, those with optimal skin elasticity tend to have better esthetic outcomes.

3.1.2 Superomedial pedicle

The superomedial pedicle (SMP) technique preserves the blood supply and innervation to the NAC from the upper and medial portions of the breast. The neurovascular supply originates from the internal mammary system. This approach allows for the repositioning of the NAC to a higher location using a rotational method.

Creating the SMP involves several precise steps (**Figure 9**) [37]. The pedicle is created such that the NAC remains attached to the breast tissue in the superior and medial quadrants of the breast. The goal pedicle length is between 8 and 18 cm, with a width of 6–8 cm [37, 38]. Excess breast tissue, fat, and skin are excised from the lower

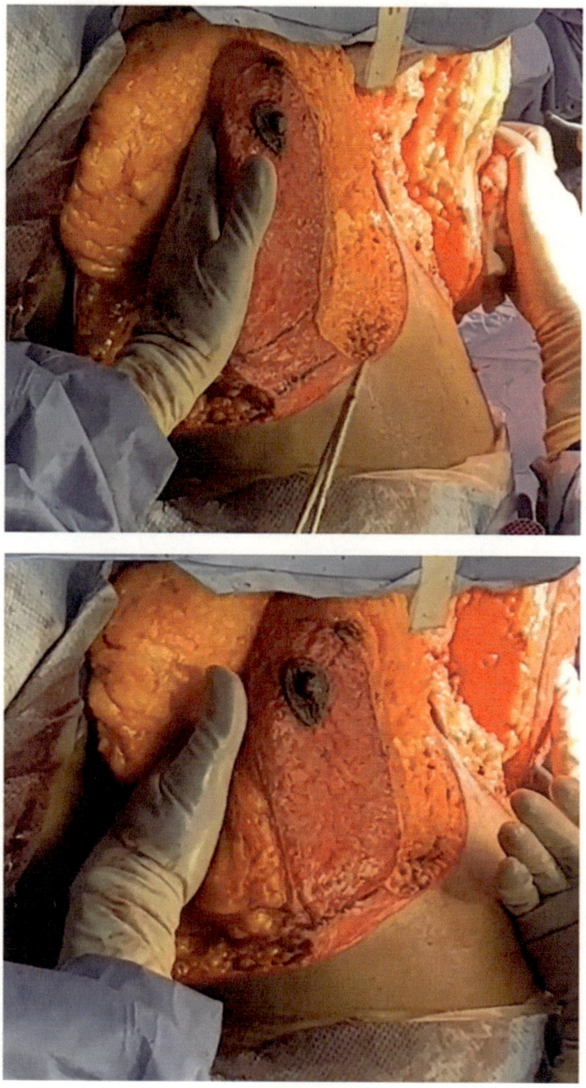

A

B

Figure 8.
The inferior pedicle is plicated to achieve a pedicle length of approximately 8 cm and decreasing the distance between the IMF and NAC.

and lateral portions of the breast. The pedicle is then rotated laterally to reposition the NAC and create a satisfactory breast shape. Stitches may be used to secure the distal aspect of the pedicle to the upper chest until sufficient scar tissue forms. The incisions are closed in layers to provide support for the pedicle. As with any reduction, drains may be placed to prevent fluid accumulation at the discretion of the surgeon [37].

The SMP technique is ideal for patients with large breasts with mild to moderate breast ptosis. It allows for substantial lifting and repositioning of the NAC [38]. The SMP often results in a more natural breast shape compared to other techniques, with a well-defined upper pole and a gentle slope toward the lower pole [37]. This method is quite versatile, making it suitable for a wide range of breast sizes and shapes, and cosmetic outcomes are generally favorable [39]. Similar to the inferior pedicle, those with good skin elasticity tend to have better esthetic outcomes, as their skin can

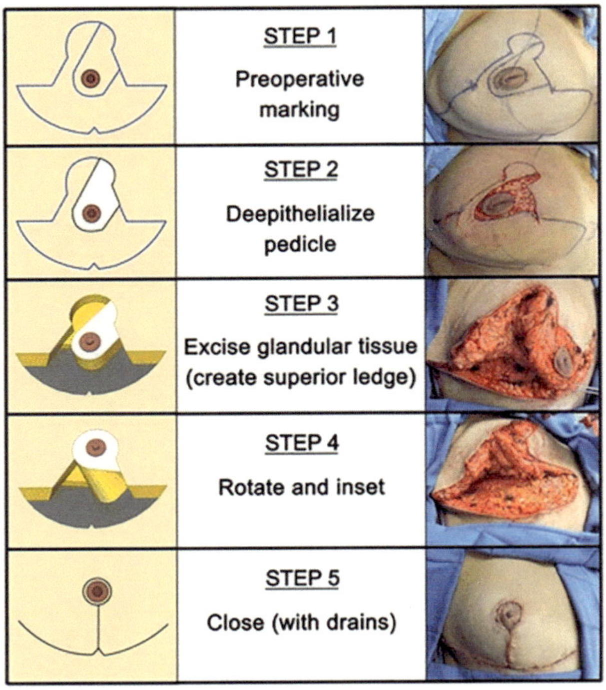

Figure 9.
Drawings and photograph of various steps within the superomedial pedicle reduction.

support the weight of the pedicle and can accommodate the stretching and reshaping more effectively. With the SMP, the NAC has a robust vascular supply from the internal mammary artery perforator and nipple loss is rare [39]. One disadvantage of this technique is that to achieve adequate pedicle rotation to NAC reseating, it is necessary to detach the distal pedicle from the underlying tissue. This sometimes requires a generous amount of undermining of the pedicle, particularly in large breasts with long pedicles. Given this degree of mobilization, blood supply to the distal aspect of the pedicle can become compromised which would affect viability of the NAC [38].

3.1.3 Superior pedicle

The superior pedicle technique preserves the blood supply and innervation to the NAC from the upper portion of the breast. The internal mammary perforators and neurovascular bundle are from the second intercostal space and are the main suppliers of this pedicle. This approach allows the NAC to be repositioned higher on the breast mound while reducing the overall breast volume.

Creation of the superior pedicle involves several critical steps (**Figure 10**) [40]. After preoperative markings and initial incisions, the pedicle is created by preserving tissue from the upper pole of the breast to the NAC. This technique utilizes a wide pedicle of 12–18 cm and a width to length ratio of 2:1 or 1:1 to minimize the risk of ischemia and necrosis [41]. Excess breast tissue, fat, and skin are excised from the lower, lateral, and medial portions of the breast (**Figure 11**) [42]. For a more generous reduction, excess tissue can be excised from the underside of the pedicle. This is safe for NAC viability as long as a pedicle thickness of at least 3 cm is maintained. The NAC is elevated and the remaining skin and soft tissue are closed in multiple layers.

DOI: http://dx.doi.org/10.5772/intechopen.1007104

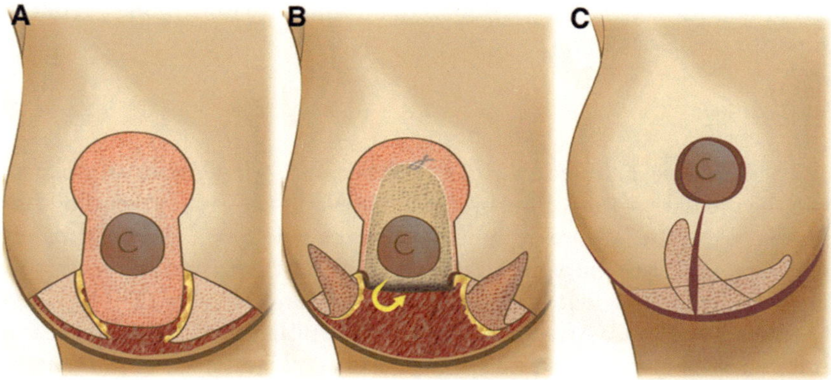

Figure 10.
Diagram of performing a modified approach to superior pedicle flap. (a) Superiorly based pedicled glandular flap dissected and both dermal flaps de-epidermized. (b) Cranial rotation to increase upper pole fullness. (c) Final result after medial fixation of the lateral triangular flap.

The superior pedicle technique offers several advantages. The superior pedicle technique is particularly beneficial for patients with moderate breast size and significant ptosis where the bulk of the excess parenchyma is below the NAC. This technique allows for significant reduction and lifting of the breast. The superior pedicle method often results in a well-defined upper pole [43]. This technique is relatively versatile and can be used in smaller and medium sized reductions. The resultant scars from a superior pedicle approach can be less extensive because the skin excision options are not limited to the conventional wise pattern and can also include vertical and periareolar patterns [41]. Major disadvantages to the superior pedicle technique include limited use in large reductions and a high risk of sensory loss at the NAC. The superior pedicle is not ideal for larger resection, particularly in patients with excess upper pole tissue, as it can be difficult to inset the pedicle [44]. The superior pedicle also has a significantly higher risk of sensory loss of the NAC, with studies demonstrating

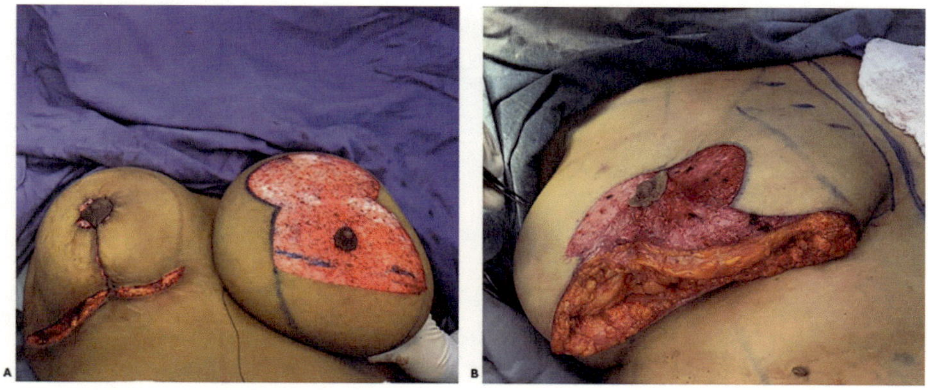

Figure 11.
Superior pedicle wise pattern excision. (A) Patient's right breast shows a completed parenchymal and skin excision and beginning of skin closure. Patient's left breast showed the pedicle which has been de-epithelialized. The round aspect of the keyhole is the anticipated new site of the NAC. The skin and soft tissue inferior to the de-epithelialized segment will be excised. (B) The inferior skin and parenchyma has been excised. The pedicle has also been debulked—the excess tissue deep to the pedicle has been excised and the pedicle is a minimum thickness of 3 cm. The NAC is then plicated to the center of the circular area.

decreased in sensation as high as 70% of women who have undergone a reduction with a superior pedicle [45, 46].

3.1.4 Medial pedicle

Medial pedicle breast reduction preserves blood supply and innervation to the NAC from the medial portion of the breast. Preservation of tissue extending from the medial breast to the NAC creates a pedicle with a retained blood and nervous supply to the NAC via internal mammary perforators and medial intercostal nerves, respectively.

Creating the medial pedicle involves several key steps (**Figure 12**) [47]. Firstly, the desired pedicle is outlined. After, the pedicle is de-epithelialized. Excess breast tissue, such as fat and skin, are excised from the upper, lateral, and inferior portions of the breast (**Figure 13**) [48]. The resultant pedicle length is approximately 4–5 cm. It is important to maintain a pedicle width of approximately 7–8 cm to ensure adequate blood supply from the third internal mammary artery [49]. The de-epithelialized pedicle is then rotated upward to reposition the NAC to a higher location [49]. Drain placement is not required to prevent fluid accumulation, though ultimately, the decision to place a drain is left to the discretion of the surgeon [50]. The incisions are closed in multiple layers [50].

The medial pedicle technique offers several advantages. This technique lifts and reshapes the breast more in comparison to the SMP technique due to elimination of the superior pedicle attachment and thus, a wider arc of rotation is available to the pedicle. Additionally, this method proves to have a high rate of sensation preservation and viability of the NAC while allowing for significant parenchymal excisions [51, 52]. The rate of

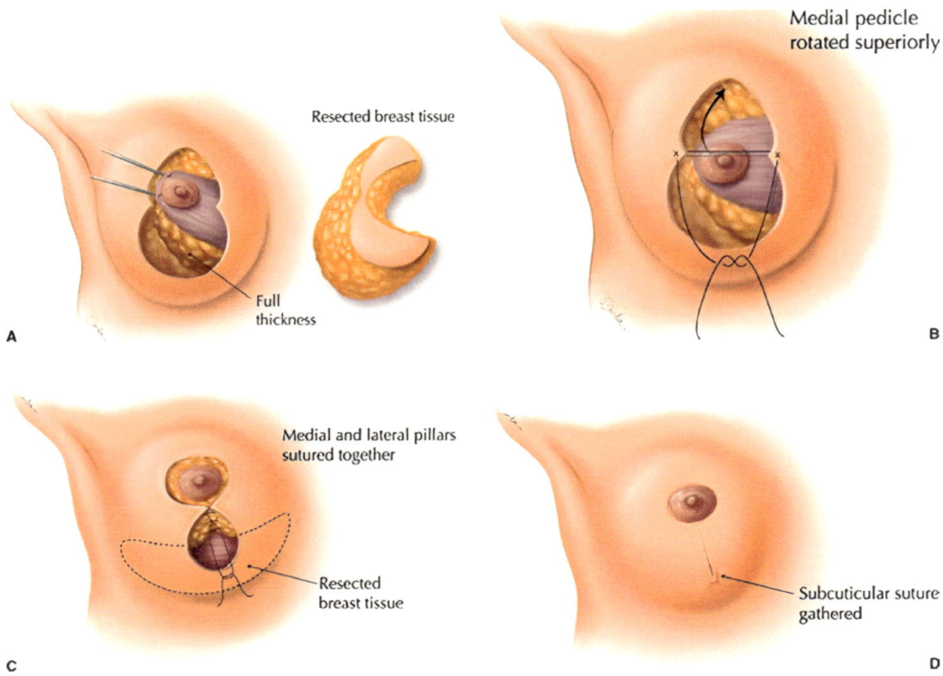

Figure 12.
Diagram of performing a medial pedicle flap. (a) Medial pedicle and skin resection pattern. (b) Rotation of pedicle. Note that the inferior border of the medial pedicle is now the medial pillar. (c) Closure of the pillars. (d). Closure of the areola and skin.

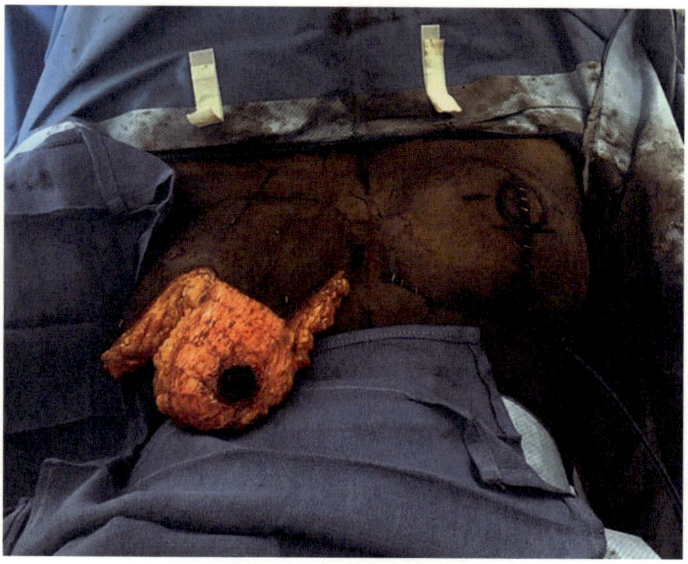

Figure 13.
Medial pedicle with wise pattern reduction. The patient's right side shows the remaining pedicle after removal of excess lateral and inferior tissue. The patient's left shows the planned skin closure around the pedicle.

pseudoptosis is lower compared to the inferior pedicle technique [30]. Furthermore, this technique is particularly beneficial for patients with pronounced medial fullness or those who desire to have greater projection of the medial aspect of the breast post-operatively. Disadvantages include limited overall breast projection and suboptimal breast shape [49, 50]. Additionally, this technique is limited in ability to remove large volumes of breast tissue unless dog ears are created to accommodate excess removal [49].

3.1.5 Central mound

The central mound technique maintains blood supply and innervation to the NAC through the central portion of the breast. This approach elevates the NAC while reducing overall breast volume.

Breast tissue extending from the NAC to the central portion of the breast is preserved, ensuring that the NAC retains its blood supply and nerve connections through the pectoralis major muscle. (**Figure 14**) [53–55]. The excess breast tissue is preferentially taken from the superolateral quadrant (**Figure 15**) [56]. The superomedial breast tissue is preserved to maintain upper breast fullness. If additional tissue excision is required, tissue is taken from the inferior medial breast. The inferolateral tissue on the mound is rotated into the space created by the superolateral resection and secured to the pectoralis fascia [54]. This re-establishes the rounded shape of the breast, narrows the base width, and fills the upper pole of the breast. The medial dermal flaps are also secured to the pectoralis muscle fascia thereby providing internal support that does not rely solely on the skin flaps [54]. Skin flaps of at least 2 cm thick are created superiorly [55]. The flaps are then closed in multiple layers around the pedicle, creating a new IMF crease [54, 55].

The central mound method results in the most natural breast shape with a well-defined upper pole and a gentle slope toward the lower pole [53]. This technique provides a balanced projection throughout the breast and preserved sensation of the NAC, even in cases of severe breast hypertrophy due to the central blood and nervous

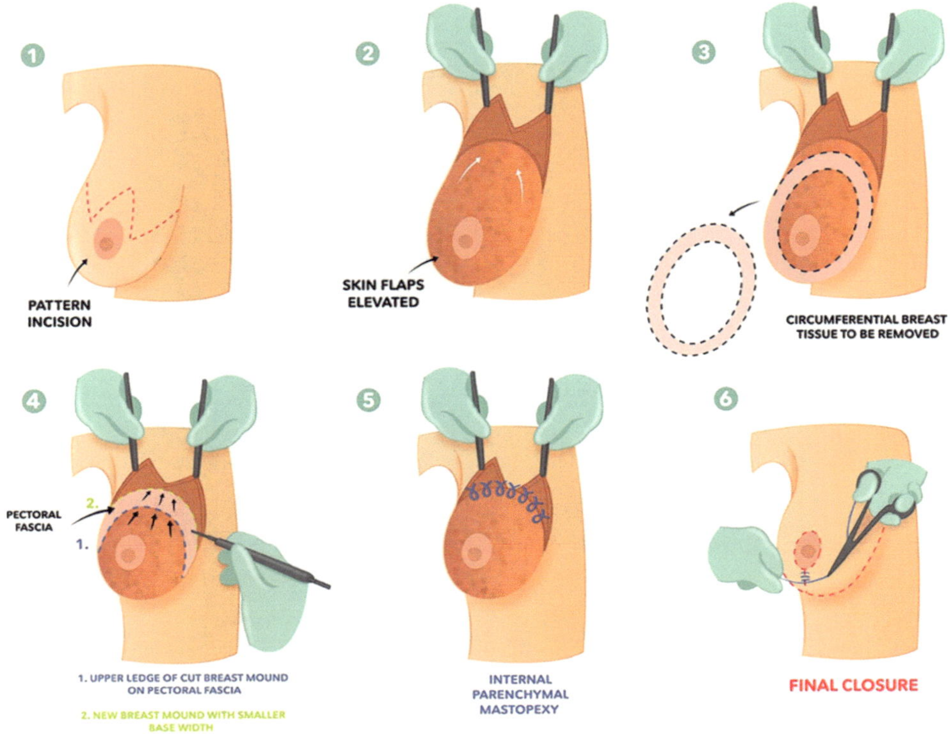

Figure 14.
Schematic depicting the central mound reduction technique. (1) A standard wise-pattern incision is marked on the patient. (2) The superior skin flaps are elevated in the plane between the breast capsule and subcutaneous tissue. (3) The desired base width is marked, and the breast parenchyma is resected to preserve the central mound cone. (4,5) The central mound pedicle is secured to the upper parenchymal ridge as an internal mastopexy. (6) Closure.

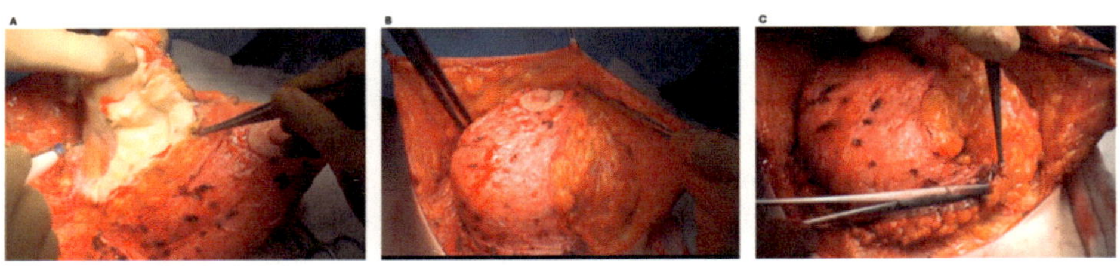

Figure 15.
Central mound pedicle (A) excision of the excess tissue in the superolateral quadrant (B) plication of the lateral tissue to the lateral upper pectoral fascia (C) securing the medical dermal flap to the medial pectoral fascia.

supply from the chest wall [55, 57]. Other advantages include the multiple sources of vascularity and possibility for extensive resection circumferentially [53]. However, the most notable disadvantage of the central mound technique includes difficulty achieving symmetry, particularly in patients with pre-existing asymmetry along either horizontal or vertical axes.

The central mound technique is especially suited for those with moderate to large breast size, even distribution of tissue and moderate ptosis who desire significant lift [55]. It is particularly useful for those seeking a more natural breast shape with a well-defined upper pole and gentle lower pole slope with balanced projection throughout the breasts.

3.1.6 Free nipple graft

Free Nipple Graft (FNG) is a technique used for patients with severe gigantomastia who require such a substantial reduction that compromised blood flow to the NAC is very likely. Most reduction techniques are centered around a pedicle of tissue in which the key objective is to maintain the blood supply to the nipple. This approach allows for more extensive tissue removal and reshaping of breast tissue.

When performing the FNG technique, the NAC is completely excised and the areola is harvested as a full thickness skin graft to be applied to the breast mound at the end of the reduction. (**Figures 16** and **17**) [58, 59].

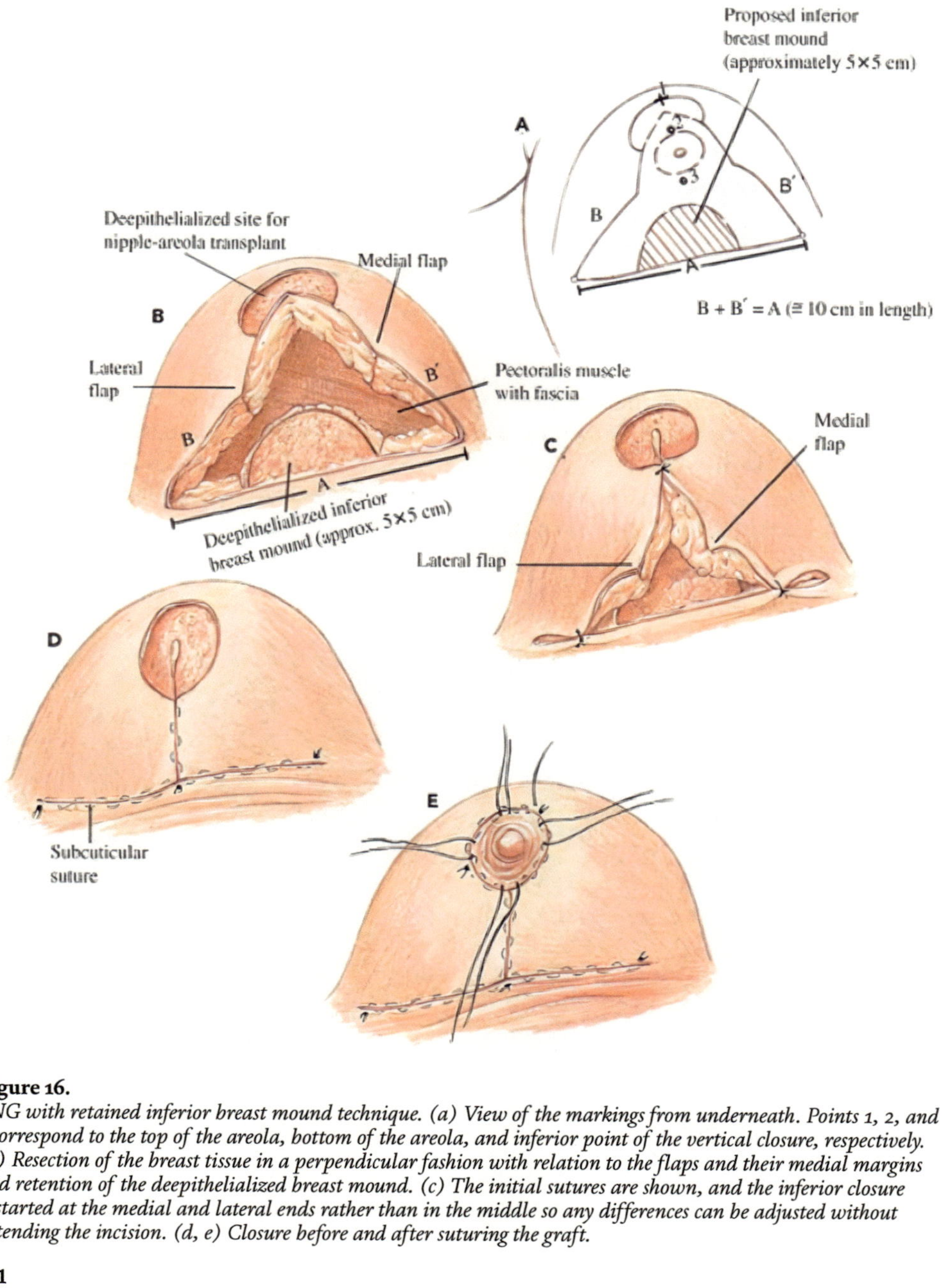

Figure 16.
FNG with retained inferior breast mound technique. (a) View of the markings from underneath. Points 1, 2, and 3 correspond to the top of the areola, bottom of the areola, and inferior point of the vertical closure, respectively. (b) Resection of the breast tissue in a perpendicular fashion with relation to the flaps and their medial margins and retention of the deepithelialized breast mound. (c) The initial sutures are shown, and the inferior closure is started at the medial and lateral ends rather than in the middle so any differences can be adjusted without extending the incision. (d, e) Closure before and after suturing the graft.

The FNG technique offers several advantages. One of the main benefits is the ability to achieve significant reduction in breast size that would not be possible with traditional pedicle techniques [60]. This method is particularly useful for patients with extremely large or pendulous breasts, where the blood supply to the NAC might be compromised if left attached during the procedure because it would be impossible to maintain the recommended length to width ratio of 3:1 while still achieving a generous reduction. By using the FNG technique, the risk of NAC necrosis is eliminated. Additionally, this technique allows for more flexibility in positioning the areola, resulting in better esthetic outcomes [61]. However, the FNG technique also has some notable disadvantages such as the loss of sensation and function to the nipple, as the nerves are severed during the removal for grafting. This results in permanent numbness and dysfunction of the nipple and areola. Additionally, the ability to breastfeed is lost [61]. Further, there is always a risk of skin graft failure.

Indications for the FNG technique are patients with markedly pendulous breasts and excessively long distance between the sternal notch and nipple. This is because the blood supply to the nipple in the native breast has a long course before reaching the NAC. After a reductive surgery, these patients have a proportionally higher risk of nipple death given the chance of blood flow compromise. Additionally, older patients or those with certain medical conditions that might impair wound healing or blood flow to the NAC are often considered for this technique.

3.2 Skin excision

Skin excision is a fundamental aspect of breast reduction procedures. This aspect of the procedure focuses on the removal of excess skin. The excision patterns include vertical, Wise pattern ('inverted T'), and periareolar. The technique utilized is determined by the amount of excess skin, the location of the excess skin, the patient's skin type, and the desired cosmetic scar outcome.

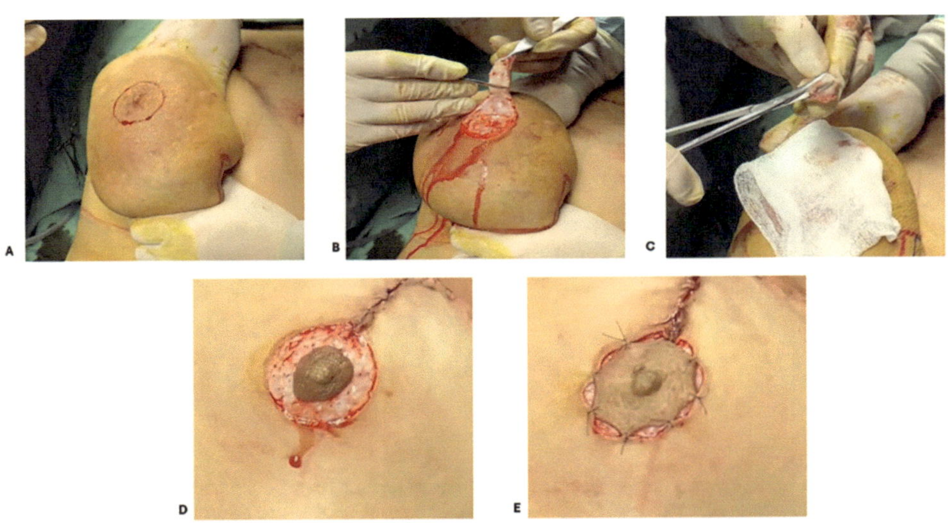

Figure 17.
Free nipple graft (A) incision around the NAC (B) harvesting the NAC graft (C) thinning the graft (D) overlay of the graft onto de-epithelialized dermis (E) securing the nipple graft with suture.

DOI: http://dx.doi.org/10.5772/intechopen.1007104

3.2.1 Vertical

Vertical breast reduction, also known as the vertical scar or lollipop incision, focuses on minimizing scarring while achieving significant reduction and reshaping of breasts.

Conducting a vertical skin excision begins with a circumferential areolar incision (**Figure 18**) [62]. First, the desired pedicle is created. Medial and lateral dissections are performed with generous undermining, resulting in the desired size of the reduced breast [62]. Next, excision of skin and soft tissue inferior to the NAC and its associated pedicle is performed. This excised tissue is usually resembles a semicircle or oblong shape and extends to the IMF (**Figure 19**) [63]. This pattern of excision resembles a lollipop [62]. Once sufficient tissue is removed, the vertical limbs are approximated and the nipple is set [62]. If there is redundant skin at the inferior

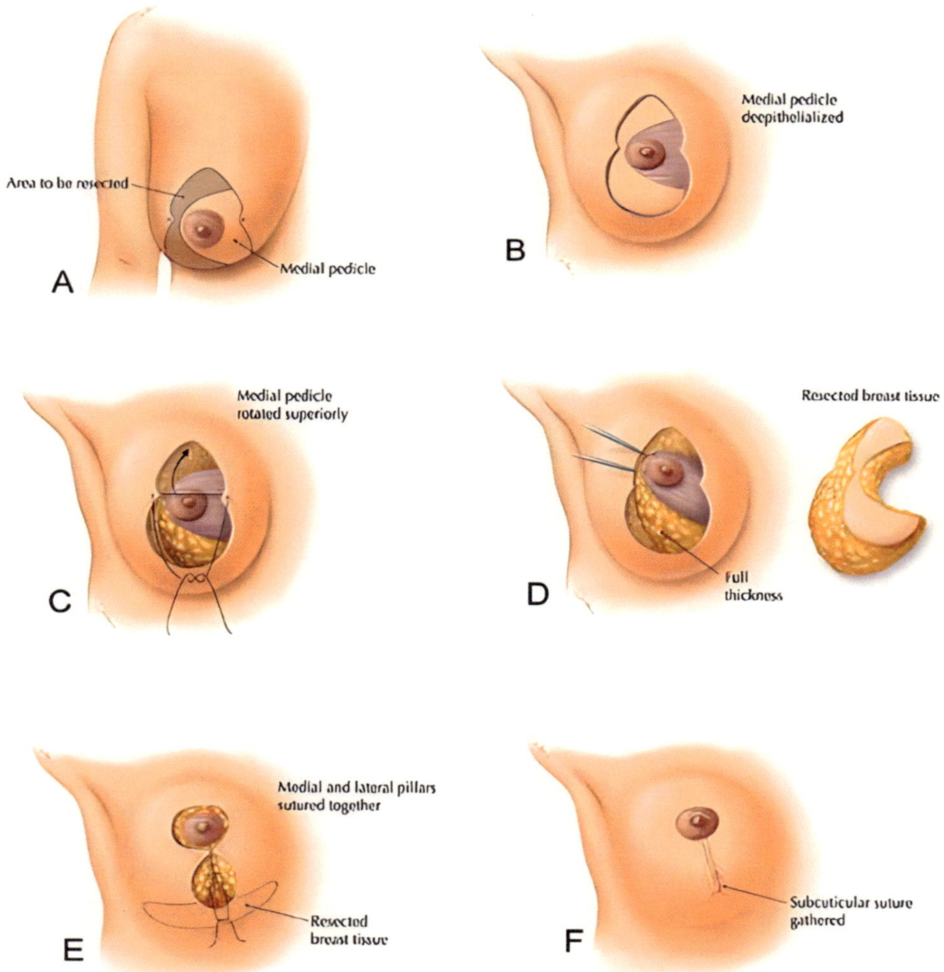

Figure 18.
A medial pedicle technique with a vertical pattern skin excision. (A) Markings. (B), Pedicle design. (C) Creation of the pedicle. (D) Parenchymal resection. (E) Closure of the vertical pillars and resection of lower pole skin and parenchyma. (F) Incision closure.

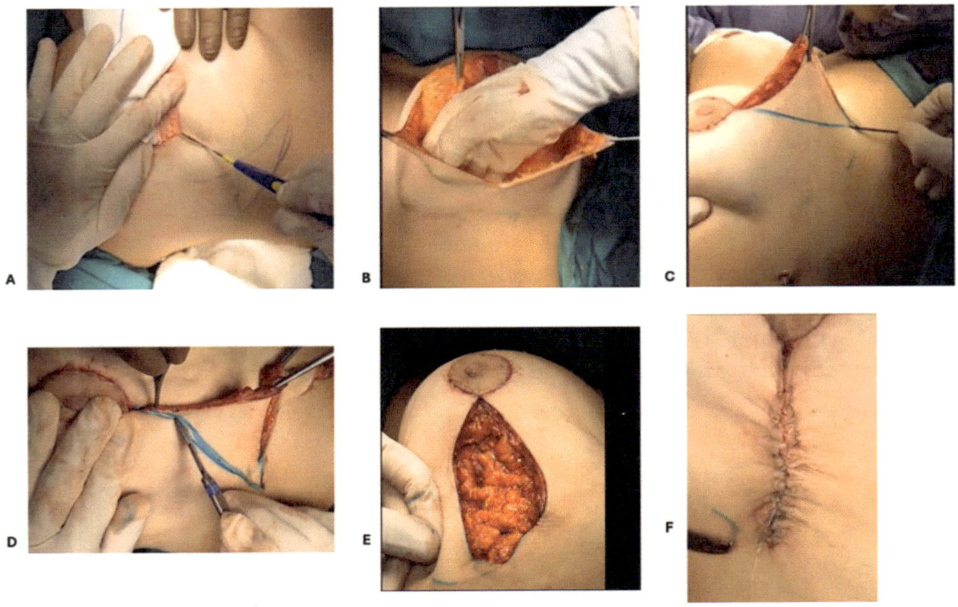

Figure 19.
Vertical skin excision (A) incision skin at the midline of the breast below the NAC to the IMF (B) create wide skin flaps and perform the parenchymal excision (C) pulling the skin taut, determine the amount of excess vertical skin can be excised (D) excise the redundant vertical skin (E) resultant defect after skin excision (F) approximate the vertical limbs.

aspect of the incision, the midpoint is secured at the IMF and the lateral dog ears are removed, creating a very small horizontal IMF scar.

Advantages of vertical skin excision include lack of an inframammary incision, reducing the surface area of scarring. This proves especially helpful in patients with a propensity of keloids or hypertrophic scars [64]. Additionally, the vertical technique allows for effective lifting and reshaping of the breast, resulting in a more natural breast shape with a well-defined upper pole (**Figure 20**) [64, 65]. The vertical scar supports the new breast shape more effectively than many other methods, reducing the risk of lower pole fullness or pseudoptosis [44, 64]. Disadvantages include possible puckering of the lower end of the scar or decreased effectiveness for extensive tissue removal of very large breasts as the limited skin excision might not provide adequate access for reduction [44, 64]. Another disadvantage includes possible visualization of the vertical incision below the level of the new inframammary fold [64].

Skin elasticity typically found in younger patient populations proves to be helpful and provides for better esthetic outcomes with more effective accommodation for reshaping alongside reduction. The vertical skin excision pattern is sufficient for patients with moderate breast hypertrophy and ptosis who desire reduction with minimal scarring, offering a balance between tissue removal, skin excision, and esthetic outcomes [64].

3.2.2 Wise pattern

Wise pattern skin excision, also known as the 'inverted T' or anchor incision, is a widely used technique which allows for significant tissue removal and dramatic reshaping.

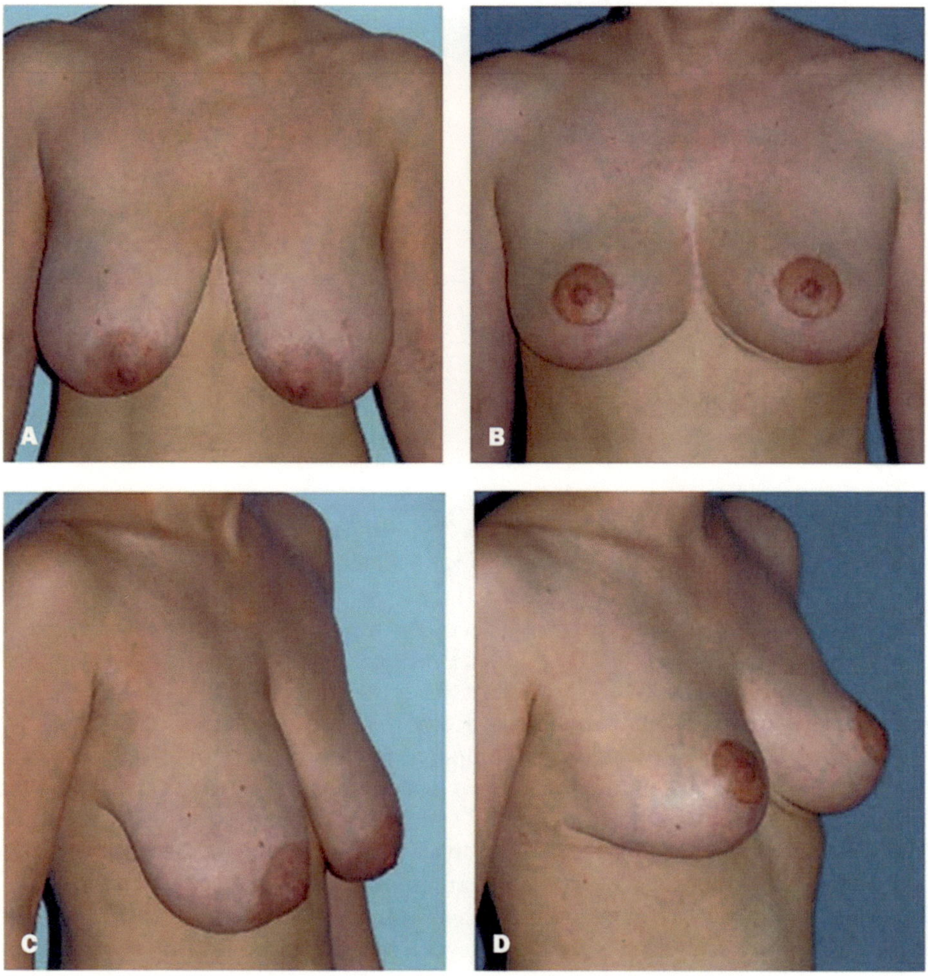

Figure 20.
(A,C) Preoperative views of bilateral ptosis. (B,D) Postoperative views of bilateral breast reduction with a vertical skin excision pattern.

Conducting a Wise pattern skin excision begins with preoperative marking (**Figure 21**) [66]. The breast meridian is measured and marked at 6–8 cm from the sternal notch and a vertical line is made down each breast. The upper breast border (UBB) is determined by manually lifting the breast and identifying where the breast projection begins. The anticipated NAC position is marked approximately 20 cm from the sternal notch along the breast meridian which should roughly equate to 8 cm from the UBB. From the NAC position, two vertical limbs are designed to make an inverted V, each limb measuring approximately 10–11 cm. The length of the limbs vary among patients. They are dependent on preoperative breast size, desired reduction outcome, and are usually longer for larger breasts. The IMF is outlined and connected to the inverted V.

Once the pedicle size and shape are deemed satisfactory, the skin and soft tissue between the inverted V and inframammary fold are removed. The skin is then brought together as depicted in **Figure 14**. The two vertical limbs are brought down and secured to the midpoint of the inframammary fold incision. The vertical limb

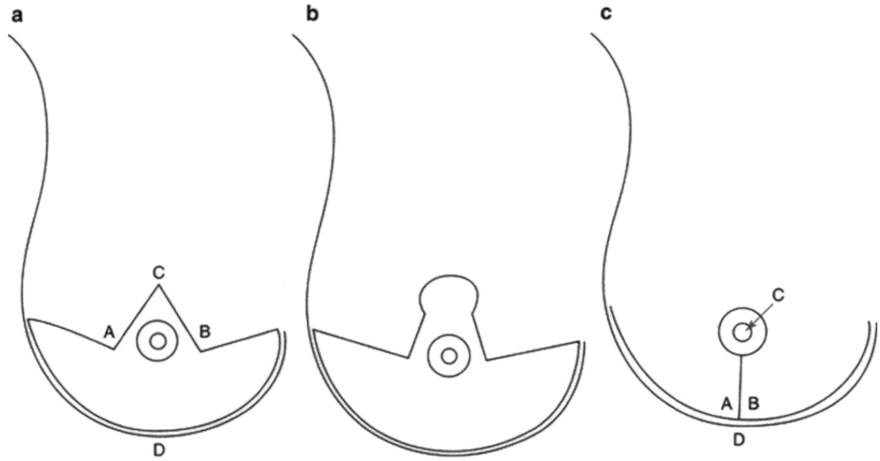

Figure 21.
Traditional markings for a wise pattern breast reduction. The points A and B are brought together to point D. (C) The new nipple position is usually centered on point C.

is then tacked closed to assist with the inset of the nipple. The nipple is set approximately 7–8 cm superior to the IMF. A keyhole is incised for the nipple.

The Wise pattern is particularly advantageous for patients with large breasts and significant ptosis, as it provides extensive access to the breasts for tissue removal and reshaping from multiple points as compared to more limited incision patterns (**Figure 22**) [67, 68]. This method allows for better control over the final breast shape and position of the NAC, ensuring optimal symmetry and proportion. Disadvantages of the Wise pattern include extensive scarring associated with the anchor-shaped incision. The horizontal scar along the inframammary fold, in addition to the vertical and periareolar scars, can be more noticeable and may be a cosmetic concern. Additionally, the extent of incision increases the risk of wound healing complications such as infection and scarring irregularities such as hypertrophic scars and keloids.

Overall, the Wise pattern skin excision is best suited for those with very large breasts and significant ptosis who require substantial reduction and reshaping but is effective for all patients desiring breast reconstruction. Additionally, those with poor skin elasticity or excess skin may achieve better esthetic outcomes with the Wise pattern, as it provides the most effective approach for removing excess tissue and manipulation of NAC positioning. Patients with significant asymmetry or complex breast anatomy may especially benefit from Wise pattern breast reduction due to the extensive alterations that may be achieved with this method.

3.2.3 Periareolar pattern

The periareolar skin pattern involves solely making an incision around the areola (**Figure 23**) [69]. This technique begins with creating a circumferential areolar incision. Parenchymal excision is performed through this incision alone. If a more extensive reduction is required, other techniques such as a vertical extension can be performed for more access to the breast tissue along with excising more excess skin.

A pronounced benefit to this approach is that the scar is well-hidden at the natural pigment transition of the breast and areola. This technique is particularly effective

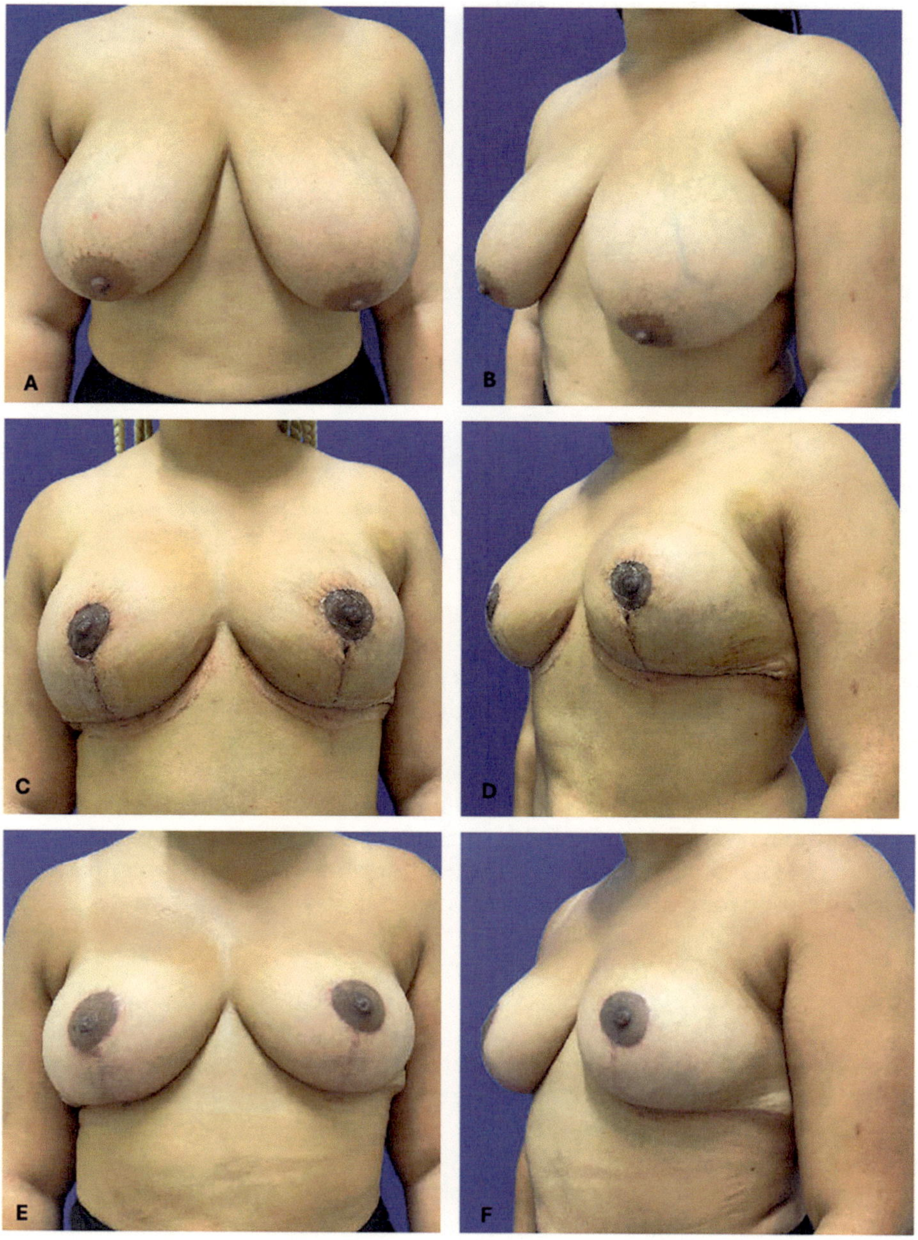

Figure 22.
Perioperative wise pattern. (A) Preoperative anterior view (B) preoperative left oblique view (C) anterior view 2 weeks post-op (D) left oblique view 2 weeks post-op (E) anterior view 6 weeks post-op (F) left oblique view 6 weeks post-op.

for patients with moderate breast size and mild ptosis who do not generally require a significant amount of skin excised and do not require a dramatic relocation of the NAC.

A drawback to the periareolar pattern is the restrictive working space. Additionally, the amount of parenchyma and skin that can be removed is limited

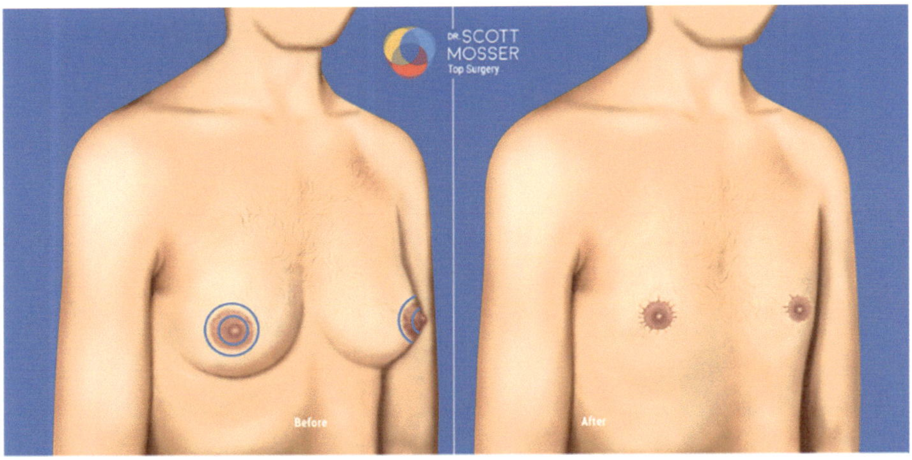

Figure 23.
Figure demonstrating location of periareolar incisions in a male patient with gynecomastia undergoing a reduction.

compared to more extensive and open excision patterns like the Wise pattern. This technique may not be suitable for patients with very large breasts or significant ptosis because it may not provide sufficient access for the necessary tissue removal and reshaping [70]. This approach can also result in changes to nipple sensation and function and can cause areolar stretching or widening over time.

Overall, the periareolar skin excision is suitable for patients with mild to moderate breast hypertrophy and minimal ptosis and minimal excess skin who desire a reduction with minimal visible scarring. This method is ideal for patients seeking a more conservative reduction with a focus on esthetic outcomes. The periareolar pattern is also a good option for patients with mild to moderate asymmetry.

4. Postoperative care

After breast reduction surgery, post-operative care is crucial to ensure optimal recovery. Inflammation and ecchymosis are common after surgery and patients are advised to wear a supportive surgical bra or compression garment to minimize swelling and provide adequate support.

During the initial recovery phase, patients are instructed to avoid strenuous activities and heavy lifting to prevent strain on the surgical incisions. Drain management is part of recovery in a few instances and drains are typically removed once daily output is less than 30 cc per day.

Follow-up appointments with the surgeon are scheduled to monitor progress, assess healing, and address any concerns. During these visits, the surgeon may provide guidance on scar management which may include the use of topical emollients or silicone sheets.

The emotional and psychological adjustment to the appearance of a patient's new breasts can also be a significant aspect of post-operative care. Patients may experience a range of emotions, from relief and satisfaction to temporary feelings of discomfort or body dysmorphia as they adapt to their new appearance. Support from healthcare professionals, as well as family and friends, can play a crucial role in recovery.

4.1 Postoperative complications

In this section, we will discuss our institution's experience with common postoperative complications after bilateral reduction mammaplasty using a cohort of 182 patients [71].

Immediate postoperative complications include excess bleeding from a transected arterial vessel. If a large hematoma forms, this may necessitate return to the operating room for hematoma evacuation and ligation of the inciting vessel. Postoperative hematoma requiring reoperation occurred in 2.75% of patients.

Other postoperative complications include seroma formation. This would be identified several weeks after surgery as breast asymmetry and notable firmness or bogginess of the affected breast. Aspiration of the seroma followed by compression is the treatment for postoperative seroma. Seroma was encountered in 0.55% of patients. Fat necrosis is a self-limiting condition in which devitalized fat solidifies. It presents like a nodule under the skin. This does not require surgical excision and will self-resolve with time. Wound breakdown is the most common postoperative complication. The most likely sites are the area under the most tension. For example

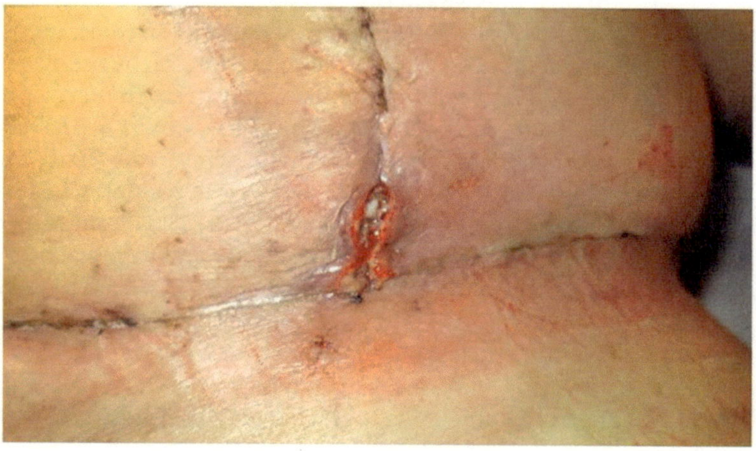

Figure 24.
This figure depicts a minor dehiscence at the T point of a wise pattern skin closure after a breast reduction.

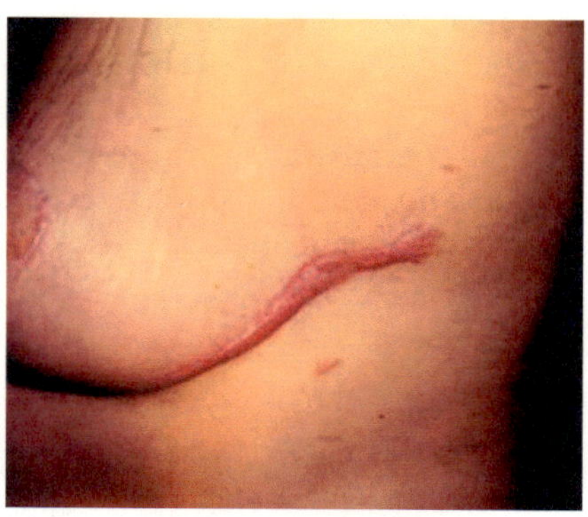

Figure 25.
Keloid of inframammary incision after a breast reduction.

in a wise pattern reduction, the 'T point,' where the two vertical limbs come together at the IMF, is the area under the most tension and where patients may develop a minor wound dehiscence (**Figure 24**) [72]. Areas where moisture is most likely to be retained are also at high risk for wound breakdown; for example, the IMF. Local wound care is usually sufficient to promote wound healing. In our cohort, dehiscence occurred at a rate of 36%. Wound healing setbacks may result in scar widening in the affected areas. Keloids were seen in 1.1% of post-operative patients (**Figure 25**) [73]. Scar revision was required in 3.3% of patients. Loss of nipple sensation occurred in 4.95% of patients and hypersensitivity was seen in 0.55% of patients. Partial and full nipple loss occurs if the blood supply to the NAC is compromised. Partial nipple lost was seen at a rate of 2.2% and full nipple loss at a rate of 0.55%. Partial and full nipple loss was managed with local wound care.

5. Nonoperative management

Non-operative management of breast hypertrophy focuses primarily on lifestyle modification including diet and exercise for weight loss. This approach aims to reduce overall body fat, including fat deposits in the breasts, potentially leading to a decrease in breast size and alleviation of associated symptoms such as discomfort and physical strain. In select cases, targeted liposuction for fat reduction can be useful.

Liposuction offers a less invasive option for managing breast hypertrophy, particularly for patients who have excess adipose tissue of the breasts but have minimal glandular hypertrophy or ptosis. This procedure involves inserting a stiff cannula through a small incision near or on the breast to evacuate excess fat. It allows for targeted fat removal, resulting in a modest reduction in breast volume. Liposuction is generally suitable for patients with optimal skin elasticity and minimal breast ptosis, given that by nature of the procedure, breast parenchyma and fat are removed but excess skin is not.

Good candidates for non-operative management include individuals with mild to moderate breast hypertrophy who are motivated to pursue weight loss through lifestyle changes. These patients should have good overall health and realistic expectations regarding the outcomes of weight loss or liposuction. They should also have adequate skin elasticity to accommodate potential changes in breast size and contour.

Conversely, poor candidates for non-operative management typically include patients with severe breast hypertrophy characterized by significant glandular tissue and ptosis. These individuals may not achieve satisfactory results through weight loss alone, as the excess skin cannot be effectively reduced without surgical intervention. Patients with poor skin elasticity or a history of unsuccessful attempts at weight loss may also be less suitable for non-operative approaches. In such cases, surgical options like breast reduction surgery may be more appropriate to achieve the desired reduction in breast size and improvement in symptoms.

6. Conclusion

In conclusion, this chapter has provided an in-depth exploration of breast reduction surgery, a crucial procedure for addressing the physical and psychological burdens of breast hypertrophy. By examining the pathogenesis, epidemiology, and anatomical considerations, this chapter has provided a solid foundation for understanding the complexities involved in surgical planning. The discussion of various surgical techniques underscores the importance of tailoring the surgical strategy to each patient's unique anatomy and desired outcomes. Furthermore, the potential complications and postoperative considerations highlight the need for planning and patient-centered care to optimize results and minimize risks. As breast reduction surgery continues to evolve, ongoing research and clinical experience will undoubtedly refine these techniques, enhancing both functional and esthetic outcomes for patients. This chapter serves as a comprehensive resource for clinicians and patients, offering valuable insights and foundational knowledge on breast reduction surgery.

Acknowledgements

The authors would like to acknowledge the support from the Frederick P. Whiddon College of Medicine and the University of South Alabama. No funding was allocated for the creation of this chapter.

Conflict of interest

The authors declare no conflict of interest.

Author details

Chandler Hinson*, Victoria Bouillon, Hallie Masters, Polly Jasper and Ronald Brooks
Frederick P. Whiddon College of Medicine, University of South Alabama, Mobile, Alabama, United States of America

*Address all correspondence to: csh2121@jagmail.southalabama.edu

References

[1] Rahman GA, Adigun IA, Yusuf IF. Macromastia: A review of presentation and management. The Nigerian Postgraduate Medical Journal. 2010;**17**:45-49

[2] Güemes A, Pérez E, Sousa R, Gil I, Valcarreres MP, Carrera P, et al. Quality of life and alleviation of symptoms after breast reduction for macromastia in obese patients: Is surgery worth it? Aesthetic Plastic Surgery. 2016;**40**:62-70

[3] Gonzalez MA, Glickman LT, Aladegbami B, Simpson RL. Quality of life after breast reduction surgery: A 10-year retrospective analysis using the breast Q questionnaire: Does breast size matter? Annals of Plastic Surgery. 2012;**69**:361

[4] Côrrea MDPD, Costa AMD, Côrrea LD, Dornelas MT, Venturelli-Júnior EP, Chaoubah A. Assessment of the quality of life in patients with breast hypertrophy before and after reduction mammoplasty. Revista Brasileira de Cirurgia Plástica. 2023;**34**:204-209

[5] Dafydd H, Roehl KR, Phillips LG, Dancey A, Peart F, Shokrollahi K. Redefining gigantomastia. Journal of Plastic, Reconstructive & Aesthetic Surgery. 2011;**64**:160-163

[6] Dancey A, Khan M, Dawson J, Peart F. Gigantomastia – A classification and review of the literature. Journal of Plastic, Reconstructive & Aesthetic Surgery. 2008;**61**:493-502

[7] Massey GG, Firriolo JM, Nuzzi LC, Pramanick T, Malloy SM, DiVasta AD, et al. Risk factors associated with severe macromastia among adolescents and young women. Plastic and Reconstructive Surgery. 2022;**150**:1212

[8] Nuzzi LC, Pramanick T, Massey GG, Walsh LR, McNamara CT, Firriolo JM, et al. The impact of combined oral contraceptives on adolescents with macromastia. Plastic and Reconstructive Surgery. 2022;**150**:731

[9] Cerrato F, Webb ML, Rosen H, Nuzzi L, McCarty ER, DiVasta AD, et al. The impact of macromastia on adolescents: A cross-sectional study. Pediatrics. 2012;**130**:e339-e346

[10] Wolfswinkel EM, Lemaine V, Weathers WM, Chike-Obi CJ, Xue AS, Heller L. Hyperplastic breast anomalies in the female adolescent breast. Seminars in Plastic Surgery. 2013;**27**:49-55

[11] Jabaiti S, Fayyad L, Isleem U. Prednisolone-induced virginal mammary hypertrophy: Case report. International Journal of Surgery Case Reports. 2019;**59**:140-143

[12] Jud SM, Brendle-Behnisch A, Hack CC, Preuss C, Arkudas A, Horch RE, et al. Macromastia: An economic burden? A disease cost analysis based on real-world data in Germany. Archives of Gynecology and Obstetrics. 2021;**303**:521-531

[13] Peters F. Entwicklungsstörungen der Mamma und deren Behandlung. Gynakologe. 1998;**31**:549-557

[14] Foreste V, Corte LD, Stradella C, Cusati B, Coco G, Stradella L. Gigantomastia during pregnancy due to Burkitt lymphoma. European Journal of Breast Health. 2021;**17**:76-80

[15] Deepinder F, Braunstein GD. Gynecomastia: Incidence, causes and treatment. Expert Review of Endocrinology & Metabolism. 2011;**6**:723-730

[16] Fagerlund A, Lewin R, Rufolo G, Elander A, Santanelli di Pompeo F, Selvaggi G. Gynecomastia: A systematic review. Journal of Plastic Surgery and Hand Surgery. 2015;**49**:311-318

[17] Gonzalez F, Walton RL, Shafer B, Matory WEJ, Borah GL. Reduction mammaplasty improves symptoms of macromastia. Plastic and Reconstructive Surgery. 1993;**91**:1270

[18] Pérez-Panzano E, Güemes-Sánchez A, Gascón-Catalán A. Quality of life following symptomatic macromastia surgery: Short- and long-term evaluation. The Breast Journal. 2016;**22**:397-406

[19] Bruhlmann Y, Tschopp H. Breast reduction improves symptoms of macromastia and has a long-lasting effect. Annals of Plastic Surgery. 1998;**41**:240

[20] Hernanz F, Fidalgo M, Muñoz P, Noriega MG, Gómez-Fleitas M. Impact of reduction mammoplasty on the quality of life of obese patients suffering from symptomatic macromastia: A descriptive cohort study. Journal of Plastic, Reconstructive & Aesthetic Surgery. 2016;**69**:e168-e173

[21] Glatt BS, Sarwer DB, O'Hara DE, Hamori C, Bucky LP, LaRossa D. A retrospective study of changes in physical symptoms and body image after reduction mammaplasty. Plastic and Reconstructive Surgery. 1999;**103**:76

[22] Rinker B, Veneracion M, Walsh CP. Breast ptosis: Causes and cure. Annals of Plastic Surgery. 2010;**64**:579

[23] See M-H, Yip K-C, Teh M-S, Teoh L-Y, Lai L-L, Wong L-K, et al. Classification and assessment techniques of breast ptosis: A systematic review. Journal of Plastic, Reconstructive & Aesthetic Surgery. 2023;**83**:380-395

[24] Pontell M, Noah H, Brown A, Rose M, Ashinoff R, Saad A. Single stage nipple-sparing mastectomy and reduction mastopexy in the ptotic breast. Plastic Surgery International. 2018;**2018**:1-9

[25] Kammath V. The Breasts - TeachMeAnatomy [Internet]. TeachMe Anatomy; 2022. Available from: https://teachmeanatomy.info/thorax/organs/breasts/ [Accessed: July 26, 2024]

[26] Mikołajczyk M, Kasielska-Trojan A, Antoszewski B. A new tool for breast anthropometric measurements: Presentation and validation for women and men. Aesthetic Plastic Surgery. 2019;**43**:1160-1170

[27] The Breasts - Learn Surgery Online [Internet]. 2020. Available from: https://learnsurgeryonline.com/the-breasts/ [Accessed: July 26, 2024]

[28] Putte P, Blockmans D, Rop C, Versyck B. Pectoral nerve block type II as the sole anesthetic for removal of a large axillary tumor: A case report. A & A Practice. 2020;**14**:e01201

[29] UCLA. Breast Anatomy [Internet]. Available from: https://www.uclahealth.org/departments/radiology/education/breast-imaging-teaching-resources/screening-mammogram/breast-anatomy [Accessed: July 26, 2024]

[30] Wong C, Vucovich M, Rohrich R. Mastopexy and reduction mammoplasty pedicles and skin resection patterns. Plastic and Reconstructive Surgery – Global Open. 2014;**2**:e202

[31] O'Grady KF, Thoma A, Cin AD. A comparison of complication rates in large and small inferior pedicle reduction mammaplasty. Plastic and Reconstructive Surgery. 2005;**115**:736

[32] Losken A. Inferior Pedicle Wise Pattern Tissue Resection and Breast Shaping. Video 2 from Safe Reproducible Breast Reduction. 2023. Available from: https://journals.lww.com/prsgo/pages/video.aspx?autoPlay=false&v=837 [Accessed: September 3, 2024]

[33] Sandsmark M, Amland PF, Abyholm F, Traaholt L. Reduction mammaplasty. A comparative study of the Orlando and Robbins methods in 292 patients. Scandinavian Journal of Plastic and Reconstructive Surgery and Hand Surgery. 1992;**26**:203-209

[34] Chang P, Shaaban AF, Canady JW, Ricciardelli EJ, Cram AE. Reduction mammaplasty: The results of avoiding nipple-areolar amputation in cases of extreme hypertrophy. Annals of Plastic Surgery. 1996;**37**:585

[35] Kankaya Y, Oruç M, Sungur N, Aslan Ö ç, Gürsoy K, Özer K, et al. Four flap suspension technique for prevention of bottoming out after breast reduction. Annals of Surgical Treatment and Research. 2016;**90**:10-15

[36] Brown RH, Izaddoost S, Bullocks JM. Preventing the "bottoming out" and "star-gazing" phenomena in inferior pedicle breast reduction with an acellular dermal matrix internal brassiere. Aesthetic Plastic Surgery. 2010;**34**:760-767

[37] Henderson PW, Chang MM, Taylor EM, Weinreb R, Rohde CH. The "superior ledge": A modification of the standard superomedial pedicle reduction mammoplasty to accentuate nipple-areola complex projection. Aesthetic Plastic Surgery. 2016;**40**:733-738

[38] Selamioğlu E, Agdoğan Ö. Mammoplasty using modified superomedial pedicle technique in severely macromastia and ptotic breasts. The Breast Journal. 2024;**2024**:7635485

[39] Brown RH, Siy R, Khan K, Izaddoost S. The superomedial pedicle wise-pattern breast reduction: Reproducible, reliable, and resilient. Seminars in Plastic Surgery. 2015;**29**:94-101

[40] Watfa W, Zaugg P, Baudoin J, Bramhall R, Raffoul W, Di Summa P. Dermal triangular flaps to prevent pseudoptosis in mastopexy surgery: The hammock technique. Plastic and Reconstructive Surgery - Global Open. 2019;**7**:e2473

[41] Arbeláez S, Arbeláez SA, Eslait RC, Lacouture CJ. Superior pedicle inverted T-reduction mammaplasty with short horizontal scar. Plastic and Reconstructive Surgery – Global Open. 2024;**12**:e5625

[42] Jaramillo R, Arias C. Breast reduction with total superior pedicle. Plastic and Reconstructive Surgery - Global Open. 2023;**11**:e4735

[43] Klinger M, Klinger F, Maione L, Lisa A, Battistini A, Giannasi S, et al. Superior pedicle breast reduction with prefiguration of final shape: A 10-year retrospective study. Plastic and Reconstructive Surgery - Global Open. 2020;**8**:e3242

[44] Hall-Findlay EJ. Pedicles in vertical breast reduction and mastopexy. Clinics in Plastic Surgery. 2002;**29**:379-391

[45] Chiummariello S, Angelisanti M, Arleo S, Alfano C. Evaluation of the sensitivity after reduction mammoplasty. Our experience and review of the literature. Annali Italiani di Chirurgia. 2013;**84**:385-388

[46] Schlenz I, Rigel S, Schemper M, Kuzbari R. Alteration of nipple and areola sensitivity by reduction mammaplasty: A prospective comparison

of five techniques. Plastic and Reconstructive Surgery. 2005;**115**:743-751; discussion 752-754

[47] Hall-Findlay E. Vertical Reducation Mammaplasty [Internet]. Available from: https://doctorlib.info/surgery/plastic/56.html [Accessed: July 26, 2024]

[48] Hinson C, Bouillon V, Brooks R. Medial pedicle wise-pattern breast reduction for gigantomastia: A single-center retrospective review. Plastic and Reconstructive Surgery - Global Open. 2023;**11**:e5170

[49] Hall-Findlay EJ. Vertical breast reduction with a medially-based pedicle. Aesthetic Surgery Journal. 2002;**22**:185-194

[50] Hunt SC, Sun Y, Azad S. A simplified approach to breast reduction using the medial pedicle. Aesthetic Surgery Journal Open Forum. 2022;**4**:ojac019

[51] Mofid MM, Dellon AL, Elias JJ, Nahabedian MY. Quantitation of breast sensibility following reduction mammaplasty: A comparison of inferior and medial pedicle techniques. Plastic and Reconstructive Surgery. 2002;**109**:2283-2288

[52] Nahabedian MY, Mofid MM. Viability and sensation of the nipple-areolar complex after reduction mammaplasty. Annals of Plastic Surgery. 2002;**49**:24-31; discussion 31-32

[53] DeLong MR, Chang I, Farajzadeh M, Nahabet EH, Roostaeian J, Festekjian J, et al. The central mound pedicle: A safe and effective technique for reduction mammaplasty. Plastic and Reconstructive Surgery. 2020;**146**:725

[54] Balch CR. The central mound technique for reduction mammaplasty. Plastic and Reconstructive Surgery. 1981;**67**:305-311

[55] Hester TR, Bostwick J, Miller L, Cunningham SJ. Breast reduction utilizing the maximally vascularized central breast pedicle. Plastic and Reconstructive Surgery. 1985;**76**:890-900

[56] Eren S, Öreroğlu AR. Modified central pedicle in breast reduction and mastopexy: The dermal suspension technique. Aesthetic Plastic Surgery. 2022;**46**:2753-2765

[57] Hagerty RC, Nowicky DJ. Integration of the central mound technique with the vertical skin takeout reduction mammaplasty. Plastic and Reconstructive Surgery. 1998;**102**:1182-1187

[58] Spear S, Jespersen MR. Breast Reduction with the Free Nipple Graft Technique [Internet]. Plastic Surgery Key; 2016. Available from: https://plasticsurgerykey.com/breast-reduction-with-the-free-nipple-graft-technique/ [Accessed: July 26, 2024]

[59] Mammadli M, Thomas M, D'silva J. Breast Reduction with Free Nipple Graft Transfer. In: Thomas M, D'silva J, editors. Manual of Cosmetic Medicine and Surgery. Singapore: Springer; 2023. DOI: 10.1007/978-981-99-3726-4_16

[60] Vazquez OA, Yerke Hansen P, Komberg J, Slutsky HL, Becker H. Free nipple graft breast reduction without a vertical incision. Plastic and Reconstructive Surgery – Global Open. 2022;**10**:e4167

[61] Colen SR. Breast reduction with use of the free nipple graft technique. Aesthetic Surgery Journal. 2001;**21**:261-271

[62] Simplified Vertical Breast Reduction: Overview, Indications, Contraindications. 2023. Available from: https://emedicine.medscape.com/

article/1818858-overview?form=fpf#a4 [Accessed: July 27, 2024]

[63] Orak F, Baghaki S. Four-flap mammaplasty. Aesthetic Plastic Surgery. 2021;**45**:1458-1465

[64] Beer GM, Spicher I, Cierpka KA, Meyer VE. Benefits and pitfalls of vertical scar breast reduction. British Journal of Plastic Surgery. 2004;**57**:12-19

[65] Kuran I, Tumerdem B. Vertical reduction mammaplasty: Preventing skin redundancy at the vertical scar in women with large breasts or poor skin elasticity. Aesthetic Surgery Journal. 2007;**27**:336-341

[66] Summerhayes C, Cutress RI, Hurren JS. Modification of the wise pattern breast reduction for therapeutic mammoplasty. In: Mugea TT, Shiffman MA, editors. Aesthetic Surgery of the Breast [Internet]. Berlin, Heidelberg: Springer; 2015. pp. 949-953. DOI: 10.1007/978-3-662-43407-9_55

[67] Kreithen J, Caffee H, Rosenberg J, Chin G, Clayman M, Lawson M, et al. A comparison of the LeJour and wise pattern methods of breast reduction. Annals of Plastic Surgery. 2005;**54**:236

[68] Cruz-Korchin N, Korchin L. Vertical versus wise pattern breast reduction: Patient satisfaction, revision rates, and complications. Plastic and Reconstructive Surgery. 2003;**112**:1573

[69] Chest Reconstruction Top Surgery Procedure Options [Internet]. Gender Confirmation. Available from: https://www.genderconfirmation.com/ftm-top-surgery-options/; [Accessed: July 28, 2024]

[70] Hammond DC. The short scar periareolar inferior pedicle reduction (SPAIR) mammaplasty. Seminars in Plastic Surgery. 2004;**18**:231-243

[71] Hinson C, Alford H, Huett W, Zeidan M, Moore R, Lee Y-L, et al. Obesity and complications in mammoplasty: A retrospective review in an obese patient population. Plastic and Reconstructive Surgery - Global Open. 2022;**10**:e4697

[72] Bota O, Schreiber M, Bönke F, Teather D, Dragu A. Wound healing in postbariatric body contouring surgery. Plastic and Aesthetic Research. 2018;**5**:30

[73] Shiffman MA. Complications of breast reduction. In: Shiffman MA, Di Giuseppe A, editors. Body Contouring: Art, Science, and Clinical Practice [Internet]. Berlin, Heidelberg: Springer; 2010. pp. 197-204. DOI: 10.1007/978-3-642-02639-3_20

Chapter 9

Axillary Breast

Niran Maharjan

Abstract

The axillary breast despite being a relatively frequent entity, the attention attributed to plastic surgery is sparse. The lack of awareness about the possibility of treatment results in underreporting. Knowledge about it has important implications for patient care; if it is not recognized for what it is, then a normal variant may be misdiagnosed as an abnormality. It can present in any form as polymastia, polythelia, or aberrant breast tissue. Though most of the swelling is asymptomatic, fear of malignancy and cosmetic reasons are the common cause of the presentation. The clinical examination along with ultrasonography of the lump is mostly enough for initiating its remedy. Either liposuction and surgical excision alone or in combination can be implemented in daycare surgery or inpatient basis. In the hands of an experienced plastic surgeon, the procedure is totally safe and is recommended as the disease processes like that of the normal breast tissue can occur.

Keywords: axillary breast, accessory breast, breast cancer, liposuction, mammary crest, pendulous mass, surgical excision

1. Introduction

Axillary breast is defined as the development of breast tissue at the axillary region due to the persistence of the mammary crest that normally regresses. This condition is also known as aberrant breast tissue, ectopic breast, extra breast tissue, or accessory breast tissue. The incidence of axillary breast in women is 2–6% while that in men is 1–3% [1, 2].

It is more common in the Asian population; the attributing factor might be either the true increased incidence or the lower threshold for presentation. In 1/3rd of the population with the axillary breast, it is present bilaterally; however, right-sided prevalence is noted [1].

Despite being asymptomatic, the axillary breast tissue can not only undergo cyclical hormonal changes but also be affected by any type of benign or malignant breast pathology. The lack of awareness about the possibility of treatment results in underreporting. Knowledge about it has important implications for patient care; if it is not recognized for what it is, then a normal variant may be misdiagnosed as an abnormality. It can present in any form as polymastia, polythelia, or aberrant breast tissue [2].

Fear of malignancy and cosmetically unappealing can easily be corrected in the form of liposuction and surgical excision alone or in combination.

2. Anatomy

2.1 Embryology

Prenatal breast development can be classified into two main processes: the formation of a primary mammary bud and the development of a rudimentary mammary gland. Around 4 to 6 weeks of gestation, mammary-specific progenitor cells are seen in the form of paired proliferation of epithelial cells in the epidermis of the thoracic region. This discrete area of proliferation extends in a line between the fetal axilla and inguinal region and forms two ridges called the mammary crests or milk lines (**Figure 1**).

Most of the mammary crest atrophies except for paired solid epithelial masses in the pectoral region at the fourth intercostal space, which form the primary mammary buds [3]. Failure of apoptosis at any region along the milk lines results in either polymastia, polythelia, or aberrant breast tissue. The persisting mammary crest at the axillary region results in the formation of an axillary breast [4].

The developed axillary breast or presence of a supernumerary breast along the milk line is addressed by the embryologic theory, which states the persistence of the tissue due to the failure of regression or displacement of the milk line. **Figure 2** depicts the regressing milk line.

However, the aberrant breast tissue beyond the milk line, such as in the face, neck, ear, lateral thigh, buttock, or knee, is not addressed by this theory. Thus, Hughes in 1950 proposed the independent migration theory, which states the migration of the nests of the primordial breast cells. Later in 1984, Craigmyle proposed the modification theory stating the aberrant breast tissue is due to the modification of the apocrine sweat glands [4].

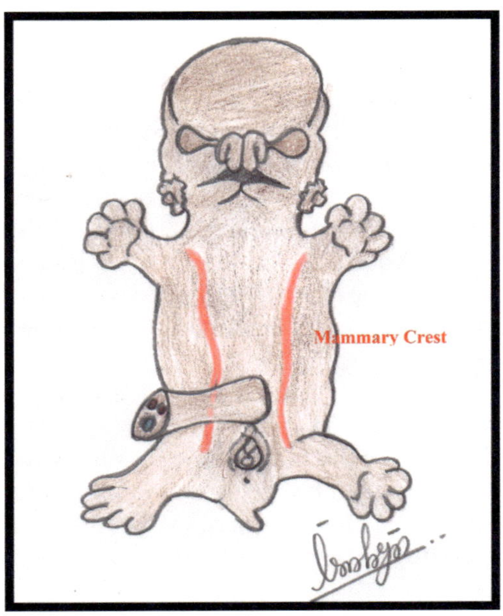

Figure 1.
Ventral view of an embryo at 28 days gestation showing mammary crests.

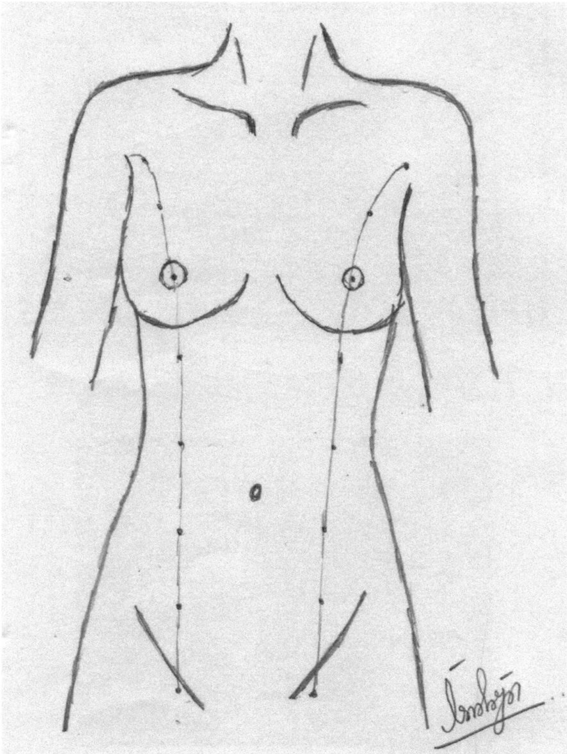

Figure 2.
The milk line as addressed by embryologic theory.

2.2 Hormone and development

The earliest stages of embryogenesis are largely hormone-independent. In the second trimester, the hormones and regulatory factors secreted by mesenchyme are important for breast development.

At 6 months of gestational age, the basic framework of the gland is established and is apparent in both boys and girls. The complex interplay between fetal, placental, and maternal hormones that have not yet been elucidated, and limited secretory activity in the late-term fetus and newborn infant may occur.

The normal gland remains quiescent from 2 years of age to puberty. Falling levels of maternal estrogens in the neonate stimulate the neonatal pituitary gland to produce prolactin, which results in unilateral or bilateral breast enlargement and/or transient secretion of milk.

At puberty, under the influence of sex hormones, in particular estrogen, the development of the breast first begins. Although the pubertal surge of estrogen is the immediate stimulus to mammary development, the action of estrogen depends upon the presence of pituitary growth hormone and the ability of growth hormone to stimulate the production of insulin-like growth factor-1 (IGF-1) in the mammary gland [3]. **Figure 3** depicts the normal development of the breast in the pectoral region with a normal axilla, while **Figures 4** and **5** demonstrate the presence of axillary breast on the right side and bilateral side with pendulous lump simultaneously.

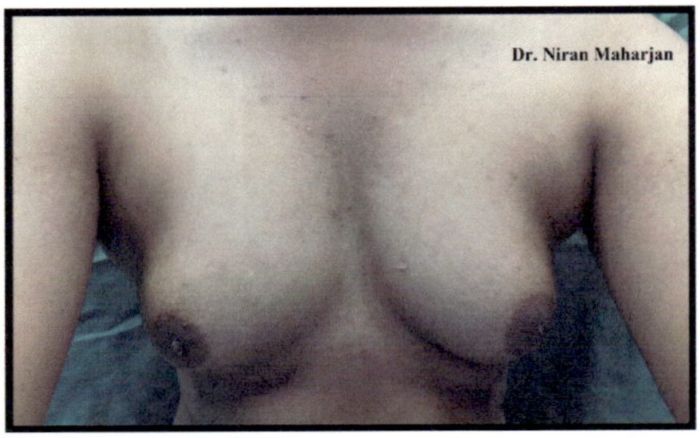

Figure 3.
Normal anatomy of breast and axilla.

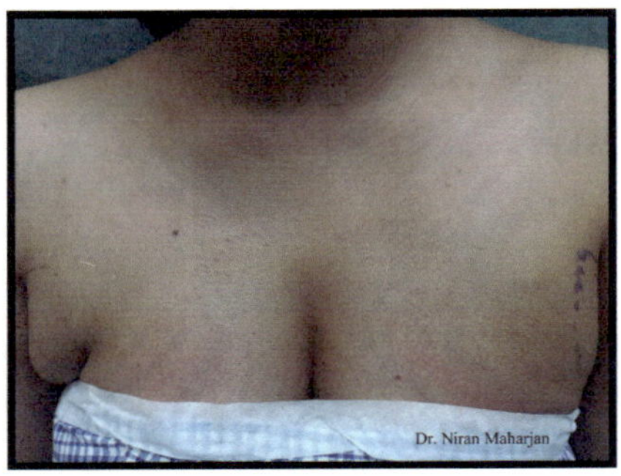

Figure 4.
Right-sided axillary breast.

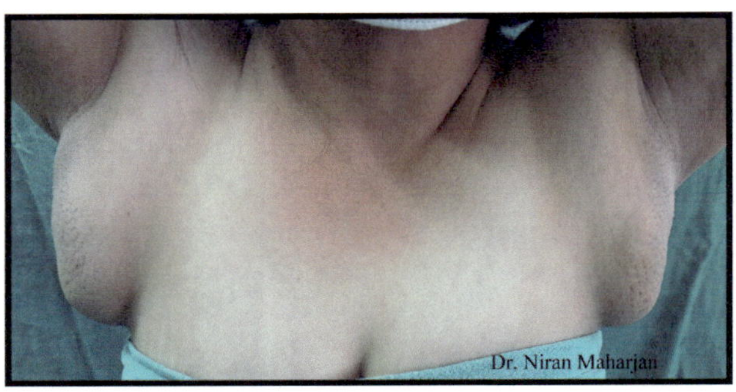

Figure 5.
Axillary breast on the bilateral side with pendulous tissue.

2.3 Applied anatomy

The axilla, an area of transition between the neck and the arm, is an irregularly shaped pyramidal space (**Figures 6** and 7) with

- 4 sides
- An apex (inlet)
- A base (floor) [5]

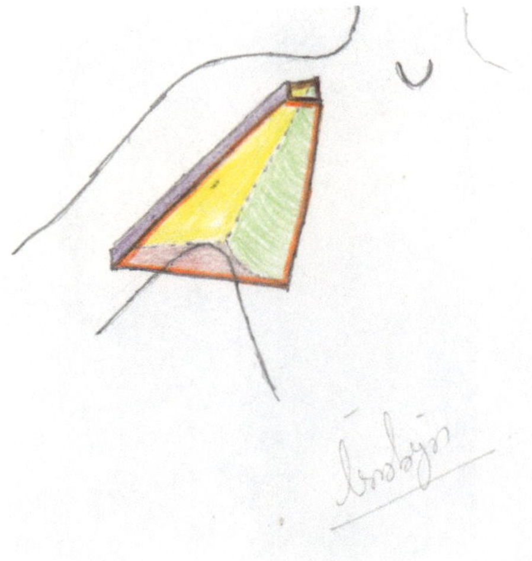

Figure 6.
Pyramidal space at the axilla.

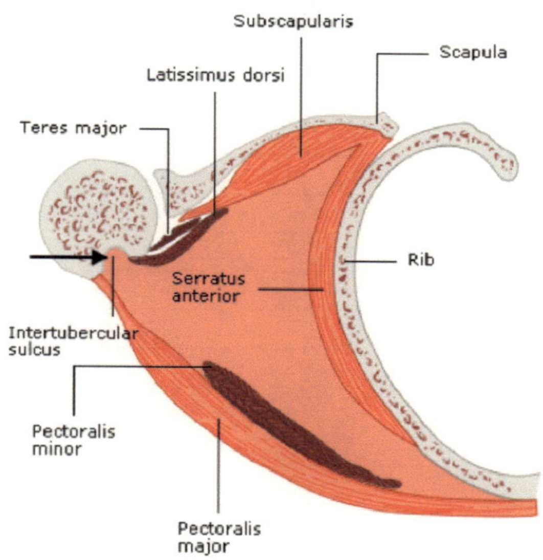

Figure 7.
Anatomical axillary space.

The salient point that every plastic surgeon should bear in mind is that the axilla is a pyramidal structure with a concave floor; thus, after the removal of the lump, it is difficult to obliterate the resultant space with the application of the pressure garment. When the arm is abducted, the neurovascular structures lying near the root are displaced downward, thus making them liable to be injured during liposuction. The esthetic landmarks of the axillar are not well discussed in the literature, but the anterior and posterior axillary folds (**Figure 8**) are the boundaries of the axilla that should not be violated to achieve an esthetically appealing result [2].

In 1915, Kajava [6] published a classification system for supernumerary breast tissue, which can be summarized as in **Table 1**. The supernumerary breast contains

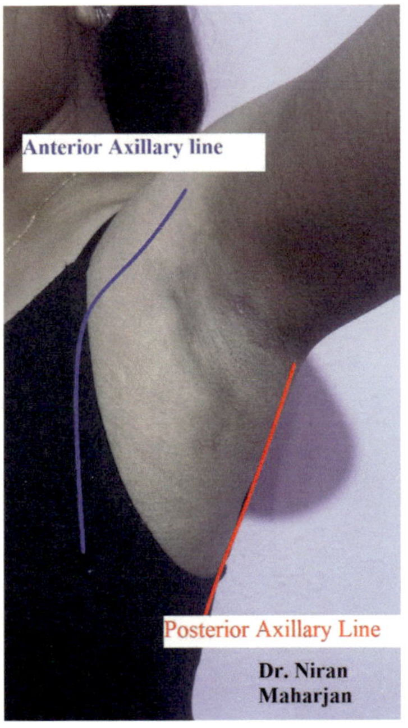

Figure 8.
Esthetic boundaries of the axilla.

Kajava Class	Areola	Gland	Nipple	Terms given
1	√	√	√	Polymastia
2	×	√	√	—
3	√	√	×	—
4	×	√	×	—
5	√	×	√	Pseudomamma
6	×	×	√	Polythelia
7	√	×	×	Polythelia areolaris
8	×	×	×	Polythelial pilosis (patch of hair)

√ → *presence of the tissue* × → *absence of the tissue.*

Table 1.
Kajava classification.

either all or part of the normal breast tissue—parenchyma, areola, and nipple. The most common clinical manifestation of axillary breast is Class 4 [4].

3. Pathophysiology

As it can present in a fully developed form or any combination of glandular, nipple, and areola, it is subjected to not only the same physiological changes, such as cyclical hormonal changes and milk secretion but also the same disease processes of aberration of normal development and involution (ANDI). Thus, the benign and malignant pathology it can carry are:

- Abscess formation
- Mastitis
- Milk fistula
- Cyclical mastalgia
- Cysts
- Fibroadenoma
- Fibroadenosis
- Hamartomas
- Phyllodes tumors
- Tuberculosis
- Duct ectasia
- Carcinoma

The incidence of axillary breast carcinoma is 0.2 to 6%. The higher incidence might be due to the stagnation in the ductal system and bears a poor prognosis due to its proximity to the axillary lymphatics and lymph nodes [1, 2, 4].

4. Clinical features

Axillary breast mostly is asymptomatic. The fear of malignancy, anxiety from the presence of a lump, pain, and tenderness, restriction of arm movement, irritation from clothing, and cosmetic problems are the presenting symptoms. Very few might present with pain along the medial arm and sticky skin causing discomfort.

Breast cancer awareness has positive and negative effects. Due to high alert, the presence of a lump that gets painful and tender on touch and also mild change in size definitely makes one think of the malignancy. Pain, swelling, and irritation along with limited movement of the arm may get worsen during puberty, menstruation, and/or pregnancy [1, 3, 7].

The lumpy armpit that gets easily visualized makes one restrict from wearing not just the sleeveless dress but even a properly fitting dress. The discomfort might hinder them from participating in social activities too.

5. Differential diagnosis

The fear that any unnatural lump in the body can be a form of cancer has dwelled deeply in the thoughts of everyone, and the credit goes to the awareness programs. When one finds a lump in their axillary region is definitely a malignancy.

Other lesions that might mimic the clinical presentations are as follows:

- Lipoma
- Axillary lymphadenopathy
- Hidradenitis suppurative
- Sebaceous cyst
- Vascular malformation [2, 8].

6. Investigation

A thorough clinical examination is mostly enough to rule out other causes of the swelling and to make a diagnosis. But without conducting an investigation, it will be almost difficult to reassure the patient. Thus, noninvasive and easily available ultrasonography can be used to support the preliminary diagnosis. When in doubt, either a mammogram or MRI can be advised. For the confirmatory diagnosis, either fine needle aspiration cytology (FNAC) or surgical incisional biopsy can be used.

7. Treatment

Reassurance or counseling might work for the asymptomatic patients who have a small negligible lump. But for those who either have symptoms or present due to fear of malignancy or moderate to severe skin laxity with visible lump, counseling or reassurance alone is never enough. For these patients, definitive treatment is the only option that must be protruded.

The known treatment modalities for taking care of this armpit swelling are either liposuction and surgical excision alone or in combination. But with recent advancements, there is the introduction of nonsurgical modalities too. As per Kurtzman et al. [7], the newer nonsurgical modalities are the use of Kybella and CoolSculpting.

Kybella (deoxycholic acid) is a prescription medicine approved in 2015 by the FDA for the treatment of double chin [9]. This synthetic medicine when injected into the submental region, breaks down fat by destroying its cell membrane. The common complications after its use are swelling, pain, numbness, and hardness, but the dreaded complication is an injury to underlying nerves and vessels [10]. Thus, the FDA has not approved its use in the axilla as the region contains important neurovascular supplies to the upper limb.

CoolSculpting or cryolipolysis is the FDA-approved noninvasive procedure that vacuums the skin above the area of fatty tissue into an applicator that freezes the fat cells to break it down as these cells are more affected by the cold temperatures than other cells. The broken-down fat cells are then removed by the body within 4 to 6 months. The complications associated with this procedure are diminished sensation in the treated area followed by swelling, bruising, redness, and localized pain [11]. However, it will not tighten the overlying skin thus skin redundancy might be more visible.

Both of the abovementioned noninvasive procedure works only if the axillary swelling is purely due to fat cell accumulation. As the most common axillary breast is

Kajava IV, the glandular portion must be addressed. Thus, invasive techniques in the form of surgical excision of the tissue along with the redundant skin or liposuction alone or in combination with glandular excision must be sought.

Surgical excision is done by placing a commonly used elliptical incision or a different one to address the pendulous skin present at the armpit so that the resultant scar can be hidden under the axilla. The markings on the skin are made prior to when the patient is in full consciousness and either on the table or before transferring to the operation theater. Patients are laid on the operation table and then are anesthetized with general anesthesia (GA). The arms are kept in an abducted position and the scalpel is run with controlled hemostasis. The excess of the skin and the glandular tissue are excised. Depending on the condition at the time of closure, either a closed drain is placed or opted for direct closure. The space is obliterated by placing a bulky dressing so that there will not be any collection underneath the skin. Collection in the form of seroma or hematoma, wound infection, and bruising are the usual complications associated with this technique. The resultant scar is generally accepted by the patients in comparison to carry on the lump.

Liposuction is usually preferred by the patients as the resultant scar is negligible in comparison to the excision technique but failure to address the glandular tissue of complete removal, thus creating a chance of leaving a remnant glandular tissue and non-address of the pendulous skin limits its choice. Thus, this can be addressed by combining the technique with the excision of the glandular tissue. But then the incision must then be lengthened. Liposuction is usually done under local anesthesia (LA), but some might prefer the GA. The Klein's solution, which is prepared by adding 100 mg of lignocaine, 10 ml of 8.4% sodium bicarbonate, and 1 ampoule of adrenaline in 1 liter of normal saline (NS), is infused in the axilla up to the lateral chest wall. The tumescent technique where more than 2 ml of the fluid is infiltrated for suctioning out half the volume is preferred by plastic surgeons. After the infiltration of the fluid, surgeons wait for at least 7 minutes for the adrenaline to show its effect. This helps to minimize the bleeding. A small stab incision of 3 to 5 mm depending on the size of the liposuction cannula is made on the axillary fold. The cannula is then attached to the suctioning apparatus of the surgeon's choice or availability. With the negative pressure exerted and the to-and-fro movements, the fat molecules are suctioned out. The to-and-fro movement is continued in a fanning shape so as to address all the swelling present on the armpit. The suctioning apparatus is turned off when the swelling has completely subsided or failed to suction out the glandular tissue, which is usually a fibrous tissue requiring the surgical excision. After confirming the hemostasis, the incision is closed, and the wound is dressed with utmost care to obliterate the space created under the skin. Complications associated are similar to the surgical excision technique but with much smaller-sized scars.

7.1 Surgeon's technique

The surgical site is prepped and draped. Klein's solution is injected with the 10 ml or 50 ml syringe till the lump turns firm. Then, we wait for 7 to 10 minutes for the adrenaline in Klein's solution to work. At the middle of the axillary fold, a stab incision with a 15 number bladed is given. The cannula is guided to the lump and then after is attached to the suctioning apparatus. The machine is turned on to generate negative pressure up to 400 mmHg; the cannula then is moved in to-and-fro movements. The maneuver is continued at one place till the presence of the lump or skin thickness gets thin as desired or there is notice of bleeding on the suctioning pipe.

The direction of the cannula is then changed, and as doing so, the fat molecules are suctioned out. From the same stab incision, which usually gets a bit stretched during the to-and-fro movement, the remaining fibrous tissue is pulled out gently and cut with sharp scissors. By remaining above the deep fascia and below the dermis, there is minimal bleeding noted. After resection of the fibrous parenchymal tissue, the cavity is irrigated with normal saline to check the hemostasis and to secure the capillary bleed. Repeating the irrigation for a couple of times and reassurance of the complete hemostasis thus achieved, the irrigated normal saline is completely drained and the incision is closed with polypropylene 6–0 sutures.

Initially, the redundant skin seems pendulous, but with due time, it shrinks; thus, the skin is repositioned and a bulky tight dressing is placed, which is changed on an alternate day basis. After removal of the suture in a week or 10 days depending on the wound condition, the pendulous skin is supported in the correct position with the use of the compression cloth and placement of the gauze pad on the underarm. A correctly implemented method aids in early recovery. It generally takes 6 weeks to 3 months for the skin to retract.

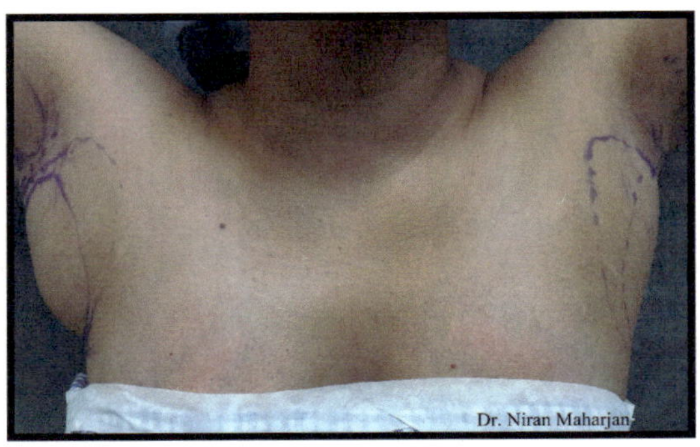

Figure 9.
Preoperative right axillary breast with markings.

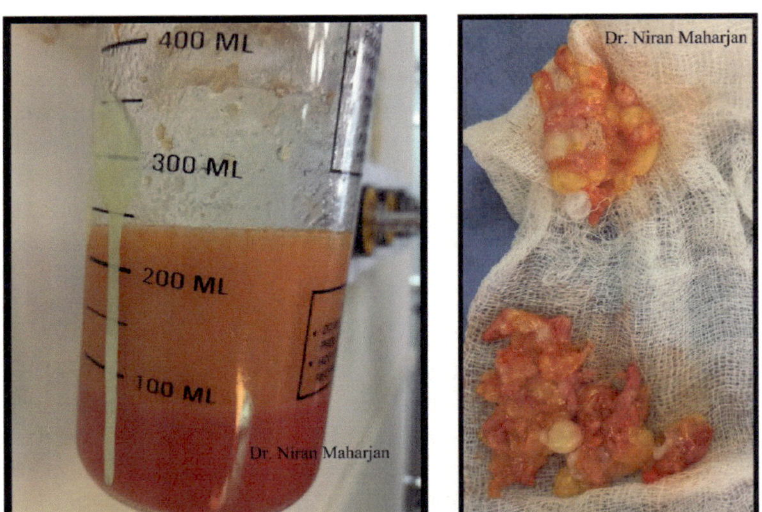

Figure 10.
Intra-op aspirated fluid along with fat and parenchymal tissue.

DOI: http://dx.doi.org/10.5772/intechopen.1007272

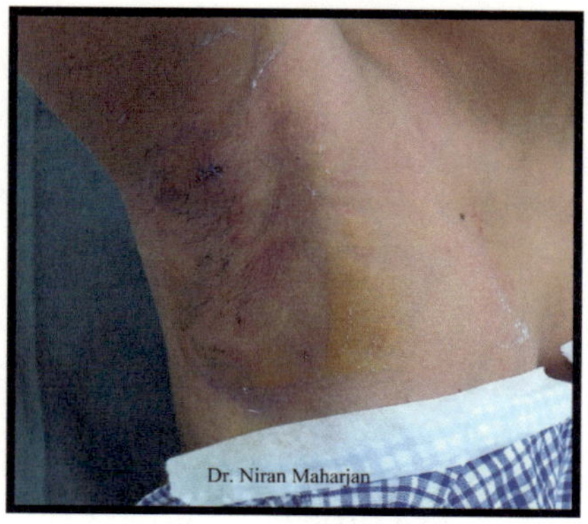

Figure 11.
5th postoperative day with the sutured wound on transverse axillary fold.

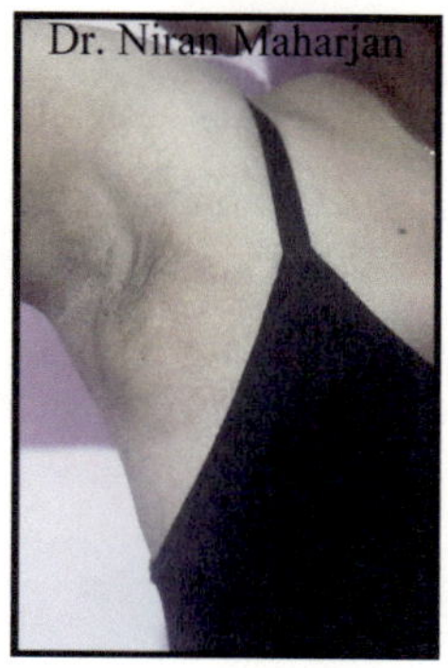

Figure 12.
35th postoperative day with retracting skin and camouflaged scar.

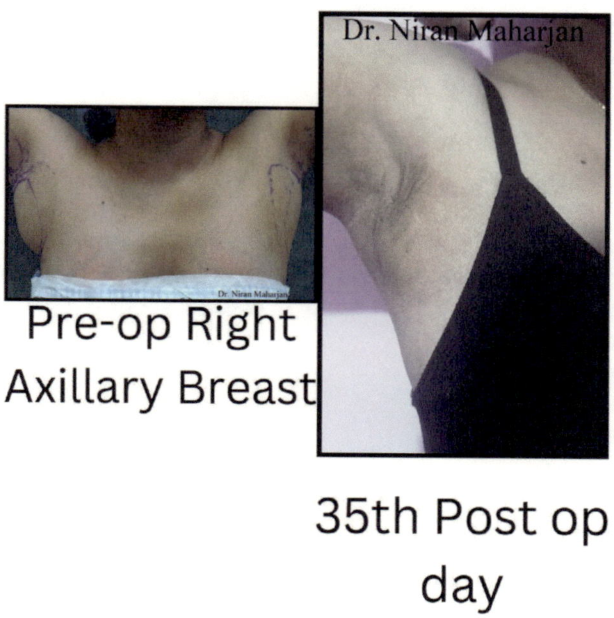

Figure 13.
Pre- and early postoperative pictures.

The limitation of incorporating this technique is the presence of a large pendulous lump as the skin recoiling may not be achievable to the desired amount.

Figures 9–13 followed below are the pictorial demonstration of the right axillary breast in the preoperative status through to the 5th postoperative week pictures for early comparison of lump status and skin retracting quality of humans.

8. Complications

The most common complication of the nonsurgical treatment is that it is not FDA approved.

The common complications associated with the interventive methods are:

- Seroma
- Hematoma
- Residual tissue
- Infection
- Intercostal brachial nerve (ICBN) injury
- Poor scar [1, 4].

9. Conclusions

The axillary breast can be treated with liposuction and excision of the glandular tissue on a daycare surgery basis. The pendulous tissue can be addressed intraoperatively with the excision of the excess tissue without jeopardizing the esthetic boundaries of the axilla thus resulting in a cosmetically pleasing resultant scar. The procedure is safe and recommended in the hands of an experienced plastic surgeon.

Acknowledgements

Without the support and guidance from my seniors, this piece of work would not have been accomplished. I am indebted to all the nursing staff of the operation theater and ward without their support my journey in taking care of the patients would not have been achieved.

Conflict of interest

The authors declare no conflict of interest.

Notes/thanks/other declarations

I would like to thank all the patients who trusted me and waited with patience before the final outcome of the desired result came.

Axillary Breast
DOI: http://dx.doi.org/10.5772/intechopen.1007272

Author details

Niran Maharjan
National Academy of Medical Sciences (NAMS), Bir Hospital, Kathmandu, Nepal

*Address all correspondence to: drnmaharjan@yahoo.com

References

[1] Down A, Barr L, Baildam AD, Bundred N. Management of accessory breast tissue in the axilla. The British Journal of Surgery. 2003;**90**(10): 1213-1214. DOI: 10.1002/bjs.4225

[2] Bhave MA. Axillary breast: Navigating uncharted terrain. Indian Journal of Plastic Surgery. 2015;**48**(3):283-287. DOI: 10.4103/0970-0358.173126

[3] Javed A, Lteif A. Development of the human breast. Seminars in Plastic Surgery. 2013;**27**(1):5-12. DOI: 10.1055/s-0033-1343989

[4] DeFilippis EM, Arleo EK. The ABCs of accessory breast tissue: Basic information every radiologist should know. AJR. 2014;**202**:1157-1162. DOI: 10.2214/AJR.13.10930

[5] Drake RL, Vogl W, Mitchell AWM. Gray's Anatomy for Students. 4th ed. Amsterdam: Elsevier; 2019. 1153 p

[6] Kajava Y. The proportions of supernumerary nipples in the Finnish population. Duodecim. 1915;**31**:143-170

[7] Kurtzman JS, Pinkasovic E, Preminger BA. Treatment options for the clinical management of axillary breast tissue. Plastic and Reconstructive Surgery. Global Open. 2023;**11**(8):e5189. DOI: 10.1097/GOX.0000000000005189

[8] Arora BK, Arora R, Arora A. Axillary accessory breast: Presentation and treatment. International Surgery Journal. 2016;**3**(4):2050-2053. DOI: 10.18203/2349-1902.isj20163571

[9] What is KYBELLA®? | KYBELLA® [Internet]. www.mykybella.com. Available from: https://www.mykybella.com/what-is-kybella

[10] Lopez LH. The Atlantic [Internet]. The Atlantic. theatlantic; 2017 [cited 2024 Oct 14]. Available from: https://www.theatlantic.com/health/archive/2017/06/kybella-the-injection-that-melts-a-double-chin/529893/

[11] Tee-Melegrito RA. What to know about CoolSculpting [Internet]. Medicalnewstoday.com. Medical News Today; 2018 [cited 2024 Oct 14]. Available from: https://www.medicalnewstoday.com/articles/322060#what-is-cool-sculpting

Chapter 10

Perspective Chapter: Mastopexy/Augmentation and Revision Aesthetic Breast Surgery

Pasquale G. Tolomeo and Angelo Cuzalina

Abstract

Breast enhancement remains one of the most frequently performed procedures in aesthetic surgery, with patients pursuing a variety of techniques to improve the shape, contour, and overall appearance of the breasts. Augmentation-mastopexy, which simultaneously corrects glandular hypoplasia or hyperplasia as well ptosis, is an essential but complex technique within a cosmetic surgeon's skill set. Achieving optimal outcomes requires careful consideration of multiple anatomical and aesthetic factors, including desired implant volume, existing breast dimensions, symmetry, nipple-areolar complex (NAC) size and placement, inframammary fold (IMF) position, and the thoracic contour. Combining mastopexy with augmentation presents technical challenges due to the contrasting objectives: mastopexy aims to tighten and elevate the breast, while augmentation involves expanding the tissue to enhance volume. These conflicting goals can complicate tissue management, vascular integrity, and implant positioning. Even with detailed preoperative planning, some cases may result in suboptimal outcomes. Potential complications include asymmetry, implant displacement, rupture, surface rippling, and capsular contracture. Addressing these issues through revision surgery demands advanced surgical acumen and experience, as it involves restoring harmony, contour, and patient satisfaction in a highly individualized manner.

Keywords: breast mastopexy, breast augmentation, aesthetic breast surgery, breast revision, implant malposition, capsular contraction

1. Introduction

Cosmetic breast surgery continues to rank among the top procedures requested by patients. According to data from the American Society of Plastic Surgeons (ASPS), breast augmentation was the second most performed cosmetic procedure in 2023, and mastopexy being the seventh most popular procedures [1]. Patients pursue a variety of interventions, ranging from implants, autologous fat transfer, lifts, reductions, or a combination of these procedures, to achieve their ideal breast aesthetics. Achieving an ideal aesthetic result depends heavily on harmony in breast size, shape, and symmetry. Importantly, the concept of beauty is inherently subjective, shaped by an individual's preference and goals. Successful breast surgery integrates both scientific principles and artistic sensibility, rooted in a comprehensive understanding of human proportions and the subtle interplay of soft tissue dynamics.

Combining mastopexy with augmentation to address both breast ptosis and glandular hypoplasia/hyperplasia is a core competency in aesthetic surgery. Achieving an optimal cosmetic result requires thoughtful control over numerous factors, including implant volume, existing breast dimensions, shape, symmetry, position and diameter of the nipple-areolar complex (NAC), inframammary fold placement, and overall thoracic contour. Common contributors to breast deflation and ptosis include pregnancy, breastfeeding, weight changes, and congenital anatomy. Over time, these factors may lead to a mismatch between the breast mound and the NAC, with the descendent of the NAC below the fold and deflating the upper pole. While mastopexy alone is more frequently performed, combining it with an augmentation introduces added complexity and is less routinely undertaken due to the detailed preoperative planning and technical precision required. Surgeons capable of harmonizing these competing variables while recognizing anatomical limitations are more likely to deliver outcomes that align with both functional goals and patient expectations.

As with any operative procedure, breast surgery carries certain risks, including asymmetry, implant rippling, displacement, deflation, and the development of capsular contracture. When complications arise or results fall short of expectations, revision breast surgery becomes necessary to restore a more aesthetic outcome. This revision procedure allows for refinement in breast shape and size, correction of prior complications, and can significantly enhance a patient's body image and self-esteem.

That said, revision procedures often present greater challenges compared to primary surgeries. Factors such as scar tissue formation, disruption of anatomical planes, and possible implant issues may increase the complexity of the revision. Risks such as bleeding, infection, and anesthesia-related complications remain, but the likelihood of these events is slightly elevated due to the altered surgical field. Because of this, aesthetic breast revision requires a surgeon with not only advanced technical proficiency but also substantial experience in managing the nuances of revisionary cases. Patients are strongly encouraged to seek out a provider with a demonstrated track record in complex breast surgery to ensure a safe process and satisfactory long-term results.

The field of breast surgery has seen continuous innovation, with new techniques and refined approaches enhancing both safety and aesthetic outcomes. As procedures become more advanced, the modern surgeon must be well-versed in a variety of operative strategies to effectively address diverse patient anatomies and expectations. Achieving reliable and lasting results requires more than technical skill, it demands a thorough understanding of the anatomical landscape. While surgical tools and methods may evolve, foundational anatomical knowledge remains essential. This understanding allows surgeons to preserve critical structures during surgery, reducing complication rates and improving the quality of postoperative results.

2. Pre-operative planning

The initial consultation is a cornerstone of successful aesthetic breast surgery. Given that many individuals seek opinions from multiple providers, establishing trust and professionalism early on is critical. During this visit, the surgeon's goals include identifying the patient's concerns, collecting a detailed medical and surgical history, conducting a comprehensive physical assessment, and offering a tailored treatment plan. This also includes outlining the benefits, risks, and limitations of proposed interventions. Importantly, this phase allows the surgeon to align expectations with realistic outcomes and educate the patient on their condition and procedural options, thereby empowering them to make informed decisions about their care.

2.1 Patient evaluation

A comprehensive pre-operative assessment is fundamental to achieving a safe and effective surgical outcome. The process begins with documenting the patient's primary concern, ideally expressed in their own words to ensure an accurate understanding of their goals. Utilizing open-ended questions encourages meaningful dialog and provides insight into their expectations. The medical review should encompass current diagnoses, a full list of medications (including dosage and frequency), allergies, and previous surgical interventions. Social factor, such as tobacco or nicotine use, are particularly relevant due to their negative effects on circulation and wound healing. Additionally, understanding the patient's occupation helps the surgeon anticipate potential limitations during the recovery period. A thorough family history, particularly regarding breast cancer, should be obtained, and for patients over 40 or those with elevated risk, preoperative imaging like a mammogram is strongly advised to ensure patient safety and comprehensive planning [2].

2.2 Patient examination

The breast examination should begin with a careful visual assessment, focusing on several critical elements. These include evaluating the quality and elasticity of the skin envelope, overall breast volume, positioning and size of the nipple-areola complex, degree of ptosis, presence of any asymmetry, and, if applicable, the location of the existing implant pocket. Aesthetic analysis is further enhanced by referencing the principles outlined by Mallucci and Branford, who highlighted four essential features in defining breast beauty: the upper-to-lower pole ratio, nipple angulation, the contour of the upper pole, and the convexity of the lower pole [3]. The surgeon should be adept at recognizing both subtle and significant differences in breast size and shape. Typically, a volume discrepancy of less than 10% is considered physiologically normal [4].

Beyond breast contour and proportions, any structural anomalies of the chest wall or spinal column must be noted, as these may contribute to visual asymmetry. A thorough palpation of the breasts and axillary regions is essential to detect any abnormal masses or lymphadenopathy, including along the supraclavicular and axillary lymph node chains.

To classify ptosis, the Regnault system is often used, which evaluates nipple position in relation to the inframammary fold (IMF) and skin envelope (**Table 1**; **Figure 1**) [5].

Regnault's classification of ptosis	
Minor ptosis (1st degree)	**Nipple at the IMF or 1 cm inferior to IMF**
Moderate ptosis (2nd degree)	Nipple inferior to IMF & superior to lower breast contour
Severe ptosis (3rd degree)	Nipple inferior to IMF & at lower breast contour
Glandular ptosis	Nipple superior to IMF & breast tissue inferior to the breast fold
Pseudoptosis	Nipple superior to IMF; breast is hypoplastic & inferior to the breast fold

Table 1.
Regnault's classification of breast ptosis [5].

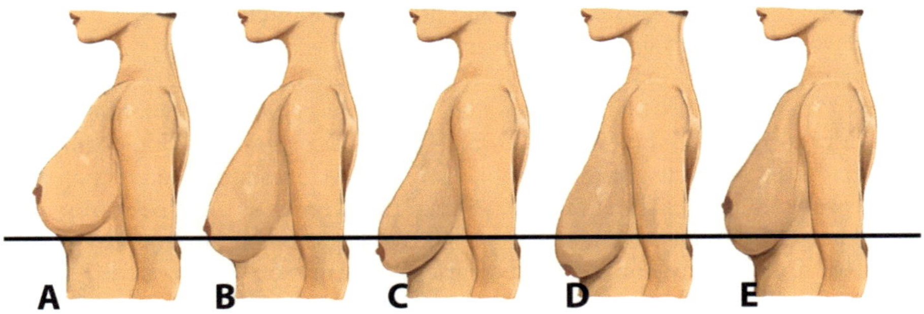

Figure 1.
Breast ptosis classification [5]. A: Normal. B: 1st degree. C: 2nd degree. D: 3rd degree. E: glandular ptosis.

The final part of the examination includes measurements and clinical photography (**Figure 2**).

Relevant dimensions include [3, 4, 6–8]:

1. Breast width (BW): midline to the anterior axillary line
2. Breast thickness (BT): upper pole thickness
3. Sternal notch to nipple (SSN-N): ideal measurement of 19–21 cm
4. Mid-clavicle to areola (MC-A): ideal measurement of 19–21 cm
5. Inter-nipple distance: ideal measurement of 19–21 cm
6. Areolar width (AW): ideal measurement of 3.5–4.5 cm
7. Nipple to inframammary fold (N-IMF): ideal measurement of 6–8 cm
8. Intermammary distance (IMD): ideal measurement of 19–21 cm from nipple to nipple
9. Ptosis: relative position of nipple to IMF

10. Mid-humeral point (MHP): mid-point between the acromion and lateral epicondyle; the ideal location of the nipple

11. Breast parenchyma size: lower pole is greater than the upper pole.

12. Skin quality

13. Parenchyma quality and elasticity

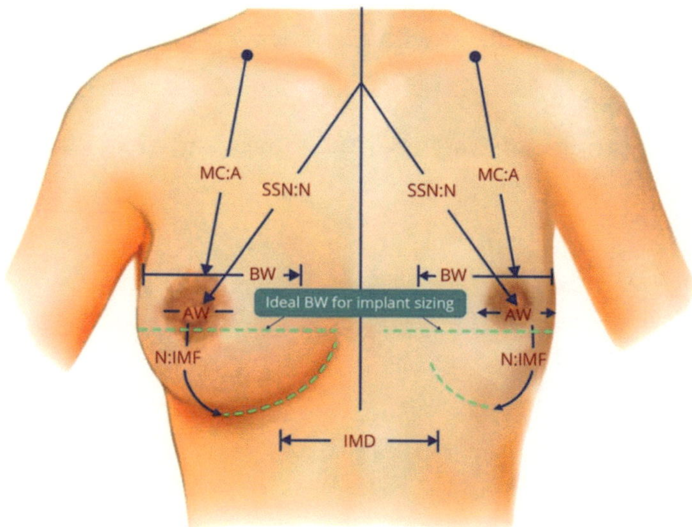

Figure 2.
Breast measurements and 'ideal' base width.

Among the key parameters in breast surgery are the breast base width, the distance from the sternal notch to the nipple, and the vertical distance from the nipple to the inframammary fold. The "ideal" or desired base width (BW) often differs from the patient's actual BW and is generally measured from the anterior axillary line to approximately 1 cm lateral to the chest midline. This desired BW is used during implant sizing to select the appropriate implant width (**Figure 2**). Precise BW ensures correct implant width to prevent issues like symmastia or lateral displacement. The nipple-to-IMF distance is particularly important in achieving desirable lower pole projection and harmonious breast proportions. Likewise, the sternal notch-to-nipple distance plays a vital role in defining the correct vertical position of the nipple-areola complex [6]. Accurate evaluation of these metrics, while staying within the breast's anatomical limits, is essential for obtaining consistent, aesthetically pleasing outcomes.

It is essential to understand that not every patient is well-suited for a simultaneous mastopexy and augmentation. These two procedures have inherently opposing goals, mastopexy involves tightening and reducing excess skin, while augmentation focuses on enhancing breast volume. When performed together, these objectives may conflict, particularly regarding the available skin envelope and vascular supply, potentially compromising the outcome. The added volume can place undue tension on the skin, which may impair arterial inflow and venous return, thereby risking reduced perfusion to the NAC.

Patients presenting with significant ptosis, constricted or tubular breast morphology, or those desiring substantial volume enhancement often achieve more favorable outcomes with a staged surgical plan. In such scenarios, separating the procedures allows for safer tissue handling and more precise contouring. Likewise, individuals with underlying health issues or those who have undergone prior breast surgeries are more likely to benefit from a phased approach. This strategy helps mitigate complications such as ischemia or NAC necrosis by allowing for improved vascular preservation and soft tissue management (**Figure 3**).

A comprehensive pre-operative assessment is essential for formulating an effective surgical plan that aligns with the patient's goals and ensures optimal aesthetic results.

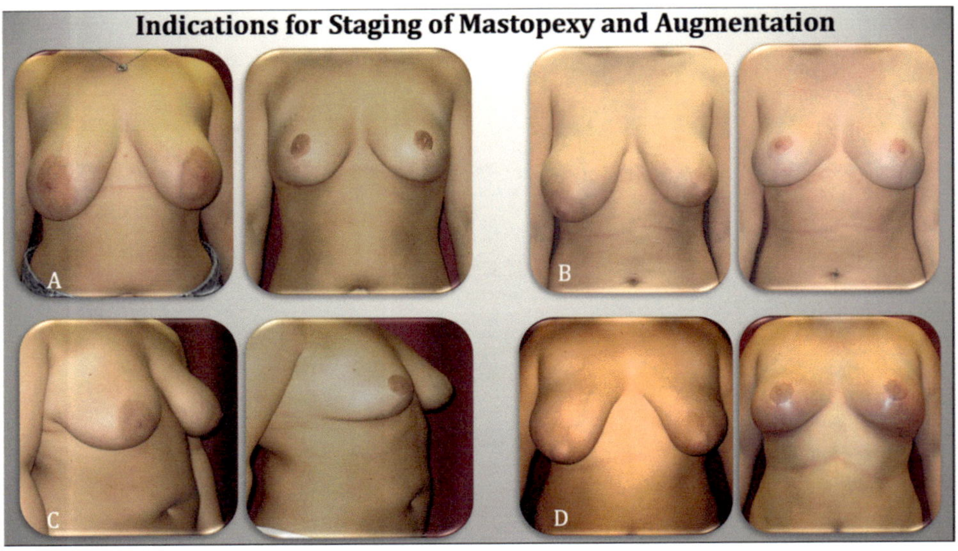

Figure 3.
Surgical staging serves to reduce the likelihood of ischemic complications affecting both the breast parenchyma and the NAC. Patients with significant breast hypertrophy and pronounced ptosis, or those exhibiting tubular or constricted breast anatomy, are at elevated risk for vascular compromise. In such cases, performing the mastopexy as a preliminary step, followed by augmentation at a later stage, offers a safer, more controlled approach. A. Dense/Asymmetric breasts with Grade 3 ptosis. B. Tubular/Constricted breasts & Grade 3 ptosis. C. Breast Reduction using Medial-Central (MC) pedicle D. Breast reduction (Right breast) & mastopexy (Left breast) with Superior-Medial Central (SMC) pedicle.

2.3 Patient discussion

It is critical to convey that no two breasts are identical, and perfect symmetry is rarely achievable, as natural variations in shape and size are the norm. The surgeon must align the patient's expectations with feasible surgical outcomes, ensuring the approach remains both safe and realistic. Open communication during the consultation is essential, with patients encouraged to clearly articulate their goals and concerns. Educating patients on the indications, limitations, and possible risks of each surgical option fosters transparency and trust, key elements in achieving a successful and satisfying aesthetic result.

3. Mastopexy incision design

The primary objective of mastopexy is to restore a breast that is well-balanced in size and shape, with results that remain stable over time. When performed in combination with other procedures, mastopexy typically includes lifting the NAC along with excision of excess skin and glandular tissue. This approach addresses ptosis while reshaping the breast to improve contour and proportion [6]. The choice of incision pattern is influenced by the extent of ptosis and the specific aesthetic goals (**Table 2**).

Mastopexy incision design	Indications	Advantages	Disadvantages
Periareolar/ Crescent	Grade I or II ptosis, NAC asymmetry	1. Subtle NAC elevation (1–2 cm) 2. Concealed scar	1. Flattened breast projection 2. Risk of scar widening
Vertical/ Teardrop	All grades of ptosis	1. Correction of ptosis & resection of excess tissue 2. Maintains NAC projection	1. Possible residual asymmetry 2. Diminished lower pole projection
Wise pattern/ inverted T	Grade II–III ptosis	1. Greater skin/parenchymal excision 2. Allows for breast reduction & lift in conjunction with augmentation	1. Increased scar presence 2. Elevated risk of wound breakdown
Multi-Planar L Scar	All ptosis grades	1. Correction of ptosis & resection of excess tissue 2. Preservation of nipple mound projection 3. Minimal Scarring	1. Decreased lateral breast projection 2. Seroma/Hematoma formation 3. Need for Surgical Drains

Various mastopexy designs and their clinical advantages [9, 10].

Table 2.
Mastopexy design.

3.1 Periareolar/crescent

Periareolar mastopexy is most appropriate for patients presenting with Grade I or II ptosis, minor NAC asymmetry, or limited skin redundancy. This method allows for elevation of the NAC by approximately 2 centimeters, offering a subtle lift without significant excision of breast tissue or skin. It is particularly useful for addressing NAC asymmetry with minimal disruption to the underlying breast structure. However, when applied to reduce the skin envelope, this technique may create a periareolar defect, increasing the likelihood of complications such as compromised wound healing, distortion of the NAC, and a reduction in breast projection [6].

A primary drawback of the periareolar mastopexy is the tendency for the periareolar scar to widen over time. To help prevent this, two techniques may be employed. First, placing the incision under maximal tension during the marking phase ensures a more predictable final NAC contour and minimizes excessive stretch during healing. Second, securing the closure with a permanent purse-string suture helps evenly distribute tension and reinforces the incision. Polytetrafluoroethylene (PTFE) is a commonly chosen material for this purpose, as it maintains suture strength and resists deformation, thereby reducing the likelihood of NAC distortion or scar expansion [6].

The crescent mastopexy represents a variation of the periareolar approach, involving the excision of circumareolar breast tissue. This technique is especially useful in patients presenting with nipple asymmetry or those needing a minimal NAC lift of approximately 1–2 cm. By selectively removing tissue in a crescent shape above the NAC, minor discrepancies in height can be corrected while limiting scarring and maintaining a subtle contour enhancement.

Benelli described a periareolar mastopexy technique that integrates reshaping of the breast parenchyma [11]. This approach is particularly helpful in managing larger breasts while employing the periareolar method. It involves excision of the surrounding skin and soft tissue around the areola. This procedure confines the incision along the areola while allowing for reshaping of the areola.

According to both the authors' experience and supporting literature, periareolar mastopexies tend to carry a higher likelihood of requiring revision due to aesthetic shortcomings, limited breast projection, and frequent recurrence of ptosis [9, 12].

3.2 Vertical-teardrop

The vertical mastopexy technique aims to elevate the NAC and address ptosis by facilitating the removal of glandular tissue, which contributes to more durable results. This method combines a periareolar incision with a vertical limb, enabling comprehensive reshaping of the breast and generally yielding more sustained aesthetic improvements than other lift approaches.

The Hall-Findlay method is a preferred technique due to its adaptable pedicle configuration, limited visible scarring, and ability to maintain breast projection. It commonly employs either a Superior-Medial-Central (SMC) or Medio-Central (MC) pedicle, both recognized for their dependable vascular inflow and drainage, which support optimal perfusion to the NAC. The procedure involves excising a wedge of tissue from the inferior breast pole, followed by approximation of the medial and lateral pillars to reinforce support beneath the NAC. This maneuver simultaneously reduces excess volume and enhances breast contour and elevation [13]. It is important to position the lower end of the vertical incision above the inframammary fold (IMF), as the IMF may shift upward over time. This placement helps prevent the scar from migrating onto the upper abdomen, which could compromise aesthetic outcomes.

When determining the appropriate implant pocket, both subglandular and subpectoral placements can be considered, especially since the vascular integrity of the 2nd and 3rd internal mammary perforators is typically maintained. This vascular preservation supports sufficient perfusion to the surrounding tissues, aiding in the overall safety and viability of the chosen placement technique [9]. Utilizing this approach, the breast initially exhibits enhanced upper pole fullness with a relatively flatter lower pole contour. Over time, typically several months, the implant gradually settles into position, allowing the inferior pole to achieve its intended projection and shape.

3.3 Wise pattern/inverted T

The Wise Pattern mastopexy, also referred to as the Inverted-T or anchor incision technique, remains one of the most comprehensive and widely utilized methods for addressing moderate to severe breast ptosis, particularly when concurrent breast reduction or augmentation is desired. This technique is particularly beneficial for patients with significant excess skin and breast tissue, offering enhanced reshaping capabilities and long-term projection control.

This approach involves a triad of incisions, periareolar, vertical, and horizontal, that together create the classic anchor shape. The periareolar and vertical incisions facilitate elevation and centration of the nipple-areolar complex (NAC), while the horizontal component allows for the excision of redundant skin and parenchyma. This facilitates restoration of an aesthetically pleasing lower pole and provides the necessary foundation for consistent NAC positioning. It also permits more precise control of the IMF distance, ensuring balanced proportions and symmetry in the final contour [12].

A key advantage of the Wise Pattern mastopexy is its adaptability in pedicle selection. Depending on the patient's breast anatomy and prior surgeries, the surgeon may choose from superior, inferior, medial, central, or combined pedicles to preserve vascular integrity while optimizing shape and projection [12]. This flexibility is critical in revision cases, where prior incisions and concern for vascular compromise may influence flap viability.

Despite its versatility, the Wise Pattern technique is not without limitations. One major concern is the potential for increased scar burden. Scars may be more visible, especially in patients with poor wound healing or keloid tendencies. Additionally, when employing an inferior pedicle, surgeons must be vigilant of the increased risk of lower pole redundancy or "bottoming out" over time. This phenomenon results from diminished structural support at the lower pole, which can compromise implant positioning and aesthetic outcomes [14].

Furthermore, in combined augmentation-mastopexy procedures, the intersection of the vertical and horizontal incision, the so-called trifurcation point, is particularly prone to wound dehiscence. This area endures higher tension due to the added implant weight, making it susceptible to delayed healing or tissue breakdown. To mitigate this, meticulous tension distribution and layered closure are recommended, along with careful selection of implant size and placement plane [9].

Overall, the Wise Pattern technique provides the highest degree of control for reshaping, lifting, and reducing the breast, particularly in cases of massive ptosis or macromastia.

3.4 Multi-planar L scar

The Multiplane L-Scar Augmentation Mastopexy, pioneered by Dr. Adel A. Bark Jr., represents a sophisticated advancement in aesthetic breast surgery. This technique aims to limit visible scarring while offering precise control over breast contour, projection, and volume. By individually addressing the skin, breast parenchyma, and muscle, the method enables tailored reshaping and improved long-term outcomes [10].

The procedure begins with the skin, marking the first phase of a triple-layered approach. An initial incision is made to expose the underlying breast parenchyma and pectoralis major. A thin dermofat flap is elevated while maintaining the subdermal vascular plexus to optimize tissue perfusion and healing. This also facilitates greater access and maneuverability for the deeper stages of dissection.

Once the skin elevation is complete, attention shifts to the parenchyma. An internal inverted-T incision is performed within the breast parenchyma to allow for repositioning and volume adjustment. The parenchyma is separated from the muscle, preserving a 2–3 cm layer of tissue to maintain blood supply and prevent recurrent ptosis.

Subsequently, the muscle is addressed in accordance with Tebbetts' method, which involves developing a modified submuscular implant pocket while conserving both medial and lateral muscular attachments [15]. The implant is then placed into this pocket, with intraoperative adjustments made for symmetry and projection. The central parenchyma is anchored to the pectoral fascia above the NAC to reinforce the upper pole and stabilize the breast mound, while the medial and lateral tissue is drawn caudally to reduce dead space. Additional contouring and approximation of the pillars are performed at this stage.

The final stage revisits the skin envelope, completing the second part of the skin strategy. Redundant skin is excised by advancing the medial and lateral flaps toward each other, often resulting in a dog-ear deformity that is corrected via a lateral L-shaped incision.

The Multiplane L-Scar Mastopexy focuses on reshaping the breast parenchyma while treating the skin as a separate entity. This technique avoids the need for a medial horizontal incision, ensuring long-term stability and optimal aesthetic results [10].

3.5 Surgeon's preference

In breast surgery, it is essential for the surgeon to establish a clear surgical plan and thoroughly inform the patient of potential complications. Obtaining prior operative reports is crucial to understanding the original planes of dissection, implant pocket selection, and pedicle design, helping to minimize the risk of further complications. When the pedicle design from previous procedures is unknown, selecting a pedicle with multiple perforators is advisable. The Superomedial-Central pedicle is often preferred for sternal notch-to-nipple distances under 30 cm, due to its robust blood supply from both medial and central sources, which enhances tissue viability and healing (**Figure 4**).

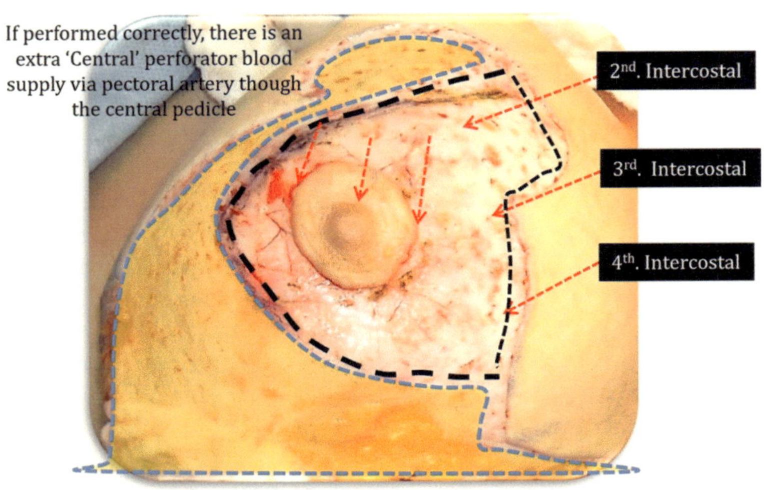

Figure 4.
Superomedial-Central Pedicle. This pedicle designs demonstrate the excellent dual blood supply to the breast and NAC via medial as well as central perforators.

DOI: http://dx.doi.org/10.5772/intechopen.1010708

The surgeon should be familiar with the range of pedicle configurations and their specific indications for use (**Figure 5**). Among these, the superior-medial (SM) pedicle, when integrated with a central (C) pedicle, offers the greatest versatility due to its extensive and reliable vascular network. This composite pedicle receives blood supply primarily from the internal mammary artery, reinforced by the 2nd to 4th internal mammary perforators (supporting the superior-medial pedicle) and the trans-pectoral perforators that branch from both the internal mammary and medial mammary vessels (supporting the central pedicle). With a base width ranging between 6 to 10 cm, this pedicle configuration ensures sufficient perfusion. However, in patients with a history of breast augmentation using a subglandular implant, the vascular integrity of the central pedicle may be compromised due to disruption of key perforators (**Figure 6**).

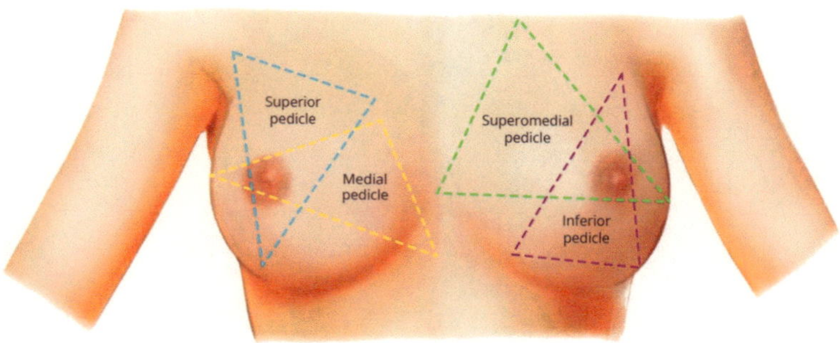

Figure 5.
Breast Pedicles. The pedicle configurations illustrate the extensive vascular support provided to the breast and NAC.

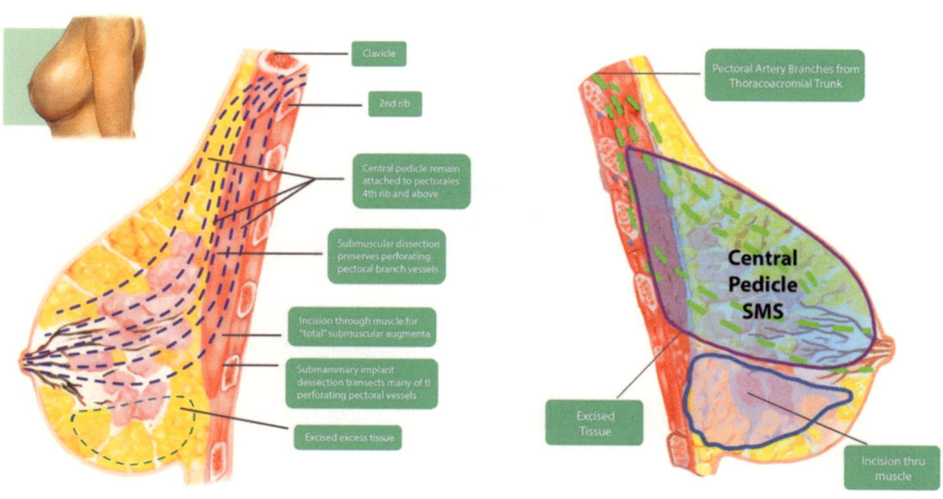

Figure 6.
Pectoral Vessels. Creating a submammary implant pocket can compromise vascular supply to the central pedicle by disrupting key perforators. In contrast, placing the implant in a total submuscular plane helps preserve these perforating branches, even when substantial excision of the inferior gland has been performed.

The selection of pedicle design remains a critical factor in complex cases. For patients presenting with pronounced ptosis or heavily pendulous breasts, often defined by a sternal notch-to-nipple distance greater than 30 cm, the medio-central pedicle offers an advantageous option. Its design allows for upward rotation of the NAC while maintaining vascular integrity and minimizing tissue strain. Vascularization is provided primarily by the internal mammary system and accompanying perforators (**Figure** 7) [16].

For cases involving mild to moderate ptosis, where the NAC lies approximately 2–3 cm below the inframammary fold, the SMC pedicle is particularly effective. This design enhances upper pole projection and breast contour by drawing vascular input from both the internal and lateral mammary arteries, along with contributions from a branch of the axillary artery. This triple-source blood supply decreases the likelihood of ischemia and supports reliable healing [16].

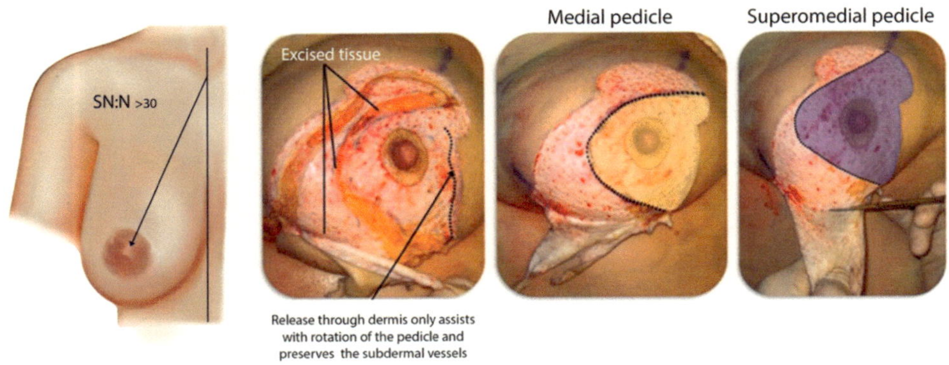

Figure 7.
The Superomedial Pedicle. The SMC pedicle is commonly selected in mastopexy procedures due to its reliable perfusion. In cases where the sternal notch-to-nipple distance exceeds 30 cm, the MC pedicle offers a favorable alternative, allowing the NAC to be rotated upward with reduced tension and minimal compromise to vascular flow.

When determining implant pocket placement, the author typically favors a total submuscular approach. This technique helps preserve the vascularity of the overlying pedicle and provides an added layer of soft tissue over the implant, which has been associated with a reduced risk of capsular contracture. Proper formation of this pocket is essential, careful muscle release is required to ensure appropriate implant positioning. Inadequate release may result in the implant sitting too high, producing exaggerated upper pole fullness and causing downward rotation of the NAC [6].

For additional soft tissue coverage, especially along the lateral and inferior implant borders, dissection beneath the serratus anterior and external oblique muscles can be performed (**Figures 8** and **9**). Over-dissection, however, should be avoided in the medial, inferomedial, and inferior zones, as this may lead to complications such as symmastia, unnatural medial contouring, or inferior implant displacement [6].

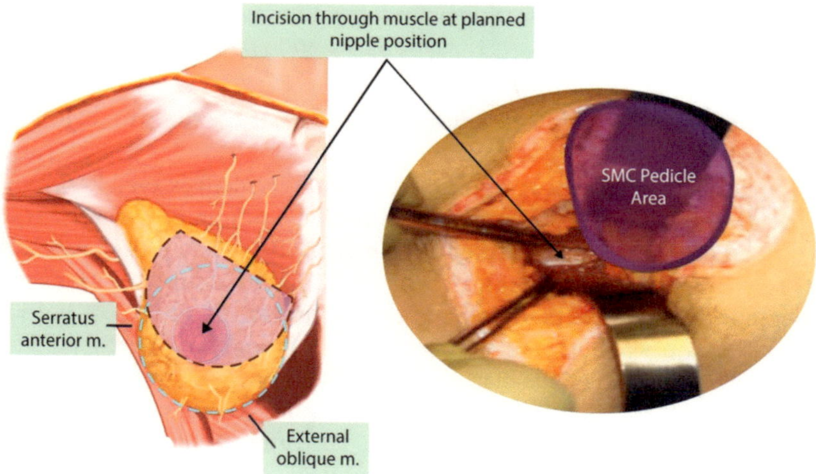

Figure 8.
The Superomedial-Central Pedicle. Employing the SMC pedicle facilitates the creation of a comprehensive submuscular pocket. This approach provides full implant coverage, offering enhanced support and protection while lowering the likelihood of inferior implant displacement or bottoming out.

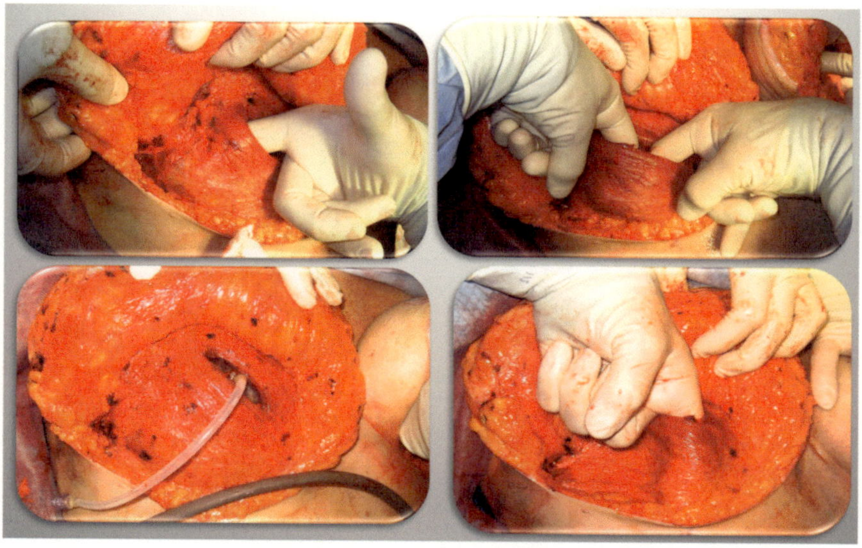

Figure 9.
Total Submuscular Pocket. Careful digital dissection enables the formation of a complete submuscular flap. Attention must be paid to avoid breaching the flap—especially in the lower portion, where it is most vulnerable to perforation.

The most conservative sequence for combining mastopexy with augmentation typically involves placing the implant first, followed by skin and parenchymal resection. This approach allows for accurate adjustment of tissue removal based on the newly added volume. However, the authors support the reverse order—performing the mastopexy before the implant placement. Conducting the lift initially enables the surgeon to carefully develop a total submuscular pocket and contour the breast tissue more effectively, leading to improved projection and symmetry. Successful outcomes require detailed preoperative planning to define resection boundaries and select the most appropriate implant, reducing the risk of excessive tissue removal and potential necrosis.

4. Complex breast (constricted, asymmetric and massive ptosis)

Certain breast deformities pose significant surgical challenges even in the absence of prior operative intervention. Complex presentations commonly include constricted or tubular breast configurations, marked asymmetry, and severe ptosis, particularly in patients following massive weight loss (MWL). These anatomic variations necessitate meticulous preoperative planning and the application of advanced, individualized surgical techniques to optimize symmetry, contour, and long-term outcomes.

Breast asymmetry should not be managed solely by augmenting the smaller breast with a larger implant. Achieving optimal symmetry requires a comprehensive approach that considers volume, shape, and NAC alignment. This often necessitates reducing the volume of the larger breast to achieve better symmetry with the contralateral side. Once native tissue volume is equilibrated, identical implant sizes can frequently be used bilaterally to maintain uniform projection and contour. In instances of marked thoracic asymmetry, such as rib cage anomalies or chest wall depression, a different implant profile or size may be necessary on the more concave side to compensate for underlying skeletal discrepancies and achieve a harmonious appearance (**Figure 10**).

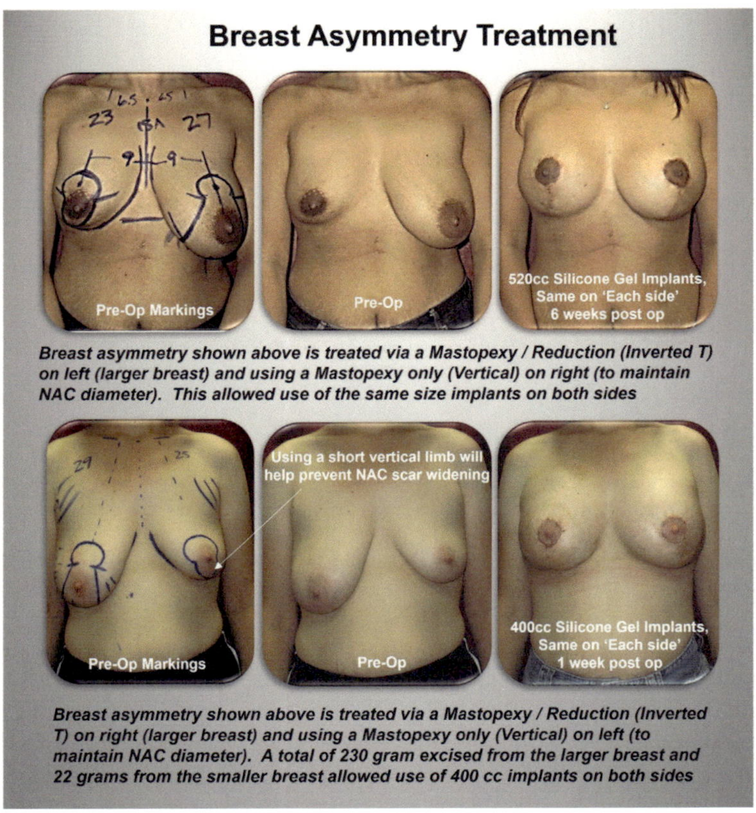

Figure 10.
Asymmetric Breast Treatment. Management of significant breast asymmetry is most effectively achieved by reducing excess tissue from the larger breast, as illustrated in the cases above. This approach facilitates the use of symmetric implant sizes on both sides, avoiding the need for disproportionately larger implants in the smaller breast.

Tubular or constricted breasts present unique technical challenges, particularly due to the risk of vascular compromise when attempting to release constricted tissues for expansion or NAC repositioning. While a periareolar or "donut" mastopexy may be appropriate in small-volume cases, it provides limited benefit in patients with larger breast volumes. These breasts often exhibit firm, fibrous tissue that necessitates more extensive release to enable proper pedicle rotation during vertical or inverted-T mastopexy procedures. This increases the risk of ischemic complications. As a result, in cases involving significantly constricted or pedunculated breasts, especially when augmentation is planned, a staged surgical approach is recommended to minimize complications and optimize outcomes (**Figure 11**).

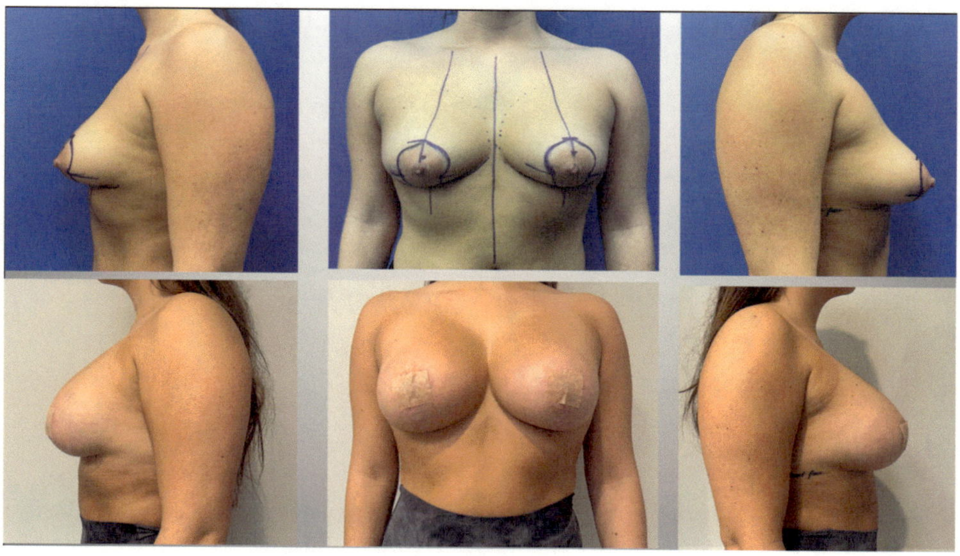

Figure 11.
Constricted or Tubular Breast Treatment. The above patient demonstrate "constricted/tubular" breast types with asymmetry. Such structural tightness poses a challenge due to limited tissue mobility and compromised vascularity. A superomedial-central pedicle mastopexy was utilized in both cases. The patient underwent a single-stage operation with concurrent implant placement.

Severe ptosis following massive weight loss presents a distinct reconstructive challenge. The residual breast tissue is typically of poor quality and offers limited structural support, rendering standalone mastopexy procedures insufficient for long-term correction. These patients often benefit from excision of as much redundant parenchyma as possible to reduce weight and mitigate the risk of postoperative deformities such as the "waterfall" or "Snoopy nose" appearance, where lax tissues descend off a fixed submuscular implant. A common surgical strategy in this cohort involves aggressive resection of stretched parenchyma and skin, followed by volume restoration with total submuscular implants. In cases involving severe ptosis or when large implants are desired, a staged surgical approach may be necessary to optimize outcomes and reduce the risk of complications (**Figure 12**).

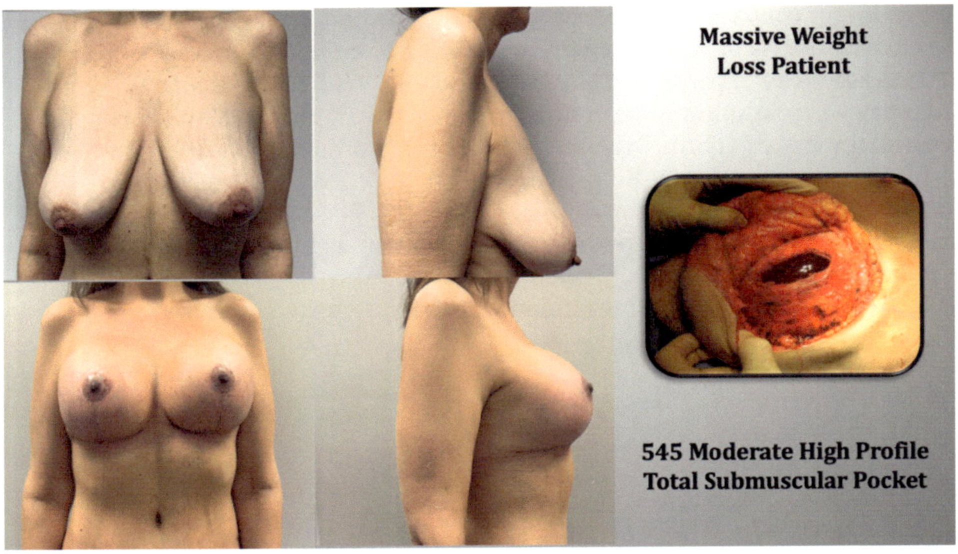

Figure 12.
Severe Breast Ptosis Treatment. Patients with a history of massive weight loss, such as the individual depicted above who lost 100 pounds, often present with significant excess breast tissue and compromised skin integrity. Surgical management typically involves excision of redundant parenchyma followed by placement of total submuscular implants to reduce the risk of implant bottoming out. This approach improves breast esthetics by increasing the implant-to-tissue ratio (more implant vs. less natural breast), thereby enhancing contour and projection. Importantly, removal of low-quality native tissue helps prevent recurrent ptosis and the development of waterfall deformities.

5. Surgical complications

5.1 Implant malposition

Breast implant asymmetry, characterized by discrepancies in size, shape, or position between the breasts, is a frequently encountered concern in aesthetic and reconstructive surgery. Implant malposition may arise from suboptimal implant selection, inadequate soft tissue support, or technical error during pocket dissection. Displacement of the implant, whether superiorly, medially, inferiorly, or laterally, often results from poorly constructed or oversized pockets and compromised native tissue integrity.

Superior implant malposition is typically the result of inadequate inferior pocket dissection, which prevents proper descent of the implant and leads to upward migration. Medial malposition, often due to over-aggressive medial dissection, may result in symmastia, characterized by the merging of the breast contours across the midline. In contrast, inferior malposition commonly arises from excessive inferior dissection, insufficient lower pole support, or the placement of overly large implants that exacerbate tissue thinning and downward displacement.

Lateral displacement, among the most prevalent forms of malposition, occurs when the implant shifts laterally into the axillary region, producing an unnatural gap between the breasts. This can lead to discomfort, visibility of implant edges, and compromised aesthetics.

Contributing factors to malposition include prior trauma, capsular contracture, or congenital thoracic wall asymmetries.

Prevention hinges on meticulous preoperative planning, including appropriate implant selection based on thoracic dimensions and ensuring balanced, controlled pocket dissection. Postoperative strategies, such as restricted physical activity and the use of compression garments, are also critical in maintaining proper implant positioning and minimizing recurrence.

5.2 Capsular contracture

Following breast augmentation, the formation of a fibrous capsule around the implant is a normal physiological response. Under typical conditions, this capsule remains pliable and contributes to maintaining implant position. However, in certain cases, an exaggerated immune reaction, often triggered by factors such as bacterial biofilm or residual hematoma, can lead to capsular contracture. This pathological response is characterized by progressive tightening and thickening of the capsule, which may result in breast firmness, contour irregularities, discomfort, and, in severe instances, pain or distortion of the breast shape.

Although the precise etiology of capsular contracture remains uncertain, several preventative strategies have been identified. Adherence to meticulous sterile technique during surgery is essential, and the use of an implant funnel can significantly reduce implant contact and contamination risk. Complete hemostasis and thorough irrigation of the implant pocket, using sterile saline and a triple antibiotic solution, are recommended to minimize biofilm development. Postoperative protocols should emphasize avoiding mechanical stress on the breasts and ensuring patient compliance with aftercare instructions. Additionally, prophylactic administration of leukotriene inhibitors such as montelukast or zafirlukast has been associated with reduced inflammatory response and a lower incidence of contracture [17]. Long-term data suggest that approximately 10% of patients may require revision surgery due to capsular contracture within 10 years, with a reduced incidence noted in those with submuscular implant placement [18].

5.3 Implant rippling/deflation

Implant rippling refers to the formation of visible folds or wrinkles along the periphery of the implant, which may become apparent beneath the skin surface. This phenomenon is particularly prevalent in patients with limited soft tissue coverage, such as those with low body fat or thin breast parenchyma. It is also more frequently observed with underfilled implants, where the edges are prone to folding.

Implant deflation typically occurs as a consequence of rupture or leakage, leading to a reduction in implant volume and alteration in breast contour. In the case of saline implants, deflation is usually apparent soon after rupture due to rapid loss of fluid, resulting in a visible change in breast size. In contrast, silicone implant ruptures may be more insidious, with no overt signs of volume loss. Contributing factors to deflation include structural fatigue of the implant shell, physical trauma, or intrinsic manufacturing flaws.

To mitigate the risks of implant rippling and deflation, it is essential to select implants of appropriate size, cohesiveness, and pocket placement.

6. Breast revision

Following a comprehensive patient evaluation, the surgeon must identify the most appropriate surgical approach to address the patient's concerns and effectively correct the underlying complication.

6.1 Post-augmentation breast ptosis

After breast augmentation, some patients may develop a "waterfall deformity," characterized by ptotic native breast tissue descending over a stationary implant [19]. Management strategies for this condition include implant removal, implant exchange, mastopexy, or no treatment.

If the patient is content with the current position, contour, and cleavage of the breasts, surgical revision may not be warranted. However, in cases where dissatisfaction persists, the treatment plan may involve either upsizing the implant or modifying the implant pocket to a subglandular plane. Caution is advised when considering subglandular repositioning in the presence of lower pole ptosis, as this may accentuate the "waterfall deformity" rather than correct it.

The most effective intervention for correcting the "waterfall deformity" is a mastopexy. This procedure is designed to enhance breast contour, re-establish symmetry, and elevate the tissue to address ptosis, ultimately yielding a more youthful and aesthetically pleasing result [6]. Mastopexy entails repositioning the NAC and excising redundant skin and parenchyma. The incision pattern selected is based on the severity of ptosis and the specific goals of the surgical plan.

6.2 Implant malposition

Implant malposition remains a frequent complication following both primary augmentation and combined augmentation-mastopexy procedures. Displacement is most commonly observed in the inferior and lateral directions. Correction typically involves surgical pocket modifications, such as capsulorrhaphy or capsulotomy, to restore appropriate implant positioning and maintain aesthetic balance.

Capsulorrhaphy is a surgical technique aimed at reinforcing and repositioning the breast implant capsule. Several modalities are employed to achieve this, including layered suture repair, application of thermal energy, and incorporation of mesh scaffolds. Spear described a multi-layered suture technique utilizing either absorbable or permanent sutures, which allows for incremental correction while minimizing focal stress on individual sutures [20]. Randquist introduced the "popcorn" method, where thermal energy is applied to the capsule to induce shrinkage and pocket reshaping [21]. GalaFLEX mesh, constructed from resorbable poly-4-hydroxybutyrate monofilament, serves as an internal scaffold reinforcing the capsule [22]. The mesh promotes host tissue integration, resulting in a well-vascularized tissue that provides structural support. Ultimately, this integration yields tissue strength that is reported to be three to five times greater than that of native tissue, thus enhancing long-term pocket stability [23].

To fix implant malposition, the author typically uses a combination of layered sutures and a "popcorn" capsulorrhaphy technique. Before surgery, the patient is evaluated while standing, and markings are made on the skin to show where the internal repair will be done. Areas that need to be released (capsulotomy) are also marked to help reposition the implant and relieve pressure on the repair.

During the procedure, the surgeon re-enters the breast through the existing inframammary incision to access the capsule. The implant is carefully removed and examined for any signs of damage or rupture. To tighten and reshape the capsule, the inner lining is scored using Bovie cautery, which produces a characteristic "pop" sound as thermal energy is applied. A capsulorrhaphy is then completed using a continuous-locking suture technique with 1 Nurolon to reinforce and secure the internal pocket.

Following completion of the capsulorrhaphy, corresponding capsulotomies are performed on the opposite side and along the anterior capsule to facilitate proper implant repositioning. Once reshaping of the pocket is finalized, it is irrigated using a triple antibiotic solution with betadine. The implant is then reinserted, and the pocket is closed. The patient is transitioned into the beach chair position to assess implant positioning and breast symmetry. After confirming adequate symmetry, the patient is returned to the supine position, and the incision is closed in multiple layers (**Figure 13A,B**).

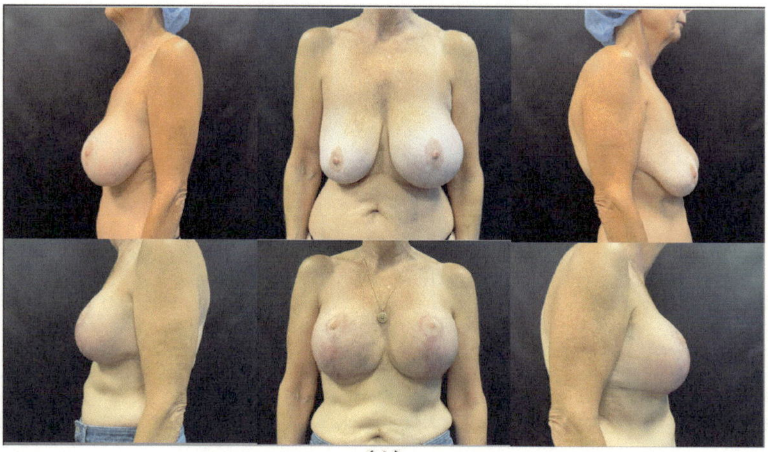

(A)

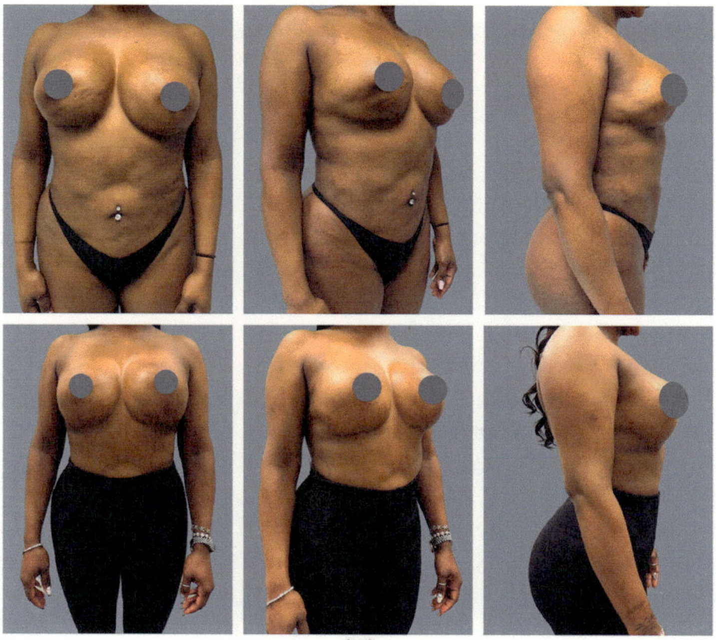

(B)

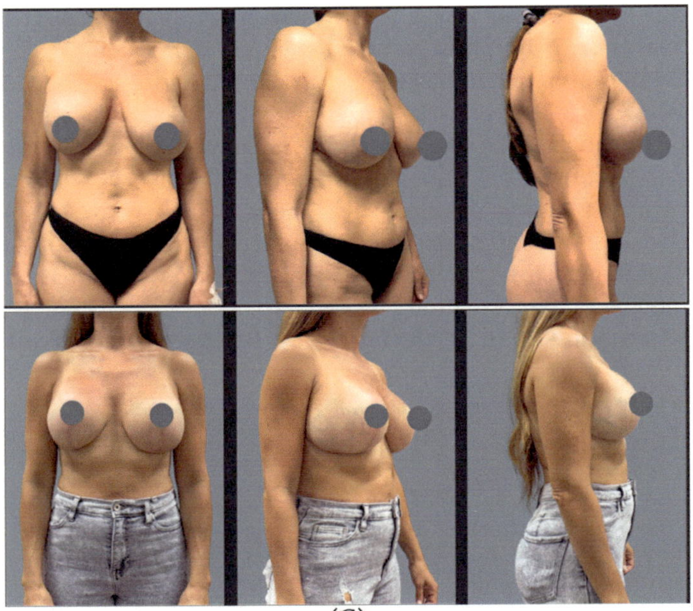

(C)

Figure 13.
(A) *Inferior Displacement of the Breast Implants and Implant Rupture. The patient presented with dissatisfaction following prior breast augmentation with saline implants. Patient experienced implant rupture of the right breast as well as bottoming out. A simultaneous mastopexy and revision augmentation were performed. To improve implant placement and elevate the breast footprint on the chest wall, a capsulorrhaphy was carried out as part of the revision procedure.* ***(B)*** *Malposition of the Breast Implants. The patient presented with dissatisfaction following prior breast augmentation with multiple revisions. Patient underwent seven revision breast surgeries to improve implant position and breast contours. A simultaneous mastopexy and revision augmentation were performed. To improve implant placement and elevate the breast footprint on the chest wall, a capsulorrhaphy was carried out as part of the revision procedure. Fat grafting was performed to address any soft tissue irregularities.* ***(C)*** *Replacement Above to Below Muscle. The patient shown is before and 3 months after switching implants from saline to silicone and changing her pocket from above muscle to a total submuscular position along with a simultaneous breast lift. This combination of techniques resulted in improved breast projection, better implant support, and enhanced cleavage. The total submuscular pocket helped prevent implant migration into the old subglandular space, offering more stable and long-lasting results.*

In instances of implant malposition within the subglandular plane, correction often necessitates explantation and creation of a new submuscular pocket. While some surgeons opt to reinforce the subglandular pocket using acellular dermal matrix (ADM) anchored to the lateral border of the pectoralis muscle, a well-constructed total submuscular pocket alone can provide adequate support. The submuscular pocket prevents implant migration into the previous pocket, often without the additional cost associated with ADM. Total submuscular placement is more readily achieved when performed with a mastopexy. However, caution is warranted in patients with a history of subglandular augmentation, as the vascular supply to the NAC may be compromised (**Figure 13C**).

In revision cases where there is a significant risk of recurrent implant malposition, mesh reinforcement can be employed to provide additional structural integrity to the breast capsule. Prior to mesh placement, fascial flaps are developed to ensure the mesh is adequately covered. GalaFLEX mesh is strategically placed over areas of weakened capsule or insufficient tissue support, then anchored to the pectoralis muscle and surrounding capsule. For enhanced stability, fixation may extend to the underlying ribs. The authors utilize a continuous 0 Vicryl suture to secure the mesh to both the rib and surrounding tissue, reconstructing a stable internal framework.

The mesh is subsequently sutured to the overlying fascial flap with the same suture technique to ensure layered soft tissue reinforcement.

In cases where soft tissue coverage is insufficient, the use of localized muscle flaps can serve as an effective method for implant coverage and correction of tissue deficiencies during breast reconstruction (**Figures 14** and **15**).

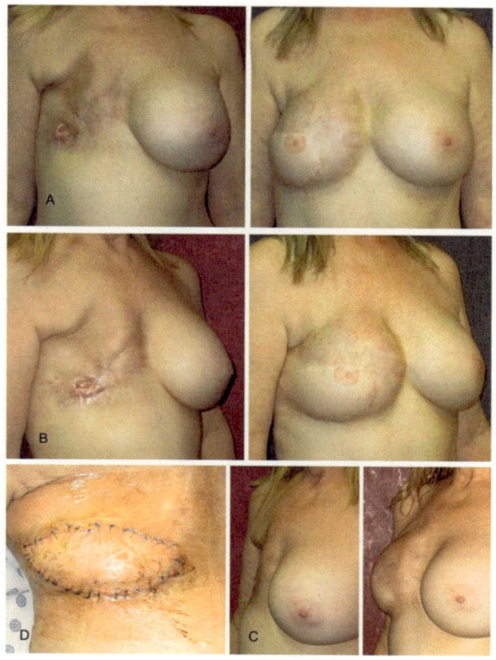

Figure 14.
Soft Tissue Reconstruction. Patient with previous mastectomy and radiation. Patient developed tissue necrosis with exposure of her rib. A latissimus dorsi flap (myocutaneous flap) was utilized to reconstruct the right breast tissue. Breast implant expanders were placed after surgery followed by final implants and nipple tattooing.

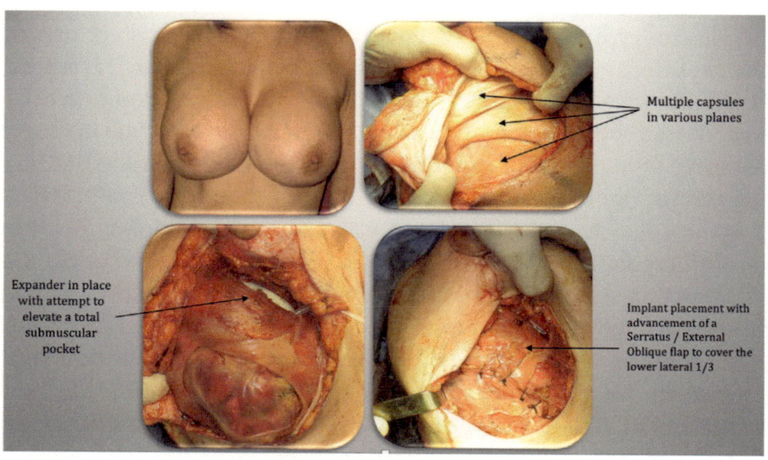

Figure 15.
Multiple Breast Revision Surgeries. The patient shown previously had a history of multiple breast augmentations, the last of which resulted in symmastia. Due to substantial damage to the overlying muscle, an inferolateral submuscular flap [was created using the serratus anterior and external oblique muscles to provide adequate soft tissue coverage for the new implant.

6.3 Capsular contracture

Capsular contracture is a condition characterized by the abnormal accumulation of fibrous scar tissue around a breast implant, which can result in firmness, discomfort, and distortion of the breast's shape. A range of factors may contribute to its onset, including a previous history of contracture, placement of implants in the subglandular plane, implant rupture (particularly with silicone), tobacco use, microbial contamination, and underlying autoimmune diseases. The progression of contracture is often insidious, with symptoms emerging months or even years after surgery, highlighting its chronic and unpredictable nature [24].

The diagnosis of capsular contracture is primarily clinical, relying on a thorough physical examination. The surgeon should evaluate the breasts for changes in symmetry, firmness, contour, and any patient-reported symptoms such as discomfort or tightness (**Table 3**) These findings help assess the severity of contracture. In certain cases, imaging studies like ultrasound or magnetic resonance imaging (MRI) can provide additional insight into the extent of capsular thickening and the integrity of the implant.

Baker Grade	Breast Description	Implant Description	Treatment
I	Soft, normal shape	Non-palpable	No treatment
II	Firm, normal shape	Palpable, not visible	Non-steroidal anti-inflammatory medications, Montelukast, capsulotomy
III	Firm, slight distortion	Palpable, visible	Capsulectomy, implant exchange
IV	Hard, severe distortion	Palpable, visible	Capsulectomy, implant exchange

Table 3.
Baker grade of capsular contracture [25, 26].

Management of breast implant capsular contracture is guided by the severity of the condition. For patients with mild symptoms, a non-surgical approach may be recommended. This typically includes regular monitoring, consistent breast massage to soften the capsule, and the use of anti-inflammatory agents such as montelukast. The goal of this conservative strategy is to alleviate discomfort and potentially slow the progression, thereby delaying or avoiding the need for surgical treatment.

In moderate to severe cases of capsular contracture (Baker Grade III/IV), surgical intervention is typically required to optimize both function and aesthetic outcomes. Treatment options may include capsulotomy, capsulectomy, implant pocket conversion, or reinforcement with ADM or GalaFLEX mesh scaffolds for additional structural support. In select cases with compromised soft tissue coverage, muscle or fasciocutaneous flaps can be employed to enhance coverage and lower the risk of recurrence [22]. Studies demonstrate a 79% success rate for reoperation with implant exchange; however, the recurrence rate remains approximately 54% [27].

In the treatment of advanced capsular contracture, surgeons often opt for en bloc removal of both the implant and surrounding capsule. This approach minimizes the risk of silicone leakage and helps reduce contamination of the implant pocket, particularly in cases where biofilm formation is suspected on the implant shell. Following explantation, the previous pocket is carefully assessed. If the original implant was positioned in a subglandular plane, a new submuscular pocket is typically created to accommodate the replacement implant and reduce the risk of recurrence. For implants previously placed in a submuscular position, the surgeon evaluates the integrity of the existing pectoralis pocket. If deficiencies are noted, reinforcement using ADM, GalaFLEX mesh, or autologous tissue flaps may be necessary to reconstruct the pocket and provide adequate support for the new implant (**Figures 16** and **17**).

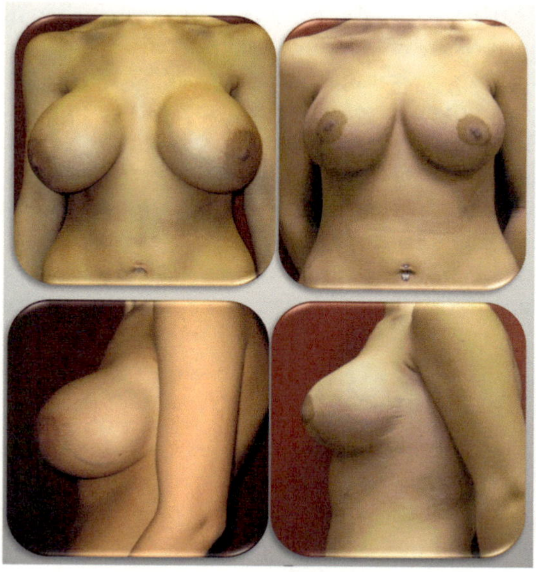

Figure 16.
Grade IV Capsular Contracture. The patient presents with Grade IV capsular contracture, characterized by significant firmness, distortion, and pain. For patients with capsular contracture who are considering simultaneous augmentation and mastopexy, must be informed of an increased risk of complications and higher likelihood of revision surgery.

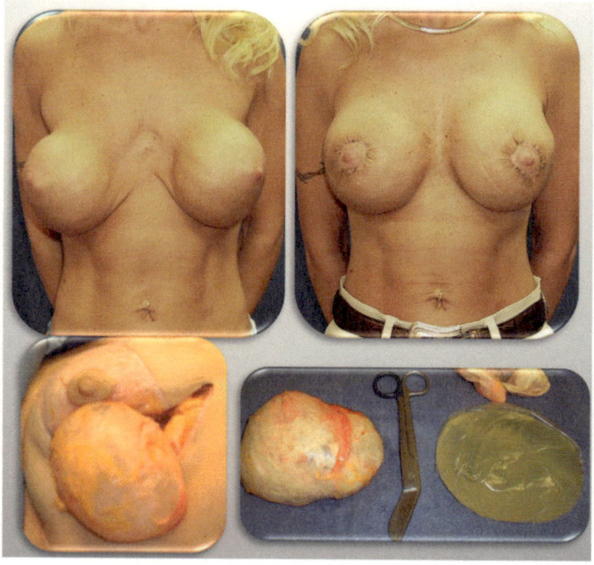

Figure 17.
Grade IV Capsular Contracture. The patient presents with Grade IV capsular contracture. Underwent an en bloc capsulectomy with simultaneous mastopexy and breast augmentation.

The use of ADM has been associated with a reduced incidence of capsular contracture in breast implant surgery. Research suggests that ADM reduces blood vessel proliferation, fibroblast activity, fibrosis, and collagen deposition, as well as attenuate the body's inflammatory response to the implant, all of which contribute to improved long-term surgical outcomes and lower complication rates [28, 29].

Before placement of the GalaFLEX mesh scaffold, soft tissue flaps are prepared in the intended area to ensure adequate coverage. The mesh is then positioned over areas of capsular weakness or tissue deficiency to reinforce the pocket. Once in place, it is anchored to the underlying pectoralis muscle and adjacent soft tissue, and in some cases, secured directly to the ribs for enhanced structural support. The author prefers using a 0 Vicryl suture in a continuous running fashion to affix the mesh securely to both the soft tissue and rib surfaces, effectively reconstructing the internal foundation. Following this, the mesh is sutured to the overlying fascial flap with a 0 Vicryl to provide an added layer of soft tissue reinforcement (**Figure 18**).

Routine postoperative and long-term follow-up is essential to monitor healing progress and detect any early signs of recurrent capsular contracture.

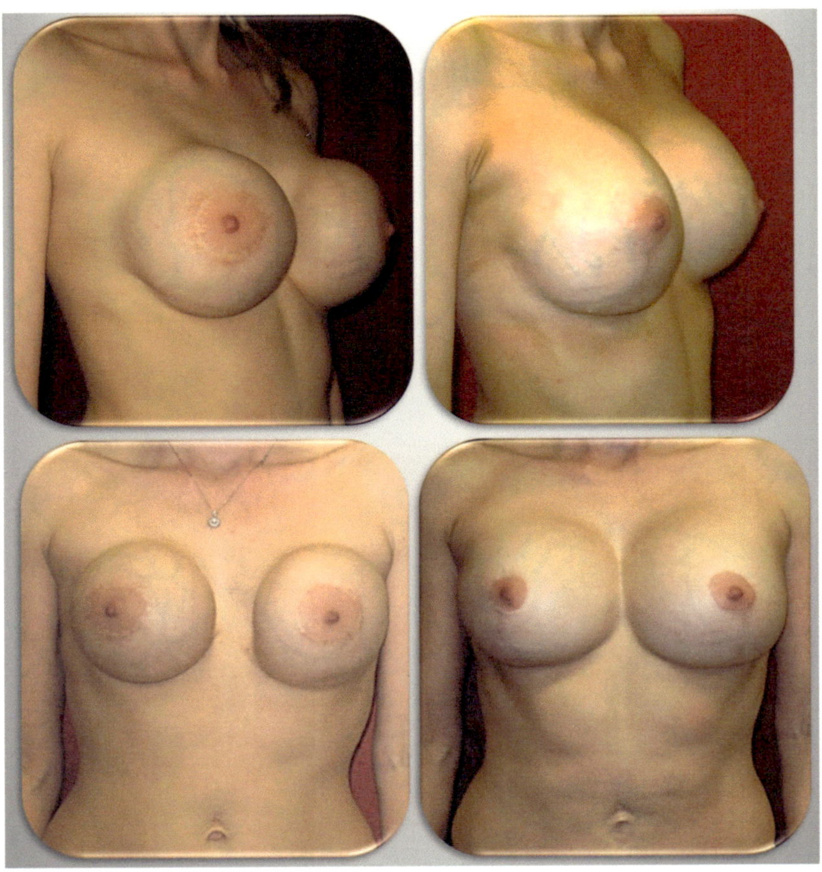

Figure 18.
Recurrent Capsular Contracture and Use of ADM. The patient presented with Grade IV capsular contracture after undergoing four prior breast augmentation procedures. On examination, residual implant pockets were identified along with a retracted pectoralis muscle and calcified capsule tissue. Surgical correction involved complete capsulectomy and pocket reconstruction using an acellular dermal matrix. The ADM was anchored to the inferior margin of the pectoralis muscle and affixed to the rib at the intended inframammary fold position. A vertical mastopexy was performed concurrently to enhance breast shape and symmetry.

6.4 Implant rippling/deflation

As previously noted, breast implant rippling refers to visible wrinkling on the skin surface due to folding or contour irregularities of the implant, particularly in patients with thin, soft tissue coverage. Surgeons should be equipped to offer both minimally invasive and surgical solutions for correction. One widely used technique is autologous fat grafting, which improves contour and increases tissue thickness over the implant. While this approach can be effective, it carries two primary considerations: the unpredictable resorption of fat over time and ongoing discussion around a potential association with increased cancer risk, though current evidence remains inconclusive and under continued investigation [30].

Research indicates that autologous fat grafts can experience resorption rates ranging from 20–90%, with an average volume retention of about 50% over time [31, 32]. Following fat grafting, patients may experience complications such as fat necrosis and the development of oil cysts, which may lead to nodule formation. It is important to counsel patients that approximately 40–60% of the transferred fat may be resorbed within 3 to 6 months, and additional grafting procedures may be necessary to reach the desired aesthetic result.

With respect to oncologic safety, current research suggests that fat grafting does not significantly increase the risk of tumor recurrence in patients who have undergone breast-conserving therapy or mastectomy [33, 34].

During fat grafting procedures, adipose tissue is harvested from a donor site elsewhere on the body and carefully injected into the breast to enhance shape, contour, volume, and soft tissue thickness. To support optimal graft survival and integration, small aliquots of fat are deposited along the pectoral and supra-pectoral planes. Surgeons should avoid injecting large volumes at once, as excessive pressure within the tissue may compromise blood supply, increasing the risk of fat necrosis and reducing graft viability. A conservative and layered technique contributes to better long-term outcomes and minimizes complications [35–37].

Implant exchange is a more involved surgical option that involves removing the current implants and replacing them with higher cohesivity silicone implants. Implant cohesiveness refers to the firmness and structural integrity of the silicone gel, which varies depending on the degree of molecular cross-linking. The more cross-linked the silicone, the firmer and more form-stable the implant becomes. Highly cohesive implants offer improved shape maintenance and are less prone to rippling, making them a viable choice, especially in patients with thin, soft tissue coverage or those undergoing revisional breast surgery [33]. The choice of implant cohesiveness should be customized to each patient's aesthetic goals and anatomical needs. Highly cohesive implants are well-suited for individuals desiring enhanced projection, upper pole fullness, and defined breast contours. In contrast, low to moderate cohesive implants offer a softer, more natural feel, while still maintaining structural integrity. Beyond their shaping capabilities, highly cohesive gel implants are associated with a lower risk of silicone leakage, thanks to their more form-stable, solid-like gel, making them a reliable option for long-term performance and durability.

When implant rippling results from subglandular placement, converting the implant to a subpectoral pocket can significantly enhance soft tissue coverage, providing improved implant support and minimizing surface irregularities. Combining pocket exchange with the use of a high-cohesivity implant as well as autologous fat grafting may deliver superior aesthetic outcomes. Although highly cohesive implants help minimize gel leakage in the event of rupture, they may be perceived as firmer to the touch, potentially compromising the natural feel of the augmented or reconstructed breast [38].

6.5 Nipple-areolar complex refinement/reconstruction

Refinement of the nipple-areolar complex plays a vital role in achieving a successful aesthetic outcome in breast reconstruction. A well-positioned, symmetrical, and proportionate NAC is often considered the focal point of breast *aesthetics*, and its reconstruction requires a high level of surgical precision. Indications for NAC revision include asymmetry, excessive size, undesirable pigmentation, or suboptimal results from previous reconstructive efforts. The objective of refinement is to recreate a NAC that is natural-looking, balanced, and proportionate, ultimately enhancing the overall harmony and appearance of the reconstructed breast.

For patients exhibiting NAC irregularities, ranging from subtle asymmetries to more pronounced deformities such as tubular breasts, a variety of mastopexy techniques can be employed to restore a balanced and aesthetically pleasing NAC. In cases of mild vertical asymmetry, a crescent lift is often sufficient to correct the discrepancy by repositioning the NAC. For tubular breast deformities with excessive projection and herniation of the NAC, a Benelli or Donut mastopexy proves particularly effective. This approach not only reduces areolar protrusion but also helps to reshape and flatten the central breast mound, contributing to a more natural contour (**Figure 19**).

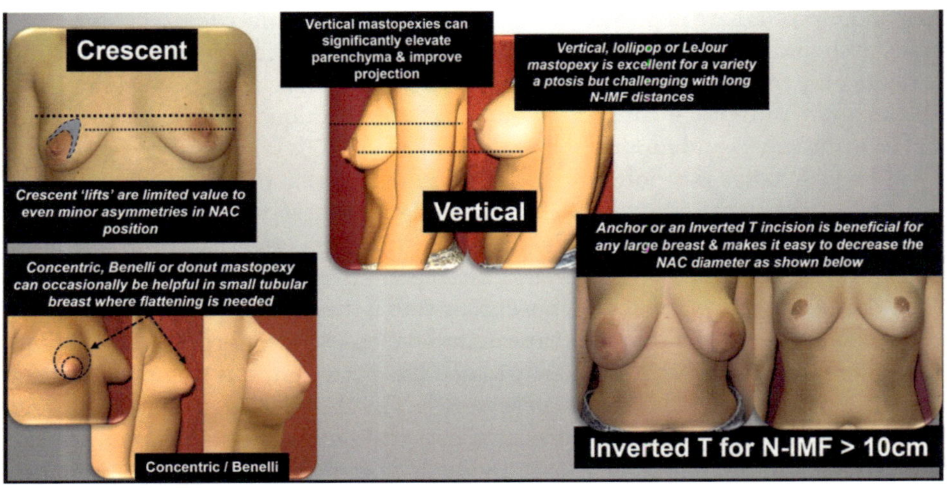

Figure 19.
NAC Asymmetry. A variety of mastopexy techniques can be utilized to correct differences between the NACs and to achieve better symmetry when the NACs appear unbalanced or mismatched in size.

Following breast reconstruction, the NAC may become disproportionate or asymmetrical. NAC widening is a common complication associated with the Benelli (donut) mastopexy, as the circular closure can concentrate tension around the areolar margin, leading to stretching over time. In contrast, a vertical mastopexy, either alone or combined with a horizontal component, allows for more balanced tension distribution across the incision. This technique not only minimizes the likelihood of NAC widening but also provides an opportunity to revise or camouflage existing periareolar or vertical scars, resulting in a more refined and aesthetic outcome (**Figure 20**).

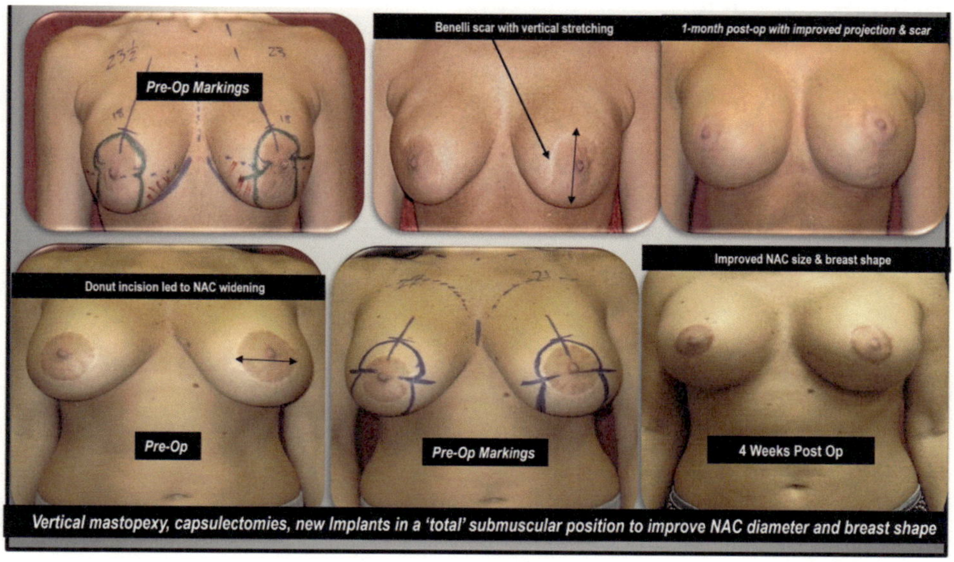

Figure 20.
NAC Refinement. Following breast reconstruction, the NAC can often appear enlarged or out of proportion to the surrounding breast tissue. Utilizing a vertical mastopexy, with or without a horizontal extension, enables the surgeon to refine the breast shape, manage preexisting scars, and limit further stretching of the NAC.

A recent advancement in optimizing post-reconstruction breast aesthetics is the artful use of NAC tattooing. Previous surgical procedures may lead to distortion, pigment changes, or even partial or complete loss of the NAC. Skilled medical tattoo artists can create highly realistic reconstructions, blending the tattoo seamlessly with surrounding skin. This process involves customizing a color palette unique to each patient, and employing shading techniques to replicate depth, texture, and dimension, resulting in an outcome that closely mimics the natural appearance of the nipple-areolar complex.

7. Conclusion

In summary, breast rejuvenation surgery is a sophisticated and continually advancing area within cosmetic surgery, demanding both technical expertise and aesthetic sensibility. Achieving optimal results in primary and revisional procedures relies on comprehensive preoperative planning, precise patient assessment, and the strategic application of surgical techniques tailored to individual anatomical and cosmetic goals. Surgeons must be well-versed in managing common complications such as asymmetry, implant malposition, and capsular contracture, especially in patients presenting with complex breast conditions. As surgical innovations and biomaterials continue to evolve, so too does the potential to deliver both functional restoration and aesthetic enhancement. Ultimately, success in breast rejuvenation stems from a collaborative partnership between patient and surgeon, grounded in clear communication and realistic expectations, to achieve satisfying and enduring outcomes.

Disclosure statement

The Authors have nothing to disclose.

Author details

Pasquale G. Tolomeo[1]* and Angelo Cuzalina[2]

1 Tolomeo Cosmetic Surgery, Fall River, MA, USA

2 Tulsa Surgical Arts, Tulsa, OK, USA

*Address all correspondence to: doctortolomeo@gmail.com

References

[1] 2023 Plastic Surgery Statistics Report. Available from: https://www.plasticsurgery.org/documents/news/statistics/2023/plastic-surgery-statistics-report-2023.pdf

[2] Breast Cancer Screening Recommendations for Women at Average Risk." Susan G. Komen®, Available from: www.komen.org/breastcancer/breastcancerscreeningforwomen.html.

[3] Mallucci P, Branford O. Concepts in aesthetic breast dimensions: Analysis of the ideal breast. Journal of Plastic, Reconstructive & Aesthetic Surgery. 2012;**65**(1):8-16

[4] Janis J. Essentials of Aesthetic Surgery. New York: Thieme; 2017

[5] Stevens W. Grabb and Smith's Plastic Surgery: Mastopexy and Mastopexy/Augmentation. 7th ed. Wolters Kluwer; 2013

[6] Nahai F, Nahai F. Art of Aesthetic Surgery. 2nd ed. Thieme Medical; 2011

[7] Atiye B, Chahine F. Metrics of the aesthetically perfect breast. Aesthetic Plastic Surgery. 2018;**42**(5):1187-1194

[8] Bolletta E, Mcgoldrick C, Hall-Findlay E. Aesthetic breast surgery: What do the measurements reveal? Aesthetic Surgery Journal. 2019;**40**(7):742-752

[9] Qureshi A, Myckatyn T, Tenenbaum M. Mastopexy and mastopexy-augmentation. Aesthetic Surgery Journal. 2018;**38**(4):374-384

[10] Bark AA Jr, Minikowski Guilherme C, Mujahed IB. U.3. multiplane L-scar augmentation mastopexy: An individualized approach to muscle, glandular tissue, and skin. Plastic and Reconstructive Surgery. 2024;**153**(4):801-809. DOI: 10.1097/PRS.0000000000010850

[11] Benelli L. A new periareolar mammaplasty: The "round block" technique. Aesthetic Plastic Surgery. 1990;**14**(1):93-100

[12] Cuzalina A, McLain L. Simultaneous Mastopexy with Augmentation. London, UK: IntechOpen; 2019

[13] Hall-Findlay E. Pedicles in vertical breast reduction and mastopexy. Clinics in Plastic Surgery. 2002;**29**(3):379-391

[14] Rohrich R, Gosman A, Brown S, Reisch J. Mastopexy preferences: A survey of board-certified plastic surgeons. Plastic and Reconstructive Surgery. 2006;**118**(7):1631-1638

[15] Tebbetts JB. Discussion: A 15-year experience with primary breast augmentation. Plastic and Reconstructive Surgery. 2011;**127**(3):1311-1313. DOI: 10.1097/PRS.0b013e318205f1aa

[16] Siy R, Khan K, Izaddoost S, Brown R. The superomedial pedicle wise-pattern breast reduction: Reproducible, reliable, and resilient. Seminars in Plastic Surgery. 2015;**29**(02):094-101

[17] Bresnick SD. Prophylactic leukotriene inhibitor therapy for the reduction of capsular contracture in primary silicone breast augmentation: Experience with over 1100 cases. Plastic and Reconstructive Surgery. 2017 Feb;**139**(2):379-385. DOI: 10.1097/PRS.0000000000003006. Epub 2017 Jan 26

[18] Headon H, Kasem A, Mokbel K. Capsular contracture after breast

augmentation: An update for clinical practice. Archives of Plastic Surgery. 2015;**42**(5):532-543. DOI: 10.5999/aps.2015.42.5.532. Epub 2015 Sep 15

[19] Frame J. The waterfall effect in breast augmentation. Gland Surgery. 2017;**6**(2):193-202. DOI: 10.21037/gs.2016.10.01

[20] Spear SL. Little JW3rd. Breast capsulorrhaphy. Plastic and Reconstructive Surgery. 1988;**81**(2):274-279. DOI: 10.1097/00006534-198802000-00026

[21] Bradley Calobrace M, Mays C, Wilson R, Wermeling R. Popcorn capsulorrhaphy in revision aesthetic breast surgery. Aesthetic Surgery Journal. 2020;**40**(1):63-74. DOI: 10.1093/asj/sjy324

[22] Williams SF, Martin DP, Moses AC. The history of GalaFLEX P4HB scaffold. Aesthetic Surgery Journal. 2016;**36**(suppl. 2):S33-S42. DOI: 10.1093/asj/sjw141. Epub 2016 Oct 3

[23] Nair NM, Mills DC. Poly-4-hydroxybutyrate (P4HB) scaffold internal support: Preliminary experience with direct implant opposition during complex breast revisions. Aesthetic Surgery Journal. 2019;**39**(11):1203-1213. DOI: 10.1093/asj/sjy276

[24] Zeplin PH, Corduff N. Influence of patient age on capsular contracture after aesthetic breast augmentation. The Canadian Journal of Plastic Surgery. 2015;**23**(2):67-69. DOI: 10.1177/229255031502300209

[25] Spear SL, Baker JL. Classification of capsular contracture after prosthetic breast reconstruction. Plastic and Reconstructive Surgery. 1995;**96**(5):1119-1123

[26] Pereira Leite L, Correia Sa I, Marques M. Etiopathogenesis and treatment of breast capsular contracture. Acta Médica Portuguesa. 2013;**26**:737-745

[27] Lardi AM, Farhadi J. Physiopathology, prevention, and treatment of capsular contracture. In: Urban C et al., editors. Oncoplastic and Reconstructive Breast Surgery. New York: Springer; 2019. pp. 601-607

[28] Moyer HR, Pinell-White X, Losken A. The effect of radiation on acellular dermal matrix and capsule formation in breast reconstruction: Clinical outcomes and histologic analysis. Plastic and Reconstructive Surgery. 2014;**133**(2):214-221. DOI: 10.1097/01.prs.0000437255.01199.42

[29] Basu CB, Leong M, Hicks MJ. Acellular cadaveric dermis decreases the inflammatory response in capsule formation in reconstructive breast surgery. Plastic and Reconstructive Surgery. 2010;**126**(6):1842-1847. DOI: 10.1097/PRS.0b013e3181f44674

[30] Gutowski KA, ASPS Fat Graft Task Force. Current applications and safety of autologous fat grafts: A report of the ASPS fat graft task force. Plastic and Reconstructive Surgery. 2009;**124**:272-280

[31] Hivernaud V, Lefourn B, Guicheux J, et al. Autologous fat grafting in the breast: Critical points and technique improvements. Aesthetic Plastic Surgery. 2015;**39**:547-561. DOI: 10.1007/s00266-015-0503-y

[32] Yin B, Zhang X, Cai L, Han X, Li F. Function-preserving fat grafting in the breast: Results based on 18 years of experience. Journal of Plastic, Reconstructive & Aesthetic Surgery. 2022;**75**(9):2996-3003. DOI: 10.1016/j.bjps.2022.04.084. Epub 2022 May 2

[33] Petit JY, Botteri E, Lohsiriwat V, et al. Locoregional recurrence risk after lipofilling in breast cancer patients. Annals of Oncology. 2012;**23**:582-588

[34] Kronowitz SJ, Mandujano CC, Liu J, et al. Lipofilling of the breast does not increase the risk of recurrence of breast cancer: A matched controlled study. Plastic and Reconstructive Surgery. 2016;**137**:385-393

[35] Delay E, Garson S, Tousson G, Sinna R. Fat injection to the breast: Technique, results, and indications based on 880 procedures over 10 years. Aesthetic Surgery Journal. 2009;**29**:360-376

[36] Khouri RK, Rigotti G, Cardoso E, Khouri RKJ, Biggs TM. Megavolume autologous fat transfer II. Plastic and Reconstructive Surgery. 2014;**133**:1369-1377

[37] Calobrace MB, Capizzi PJ. The biology and evolution of cohesive gel and shaped implants. Plastic and Reconstructive Surgery. 2014;**134**:6S11S

[38] Handel N, Garcia ME, Wixtrom R. Breast implant rupture: Causes, incidence, clinical impact, and management. Plastic and Reconstructive Surgery. 2013;**132**:11281137

Chapter 11

Perspective Chapter: Comprehensive Overview of Breast Reduction Surgery – Techniques, Outcomes, and Global Perspectives

Engin Selamioğlu

Abstract

Breast reduction surgery, or reduction mammoplasty, is a procedure aimed at alleviating physical discomfort and enhancing body image by reducing the size and weight of large breasts. This chapter provides a comprehensive overview, starting with common patient complaints such as chronic pain, skin irritation, and postural problems, as well as psychological issues like body image concerns and social anxiety. Pre-operative imaging techniques, including mammography, ultrasound, and MRI, are discussed to ensure thorough assessment. Detailed pre-operative planning and marking are crucial for successful outcomes. The surgical techniques covered include various incision patterns and tissue removal methods, with a focus on preserving nipple-areola complex sensation through different pedicle types. Potential complications, such as hematoma, infection, and scarring, are outlined along with strategies for mitigation. Post-operative care emphasizes the importance of supportive garments, activity restrictions, and scar management. This chapter aims to equip medical professionals with the knowledge required for performing breast reduction surgery and managing patient care effectively, ensuring both physical and psychological benefits for the patient.

Keywords: breast reduction surgery, chronic shoulder pain, skin irritation, pre-operative imaging, complications, scar management

1. Introduction

The subject of breast reduction plastic surgery—also known as reduction mammoplasty—is quite a significant one, considering the number of women (and some men!) who have undergone or will undergo this operation. Why is that? Well, because large breasts can be a real pain and awkwardness for those who have them and because "reducing" them can relieve both physical and psychic torment in such persons [1, 2].

2. Breast reduction surgery: A global perspective

The condition known as macromastia brings many sufferers immense chronic pain in the back, neck, and shoulders. This is because their unusually large breasts are a huge weight for their bodies to carry. Studies have shown that an astonishing 85% of women seeking breast reduction report severe pain in these areas—not only directly under their breasts but also on either side and at the top of their chests [3].

Moreover, almost all globally, women who undergo breast reduction report that they feel infinitely more relieved from chronic pain after surgery. Whether this relief takes the form of methodology or moot point—members of both genders are quick to opine when asked—the suffering these individuals endure makes them nothing short of superheroes in my book.

Having large breasts can lead to persistent skin irritation and infections in the fold underneath them. This is called intertrigo. It happens when the skin in that area gets rubbed excessively and meets moisture, which causes a kind of dermatitis that develops into a chronic infection. Studies have found that fully 60% of women with macromastia (breasts larger than average) get these infections recurrently—an experience that is not only itchy and uncomfortable but also potentially dangerous, given the ease with which bacteria can work their way deep into the skin via those folds [4, 5].

Many women with large breasts find that the deep creases under their shoulders, where the bra straps fall, become a common site for skin tags. Why does this happen? Because a bra strap does not stretch, it cuts into the skin with every move the unrestrained breast makes. This also happens because we do not often think about putting on our breasts when we apply our bras. General Ian Harris, FRCS (a surgeon), details in One Hundred Semiconductor Epitaxial Wafers Later how severe a problem shoulder pain and nerve compression can be for women with macromastia. He states that a recent study reveals that 70% of such women suffer from chronic and debilitating shoulder pain—an average annual cost to the society of over $13 billion—at least as documented within the United States [6].

Many women with large breasts find that discomfort and pain related to breast motion limit their ability to engage in exercises, sports, or even go for a run. Nevertheless, these are powerful ways of maintaining our overall health—physically, socially, and psychologically. On a global level, over 75% of women considering breast reduction express limited physical activity as one of their primary motivators. Why should this be the case?

The weight of large breasts can push the chest forward and force women to slump, creating short, tight muscles on either side of their spine. This can pull their upper back down into a kyphosis, or hump, that can make them appear round-shouldered—a condition associated with chronic back pain and muscle spasms [6, 7].

Significant psychological and social impacts can result from macromastia. For many women, the condition holds somewhat harmful implications for their lives because of the direct relation between large breasts and self-esteem.

Breasts are a very significant part of women's bodies—almost to the point where they can make or break a woman's body image. Nevertheless, these essentially goofy things called breasts, with 80% of women reporting dissatisfaction with their breast size or shape (most often to the extent that they feel unfit), play a nearly invisible role in the conversation about this issue. The only thing even close to providing some background noise on this issue is what happened recently when Sherri Shepherd sought help for her massive breasts from "The View."

For women over 40 and those with a family history of breast cancer, mammography is the most effective tool for diagnosing breast cancer in its early stages. However, there is a flip side: Mammography screeners may sometimes tell mastectomy candidates that they have breast cancer when nothing is wrong [8].

Breast ultrasound is most useful for younger or dense breast tissue patients. It gives a clear, detailed picture of the internal structure of the breasts, making it easy to identify any abnormalities. This task can be tricky, if not impossible, with a mammogram [9, 10].

Part of what makes ultrasound so safe and simple is that there is no exposure to X-rays. In fact, worldwide, 70% of breast reduction (reduction mammominus simplified-disappearance) involves pre-operative ultrasound.

For individuals at high risk for breast cancer or with complex breast anatomy, magnetic resonance imaging (MRI) may be the imaging modality of choice. It affords exquisite visualization of the breast, aiding surgeons in a critical stage of workflow—just ahead of "the big reveal," when decisions about whether and how much to excise are made. Today, on this blog, we bring you three stories from around the world illustrating how MRI is used for these critical decisions.

The first contact with a patient usually involves an initial consultation. In this evaluation, our experienced breast plastic surgeons conduct a thorough medical history and physical exam to assess each individual's qualifications for surgery.

When performing this evaluation, we consider three main aspects: the size and shape of the breasts; in assessing these, we look not just at the absolute size but also at how much reduction is needed and how symmetrical (or nearly so) the breasts are. We also evaluate skin quality—a key consideration because it can result either in natural-looking folds after your breast surgery or substantial scarring that can be very visible—along with skin elasticity (which should not be confused with sagging) [10].

It is essential to mark the body accurately and entirely before a mastectomy, with some form of pre-operative surgery marking. This is not an advisory service; it is a mandatory part of the safe delivery of breast cancer surgery. Globally, this seems to be a consensus that should be widely adopted. In my practice, I find it helpful to use three types of pre-operative markings that allow me both to plan and perform the operation safely and reasonably efficiently: midline chest markings for symmetry (95% of surgeons use these), inframammary fold markings (90% use those), and trans-nipple markings for the creation of new nipple tattoos at the level either of or slightly above the natural inframammary crease—tattoos that replace missing nipples in most instances during reconstructive breast surgery (85% usage).

Breast reduction is a safe and effective procedure used to reshape one or both breasts. The process typically begins with the patient being administered general anesthesia, ensuring they are unconscious and cannot feel any pain throughout the operation. This helps minimize any distress the individual may experience during what could amount to several long hours of surgery, depending on how much tissue needs to be removed [11].

Healthcare providers use several incision patterns for breast reduction. They are based on the type and amount of tissue to be removed, as well as the individual's breast anatomy—especially the extent of stretch marks and previous scars. These help determine which incision technique might work best for a particular patient [12].

The most common is the inverted T or anchor incision, which offers the "best concealability." This includes not only an incision surrounding the areola but also two additional arms that extend downward toward—but not all the way to—the crease where the breast meets the body; this helps to minimize vertical pull on the skin during a person's natural upward trajectory of the breasts when she stands up or raises her arms.

Incisions in this area can result in some very conspicuous scar tissue—upwardly extending scars that can look like widow's peaks.

I removed excess breast tissue, fat, and skin during a breast reduction. After removing these excesses, the doctor can then reposition what is left to create an esthetically pleasing contour for the breast. Sometimes liposuction is used with other techniques to achieve this end—and 40% of the time.

The nipple-areola complex is relocated to a higher, and therefore more natural, position on the breast. In doing so, it is crucial not to impair blood supply and sensation to this part of the breast. The type of pedicle (a flap of tissue that carries the complex up to its new home) used in mastopexy or breast reduction may vary depending upon many factors, like how large or small the breasts are, how much tissue needs to be removed, and whom you choose to perform the procedure.

Overall, when performed correctly with surgeons using any number of techniques—including those that involve direct attachment—breast enlargement through lipo-filling can result in very sustainable, natural-looking results.

The nipple-areola complex remains attached to a pedicle of superiorly based tissue. This technique occasionally referred to as the "nipple-sparing mastectomy," maintains both sensation and blood supply to the nipple.

When performed correctly, this technique carries an acceptable risk of complications—87%, according to one major review. Still, some value can be found in examining how this procedure is performed and what sort of results might be expected.

To help my listeners understand what I am saying, I have drawn diagrams illustrating the inferior breast-tissue pedicle we have discussed and these three other types.

A reliable outcome for important breast drooping (ptosis) can be expected with an inferiorly based pedicle that preserves the nipple-areola complex. A commonly used technique for turning this concept into reality is illustrated here with a diagram that shows just how it has been done. When techniques are discussed, they are sometimes accompanied by statistics about the percentages of plastic surgeons using which techniques and in what parts of the world. Here, we will delve a bit into both the concept and the technique to understand better why one might opt for using an inferiorly based nipple-areola complex as part of a mastopexy or breast uplift procedure (**Figure 1**).

The medially based tissue pedicle is a great way to keep the nipple-areola complex intact during breast reduction (**Figure 2**). It is a thin shelf of fat and areolar skin that attaches to the inside of the breast, under the nipple, and projects forward. When you look at illustrations of this technique, I think it is essential patients understand what will be done in their operation—you can get a sense both for how unique this part of the female physique is and just how much variation there is from person to person, even within our Western cultural criteria for what constitutes an ideal NAC (**Figure 3**).

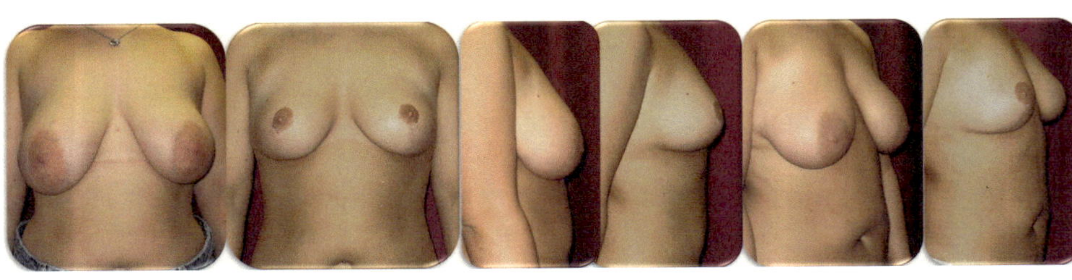

Figure 1.
A 20-year-old female showing three views before and 6 months following an inferior pedicle breast reduction/lift. She had a classic inverted T-type incision. Because her right breast was larger the left preoperatively, extra tissue was removed from the right compared to the left to help improve symmetry (all photos courtesy of Dr. Cuzalina).

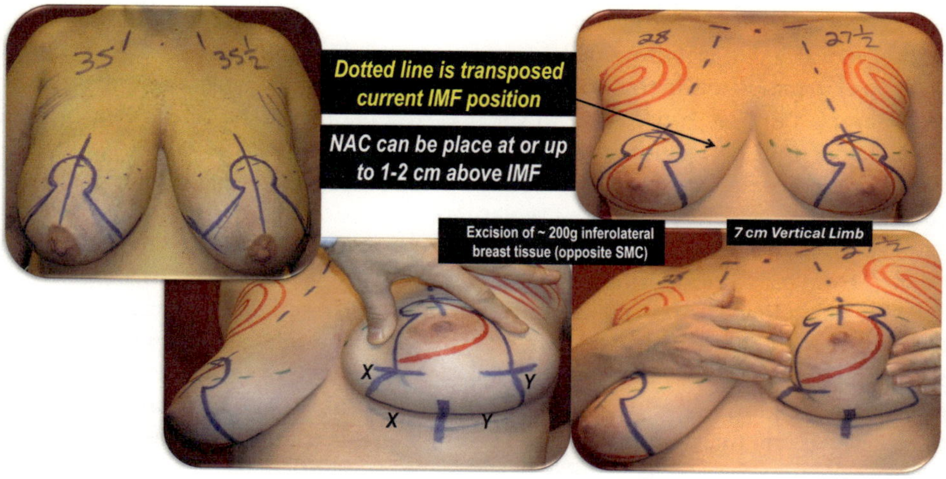

Figure 2.
The figures above demonstrate marking and vertical limb length specifically when using a medial-central pedicle or superomedial central pedicle. An inferior pedicle technique bottoms out more so the vertical limb length should be closer to 5 cm. The central portion of the pedicle is important because the pectoral branches off the thoracoacromial artery and provide blood supply to the pedicle besides the medial perforators. Other markings include areas planned for liposuction typically in the anterior axilla and lateral breasts areas (all photos courtesy of Dr. Cuzalina).

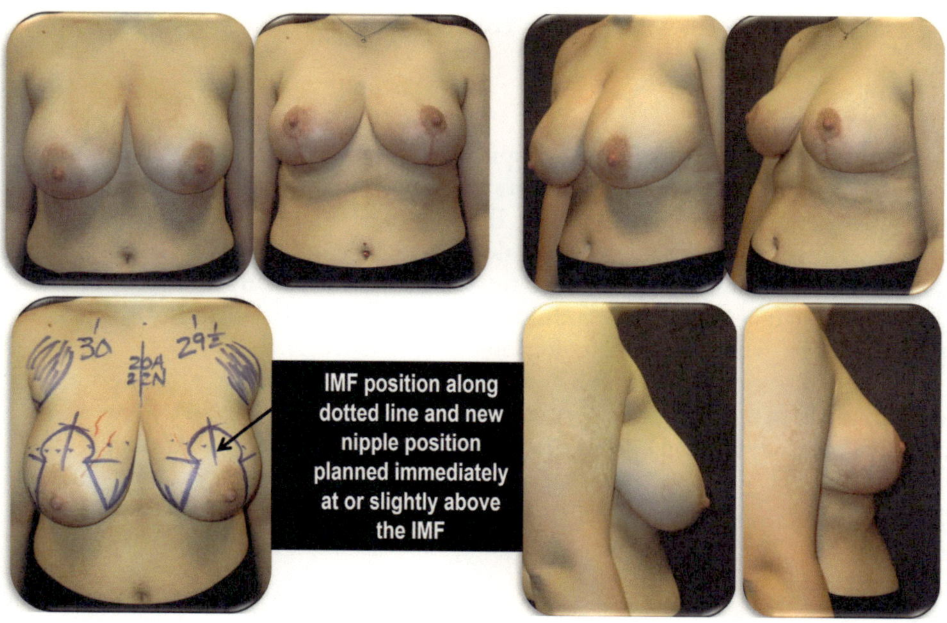

Figure 3.
A young female showing three views before and only 4 weeks following a medial pedicle breast reduction/ lift. She had a classic inverted T-type incision. The markings shown record her SN-N distance preoperatively and the inverted T-type pattern and dotted lines along her current inframammary fold location. Her planned nipple position is marked at 22 cm, and the top of her new areolar positon is at 20 cm (all photos courtesy of Dr. Cuzalina).

Globally speaking, let us say about 15% of women who want breast reduction use this method. Is it still right for you?

As an alternative to the traditional superior pedicle, this flap attaches the nipple-areola complex to tissue on the side of the breast. It is appropriate for specific, unique breast shapes and sizes and is indicated for cases where individual anatomy calls for it. Like all reconstruction techniques, this one is not without risk: complications can occur. Nonetheless, flapless nipple-areolar reconstruction makes breasts look whole again. All Prostate Cancerasca Handbook illustrations depict each step of "the lateral pedicle," from preparation through closure.

Breast reduction by Laboratories of Plastic Surgery Description: The principal object of the breast reduction technique is to reduce the size and weight of a hypertrophied breast. Severe cases may require a more extensive procedure during which some portion of the breast is pedunculated or attached by a stalk to another part of the same breast; in such cases, it is said that an "areolar flap" or "nipple-areola complex" has been raised.

(After the American Society of Plastic Surgeons) Illustration: Here, we have shown what the 11-loupe magnification might look like if we were performing such an operation.

Complications from surgery can sometimes happen, but many can be avoided with proper planning and care. Some complications that can occur directly after a breast reduction are significant bleeding inside the breast, which in rare cases might require the patient to come back into the operating room to have it controlled. Breathing problems associated with obesity or sleep apnea may not be immediately relevant to breast reduction but affect patients who may undergo this procedure. Even though these issues are relatively unheard of as causes for breast reduction, they do underscore the importance of your doctor knowing about all your health aspects before you undertake major surgery—Redefining "complications," p. 135.

2.1 Long-term results

Complications can and do occur despite efforts to minimize them. Scarring is one such complication. While some scarring is unavoidable, the appearance of scabs and subsequent scars can be minimized through careful suturing and postoperative scar care. However, noticeable scarring does occur in about 15% of breast reduction cases—meaning it might happen to your teenager now if you urge her to have the surgery at my suggestion (or your child's decision), and global visibility obscures an appreciation for what a good outcome looks like (**Figure 4**).

Nipple sensation often remains a concern because nerve damage during surgery can result in temporary or permanent changes. About one in five women who have breast reduction undergo nerve damage that leads to altered nipple

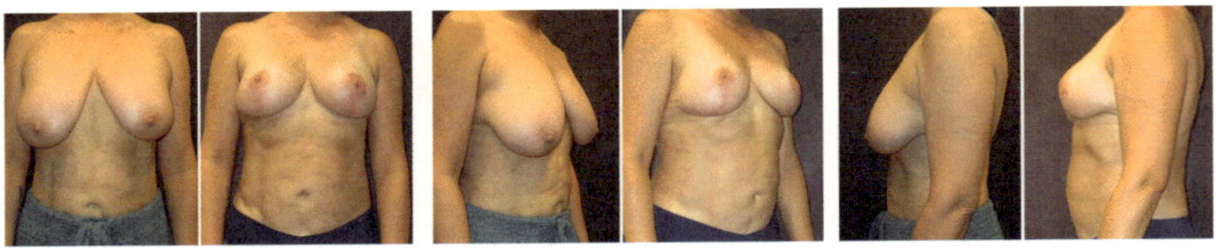

Figure 4.
A 53-year-old female showing three views before and 6 months following a superomedial pedicle breast reduction/lift. She had a classic inverted T-type incision. Because her right breast was almost one bra cup size larger preoperatively, approximately 132 g extra was removed from the right compared to the left to help improve volume symmetry (all photos courtesy of Dr. Cuzalina).

sensations—fortunately, it is not usually a severe development, although it can sometimes be quite annoying to the woman experiencing it.

There are specific risks associated with DIEP flap breast reconstruction. While they are rare, they can and do happen—especially to smokers or individuals with poor blood circulation. Careful planning on the surgeon's part and good postoperative care can help alleviate these complications. Nipple necrosis is one such risk; it is a severe, uncommon complication that usually occurs in 0.5% of patients who have this procedure—and for my patients, I use nipple-sparing techniques to minimize that risk even further.

Fat necrosis is another rare but significant risk for recipients of DIEP flap breast reconstruction. In its extreme form, fat death leads to lumps beneath the skin that refuse to go away unless more surgery intervenes.

Optimal recovery after surgery is ensured by proper postoperative care. The initial phase centers around the body's immediate recovery, with a few critical tasks to perform in order to keep the surgical site healthy. These are putting on dressings (which act as a barrier that protects the surgically repaired area) and managing fluids (either through drainable avenues or avoiding them altogether). About 95% of all surgeries involve using drains.

This phase also sees attempts made at managing something else—a lot has been said about this, but it is worth reiterating: effective pain management is not an option—it is mandatory if one hopes to get on an access road back to good health after surgery. Pain subjects patients (and their support people) to reduced tolerance for other kinds of hassles during recovery; it engages the brains of both the recently operated-on person and those close to them, adequately preparing for other trials along the access road leading back home.

The recovery period is a time of healing and comfort. During this phase, the body rebuilds itself; scars formed and the area around the incision heal. The breasts maintain their shape during this time, too. One thing that is often overlooked but is very important to breast reformation efforts is access to emotional support.

Incidence rates globally: 85% of patients are told to wear a bra for added comfort during healing. Subsequent activity changes (reducing "up," "down," and "across," or lateral movements) enable better blood flow, which enhances healing on two fronts: within the breasts themselves and in the skin directly above them—the skin into which stitches will be placed. In my next life, I'm going after an incision-free NABA surgery!

The long-term care of breast cancer patients requires ongoing monitoring to ensure that the disease does not recur. The appearance of scars is one aspect of a woman's life after breast cancer that can be a concern. Several treatments are available to improve and even out the scarred area. These may include silicone sheets or gels, cortisone creams to reduce redness and hardness, or massage techniques to help break up fibrotic tissue and improve healing.

There are many different methods for improving the appearance of scars—so much so that some people find it hard to believe they are being told about only two or three at a time. After we looked at how often these techniques are used, in 70% of cases, they are applied in this way globally [13].

The life-enhancing potential of breast reduction surgery cannot be overstated for both the immediate and long-term benefits it confers. Not only can this type of plastic surgery ease the severe discomfort that larger breasts can inflict on a woman's daily life but it also opens up new possibilities for improved body image, allowing women to see themselves in a more favorable light. From what I have gathered through my research, here are some key points about how breast reduction is performed and with what minimum of risk [13, 14].

In terms of pre-operative planning, an important part—may be the most important part—that plastic surgeons undertake is detailed sizing of the breasts. Why? To ensure that in the unforgiving world of 3-D sculpting, every patient's imagined ideal outcome is not only achievable but safe for the patient, not something that carries any risk worthy of mention, signals up sufficient safety rituals toward this end.

Acknowledgements

The author acknowledges the use of Grammarly (AI tool) for language polishing of the manuscript.

Author details

Engin Selamioğlu
Haliç University, Istanbul, Turkey

*Address all correspondence to: doktorengin@hotmail.com

References

[1] Manahan MA, Buretta KJ, Chang D, Mithani SK, Mallalieu J, Shermak MA. An outcomes analysis of 2142 breast reduction procedures. Annals of Plastic Surgery. 2015;**74**(3):289-292. DOI: 10.1097/SAP.0b013e31829d2261

[2] Cunningham BL, Gear AJ, Kerrigan CL, Collins ED. Analysis of breast reduction complications derived from the BRAVO study. Plastic and Reconstructive Surgery. 2005;**115**(6):1597-1604. DOI: 10.1097/01.prs.0000160695.33457.db. Erratum in: Plast Reconstr Surg. 2005;116(1):361

[3] Iwuagwu OC, Platt AJ, Drew PJ. Breast reduction surgery in the UK and Ireland—Current trends. Annals of the Royal College of Surgeons of England. 2006;**88**(6):585-588. DOI: 10.1308/003588406X130598

[4] Canelo-Aybar C, Taype-Rondan A, Zafra-Tanaka JH, Rigau D, Graewingholt A, Lebeau A, et al. Preoperative breast magnetic resonance imaging in patients with ductal carcinoma in situ: A systematic review for the European Commission Initiative on Breast Cancer (ECIBC). European Radiology. 2021;**31**(8):5880-5893. DOI: 10.1007/s00330-021-07873-2. Epub 2021 May 30. Erratum in: Eur Radiol. 2022;32(6):4333. DOI: 10.1007/s00330-021-08489-2

[5] Lonie S, Sachs R, Shen A, Hunter-Smith DJ, Rozen WM, Seifman M. A systematic review of patient reported outcome measures for women with macromastia who have undergone breast reduction surgery. Gland Surgery. 2019;**8**(4):431-440. DOI: 10.21037/gs.2019.03.08

[6] Sapino G, Haselbach D, Watfa W, Baudoin J, Martineau J, Guillier D, et al. Evaluation of long-term breast shape in inferior versus superomedial pedicle reduction mammoplasty: A comparative study. Gland Surgery. 2021;**10**(3):1018-1028. DOI: 10.21037/gs-20-440. Erratum in: Gland Surg. 2021;10(5):1840. DOI: 10.21037/gs-2020-04

[7] Kemaloğlu CA, Özocak H. Comparative outcomes of inferior pedicle and superomedial pedicle technique with wise pattern reduction in gigantomastic patients. Annals of Plastic Surgery. 2018;**80**(3):217-222. DOI: 10.1097/SAP.0000000000001231

[8] Blomqvist L, Eriksson A, Brandberg Y. Reduction mammaplasty provides long-term improvement in health status and quality of life. Plastic and Reconstructive Surgery. 2000;**106**(5):991-997. DOI: 10.1097/00006534-200010000-00005

[9] Ozbey R, Cansel N, Firat C, Baydemir MB. Factors affecting patient satisfaction in breast reduction surgeries: A retrospective clinical study. Aesthetic Plastic Surgery. 2021;**45**(6):2658-2664. DOI: 10.1007/s00266-021-02354-9. Epub 2021 Jun 1

[10] Meretsky CR, Polychronis A, Schiuma AT. A comparative analysis of the advances in scar reduction: Techniques, technologies, and efficacy in plastic surgery. Cureus. 2024;**16**(8):e66806. DOI: 10.7759/cureus.66806

[11] Tanas Y, Tanas J. Comparative outcomes of superomedial and inferior pedicles in breast reduction and mastopexy: A meta-analysis of 5123 breasts. Aesthetic Plastic Surgery. 2024. DOI: 10.1007/s00266-024-04389-0

[12] Giorgi Rossi P, Djuric O, Navarra S, Rossi A, Di Napoli A, Frova L, et al. Geographic inequalities in breast cancer in Italy: Trend analysis of mortality and risk factors. International Journal of Environmental Research and Public Health. 2020;**17**(11):4165. DOI: 10.3390/ijerph17114165

[13] Derebaşınlıoğlu H, Karaca SN. The importance of preoperative imaging methods in reduction mammoplasty. Journal of Plastic, Reconstructive & Aesthetic Surgery. 2022;**75**(4):1424-1430. DOI: 10.1016/j.bjps.2021.11.073. Epub 2021 Nov 29

[14] Simpson AM, Donato DP, Kwok AC, Agarwal JP. Predictors of complications following breast reduction surgery: A National Surgical Quality Improvement Program study of 16,812 cases. Journal of Plastic, Reconstructive & Aesthetic Surgery. 2019;**72**(1):43-51. DOI: 10.1016/j.bjps.2018.09.002. Epub 2018 Sep 20. Erratum in: J Plast Reconstr Aesthet Surg. 2019;72(8):1434-1435. DOI: 10.1016/j.bjps.2019.04.002

Chapter 12

Mastopexy with Augmentation Mammoplasty

Morgan L. Fish, Rebecca Kelley, Marco Swanson, Alanna Fostyk and Mark A. Foglietti

Abstract

Mastopexy with breast augmentation is one of the more complex body contouring procedures causing even the most experienced plastic surgeons to approach this procedure with caution. The competing forces inherent to each procedure contributes to unpredictability, potential complications, and patient dissatisfaction. Preoperative planning is imperative including assessment of ptosis and elicitation of patient goals. Classically a subpectoral approach with mastopexy tailored to the degree of skin laxity has been described; subglandular augmentation with mastopexy may avoid sequelae of submuscular implant placement particularly in the aging breast. With careful execution, augmentation mastopexy has the ability to produce excellent results while minimizing complications when performed in either a simultaneous or staged fashion. Herein, various techniques for augmentation and mastopexy are described including pearls and pitfalls. Finally, the preferred technique executed by senior author (M.A.F.) is explained in detail.

Keywords: mastopexy, breast augmentation, breast lift, body contouring, esthetic surgery

1. Introduction

Augmentation mastopexy is arguably one of the most difficult esthetic surgeries performed by plastic surgeons. The opposing forces inherent to this operation, tightening of skin envelope to address ptosis with simultaneous stretching of skin and parenchyma for augmentation, lessen predictability and may contribute to higher rates of complications and patient dissatisfaction [1–3]. Despite this, with careful patient selection, attention to detail, and surgical execution, excellent surgical results are achievable.

2. Background

Since first described by Gonzales-Ulloa in 1960 and Regnault in 1966, various surgical approaches have been developed [3, 4]. Traditional mastopexy techniques including periareolar, vertical, and inverted T patterns with a combination of augmentation modalities including implants and auto augmentation have been utilized.

Historically, submuscular, or more commonly subpectoral, implant placement has been considered the standard approach. As trends in breast augmentation have evolved so have trends with augmentation mastopexy. Varying techniques utilized in augmentation mastopexy will be described below including the pitfalls associated with each approach.

3. Preoperative assessment

3.1 Patient evaluation

As with any surgical procedure, thorough preoperative patient evaluation, including a detailed history and focused physical examination, is essential. It is important to elicit history of diabetes, weight loss, smoking status, use of immunosuppressive medications, and prior radiation as these may predispose to risk factors such as delayed wound healing. It is paramount to explore and document any previous breast surgery to determine any disruption to the normal circulation of breast parenchyma and nipple-areola complex, increasing the risk of tissue necrosis [5, 6].

During the preoperative consultation, patient goals and expectations are discussed. It is important to determine if a mastopexy alone would suffice or if the patient desires increased volume or upper pole fullness which would warrant implant placement. In cases of mild ptosis, an implant alone may be adequate to provide a modest lift in patients that desire augmentation. As always, pre-existing asymmetries should be brought to light as these may persist despite attempts for correction at the time of surgery.

The ideal patient for augmentation mastopexy has a normal BMI, non-smoker, with excess breast skin and relatively deficient breast volume. There have been numerous algorithms and special tests described to determine if a patient will benefit from augmentation alone, mastopexy alone, versus augmentation mastopexy [7–9]. In the senior author's experience, in patients with excess skin compared to breast volume, augmenting the breast in addition to mastopexy provides the optimal result. Reducing the skin envelope while using an implant to restore upper pole fullness allows for creation of an ideal breast footprint.

3.2 Physical examination

Physical examination includes body mass index and breast analysis. Standard breast evaluation is performed with the patient in an upright position. First, the degree of ptosis is visually determined using Regnault classification [10]. The Regnault classification is a widely used system in which the degree of breast ptosis is determined based on the nipple position in relation to the inframammary fold (IMF). Grade 1 is defined as mild ptosis with the nipple at the level of the IMF. Grade 2 describes moderate ptosis where the nipple is positioned below the level of the IMF but not at the most dependent part of the breast. Grade 3 represents severe ptosis where the nipple is positioned below the IMF and at the most dependent portion of the breast. Pseudoptosis is characterized the nipple at or above the level of the IMF with the majority of breast parenchyma positioned below the level of the IMF [10, 11].

Next, measurements of the breast are obtained including base width, sternal notch to nipple, nipple to inframammary fold, nipple diameter, and inter nipple distance [11, 12]. Obtaining these objective measurements helps highlight any asymmetries and is essential in choosing the appropriate implant.

Breast skin quality and parenchyma should be noted including presence of any striae, thin skin, and relationship of skin excess to parenchyma volume [6]. The soft tissue pinch test is a useful adjunct to assess the soft tissue coverage. This is performed by pinching an area of the breast above the nipple areolar complex between the thumb and index finger. Classically, soft tissue pinch less than 2 cm is an indication for subpectoral implant placement to avoid implant visibility and rippling [13].

4. Surgical planning

Various measurements are taken into account when determining whether to perform augmentation-mastopexy simultaneously or in a staged manner. Vertical excess, defined as the difference between the desired nipple to IMF position measured under stretch from the new nipple position and the current IMF, degree of nipple elevation required, available breast tissue, and skin quality are all factors that may affect predictability and complication rate and are therefore important considerations during the decision-making process [7, 14, 15].

5. Techniques

5.1 Mastopexy

The main factors influencing the selection of mastopexy technique are degree of ptosis and skin excess. This decision is often finalized in the operating room after the implant is placed and the residual excess may be assessed. The most commonly used techniques are periareolar, vertical and wise pattern each with their own advantages and disadvantages (**Table 1**) [11, 16].

Periareolar technique can be utilized on patients with minimal ptosis (Grade 1 or 2). There are variations of this technique including crescent mastopexy, circumareolar or "donut" mastopexy, and Benelli procedures. Crescent mastopexy is performed by designing an eccentric oval circumferentially around the areola preferentially excising

Mastopexy type	Indications	Advantages	Disadvantages
Periareolar	Grade I or II	• Minimal scar burden hidden along areolar border	• Widened scar • NAC deformity • Deprojection of the breast
Vertical (Hall-Findley)	Grades I-III	• Ptosis correction • Augments structural support with pillar unification	• Delayed final results • Elongation of NAC to IMF distance • Scar migration on to chest wall
Wise pattern	Grades I-III	• Adaptive technique • Excellent in cases of poor skin quality	• Scar burden • Breakdown at T junction • Bottoming out

Table 1.
Mastopexy techniques with indications and clinical implications.

tissue superior to the NAC to elevate the nipple [11]. Alternatively, a circumareolar or "donut" mastopexy is performed by designing a circular incision around the NAC. This can be utilized to modestly elevate the NAC (no more than 2 cm) and address enlarged areolar diameter. It is recommended not to exceed 7 cm diameter of the outer incision and maintain outer diameter to inner diameter ratio of 2:1 [16–18]. Lastly the Benelli procedure utilizes this same circumferential periareolar approach with the addition of parenchymal repositioning. This is achieved by performing extensive skin undermining, exposing the parenchyma, which is then incised creating medial and lateral flaps that are repositioned and overlapped at the midline [19, 20]. Although the Benelli procedure allows for decreased scar burden compared to other mastopexy techniques the breasts commonly have a narrow, coned appearance post operatively [16–18]. This technique also mandates a submuscular approach be utilized when combined with augmentation due to the wide undermining and parenchymal manipulation [11, 21]. Each variation of periareolar mastopexy carry the risk of pleating, widened scar, and deprojection of the breast [17].

Vertical mastopexy adds an additional vertical component down the meridian of the breast. This technique increases the ability to raise the nipple areolar complex and resect excess skin. There are a few variations of the vertical scar mastopexy. The most commonly used are short-scar periareolar inferior pedicle reduction (SPAIR) and Hall Findlay technique. Originally described by Hammond, the SPAIR technique transposes the nipple superiorly via an inferior pedicle technique [21, 22]. Due to the wide undermining of this approach traditionally employs it is not customary to use an implant [11]. Alternatively, the Hall Findlay approach can be utilized with an implant. This technique transposes the nipple on either a superior medical or medial pedicle. Since the blood supply to the nipple for this technique is the 2nd or 3rd internal mammary perforators, an implant can safely be placed in either the submusclar or subglandular plane [11, 23, 24].

The wise pattern or inverted T mastopexy is known to easily address those patients with severe ptosis and vertical excess. Similar to the previously described mastopexy techniques, this approach utilizes periareolar incisions and vertical limbs with the addition of horizontal limbs carried out both medially and laterally at the level of the inframammary fold [23, 25]. In the senior author's experience, this technique can easily be used in a skin only fashion. When performed as skin only an implant can be placed submuscular or subglandular as perforators to the nipple have remained in continuity. Patients often voice concern about the addition of a horizontal scar, however this is easily hidden in the inframammary fold.

5.2 Pocket selection

5.2.1 Subpectoral

Submuscular and dual plane techniques are traditionally considered standard of care due to the safety profile. Placement of the implant in a subpectoral pocket, or partial subpectoral in the case of dual plane technique, provides relative protection of the implant in cases of wound breakdown, as well as vascular preservation and soft tissue coverage affording a more natural result in very thin patients. As the implant remains fixed under the pectoralis major muscle, upper pole fullness is maintained overtime with use of a subpectoral pocket. Immediately postoperatively, this pocket will result in a high riding appearance of the implants which take time, often months, to settle and drop into the appropriate position. As will subpectoral augmentation, there is a risk for animation deformity where the implants become displaced with activation of the pectoralis muscle. In the long term, as breast ptosis occurs, there is also a risk of developing waterfall deformity where the soft tissue parenchyma cascades off the implant, which remains in the upper pole of the breast, creating an unnatural appearance.

5.2.2 Subglandular

Subglandular breast augmentation has become more common and produces excellent results in the appropriate patient (e.g. **Figures 1–3**). The rise in subglandular augmentation has paralleled the rise in prepectoral implant-based breast reconstruction,

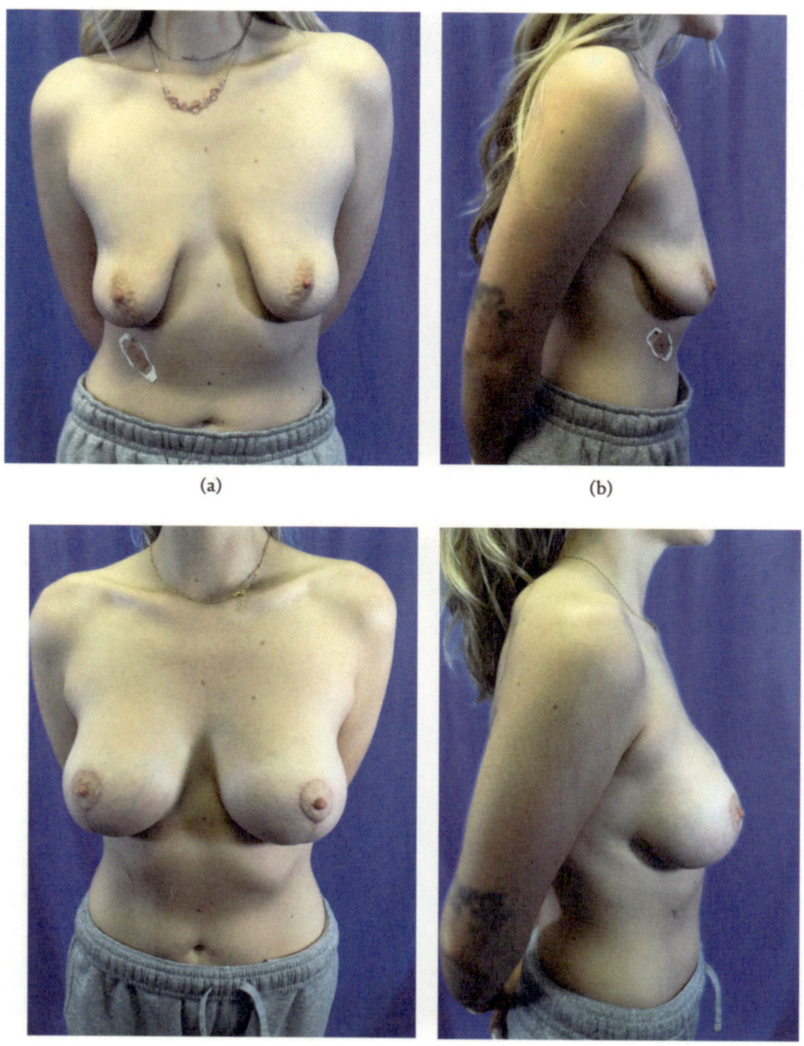

(a) (b) (c) (d)

Figure 1.
Twenty year old female patient who underwent simultaneous augmentation-mastopexy; (a-b) preoperative photo demonstrating grade II ptosis and upper pole deflation; (c-d) 2 months post operative subglandular augmentation with 325 cc full profile silicone implants and wise pattern mastopexy.

which has demonstrated the relatively safety and effectiveness of prepectoral procedures. The safety of prepectoral implant placement has been demonstrated in direct to implant reconstructive cases during which the implant is placed subcutaneously under freshly devascularized soft tissue with similar complication profile relative to subpectoral placement. Still, many surgeons approach with caution or choose to avoid utilizing the subglandular pocket in esthetic augmentation out of concern for increased

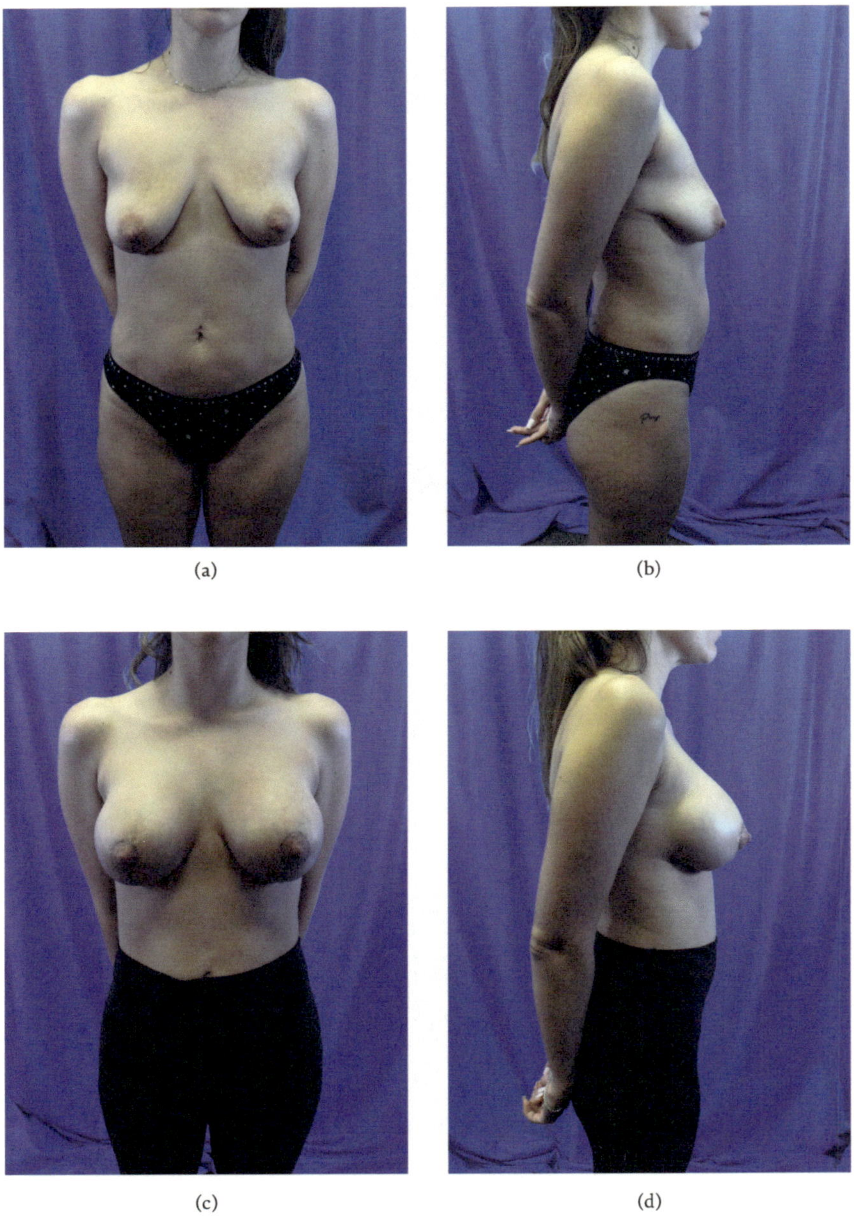

Figure 2.
Thirty five year old female patient who underwent simultaneous augmentation-mastopexy; (a-b) preoperative photo demonstrating grade II ptosis and breast asymmetry; (c-d) 2 weeks post operative subglandular augmentation with 345 cc full profile silicone implants and wise pattern mastopexy with implants in a natural position in the immediate post operative period.

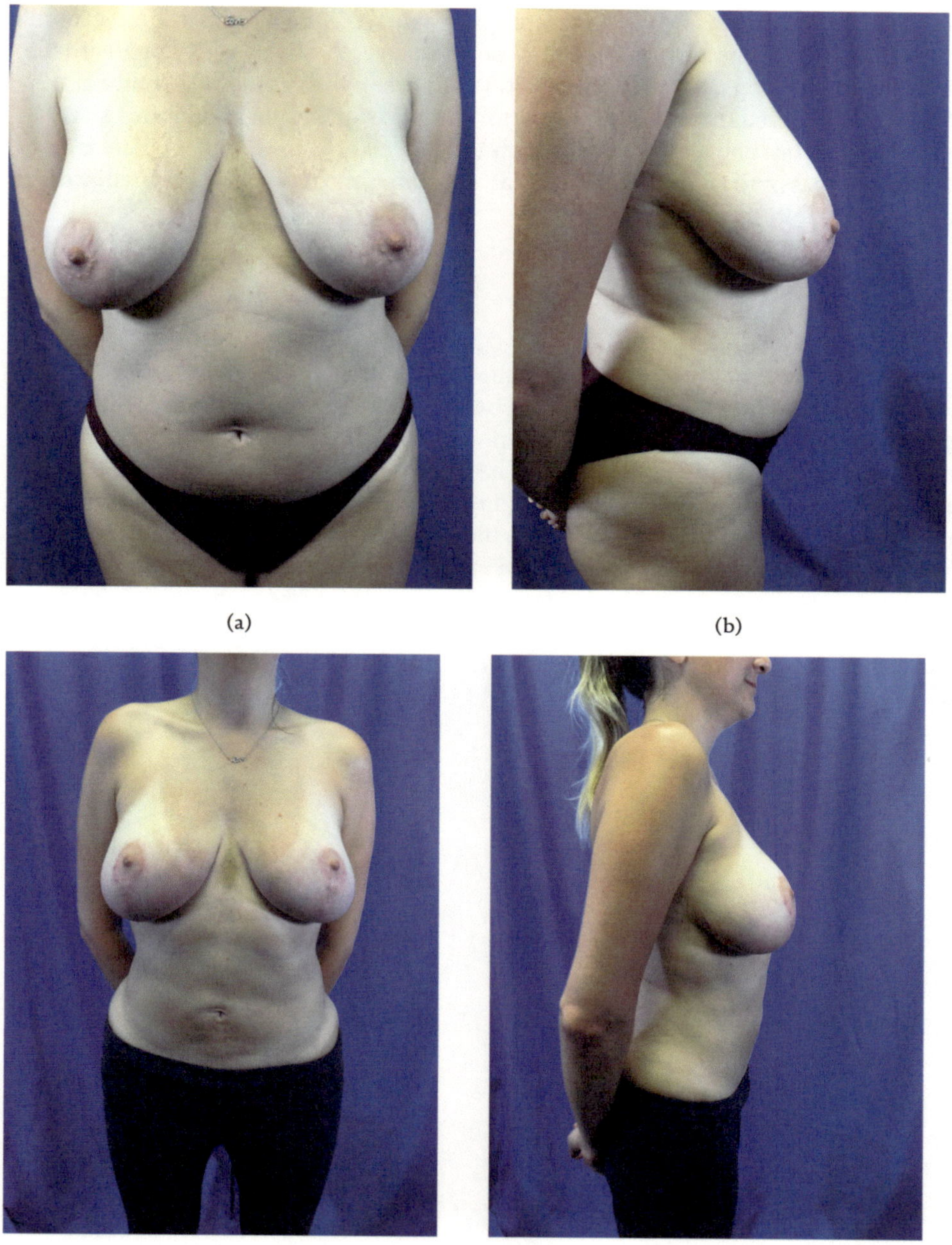

(a) (b) (c) (d)

Figure 3.
Thirty seven year old female patient who underwent simultaneous augmentation-mastopexy; (a-b) preoperative photo demonstrating grade II ptosis; (c-d) 5 months post operative subglandular mastopexy augmentation with 200 cc full profile silicone implants and wise pattern mastopexy.

incidence of capsular contracture and potential risk for implant exposure in the case of augmentation mastopexy. The subglandular pocket has the advantage of providing excellent immediate postoperative results as the implant is in the appropriate position and there is no need to wait for the implant to drop. This pocket also eliminates potential for animation and minimizes surgical pain. As aging occurs, the subglandular implant tends to maintain a more natural position and effectively ages along with the ptotic breast offering a long-lasting result. With these observations, the senior author (M.A.F.) has altered his practice now performing mastopexy augmentations almost exclusively in the subglandular rather than the subpectoral plane, unless there is a compelling reason to favor the later such as very thin soft tissue coverage predisposing to implant visibility.

6. Operative sequence

The senior author's preferred technique for simultaneous augmentation-mastopexy is to use the subglandular implant pocket and tailor the mastopexy technique to the patient's needs (**Figure 4**). A goal photo is routinely chosen by the patient and reasonable expectations are discussed. The patient is routinely marked in the preoperative holding area in the upright position. Following induction of general anesthesia, the patient is prepped and draped in the usual sterile fashion and prophylactic IV antibiotics are administered. A 4.5 cm incision is designed in the inframammary creased centered at the nipple. The incision is made and dissection carried down with cautery to identify the plane above the pectoralis muscle. The subglandular pocket is dissected according to preoperative markings followed by placement of a

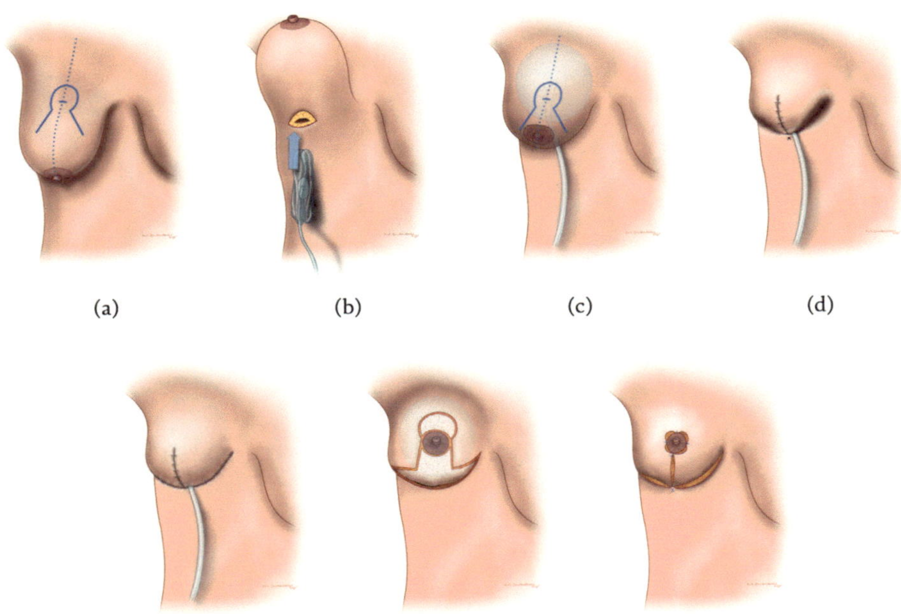

(a) (b) (c) (d)

(e) (f) (g)

Figure 4.
Operative sequence of subglandular augmentation-mastopexy; (a) preoperative mastopexy markings which are used as a guideline and adjusted following implant placement; (b) a subglandular pocket is dissected via IMF incision and saline sizer is placed; (c) the sizer is filled to the anticipated implant volume and adjusted to align with the patient's goals; (d) once and implant size is selected, a vertical mastopexy is tailor-tacked; (e) medial and lateral horizontal extensions are added; (f) incisions are made and the entire skin pattern is deepithelialized then scored along the incisions and periareolar; (g) NAC is advanced into position and incisions are closed.

saline sizer which is inflated to the anticipated implant volume. The patient is then sat in the upright position and implant volume is adjusted as needed. The patient is then returned to the supine position. A vertical mastopexy is performed which serves to contour the breast mound. Vertical skin excess is estimated by pinch, then marked and tailor tacked. Medial and lateral horizontal extensions are marked if needed based on esthetic contour and the distance from the inferior border of the areola to the IMF in order to prevent migration of the vertical scar onto the chest wall. Following confirmation of symmetry, the NAC is outlined with a cookie cutter, incisions are confirmed and made, then the entire skin pattern is de-epithelialized. The dermis is scored until subcutaneous fat is visible along the entire pattern approximately 1–1.5 cm from the skin edge to prevent thermal injury. Periareolar scoring is essential to achieve NAC elevation without undue tension. The sizer is then removed and hemostasis is confirmed. A round smooth silicone permanent breast implant is placed and all incisions are closed, then dressed with Steri-strips and a surgical bra. The patient is discharged home the same day. This technique has produced excellent immediate postoperative and long-term results.

7. Complications

Many surgeons approach simultaneous augmentation-mastopexy with caution or choose to stage the procedures altogether to avoid NAC vascular compromise and wound healing complications which could potentially lead to implant exposure. In reality, the incidence of these complications is relatively low [26]. Overall complication rate is estimated to be approximately 13% with the most commonly cited complication being recurrent ptosis [26]. Recurrent ptosis results in a waterfall deformity which is characterized by the breast parenchyma falling off the implant which remains in the upper pole underneath the pectoralis muscle (**Figures 5** and **6**). In patients who require subpectoral implant placement, some surgeons advocate for excision of

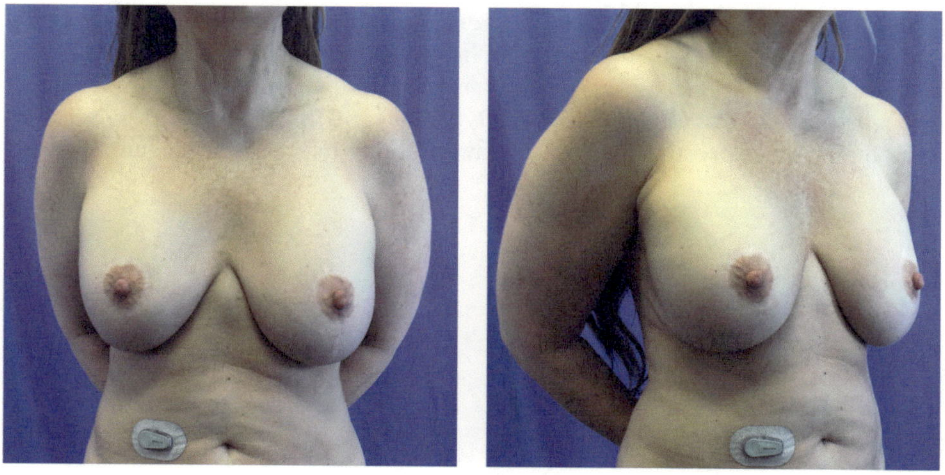

(a) (b)

Figure 5.
(a-b): 56 year old female who underwent subpectoral augmentation-mastopexy at an outside facility with 350 cc saline implants. She presented with recurrent breast ptosis and waterfall deformity.

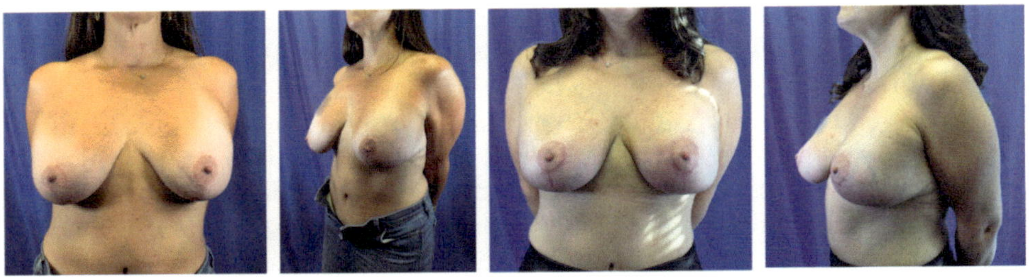

(a) (b) (c) (d)

Figure 6.
(a-b) 51 year old female who is 7 months status post subpectoral augmentation-mastopexy with 485 cc full profile silicone implants which resulted in waterfall deformity; (c-d) 2 months post operative revision mastopexy, capsular revision and replacement of previous implants.

the lower pole and increasing implant size accordingly at the index surgery in order to remove the natural weight of the breast lessening the tendency of soft tissue to slide off the implant [27]. Secondary correction of waterfall deformity requires redo mastopexy with or without pocket change. In the senior author's experience, subglandular implant placement at the time of mastopexy may reduce the risk of waterfall deformity which is often seen after subpectoral implant placement once ptosis recurs and may be addressed with redo mastopexy with or without pocket change. Capsular contracture should be discussed with all patients undergoing breast augmentation with implants with or without mastopexy and subglandular placement may increase this risk. Like any esthetic procedure in plastic surgery, patient dissatisfaction may arise despite a well-executed surgical procedure without postoperative complications.

8. Conclusion

Mastopexy with breast augmentation is indicated for patients with breast ptosis who desire a lift with added upper pole fullness. These procedures may be performed simultaneously or in a staged fashion. Various techniques exist and plastic surgeons performing esthetic breast surgery should have thee in their repertoire. Complications and unfavorable sequelae may occur, therefore careful preoperative planning and thorough patient counseling is essential. Overall, augmentation-mastopexy is an essential procedure in esthetic surgery with the ability to produce excellent results.

Author details

Morgan L. Fish[1], Rebecca Kelley[1], Marco Swanson[1], Alanna Fostyk[2] and Mark A. Foglietti[2*]

1 Cleveland Clinic Foundation, Cleveland, OH, USA

2 Foglietti and Fostyk Plastic Surgery, Cleveland, OH, USA

*Address all correspondence to: Mafoglietti@aol.com

References

[1] Abdelkader R, Raafat S, Sakr W, Abdelaziz M, El Noamany S. Augmentation mastopexy: A five-step standardized strategy approach. Plastic and Reconstructive Surgery. Global Open. 2022;**10**(6):e4349. DOI: 10.1097/GOX.0000000000004349

[2] Spear SL. Augmentation/mastopexy: "Surgeon, beware". Plastic and Reconstructive Surgery. 2006;**118** (Suppl. 7):133S-135S. DOI: 10.1097/01.PRS.0000072225766189.3E

[3] Ali B, Choi EE, Barlas V, et al. Perioperative safety of combined augmentation-mastopexy: An evaluation of national database. Annals of Plastic Surgery. 2021;**87**(5):493-500. DOI: 10.1097/SAP.0000000000003022

[4] Spear SL, Pelletiere CV, Menon N. One-stage augmentation combined with mastopexy: Aesthetic results and patient satisfaction. Aesthetic Plastic Surgery. 2004;**28**:259-267. DOI: 10.1007/s00266-004-0032-6

[5] O'Dey DM, Prescher A, Pallua N. Vascular reliability of nipple-areola complex-bearing pedicles: An anatomical microdissection study. Plastic and Reconstructive Surgery. 2007;**119**(4):1167-1177. DOI: 10.1097/01.prs.0000254360.98241.dc

[6] Pferdehirt R, Nahabedian MY. Finesse in mastopexy and augmentation mastopexy. Plastic and Reconstructive Surgery. 2021;**148**(3):451e-461e. DOI: 10.1097/PRS.0000000000008303

[7] Chapman J, Birch T. Augmentation mastopexy-An algorithm to demystify surgical planning. Aesthetic Plastic Surgery. 2023;**47**(5):2194-2196. DOI: 10.1007/s00266-023-03337-8

[8] Parsa AA, Jackowe DJ, Parsa FD. A new algorithm for breast mastopexy/augmentation. Plastic and Reconstructive Surgery. 2010;**125**(2):75e-77e. DOI: 10.1097/PRS.0b013e3181c725fb

[9] Spear SL, Giese SY. Simultaneous breast augmentation and mastopexy. Aesthetic Surgery Journal. 2000;**20**(2):155-164. DOI: 10.1067/maj.2000.106474

[10] Regnault P. Breast ptosis. Definition and treatment. Clinics in Plastic Surgery. 1976;**3**(2):193-203

[11] Qureshi AA, Myckatyn TM, Tenenbaum MM. Mastopexy and mastopexy-Augmentation. Aesthetic Surgery Journal. 2018;**38**(4):374-384. DOI: 10.1093/asj/sjx181

[12] Penn J. Breast reduction. British Journal of Plastic Surgery. 1955;**7**(4):357-371. DOI: 10.1016/s0007-1226(54)80046-4

[13] Maxwell GP, Gabriel A. Breast augmentation. In: Plastic Surgery. Breast. Vol. 5. Philadelphia, PA: Elsevier; 2013

[14] Lee MR, Unger JG, Adams WP. The tissue-based triad: A process approach to augmentation mastopexy. Plastic and Reconstructive Surgery. 2014;**134**(2):215-225. DOI: 10.1097/PRS.0000000000000387

[15] Sanniec K, Adams WP. The tissue-based triad in augmentation mastopexy: Single-stage technical refinements. Aesthetic Surgery Journal. 2019;**39**(12):1331-1341. DOI: 10.1093/asj/sjz006

[16] Hidalgo DA, Spector JA. Mastopexy. Plastic and Reconstructive Surgery.

2013;**132**(4):642e-656e. DOI: 10.1097/PRS.0b013e31829fe4b4

[17] Ramanadham SR, Rose JA. Breast lift with and without implant: A synopsis and primer for the plastic surgeon. Plastic and Reconstructive Surgery. Global Open. 2020;**8**(10):e3057. DOI: 10.1097/GOX.0000000000003057

[18] Spear SL, Kassan M, Little JW. Guidelines in concentric mastopexy. Plastic and Reconstructive Surgery. 1990;**85**(6):961-966. DOI: 10.1097/00006534-199006000-00023

[19] Benelli L. A new periareolar mammaplasty: The "round block" technique. Aesthetic Plastic Surgery. 1990;**14**(2):93-100. DOI: 10.1007/BF01578332

[20] Rohrich RJ, Thornton JF, Jakubietz RG, Jakubietz MG, Grünert JG. The limited scar mastopexy: Current concepts and approaches to correct breast ptosis. Plastic and Reconstructive Surgery. 2004;**114**(6):1622-1630. DOI: 10.1097/01.prs.0000139062.20141.8c

[21] Hammond DC, Alfonso D, Khuthaila DK. Mastopexy using the short scar periareolar inferior pedicle reduction technique. Plastic and Reconstructive Surgery. 2008;**121**(5):1533-1539. DOI: 10.1097/PRS.0b013e31816c3b0b

[22] Hammond DC. Short scar periareolar inferior pedicle reduction (SPAIR) mammaplasty. Plastic and Reconstructive Surgery. 1999;**103**(3):890-902. DOI: 10.1007/3-540-27218-6_6

[23] Hall-Findlay EJ. Pedicles in vertical breast reduction and mastopexy. Clinics in Plastic Surgery. 2002;**29**(3):379-391. DOI: 10.1016/s0094-1298(02)00008-1

[24] Hall-Findlay EJ. Vertical breast reduction. Seminars in Plastic Surgery. 2004;**18**(3):211-224. DOI: 10.1055/s-2004-831908

[25] Ship AG, Weiss PR, Engler AM. Dual-pedicle dermoparenchymal mastopexy. Plastic and Reconstructive Surgery. 1989;**83**(2):281-290. DOI: 10.1097/00006534-198902000-00014

[26] Khavanin N, Jordan SW, Rambachan A, Kim JY. A systematic review of single-stage augmentation-mastopexy. Plastic and Reconstructive Surgery. 2014;**134**(5):922-931

[27] White CP, Peterson BD. Augmentation mastopexy with surgical excision of the lower pole to avoid waterfall deformity: A surgical technique and nipple areolar complex case series. Plastic Surgery. 2021;**29**(2):103-109. DOI: 10.1177/2292550320933662

Chapter 13

Abdominoplasty Surgical Techniques

Andrew Sohn and Sebastian Gutierrez de Pineres

Abstract

This chapter offers a comprehensive exploration of abdominoplasty, focusing on the various types of techniques and the critical criteria for patient selection. It emphasizes the factors that influence the choice of surgical approach, ensuring optimal outcomes for different patient profiles. A detailed examination of abdominal anatomy is provided, as understanding this anatomy is essential for safe and effective surgical intervention and satisfactory outcomes. The chapter categorizes different abdominoplasty techniques, including the traditional approach, reverse abdominoplasty, high lateral tension, Fleur de Lis, and corset body lift. It details the specific indications, markings, surgical steps, and potential complications for each approach. Finally, the authors address comprehensive postoperative care guidelines to enhance recovery and minimize risks. Through this multifaceted discussion, the aim is to equip cosmetic and plastic surgeons with the knowledge needed to make informed decisions in the field of abdominoplasty.

Keywords: traditional abdominoplasty, mini abdominoplasty, Fleur de Lis, reverse abdominoplasty, corset abdominoplasty

1. Introduction

Abdominoplasty, commonly known as a tummy tuck, is a surgical procedure performed either alone or in combination with other procedures to address issues involving the skin, underlying fat, and muscles of the abdomen. Cosmetic surgeons performing abdominoplasty have recognized that variations in abdominal contour and presenting conditions require modifications to the surgical approach. For instance, patients with fat deposits and good skin quality may achieve excellent results with liposuction alone, which involves minimal scarring and morbidity compared to a full abdominoplasty. However, patients who have undergone full-term pregnancies or significant weight loss typically require a full abdominoplasty, with potential modifications tailored to their specific needs. These modifications aim to address individual concerns and provide a more personalized approach to the procedure.

2. Types of abdominoplasty

1. Traditional abdominoplasty:

   - The original technique, introduced in the 1960s, involved a long incision and a more invasive approach. Modern techniques prioritize minimal scarring, reduced blood loss, and faster recovery times.

2. Mini abdominoplasty:

   - A modified version of the traditional procedure designed for patients with less significant skin laxity and fat deposits limited to the area below the umbilicus.

3. Extended/lateral tension abdominoplasty:

   - This variation targets the love handles, lower back area, lateral hips, and upper thighs, providing a more comprehensive body contouring solution.

4. Fleur-de-lis abdominoplasty:

   - A modification of the traditional procedure to remove excess circumferential skin and fat from the abdomen. The incision is shaped like a fleur-de-lis, with a vertical component in the midline and two lateral extensions resembling the petals of the fleur-de-lis symbol.

5. Reverse abdominoplasty:

   - Also known as an "upper tummy tuck", this procedure targets the upper abdomen, focusing on the area above the umbilicus to remove excess skin and fat and improve contour.

6. Liposuction only:

   - A viable alternative to abdominoplasty that removes excess fat from the abdominal area but does not address excess skin or muscle laxity.

These advancements have made abdominoplasty a safer, more effective, and personalized procedure for individuals seeking to rejuvenate their abdominal appearance.

3. Patient selection and criteria

Traditionally, abdominoplasty was primarily sought by women who wanted to regain their youthful appearance post-pregnancy and after subsequent weight loss. However, abdominoplasty has been increasingly sought by both men and women due to rising obesity rates, bariatric surgery, and the use of GLP-1 receptor agonists. Women post-pregnancy benefit from addressing muscle separation (diastasis recti) and skin laxity to restore pre-pregnancy contour. Individuals with significant weight loss may require extensive procedures to remove excess skin and fat, alleviating skin irritation and discomfort. Gastric surgery patients often need abdominoplasty to address excess skin and improve body contour post-surgery.

4. Factors influencing surgical approach

1. Location of dat:

    - Patients with localized fat deposits in the lower abdomen might be candidates for a mini abdominoplasty, which involves a smaller incision and focuses on the area below the umbilicus.

2. Skin laxity:

    - The degree of skin laxity is a critical factor in determining the type of abdominoplasty. Extensive skin laxity might require a full abdominoplasty to remove excess skin and tighten the abdominal muscles.

3. Dermal breakdown and muscle separation:

    - Patients with dermal breakdown or significant scarring may require a more complex procedure, such as a fleur-de-lis abdominoplasty, which can address extensive circumferential skin and fat removal. Muscle separation, common post-pregnancy, is typically corrected during a full abdominoplasty.

4. Type of procedure:

    - Traditional abdominoplasty: A comprehensive approach for extensive skin laxity and muscle repair.

    - Mini abdominoplasty: Suitable for minor skin laxity and fat deposits below the umbilicus.

    - Extended/high lateral tension abdominoplasty: Addresses love handles, lower back, lateral hips, and upper thighs for more comprehensive body contouring.

    - Fleur-de-lis abdominoplasty: Ideal for patients with significant circumferential skin and fat removal needs.

    - Reverse abdominoplasty: Focuses on the upper abdomen, removing excess skin and fat above the umbilicus.

    - Liposuction only: An alternative for patients with good skin quality but excess fat, without addressing skin laxity or muscle separation.

5. Patient selection criteria for abdominoplasty

- Age:

    - 18–65 years old.

- Health status:
    - Good overall health, free of chronic diseases.
- Body Mass Index (BMI):
    - Ideal: <30.
- Acceptable: 30–35.
    - High-risk: >35.
- Smoking status:
    - Non-smoker or willing to quit.
- Pregnancy status:
    - No current or planned pregnancy.
- Weight stability:
    - Stable weight for at least 6 months.
- Abdominal anatomy:
    - Excess skin and fat.
    - Muscle separation (diastasis recti).
    - Bulging or protruding abdomen.
- Realistic expectations:
    - Understanding of the procedure's limitations and expected outcomes.
- Motivation:
    - Personal desire for improvement, not driven by external pressures.
- Psychological stability:
    - Emotionally stable, with no significant mental health concerns.
- Previous surgeries:
    - No significant abdominal scarring or hernias.
- Post-gastric surgery:

    At least 1–2 years post-op, with stable weight and no complications.

These criteria help ensure a safe and successful abdominoplasty procedure. Your plastic surgeon may have additional or modified criteria based on individual circumstances.

6. Anatomy

A thorough understanding of abdominal anatomy is essential for performing abdominoplasty. This knowledge encompasses the layers of soft tissue, vascular structures, and blood supply to the abdominal tissues and umbilicus, as well as the separation and laxity of the fascia and muscles. Such anatomical insight, coupled with a detailed clinical examination, allows surgeons to develop a treatment plan tailored to each patient's unique needs. This expertise aids in determining optimal incision locations, flap elevation, and tissue removal, particularly in patients with minimal skin laxity or a history of prior abdominoplasty. This understanding is also crucial when combining procedures such as liposuction with abdominoplasty to ensure both esthetic and functional outcomes.

7. Skin

The abdominal wall is composed of seven distinct layers: skin, subcutaneous fat, Scarpa's fascia, subscarpal fat, the anterior rectus sheath, muscle, and posterior rectus sheath. These layers work together to support abdominal organs, protect internal structures, and facilitate movement. The skin serves as a protective barrier and sensory interface, while Camper's fascia contains superficial adipose tissue. Scarpa's fascia, a dense connective tissue layer, separates the superficial and deep adipose tissue, providing structural support. Below this lies the muscular layer, surrounded by the anterior and posterior rectus sheaths.

Skin quality in the abdominal region varies based on genetics, age, pregnancy history, and weight fluctuations, all of which affect its elasticity and response to surgical procedures. Skin elasticity, primarily determined by genetics and collagen production, dictates how well the skin can stretch and retract. Factors such as aging, significant weight changes, and pregnancy impact abdominoplasty outcomes by influencing skin tension and redundancy.

Body Mass Index (BMI) affects how the skin responds to weight changes. Higher BMI, indicative of increased body fat, can stretch the skin, reducing its elasticity. After weight loss, the skin may not fully retract, resulting in sagging and loose skin, especially in the abdomen.

Younger individuals generally have more elastic skin and better accommodating changes such as weight gain. In contrast, prolonged stretching, as seen with pregnancy or significant weight fluctuations, diminishes skin elasticity, leading to sagging and loose skin, particularly in the abdomen. Pregnancy presents additional challenges to abdominal skin elasticity and muscle tone, potentially leading to diastasis recti, where the abdominal muscles separate. While postpartum exercises can strengthen muscles, excess skin, and muscle laxity may persist, prompting consideration of abdominoplasty to restore shape and firmness.

Stretch marks (striae) result from dermal breakdown due to rapid changes like weight fluctuations and pregnancy. During abdominoplasty, stretch marks below the umbilicus may be removed, while those above typically remain. Various treatments exist to reduce their appearance, but complete elimination is challenging. Understanding these factors helps manage expectations regarding abdominoplasty outcomes.

Abdominoplasty addresses these issues by removing excess skin and fat and tightening muscles to restore a contoured abdomen. Patients with higher BMIs may require more extensive surgical techniques due to greater skin laxity.

8. Fat

The abdominal adipose layer is divided into superficial and deep layers by Scarpa's fascia. Scarpa's fascia, situated deep within the abdominal wall, is composed of dense, relatively avascular fibrous connective tissue, providing structural support and separating deep adipose tissue and muscles from subcutaneous fat [1].

The superficial fat layer is typically thicker and denser, with a robust vascular supply from the subdermal plexus and underlying perforators from the musculocutaneous system. In contrast, the deep layer of adipose tissue is less dense and receives its blood supply primarily from musculocutaneous perforators. When considering lipectomy or liposuction during abdominoplasty, it is crucial to understand that the blood supply to deeper fat is separate from the skin's supply. Liposuction deep into Scarpa's fascia and skin excision can be performed safely without compromising skin vascularity. However, thinning the fat layer superficial to Scarpa's fascia can lead to vascular compromise and skin necrosis.

In surgical contexts, Scarpa's fascia is often referenced for deeper dissection to achieve optimal esthetic outcomes while minimizing complications. Understanding its role in fat layer dissection is crucial for preserving abdominal contour and stability (**Figure 1**).

9. Muscle

The abdominal wall muscles, including the rectus abdominis, external oblique, internal oblique, and transversalis abdominis, each plays unique roles in function and movement. The rectus abdominis muscle, commonly referred to as the "six-pack," is positioned centrally and runs vertically along the abdomen from the pubic bone to the sternum. It provides structural support to the anterior wall, flexes the lumbar spine, and stabilizes the pelvis.

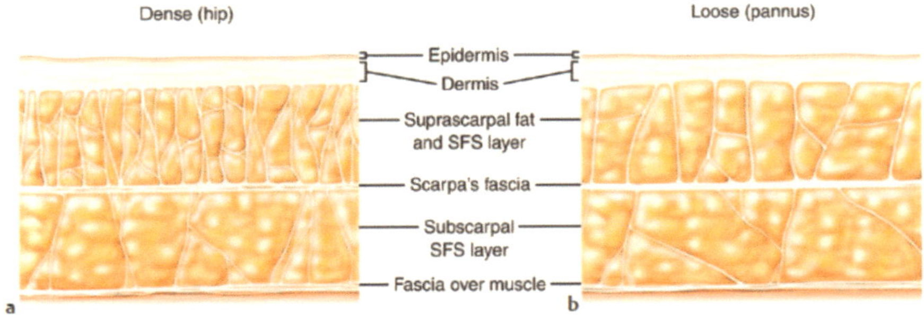

Figure 1.
Layers of the abdominal wall [2].

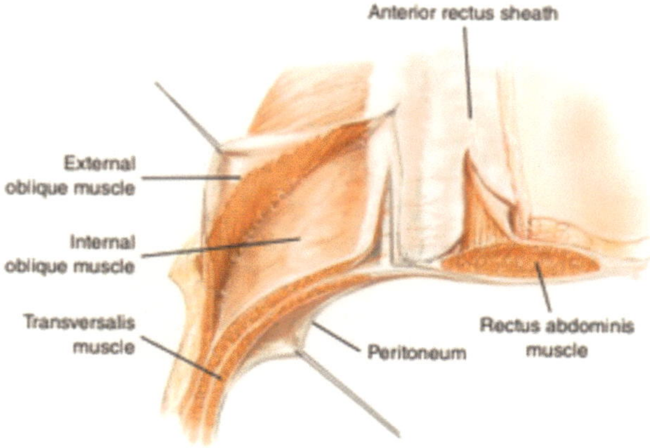

Figure 2.
Soft tissue layers of the abdominal wall [2].

Surrounding the rectus abdominis is the external oblique, internal oblique, and transversus abdominis muscles, which together support trunk rotation, flexion, and compression of abdominal contents.

The rectus abdominis is enclosed within the rectus sheath, formed by the aponeurosis of the transversalis abdominis and the two oblique muscles. These aponeuroses envelop the rectus abdominis, forming anterior and posterior sheaths that fuse in the midline to create the linea alba. Pregnancy and significant weight fluctuations can stretch the linea alba, causing rectus diastasis, which may require surgical repair for optimal abdominoplasty results.

The arcuate line, located approximately halfway between the umbilicus and the pubic symphysis, represents a transition point. Above this line, distinct anterior and posterior rectus sheaths exist; below it, aponeuroses from the internal oblique and transversalis join those from the external and internal obliques to form a single anterior rectus sheath, with no posterior sheath.

The peritoneum lines the abdominal cavity and covers abdominal organs, reducing friction and facilitating smooth organ movement during digestion and other bodily functions. Understanding the complex anatomy of the abdominal wall is crucial for diagnosing conditions, planning treatments, and ensuring optimal outcomes in surgical procedures like hernia repairs and abdominoplasty (**Figure 2**) [3].

10. Vascular supply

The blood supply to the abdominal wall originates from multiple sources, ensuring proper nourishment and function. The intercostal arteries, branching from the thoracic aorta, extend from the rib cage into the abdominal wall, supplying both skin and underlying tissues. The lumbar arteries, from the abdominal aorta, supply the posterior wall's skin and subcutaneous tissue. The superficial epigastric and circumflex iliac arteries, originating from the femoral artery, supply the lower abdomen and groin, critical during abdominoplasty.

The abdominal muscles receive blood from several key arteries. The superior epigastric artery, a continuation of the internal thoracic artery, descends into the rectus sheath, supplying the upper rectus abdominis muscle and overlying skin.

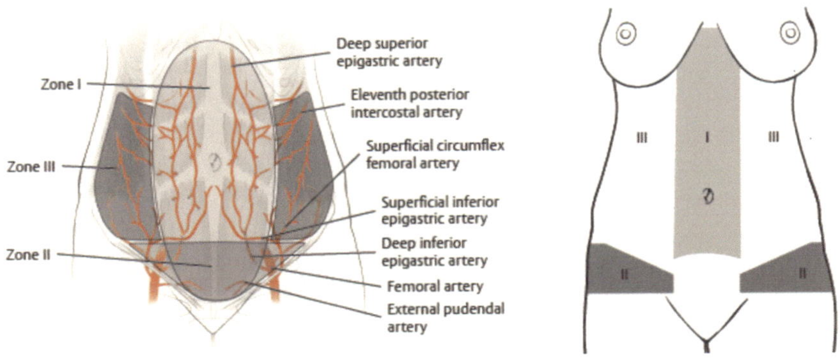

Figure 3.
Huger vascular zones [4].

During surgery, maintaining blood flow from this artery is essential for the viability of upper abdominal tissue. The inferior epigastric artery, branching from the external iliac artery, ascends within the transversalis fascia, entering the rectus sheath to supply the lower rectus abdominis, anastomosing with the superior epigastric artery. Preserving this artery ensures adequate blood supply to the lower abdominal wall. The deep circumflex iliac artery, also from the external iliac artery, runs along the iliac crest, supplying lower wall muscles, including the internal oblique and transversus abdominis, by penetrating their muscular layers. The intercostal and lumbar arteries provide additional blood flow to the lateral and posterior wall muscles, including the internal and external obliques and transversus abdominis, by traveling between muscle layers and giving off perforating branches (**Figure 3**) [5].

During abdominoplasty, elevating skin and fat flap may disrupt the blood supply. Although numerous anastomoses between arteries create a rich blood supply and collateral circulation, careful planning of incision lines and flap elevation is necessary to preserve key vessels, especially perforating branches that supply critical blood flow to the skin. By maintaining the integrity of these vessels, surgeons can help ensure proper healing and reduce the risk of complications such as flap necrosis. Understanding the vascular anatomy and the importance of these vessels is crucial for successful and safe surgical outcomes in abdominoplasty procedures.

11. Nerves

Sensation of the anterolateral abdomen is provided by the anterior branches of the spinal nerves T7–12 and L1. The anterior branches of the spinal nerves T7-T11 also known as intercostal nerves, after emerging from the intercostal muscles, travel between the internal oblique and transversalis muscles to penetrate the posterior rectus sheath, innervating the skin. The anterior branch of T12, the subcostal nerve, and the anterior branch of the L1, the spinal nerve are divided The lateral cutaneous nerves perforate the intercostal muscles at the midaxillary line and travel within the subcutaneous plane. The T7 to T9 nerves predominantly return sensation from the inferior portion of the lateral thoracic wall above the umbilicus. The T10 innervates around the umbilicus while T11 to T12 nerves predominantly return sensation from the lateral anterolateral abdominal wall below the umbilicus [6]. During

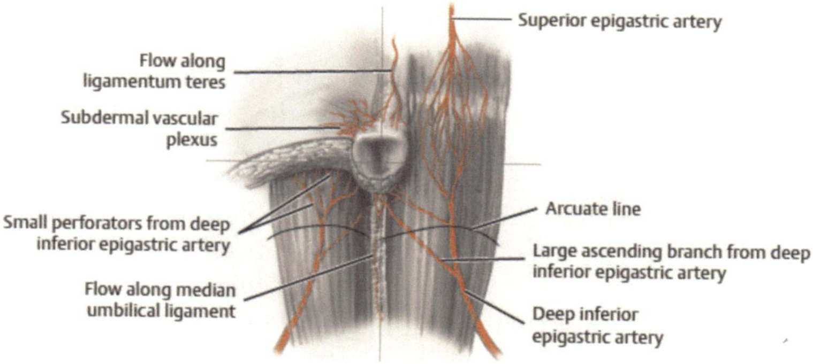

Figure 4.
Blood supply to the umbilicus [4].

abdominoplasty, a rearrangement of abdominal wall nerves can occur where dermatomes T5-T12 move inferiorly. Dermatomes T5-T9 become magnified in the abdominal wall and T10-T-12 are generally resected with the skin. This change in dermatome location is of profound importance for patients undergoing spinal anesthesia.

12. Umbilicus

The umbilicus, or navel, is a scar on the abdomen marking the site of the former umbilical cord attachment. Located on the anterior abdominal wall near the level of L3-L4 vertebrae, it is formed by the obliteration of umbilical vessels and the urachus, surrounded by skin and underlying connective tissue, with a central depression. Beneath the skin lies a rich subdermal plexus that plays a crucial role in the blood supply, receiving contributions from the deep inferior epigastric arteries, branches of the external iliac arteries [1]. The ligamentum teres (a remnant of the fetal umbilical vein) runs from the umbilicus to the liver, adding to its anatomical significance.

Esthetically, a pleasing umbilicus is typically small, vertically oval-shaped, and positioned midline on the abdomen, with a slight inward contour and moderate depth. Symmetry with the surrounding abdomen is crucial for esthetic balance. Features that contribute to an appealing umbilicus include a vertical shape, slightly superior hooding, shallow depth, and a well-defined lower margin. The surrounding skin should be taut and harmonious with the abdominal musculature. Excessive protrusion, retraction, or irregularities can detract from its appearance, emphasizing the importance of a well-defined navel in overall abdominal esthetics. Understanding the anatomical structure and vascular supply of the umbilicus is essential in abdominoplasty to preserve its blood supply and achieve a natural appearance post-surgery (**Figure 4**).

13. Patient education

Patient education and informed consent are crucial components of the abdominoplasty process, ensuring that patients have realistic expectations and are prepared for postoperative care. Patients should be informed that not all excess skin may be removed, and abdominal protrusion might still be present depending on factors such as intra-abdominal fat, scarring, and potential flap necrosis. It is essential to discuss these limitations openly so patients have a clear understanding of the likely outcomes.

Prior to surgery, patients are instructed to follow several key preoperative measures: stopping smoking 2–3 weeks before and after the procedure to enhance healing, adhering to a high-protein diet to support tissue repair, and starting a bowel program to avoid constipation, which can complicate recovery. Patients are also advised to shower with antiseptic soap before the operation and follow specific wound care instructions to minimize the risk of infection.

During the surgery, anti-clot measures are implemented, including the use of compression stockings and intermittent pneumatic compression devices, both intraoperatively and postoperatively, to reduce the risk of deep vein thrombosis (DVT) and pulmonary embolism. Postoperative instructions include the use of an abdominal binder to support the healing area, proper care of any drains placed to remove excess fluid, and pain management with medications, including the potential use of exparel for long-acting pain relief. Patients should anticipate taking 1–2 weeks off from work, with a gradual return to light duties over the following 6 weeks.

To prevent complications and promote recovery, patients are encouraged to engage in light ambulation and leg exercises to reduce the risk of DVT and embolism. Swelling and bruising are common and typically resolve within 2–3 weeks, though some residual swelling may persist for up to 3–6 months. Drain removal is usually performed 1–2 weeks postoperatively. Overall, patient education plays a pivotal role in preparing individuals for the procedure and ensuring adherence to postoperative care, ultimately contributing to a smoother recovery and better surgical outcomes.

14. Procedure selection

Procedure selection for abdominoplasty involves careful consideration of skin tone, the amount of excess skin and fat, and individual patient needs. For patients with mild excess fat but good skin tone and no significant skin laxity, liposuction alone or combined with endoscopic diastasis repair may be sufficient. This approach is ideal for those seeking contour improvements without extensive skin removal. When patients present with excess fat primarily below the umbilicus and some skin laxity, a mini abdominoplasty combined with diastasis repair can address both concerns effectively, offering a less invasive option than a full abdominoplasty.

For individuals with significant fat deposits and excess skin, a traditional abdominoplasty with or without liposuction is generally recommended. This procedure removes excess skin and fat from the abdominal area, providing a more dramatic contour improvement. In cases where there is extensive excess skin laterally and around the back, especially after massive weight loss, a circumferential abdominoplasty may be necessary. This technique, also known as a body lift, addresses the skin around the entire torso, improving overall contour and tightening the abdomen.

Patients with excess skin in lateral abdominal areas, hips, thighs, pubis, and anterior medial thighs might require a lateral tension abdominoplasty. This technique focuses on tightening and lifting the lateral aspects of the abdomen and thighs, often following significant weight loss. For those with extensive excess skin in both vertical and horizontal dimensions, particularly in the upper midline region, a fleur-de-lis abdominoplasty may be indicated. This advanced technique allows for substantial skin removal and contouring in multiple directions, addressing complex cases of skin redundancy and offering significant esthetic enhancement.

Each surgical approach is tailored to the patient's unique anatomy and goals, ensuring optimal results and addressing specific areas of concern. By selecting the appropriate procedure, surgeons can effectively manage excess skin and fat, improve abdominal contour, and enhance overall patient satisfaction.

15. Abdominoplasty

15.1 Surgical techniques

15.1.1 General overview

Management of excess skin

- The goal is to remove skin and fat that extends from *above the umbilicus down to pubis* and extending laterally enough to prevent dog ears from forming. All while maintaining the scar as low as possible.

Management of excess fat

- Perform liposuction

Management of abdominal wall

- Repairing tendency to demonstrate diastasis or reinforce the lateral musculofascial envelope – > the waist can be narrowed.

Management of the umbilicus

- By definition- abdominoplasty will translocate the umbilicus. — As opposed to the panniculectomy procedure, where a wedge of skin and fat simply is removed from the lower abdomen without translocation of the umbilicus.

- The basics: Create mild umbilical depression with a hidden scar properly positioned in the midline of the abdomen.

16. Full abdominoplasty

The patient presents with enough redundancy of skin and fat in the anterior abdominal wall that the resection pattern can occur above the umbilicus. This allows the scar to be positioned low along the abdominal wall while also allowing for transposition of the umbilicus (Foad). Abdominal wall plication is used classically. This is usually performed to correct the musculofascial laxity and diastasis recti deformity that many patients are concerned about. There are isolated areas of fat deposition where liposuction is performed prior to making any surgical incisions while ensuring that the supply to the eventual abdominoplasty flap is not violated as this could result in eventual complications of skin necrosis and failed procedure.

16.1 Patient marking

Demonstration video available to download at the end of the chapter.

16.2 Surgical technique

16.2.1 Selective liposuction and management of excess fat

After tumescent anesthesia is delivered to the lower and lateral abdomen we then focus on selective liposuction. Liposuction in the lateral abdomen is performed to facilitate flap eventual redraping while preserving the perforating blood supply from the deep epigastric vessels and lateral perforators.

16.2.2 Incision and dissection

10-blade was used to make the lower abdominal incision through the skin, subcutaneous tissues, and Scarpa's fascia down to approximately the rectus abdominal fascia. Sharp dissection with Bovie electrocautery is performed and carried to the umbilicus. Care must be taken to ensure that the umbilicus remains in place and attached to the stalk while avoiding inadvertent amputation. Sharp dissection is performed around the umbilicus with #11-blade and Bovie electrocautery. The abdominoplasty flap dissection continued with selective undermining along the midline from the umbilicus to the xyphoid process while maintaining hemostasis and preserving the lateral perforators.

16.2.3 Management of excess skin and abdominal wall

The table is then bent into a 30-degree angle and the abdominal flap is retracted inferiorly to determine the amount of excess skin to be excised. Using a hand-over flap, the surgeon's fingers bring the superior aspect of the flap to meet the inferior skin edge. This allows recognition of excess skin to be excised.

A 10-blade is then used to excise the skin and amputate the excess tissue. It is important to note that the umbilicus was kept intact at the stalk. The patient is returned to a non-inclined position. A 2 PDO suture is used to plicate from the xiphoid process to the pubic bone. A fully perforated JP drain is placed flat through the suprapubic flap.

A 2-Vicryl suture is used to suture the Scarpa's fascia of the inferior flap to the rectus fascia to prevent superior migration of the Mons. 0-monocryl suture was then used to center the inferior flap at the midline. Several key sutures are placed using 2 Vicryl to approximate Scarpa's to Scarpa's fascia tacked to the underlying rectus fascia. Then, 0-Monocryl was used to reapproximate the remaining Scarpa's to Scarpa's fascia along the abdominal flap. A 3-0 Monocryl is used to reapproximate the subcutaneous layer. Prior to the complete closure of deep layers, a flat JP drain was placed along the inferior aspect of the abdomen.

Starting from the later edges, staples are used to reapproximate the lateral component of the skin edges and move medially just lateral to an imaginary vertical line over the inguinal fold. Approximating the lateral edges of the skin first helps avoid dog ears. We then use a 3-0 monoderm quill to reapproximate the abdominal flap incision at the subcuticular level from the midline of the abdominal incision to two-thirds the length of the incision laterally. Prior to the closure of the incision, it is important to identify the location of the umbilicus to recreate its opening and umbilical depression.

16.2.4 Management of the umbilicus

An incision was then made with a #10-blade to create the new umbilical position. Dissection was carried out to identify the previously dissected umbilicus. Once identified, the umbilicus was then secured to its new position using 2-0 Vicryl. The umbilicus is packed with xeroform dressing and covered with Robbins tape.

Pearls

- The upper pannus is a window shade that is pulled downward after undermining.
- The lower incision will ride up to meet it simply as a result of elasticity.
- The scar will be several cm above the lower mark.
- Closure should be started at the lateral edges of the wound to mitigate the formation of dog ears.
- Avoid marking the lower aspect of the incision directly over the pannus fold as it will cause postoperative un-anesthetic break over the scar, negating the surgery cosmetic goals.
- If possible, exparel should be given to all patients to reduce postoperative pain.

17. Reverse abdominoplasty

Reverse abdominoplasty is particularly relevant in patients with primarily or residual excess upper abdominal skin. This approach can be very synergistic when combined with a Wise pattern type of breast surgery.

Residual skin is a complication not really unique to the HLTA. In fact, there is a good argument that because this technique has a more oblique vector of pull, it can efface more of this redundancy. However, the patient with significant excess (a second pannus) should be informed preoperatively of its probable persistence. Only a fleur-de-lis or reverse abdominoplasty can treat this zone definitively and should otherwise be considered in the first place [2].

18. Fleur De Lis abdominoplasty

18.1 Indications

Consider Fleur De LI if there is excess circumferential skin at the waist or if there is excess skin with concomitant previous subcostal or midline scars. It is appropriate for patients who require aggressive treatment of excess skin throughout the abdomen and trunk but particularly at the upper pole of the abdomen and lower chest, waist, hips, and thighs.

The trade-off with this approach is the full midline scar that is required for more complete skin resection.

If the patient desires to avoid the midline scar, an alternative approach could be a traditional abdominoplasty or High Lateral Tension Abdominoplasty (HLTA) followed by reverse abdominoplasty in a second-stage surgery [2].

Another indication of the Fleur De Li abdominoplasty approach is when a patient has previous abdominal scars whereby the position of the previous incision may have already compromised blood supply from perforator vessels near the costal margins that are normally carefully preserved during formal abdominoplasty.

When combined with an HLTA the upper abdominal zone is addressed with direct excision, and there is an indirect corset effect on the entire anterolateral chest, flank, and back. This combination can address the pannus but also residual excess skin rolls. This is very beneficial in massive weight loss patients.

- In some circumstances, when adequate resection of skin following the Fleur de li approach is completed, most of the anterior abdominal wall is exposed and the peripheral "waistcoat" skin, lying in the wings, advances to close the defect [2].

18.2 Markings

Marking is performed with the patient in a standing position with hands held at their sides. The markings for a standard abdominoplasty are performed, extending laterally as indicated.

Once the upper traditional abdominoplasty incision line is marked, the redundant soft tissue in the midline abdomen is pinched together in a vertical fashion to allow visualization of approximate excess tissue to be removed. The vertical marking is from the xiphoid down to the upper abdominoplasty incision marking previously made (**Figure 5**).

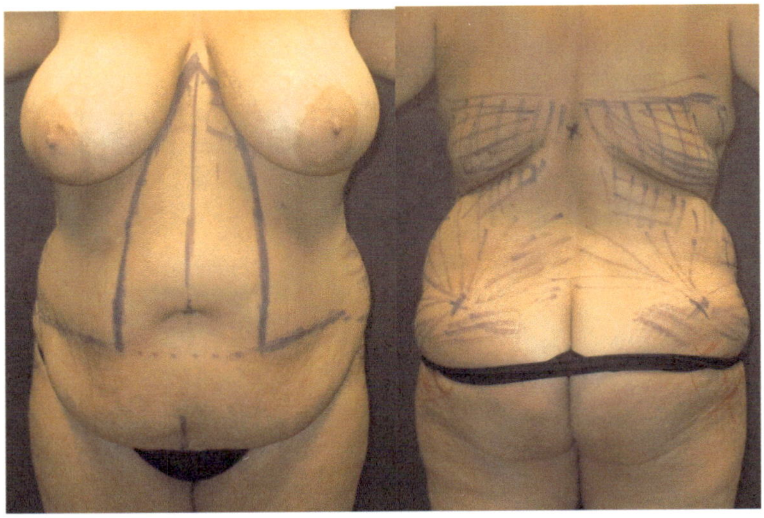

Figure 5.
Fleur De Lis preoperative markings including associated liposuction to back and hips.

18.3 Surgical technique

An incision is begun at the level of the xyphoid process in the upper abdomen through the skin, subcutaneous tissues, and Scarpa's fascia down to the rectus abdominis fascia (**Figure 6**).

A pre-rectus fascia dissection is carried inferiorly to the level of the umbilicus. Careful attention is directed toward identifying potential abdominal hernias that may require repair.

The suprapubic (lower abdominal) incision is then created approximately 7 cm superior to the vaginal cleft. This dissection is taken to the level of the rectus abdominis fascia. It is important to make every attempt to have the lateral extent of this incision at the same height to improve symmetry.

A periumbilical incision is created to free the umbilicus from the abdominal flap but attached to abdominal stalk.

In a 30-degree fixed position the abdominal flap is stretched inferiority to assess excess tissue and this is then excised. A 2-0 PDO quill suture was used to plicate from the xiphoid process to the pubic bone to address areas of severe rectus muscle diastasis. Layered closure as previously described in the traditional abdominoplasty section is performed and the umbilicus is secured to a new position with 3-0 Monocryl (**Figure 7**).

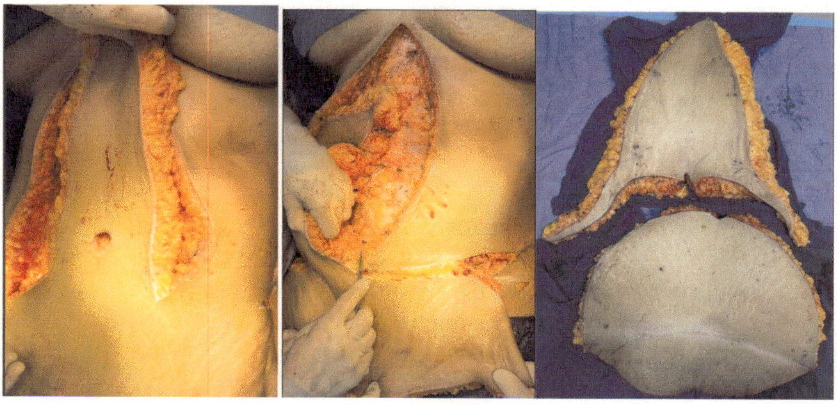

Figure 6.
Vertical and horizontal dissection of Fleur De Lis incision design and corresponding resected abdominal fat.

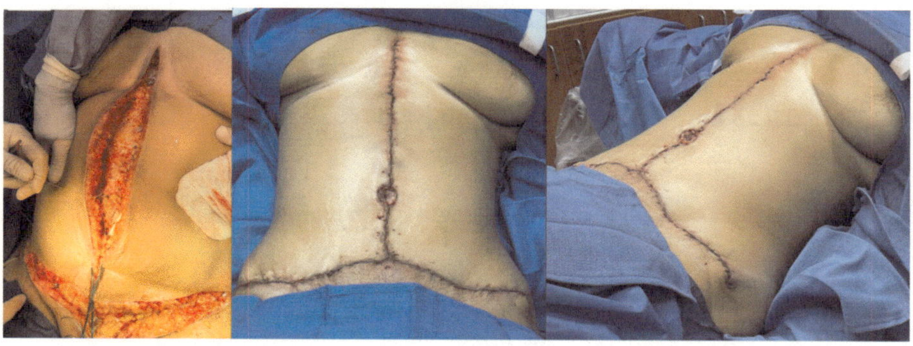

Figure 7.
Fleur De Li closure.

18.4 Problems and complications

Fleur De Li's abdominoplasty approach can have many of the same complications as a full abdominoplasty. However, this technique has a specific risk of having a midline scar that extends too far superiorly, leading to symmastia if the patient is having simultaneous breast augmentation surgery.

To avoid this, the surgeon must begin the superior aspect of the incision no higher than the inferior portion of the xiphoid process and avoid the impulse to chase excess skin found in the chest. Additionally, when performing a vertical incision, care to ensure both sides of the vertical component of inverted T are symmetrical is pivotal to prevent a curved vertical scar. If this is noted during surgery, an attempt to correct should be made by respecting necessary skin from one side or the other.

Pearls:

- The effects of the Fleur de Li technique can be the most dramatic given the recruitment of skin from the lateral trunk and correction made at the waist, back, and flank folds [2].

- The wide exposure of the fascia, especially in the epigastric region, allows powerful correction of abdominal wall deformity that may be constrained by traditional or HLTA's narrow tunnel of dissection.

- Despite extensive dissection, flap ischemia is not a major concern since segmental lateral perforators and large perforator vessels near the costal margin are preserved.

19. High lateral tension abdominoplasty

Generally: A successful result has to demonstrate the greatest degree of safety with zero tolerance complications, (2) give maximal esthetic results, (3) and must be consistent and reliable (Regardless of patient "Deformities" [2].

- Excess pubis should be corrected by excision rather than be used to close an exaggerated abdominal skin excision.

Consider laxity of the buttocks, the anterolateral and medial thigh, *as well as the mid and lower abdominal laxity.* Otherwise, the tissues below the incision may appear distractingly untreated

- Traditional abdominoplasty does not fully address excess skin laterally at the hip and thigh.
    - With the HLTA approach, the surgeon can achieve true body lift through an anterior incision only.
    - HLTA addresses excess lateral skin at the hip and thigh through the oblique incision vector whereby the emphasis is placed on resecting lateral redundancy of tissue in the hip, thigh, and buttock instead of the medial region to realize a superior correction of laxity [7].

- HLTA addresses skin at the epigastrium that the traditional abdominoplasty is unable to use for closure or removal.

HLTA approach takes advantage of proposed vectors of skin laxity of the abdomen depicted in **Figure 8** and allows designed incision to more efficiently treat redundant skin. This is particularly beneficial in patients with massive weight loss where the obvious suprapubic pannus is accompanied by excess fat and skin in the subcostal, lateral chest, hips, and anterolateral thighs.

With greater central tension, the mid portion of the final scar rises, resulting in a relatively horizontal scar orientation, even if the lateral initial incision did curve superiorly. With higher lateral tension, the scar remains low in the center and rises laterally [8].

19.1 Marking

With the patient in a standing position, with a wall as support which may be necessary during the traction-assisted process. Make suprapubic marking at a point 5–7 cm above the vaginal cleft or base of the penis [2].

A lateral vertical marking is made at the most lateral extent of the excess skin/ pannus.

The original authors of HLTA describe creating a closure marking whereby the pen is moved superolaterally from the suprapubic mark to meet somewhere along the lateral mark. This line usually rests between the inguinal and abdominal wall gullies (Foad). In a post-massive weight loss patient with extensive excess skin, it may be useful to extend the marking to include the design of the posterior body lift.

Defining the lower margin of excision:

The marking pen is placed over the line of future closure, and this position is maintained while pulling excess tissue vigorously upward until taut. When this skin is tensed superiorly, the skin below the pen is marked. This maneuver is performed across the width of the abdomen [8].

Estimating the upper margin of excision:

By pinching excess skin with thumb on the lower incision and fingers at the superior extent of the excess, while maintaining the premarked final closure line at the middle of the skin roll. These markings begin laterally and extend medially.

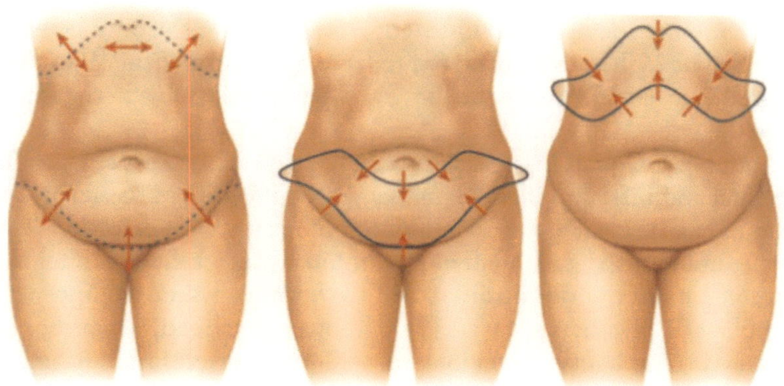

Figure 8.
Vectors of skin laxity of the abdomen [2].

To determine if the umbilicus should be floated inferiorly, the surgeon must note moderate excess skin below *and* above the umbilicus. In our practice the umbilicus is usually circumscribed at the skin, the stalk is left in place and the opening is recreated once the flap is positioned.

19.2 Operative technique

The principles described in the previous sections are similar. Lateral perforators are maintained, and there is minimal liposuction in the midline region in cases where the flap requires midline tunneling above the umbilicus. Umbilicus should be about 9–12 cm above pubis superior margin.

Rectus diastasis is corrected by plication of midline abdominal wall fascia with additional oblique or horizontal vector plication when indicated at the anterolateral abdominal wall to narrow waist and flatten appearance [2].

Excision of excess skin is made and layered closure with deeper fascial sutures with minimal skin tension is performed. All patients have a drain which is removed when output is less than 50 ccs per 24-hour period.

20. Mini abdominoplasty

20.1 General/preoperative evaluation

There are circumstances when there is minimal to moderate excess adipose, normal skin elasticity, but minimal skin laxity of the lower abdomen, making it unsafe to remove all the skin between the umbilicus and the pubis and still be able to achieve primary closure. In this situation, the upper incision of an abdominoplasty would have to be *below* the umbilicus–thus obviating the possibility of umbilical translocation, resulting in a scar that would be higher on the abdomen. This would be unaesthetic. To overcome this, a mini-abdominoplasty is performed whereby the redundant skin and fat of the lower abdomen are removed, the fascia of the lower abdomen can be plicated, and liposuction of the hip and abdomen can be performed as needed.

Another common situation when this procedure can be considered is when the umbilicus is located higher in the abdominal wall than what is considered to be esthetic. Some authors use a proportion of 1: to 1.6 or 1.5 as an esthetic proportion of the lower abdomen to the upper abdomen in relationship to the umbilicus [9]. Proportions of 1–1.4 or higher are considered to have a high umbilicus [9]. Other sources report the umbilicus should be 14 cm above the symphysis pubis in the midline or 10 cm above the pubic hair [2].

A high umbilicus in combination with little to moderate excess skin in the supraumbilicual and infraumbilical segments with mild adipose tissue excess in abdomen and flanks can be treated with mini-abdominoplasty with resection of skin inferior to the umbilicus, detachment of the umbilical pedicle and reattaching it with a bolter suture in a more inferior position, and performing associated liposuction to flanks and indicated plication of fascia [9]. Although described, the authors have never performed this surgery in conjunction with the mini abdominoplasty.

It is important to identify an umbilical hernia that can be repaired during surgery. Diastasis should be noted and planned for repair with musculofascial tighterning.

20.2 Marking

Guidelines to mark follow those of previous discussions. The superior incision is the predicted incision and it is below the umbilicus. The inferior committed incision is measured approximately 5–7 cm above the vaginal cleft in an effort to maintain the incision low. Hips and flanks are marked for liposuction.

If the patient has a previous low suprapubic scar, it should be included in the tissue to be excised.

20.3 Operative technique

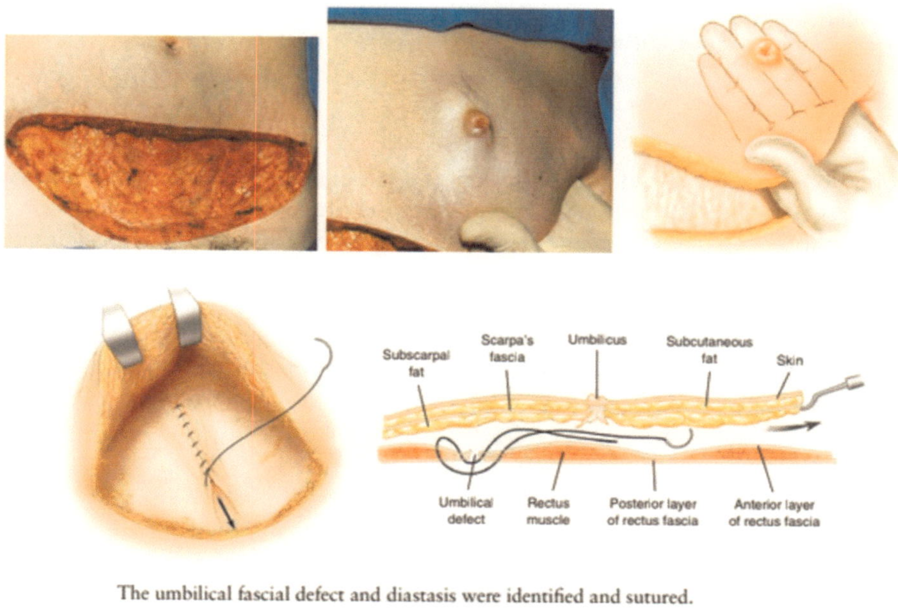

Figure 9.
Mini abdominoplasty dissection and simultaneous floating umbilicus permitting superior midline tunneling for midline rectus diastasis correction.

21. Reverse abdominoplasty

21.1 Overview and indications

Reverse abdominoplasty has been described by some to be a procedure best utilized in combination with other techniques previously discussed. It addresses the superior abdominal fat and redundant tissue that is left when other forms of abdominoplasty techniques do not achieve maximum results in this area (**Figure 9**).

It is used in isolation when patients have skin excess and abdominal protuberance primarily in the upper pole of the abdomen [2]. This technique will also address major stria or surgical scars that are confined to the superior abdomen. This approach can be used in conjunction with inframammary incisions when performing mastopexy, or a

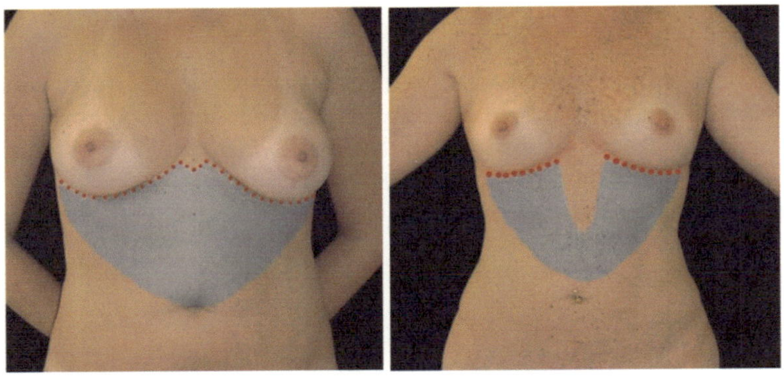

Figure 10.
Unification of Incision at the midline in a group with severe supraumbilical laxity (Left). Moderate supraumbilical skin laxity and no diastasis of underlying rectus muscle permitting two separate inframammary fold incisions [10].

combination mastopexy and augmentation. If a patient has previous inframammary incisions/scars the surgeon should also consider the procedure.

Some authors characterize candidates for this procedure in two groups: Patients with larger amounts of skin to be resected at the upper pole of the abdomen that will require unification of incision at the midline and a second group with moderate supraumbilical skin laxity and no diastasis of the underlying rectus muscle that will permit two separate inframammary fold incisions without unification at the midline (**Figure 10**) [10].

21.2 Marking

The degree of laxity in the upper pole of the abdomen will help dictate whether the incision should be unified at the midline or if two separate inframammary incisions will be sufficient to address the entirety of the skin laxity [10].

The patient is marked in the supine position. The upper margin of resection is outlined initially. The mark should start as far lateral as the skin demands, while maintaining the final closure within the bra strap line [2]. The marks continue medially and meet at the epigastrium with "V" shape.

Excess skin at the upper pole of the abdomen is pinched and pulled superiorly to determine the approximate inferior line of redundancy. Maximum tautness during this pinch maneuver will determine the extent of skin resection [2].

21.3 Operative technique

We infiltrate the patient with a tumescent solution. The upper incision is made and the abdominal flap is elevated to the level of the rectus fascia. The inferior extent of the flap is made several centimeters above the umbilicus to avoid potential excessive advancement.

The inframammary fold is marked on the abdominal wall so the skin excision is appropriately estimated. This should be done with the patient in the upright position. If done supine, the fold can rise unnaturally by several centimeters and the eventual crease could be sutured too high [2].

Using Kocher clamps, we then provide upward and slightly lateral traction to determine the degree of excess skin to be excised. The resultant abdominal flap is then sutured to the planned location of the inframammary fold in the abdominal wall by capturing deep fascia at both ends using 2 Vicryl and then closing the remaining layers sequentially to achieve tension-free closure.

If performing simultaneous breast surgery, it is preferable to perform reverse abdominoplasty first to create a solid base on which the breast can be built.

One, 10 mm flat JP drain is placed before closure.

21.4 Complications

The most common complication with this technique is excessive advancement of the umbilicus superiorly. To avoid this, the inferior extent of the flap should finish several centimeters above the umbilicus. Another technique to halt the unwanted superior advancement of the umbilicus is to suture the umbilical stalk to the rectus fascia.

22. Body lift-corset

22.1 Overview

Post-massive weight loss patients provide the surgeon with complex and varied challenges. With the advent of bariatric surgery and now with the use of GLP-1 inhibitors, cosmetic surgeons should be comfortable providing options to patients who wish to complement their weight loss journey with a more esthetic contour.

The corset body lift procedure as described by Alexander Moya provides versatility of addressing multiple skin rolls in the upper, mid, and lower abdomen and can be used in patients who may have a BMI > 30. It is a good alternative for patients who would like to address a significant amount of abdominal laxity and value an improved contour over the extent and location of scars.

This procedure comprehensively addresses the contour of the entire vertical abdominal wall and indirectly addresses the posterior waistline to provide a 360° improvement.

22.2 Markings

All markings are performed supine after the patient has been prepped and prior to the tumescent solution to avoid infiltration from affecting incisional markings. Pre-operative reference lines consist of the vertical midline (1), the lower chest (2), and the pubic line (3) (**Figure 11**).

22.3 Operative technique

The incisional markings are infiltrated with the tumescent solution and the incision begins along the subcutaneous tissues previously outlined (**Figure 12**).

Vertical Closure of the remnant defect follows diastasis. See **Figure 13**.

Attention is then placed at resecting the redundant lateral chest skin. Again, utilizing the tailor tacking technique, the excess later chest skin is marked by pulling the

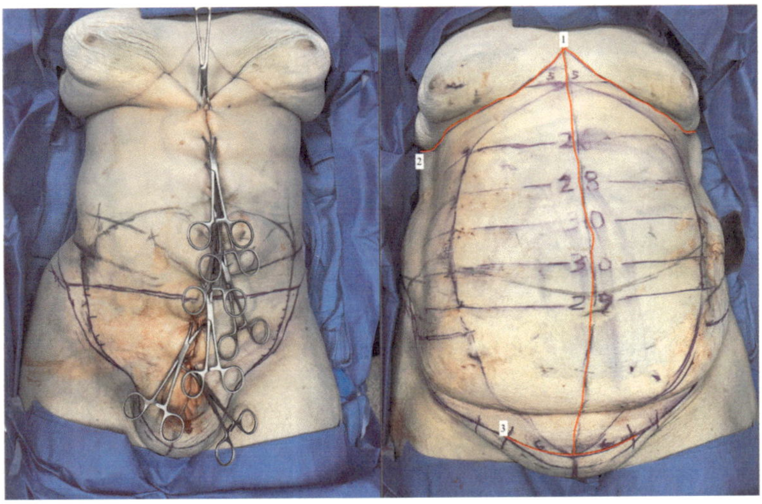

Figure 11.
Using tailor tacking technique, excess skin is approximated to help determine the extent of abdominal skin resection to be performed. Several transverse hash lines are drawn to aid in closure and they are maintained equidistant from the midline to ensure a straight vertical scar. A large vertical ellipse is outlined by connecting the midpoint of the lower chest, the lateral skin marks, and the midpoint of the reference line.

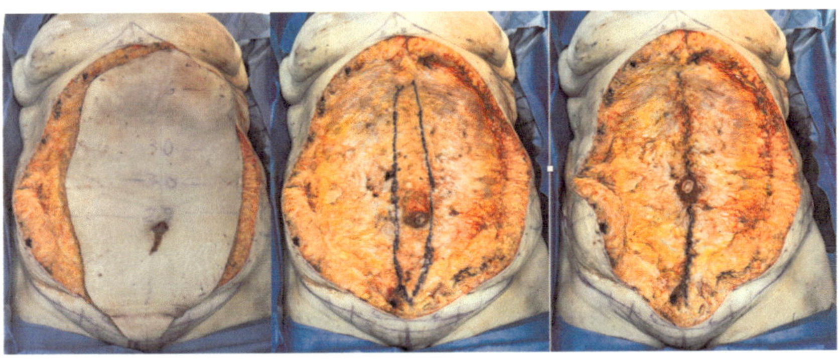

Figure 12.
(A) Vertical ellipse is incised with scalpel and Bovie electrocautery subsequent to release of umbilicus from the skin. Dissection is carried down to abdominal chest fascia circumferentially to excise the ellipse of skin and adipose. (B) Abdominal rectus muscle diastasis is visualized and outlined. (C) #2 Quill PDO suture is utilized for plication along the entirety of the vertical diastasis ensuring abdominal stalk is not strangulated and maintained with its remnant blood supply.

inferior tissue up to the lower chest reference line. The final resection outline incorporates the recreation of the IM folds (Moya). See **Figure 14**.

The next portion of the surgery focuses on performing lower trunk resection to remove the lower midline dog ear created by the vertical closure and resect the redundant lower waistline skin. This is performed while flexing the patient to maximize the removal of excess skin (**Figure 15**).

23. Complications and management

Like any other surgery, abdominoplasty does not come without risks.

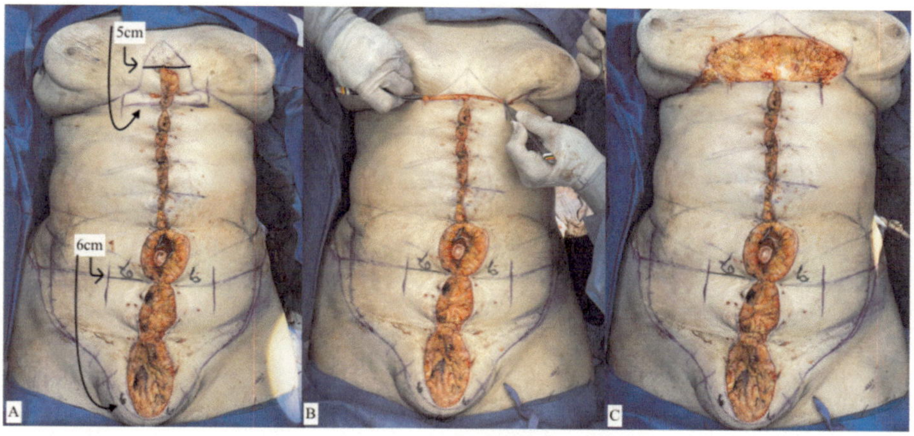

Figure 13.
(A) Sccarpa's fascia has been re-approximated with #0 Monocryl along the vertical defect while pushing skin edges together to reduce tension along the closure. This layer is reinforced using #2 PDO. Arrows point at the corresponding upper and lower matching transverse lengths made to match the lower chest reference line and lower abdomen reference lines respectively (B) Upper dog ear inferior resection margins assessed using tailor tacking technique (C) Upper dog ear resected.

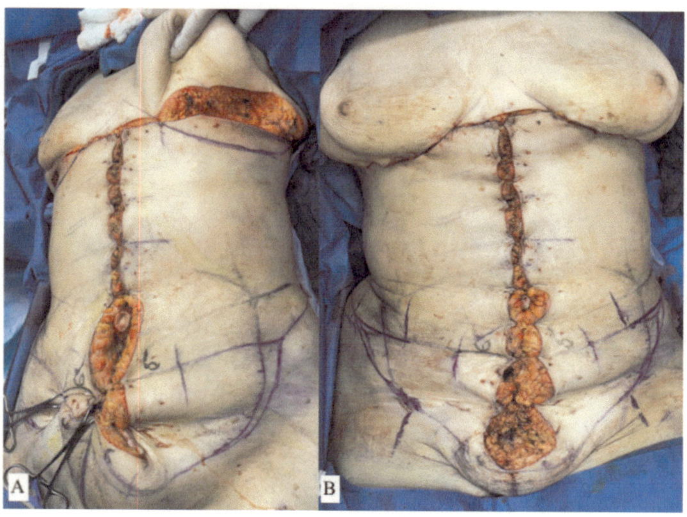

Figure 14.
(A) Lateral excess chest skin marking. This resection can extend from one scapula to the other depending on the amount of redundant skin. Dissection is carried in perpendicular to the chest wall along the lower chest reference line to aid in identifying the position of IM fold during closure. Dissection is carried down along the inferior resection margin in an oblique fashion to the skin (away from the upper abdominal flap edge to aid preservation of vascularity of the skin edges. (B) Redundant skin was excised and IM fold has been recreated by suturing deep layer abdominal flap to chest wall followed by superficial layered closure.

23.1 DVT/thromboembolism

One of the most severe potential complications with this procedure is the development of deep vein thrombosis and associated thromboembolism. Factors that contribute to increased risk of thromboembolic events (VTEs) include advancing age, prolonged operative time, elevated BMI, previous history of cancer, previous history of DVTs, or clotting disorders [2].

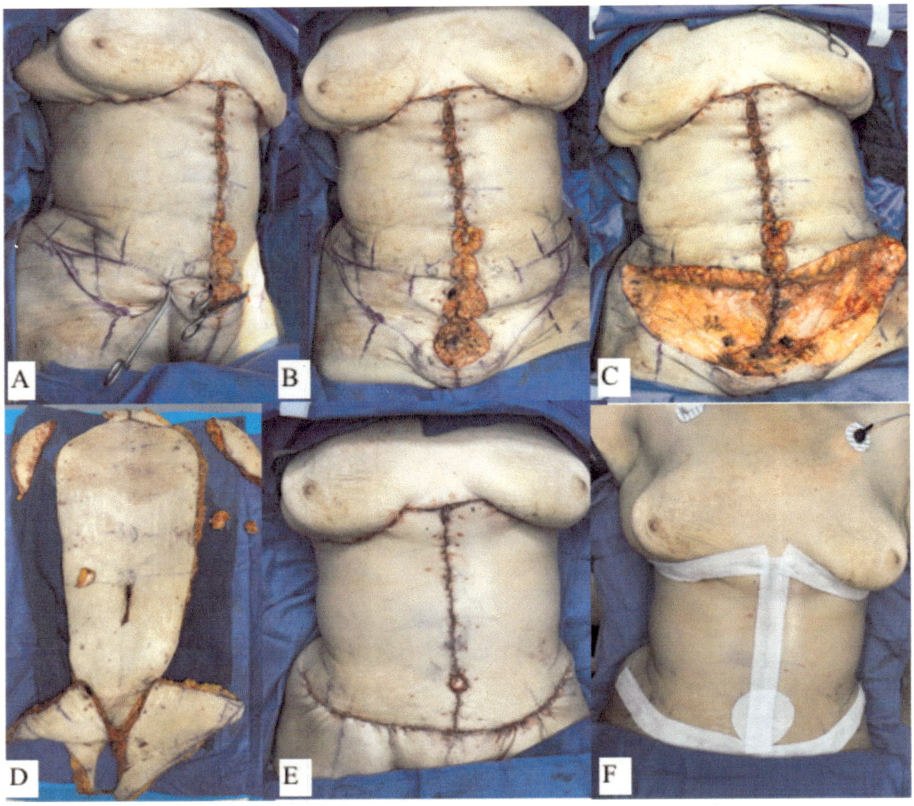

Figure 15.
(A) A tailor-tacking technique is used to identify the lower transverse lines along the abdominal flaps. The overall transverse length is made to match the pubic reference line (B) The lower waistline is addressed by marking the position of the lateral incision. In this case, they are placed high on the hips to enhance the abdominal-to-hip contour (C) Resection is completed. (D) 13 lbs. of skin removed (E) Closure follows the same layered closure of previous incisions starting with deep fascial 0 Monocryl, #2 PDO, #2-0 Quill, #3-0 Quill. Umbilicus is inset with 4-0 Monocryl Suture. A drain is placed (F) Robins tape along incisions.

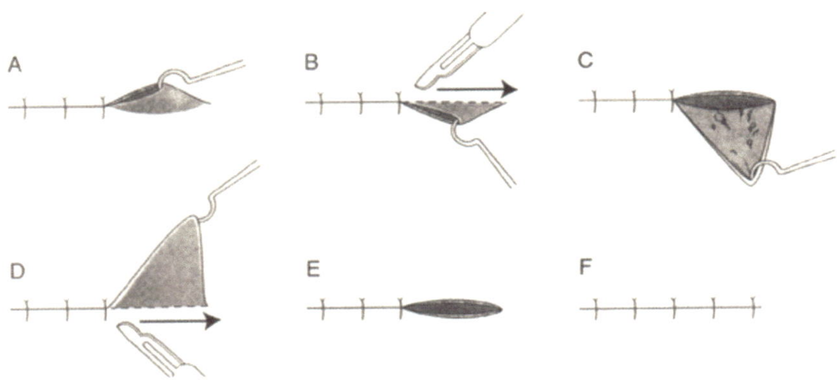

Figure 16.
Dog ear correction technique [11].

- *Management*: Preventive measures are the best course of action to address this potential risk. However, there is no current clear consensus in the literature regarding the course of time of chemoprophylaxis or whether it should be given preoperatively or postoperatively. In our practice, we measure preoperative hemoglobin and hematocrit and then take this lab value postoperatively as well. This helps us make decisions about the administration of chemoprophylaxis postoperatively. If post-op H/H is within the allowable decrease and the patient is not otherwise showing signs or symptoms of postoperative anemia, we administer 1x chemoprophylactic dose of enoxaparin. Lower Extremity compression socks or pneumatic compression devices are also used in those patients that stay in our facility overnight. Ultimately, it is up to each individual surgeon to assess the risk of each patient who presents for abdominoplasty and determine the use of mechanical and chemoprophylaxis when appropriate.

- Ambulation in the same day of surgery is encouraged and is a regular part of our postoperative abdominoplasty regimen

23.2 Dog ear formation

One of the most common complications in abdominoplasty surgery is the formation of a dog ear at the ends of the lower abdominal scar. To prevent the formation of a dog ear, the surgeon should plan to extend incision/scar as much as possible laterally along the relaxed skin tension lines to maximize a smooth postoperative contour.

- *Management*: If the dog ear does, in fact, form, it can be re-excised under local anesthesia if the area is small or under sedation if the procedure is more involved. (**Figure 16**, demonstrates one technique to manage dog ear complication).

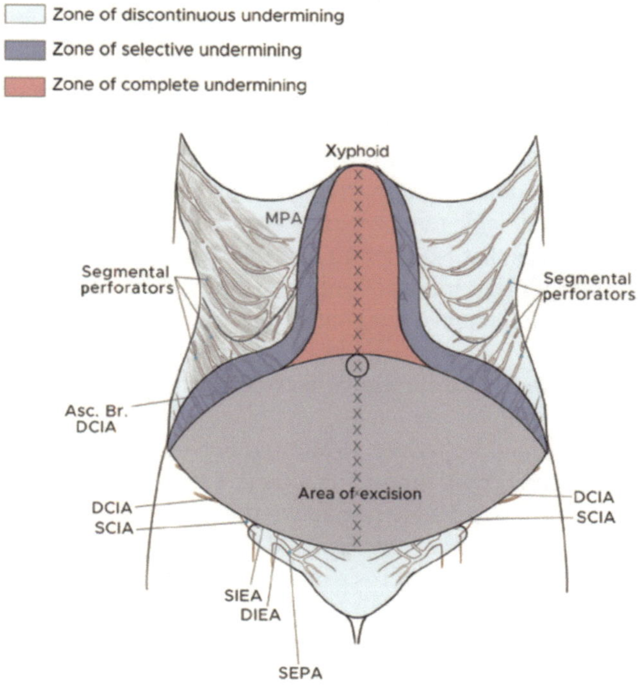

Figure 17.
Undermining should be tailored to esthetic goals while limiting disruption of blood supply from the underlying abdominal wall [12].

- Lateral dog ears can be best avoided intraoperatively by starting out with lateral closure first. Creating a perfect contour at the lateral edges and then adjusting as closure proceeds medially is one way to manage this complication. Another technique is to extend the incision laterally to maximize a straight-line closure.

23.3 Seroma

Fluid accumulation in the dissection spaces to an extent that it causes noticeable fluid waves across the lower abdomen. If the volume of this fluid is excessive, it can cause patient discomfort, pain, and a noticeable unaesthetic appearance. If not addressed, over time, the body may naturally seal off the accumulation of fluid and a formation cyst or abscess can form if infected.

- *Management:* Abdominal drain is an important component to prevent the formation of a seroma. However, if seroma forms subsequent to drain removal, serial aspirations, until seroma resolves, provide adequate treatment. In rare cases, it becomes necessary to temporarily place another drain.

- An abdominal binder in combination with the drain helps prevent seroma formation.

- We limit midline liposuction to the area above the xiphoid region to preserve lymphatics located superior to deep fascia and sub-scarpal. Tourani et al. found that lymphatic drainage of the lower abdomen also lies superficial to Scarpa's fascia in 8 hemi-abdomen specimens from four cadavers. However, a systematic review of four studies (including 630 patients) found that preservation of the Scarpa's fascia (and cutaneous tissues *deep to this layer*) was associated with significantly decreased seroma rate, time to drain removal, drain output, and hospital stay [12]. All of our abdominoplasty patients receive a postoperative day 1 manual lymphatic massage included as part of their surgery packet and are encouraged to continue lymphatic massages at least once a week for 6 weeks after surgery. In our experience, this significantly helps reduce postoperative lymphedema and thereby seroma formation. The physiologic mechanism of lymphatic massage remains unclear, but some sources propose that MLD promotes a decrease in distal lymphatic pressure, enhancing uptake, or that manual lymphatic drainage improves accessory lymphatic routes that enhance lymphatic reuptake [13].

23.4 Delayed wound healing/dehiscence/ischemia

This can be a difficult complication to address depending on the size of the tissue involved. Most of the time, poor wound healing is a result of decreased blood supply to a particular area. The wound edge just above the mons pubis is far from the peripheral blood supply that enters the skin and the soft tissues. This may lead to signs of ischemia that may progress to necrosis over the course of several days.

- *Management:* If an area of poor wound healing is less than 2 cm, the area can often be left to heal by secondary intention [2]. Larger areas are best managed with wet-to-dry dressing changes over a course of 1–2 weeks to allow the wound margins to demarcate. Once the margins are well demarcated, a decision to debrided any necrotic tissue is performed. All non-viable tissue should be removed because it serves as a nidus for infection and impairs wound healing [14]. Daily dressing changes are continued with frequent inspection to ensure adequate healing is taking place. If the wound allows it, retention-type sutures can be placed laterally to reduce the overall size of the defect and facilitate a more rapid closure. In certain cases, a negative pressure wound vac may be useful to allow for faster healing by secondary intention.

- During the elevation of the abdominoplasty flap, superficial inferior epigastric and superficial circumflex iliac artery systems are divided with the creation of the low transverse incision.

- We follow Saldanha's technique of abdominoplasty with selective undermining between the medial borders of the rectus and discontinuing undermining with liposuction in the lateral abdomen to facilitate flap redraping while preserving the perforating blood supply from the deep epigastric vessels. Blood supply to the skin and subcutaneous flap is from intercostal and subcostal segmental perforators. We maintain a minimum flap thickness of 2–3 cm to maximize subdermal plexus preservation (**Figures 17** and **18**) [12].

- Preventive measures to avoid wound breakdown are employed by reducing tension at wound edges. Two key, 2 Vicryl sutures are typically placed medial to inguinal fold and lateral to the midline on each side to approximate Scarpa's to Scarpa's tacked to the underlying rectus fascia. 0-monocryl is then used to reapproximate the remaining Scarpa's to Scarpa's fascia of the abdominal flap

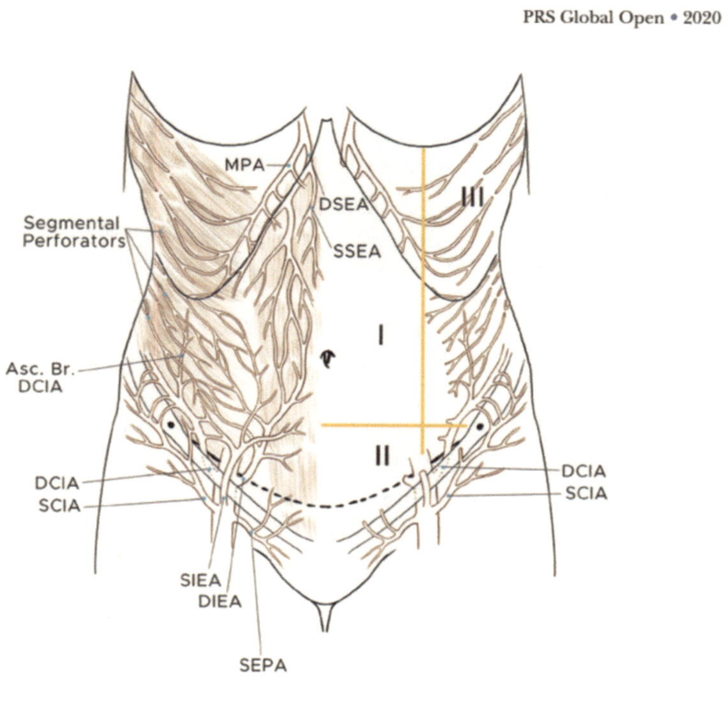

Figure 18.
Illustration of Abdominal wall supply according to Huger zones (I, II, III). The right hemi-abdomen represents preoperative anatomy. The left hemi-abdomen represents an expected disruption of the perforating blood supply to the skin and subcutaneous tissue during abdominoplasty [12].

lateral to the inguinal fold. A 3-0 monocryl is then used to approximate the deep dermal layer and a 3-0 monoderm quill is then used in subcuticular fashion. Additionally, ensuring that the patient is in a 30° position when deciding on a superior cut is important to avoid excessive tension.

23.5 Hypertrophic scar

- Can be mitigated by careful closure of deeper tissues. Performing reapproximation of deeper tissues limits widened depressed scars. As mentioned previously we employ key fascial sutures to ensure minimal tension to superficial skin layers.

- The literature supports the use of intralesional triamcinolone acetonide +5-fluorouracil (5-FU) which has been shown to decrease pigmentation significantly faster compared to the administration of intralesional 5-FU or triamcinolone alone [15]. Therefore, we use small volumes of this combination of drugs in areas that may benefit.

- Even though we do everything possible to perform adequate tissue handling and promote postoperative care conducive to minimal scarring, some patients will inevitably form an unaesthetic scar which is revised by excision of skin, and creation of a sharp 90° wound edges with layered closure to support an esthetic result [2].

23.6 Umbilical deformity/necrosis

- We perform rectus plication superior and inferior of umbilicus from xiphoid down to superior pubis. The umbilical stalk is tethered at 6, 3, 9, and 12 o'clock to assist the creation of a pleasing umbilical depression. We avoid excessive tightening of the surrounding rectus fascia in this region of plication. Additionally, we avoid excessive defatting of the periumbilical fat and maintain a wider fatty base to ensure a pyramidal shape to the periumbilical fat.

- If ischemic changes were to ensue, immediate release of superficial dermal sutures should be performed to remove tension. If ischemia occurs, demarcation would be allowed to take place followed by debridement of eschar formation and secondary healing with regular dressing changes to allow stabilization of the wound (Foad).

- To help with the creation of umbilical depression, the senior author sometimes places a small marble or xeroform for a period of time to allow healing in the adequate shape.

23.7 Hematoma

- Meticulous attention to ensuring hemostasis during abdominal flap elevation helps prevent hematoma formation.

- All of our abdominoplasty patients receive abdominal binder; stay in our in-house suite and are examined postoperatively on the day of surgery and then again on the first postoperative day to recognize hematoma.

23.8 Contour irregularity/abdominal wall relaxation

- Epigastric bulging subsequent to abdominoplasty can occur when inadequate plication of rectus muscle in the superior abdominal wall occurs near the xiphoid. To avoid this, we undermine the flap in the midline up to xiphoid to allow complete access for full superior plication.

24. Postoperative care

24.1 Abdominal support and incision care

- Abdominal binder is worn 24 hours a day for 1 week. After 1 week, the binder is replaced with a "faja" best fitted to the patient, which is generally worn for 6 weeks. After 6 weeks, the patient may choose to stop wearing the "faja".

- Robbins tape is left on for 1 week. At the 1 week postoperative appointment, the tape is replaced with brown paper tape which is left in place for up to five more weeks. Silicone tape is then recommended to be worn whenever feasible for the next 3 months.

24.2 Activity/restrictions

- Week 1:

    - No lifting >10 lbs. Remain flexed at the hip for the first 3 days after surgery. On postoperative day 4, patients may gradually increase extension at the hip when ambulating until they feel tension and holding that position for 30 s, then releasing the tension and re-bending at the waist. This is repeated throughout the day until patients are able to be fully erect.

    - Daily showering using hibiclens soap is allowed.

    - Should avoid heating pads, hot showers, or sunbathing until sensation in abdominal skin is regained to avoid potential burns.

    - Diet should include a minimum of 100 grams of daily protein and plenty of fluids (64 oz./day)

    - Prophylactic antibiotics are continued for 5 days

    - Pt should document drain output- removal when <50 cc/24 hours.

- Week 2:

    - Maintain the same activity restrictions as week 1.

- Week 3–6:

    - Light lower extremity exercises, like walking are permitted. Avoid abdominal muscle exercises for 3 months to protect abdominal wall plication.

25. Cases

25.1 Traditional abdominoplasty case 1

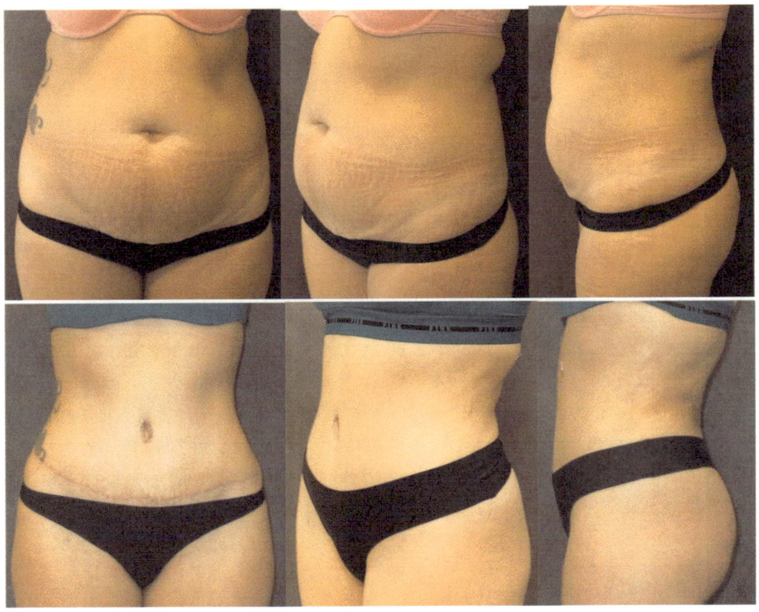

Pre Op: 37F, Weight: 162 lbs., Height: 64″, BMI: 27.8.
Surgery:

- Full Abdominoplasty with associated liposuction to abdomen, waist, and hips.
- Total Fat Removed after Liposuction: 2300 ccs
- Excised Skin Weight: 2.3 lbs.

Post Op Photos: 6 weeks.

25.2 Traditional abdominoplasty case 2

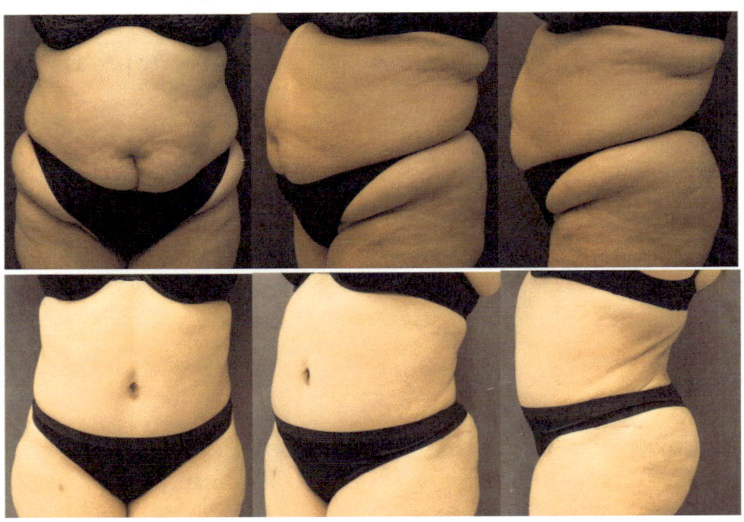

Pre Op: 43F, Weight: 202 lbs., Height: 63″, BMI: 35.8.
Surgery:

- Full Abdominoplasty with associated liposuction to abdomen, waist, hips, and back roll

- Total Fat Removed after Liposuction: 5000 (5300) ccs

- Excised Skin Weight: 5.6 lbs.

Post Op Photos: 6 months.

25.3 Traditional abdominoplasty case 3

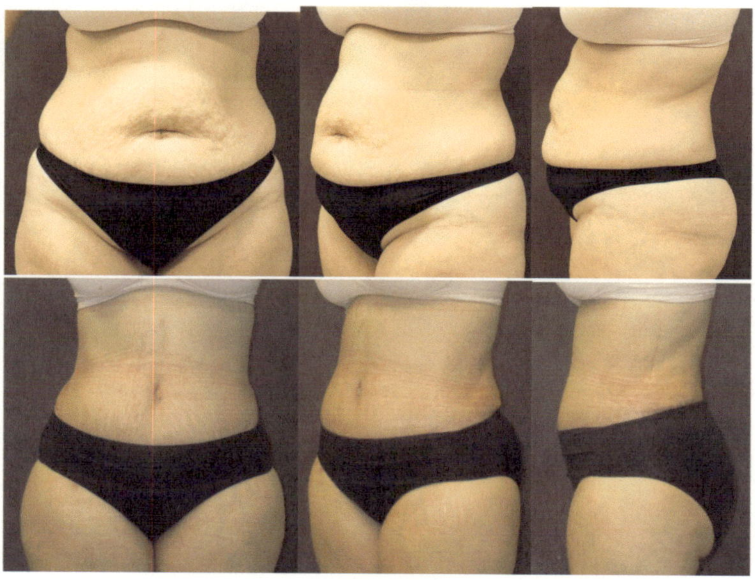

Pre Op: 51F, Weight: 145 lbs., Height: 64″, BMI: 24.9.
Surgery:

- Full Abdominoplasty with associated liposuction to abdomen, waist, and hips.

- Total Fat Removed after Liposuction: 1600 ccs

- Excised Skin Weight: 3 lbs.

Post Op Photos: 8 weeks.

25.4 Traditional abdominoplasty case 4

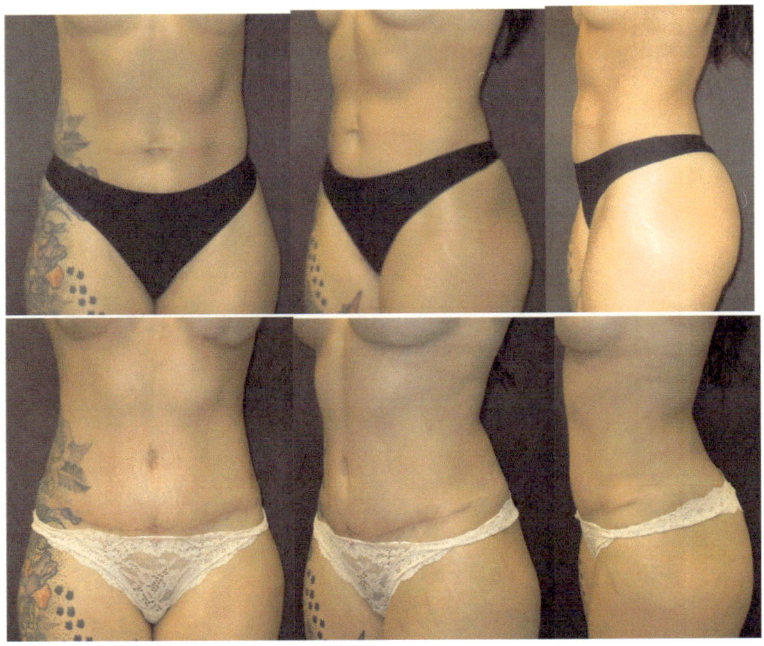

Pre Op: 33F, Weight: 138 lbs., Height: 62″, BMI: 25.2.
Surgery:

- Full Abdominoplasty with associated liposuction to abdomen, waist. (Subcutaneous mastectomy and breast augmentation with silicone implants)
- Total Removed Fat after Liposuction: 200 ccs
- Excised Skin Weight: 1 lbs.

Post Op Photos: 6 weeks.

25.5 Traditional abdominoplasty case 5

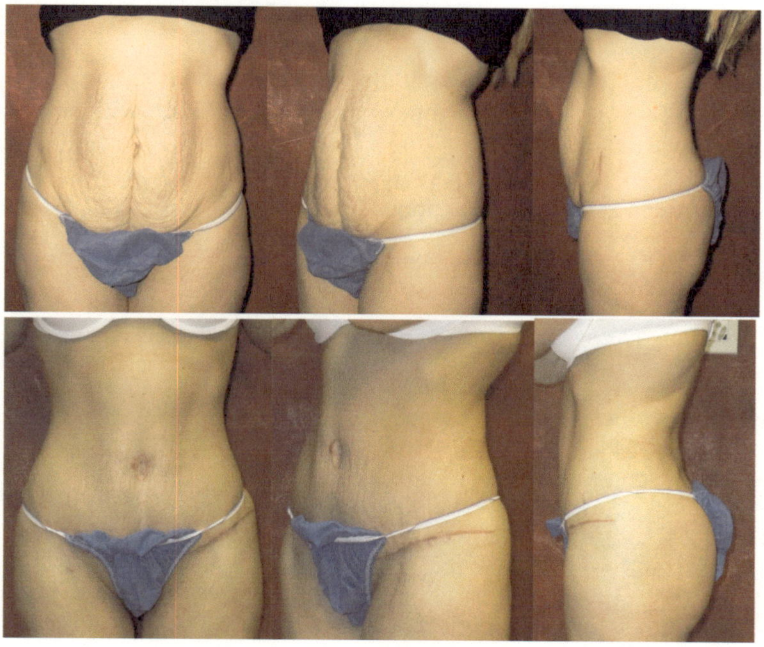

Pre Op: 45F, Weight: 116 lbs., Height: 63″, BMI: 20.5.
Surgery:

- Full Abdominoplasty with associated liposuction to abdomen, waist, and hips.
- Total Removed Fat after Liposuction: 950 ccs
- Excised Skin Weight: 1.8 lbs.

Post Op Photos: 8 weeks.

25.6 Traditional abdominoplasty case 6

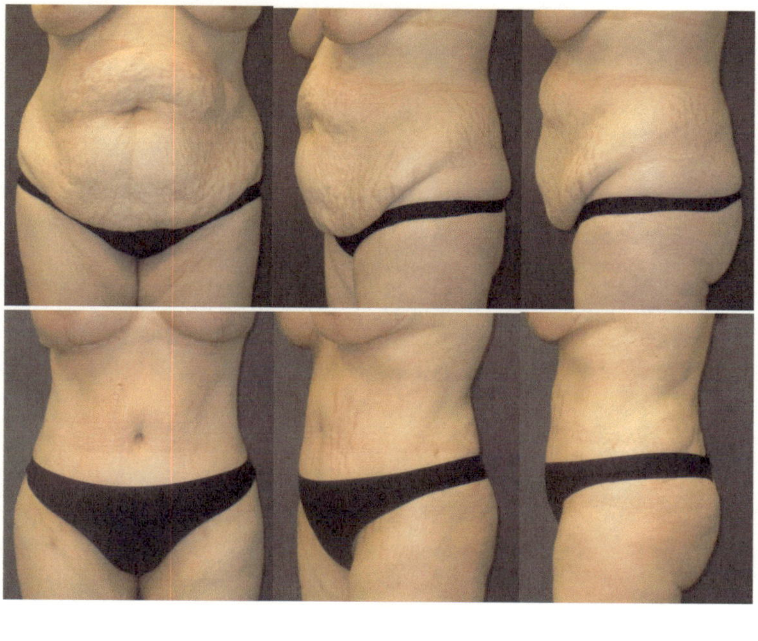

Pre Op: 48F, Weight: 185 lbs., Height: 69″, BMI: 27.3.
Surgery:

- Full Abdominoplasty with associated liposuction to abdomen, waist, hips, and thighs. Simultaneous Breast Mastopexy and Augmentation with silicone implants. J plasma to thighs.

- Total Removed Fat after Liposuction: 4600 ccs

- Excised Skin Weight: 7 lbs.

Post Op Photos: 12 weeks.

25.7 Traditional abdominoplasty case 7

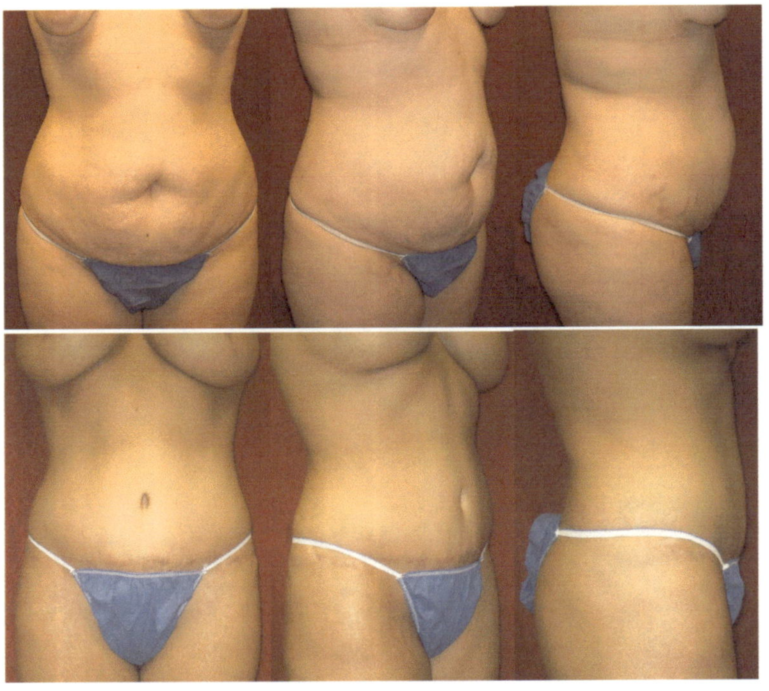

Pre Op: 26F, Weight: 168 lbs., Height: 68 BMI: 30.7.
Surgery:

- Mini Abdominoplasty with associated liposuction to abdomen and waist.

- Total Removed Fat after Liposuction: 2200 cc

- Excised Skin Weight: 1.25 lbs.

Post Op Photos: 6 weeks.

25.8 High lateral tension/extended abdominoplasty case 7

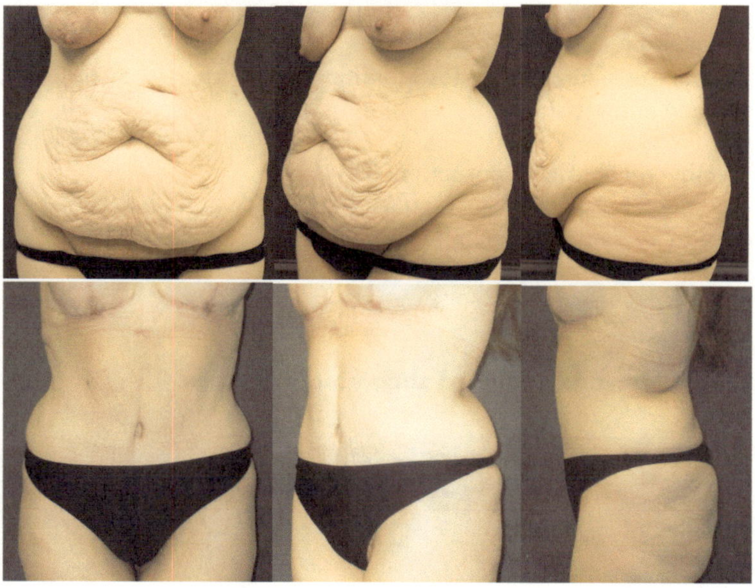

Pre Op: 34F, Weight: 142 lbs., Height: 62″, BMI: 26.0, status post previous 120 lbs. weight loss.
Surgery:

- High Lateral Tension/Extended Abdominoplasty with associated liposuction to abdomen and waist after massive weight loss.
- Total Removed Fat after Liposuction: 400ccs
- Excised Skin Weight: 6.8 lbs.

Post Op Photos: 6 months.

25.9 High lateral tension/extended abdominoplasty case 8

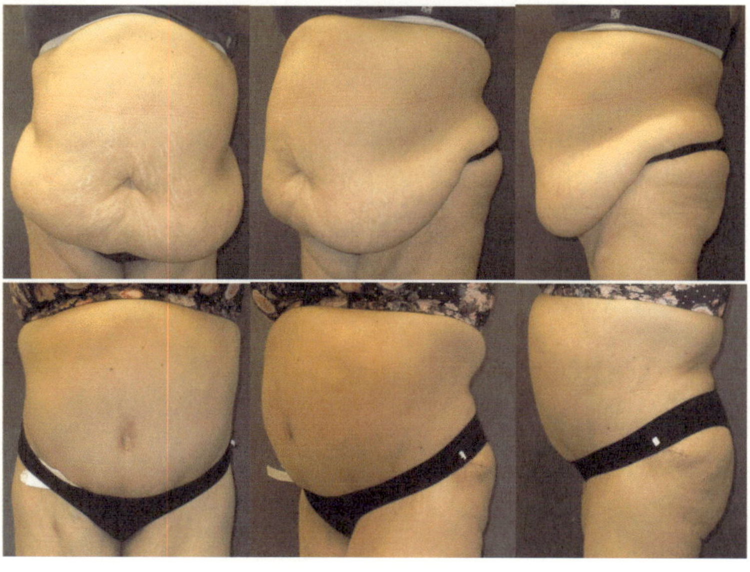

Pre Op: 52F, Weight: 206 lbs., Height: 63″, BMI: 36.5.
Surgery:

- High Lateral Tension/Extended Abdominoplasty with associated liposuction to the abdomen and waist.
- Total Removed Fat after Liposuction: 3200 ccs
- Excised Skin Weight: 11.5 lbs.

Post Op Photos: 8 weeks.

25.10 High lateral tension/extended abdominoplasty case 9

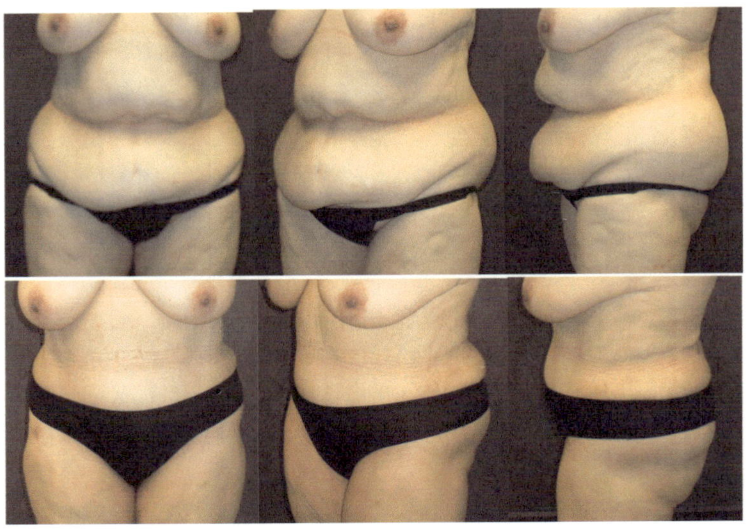

Pre Op: 68F, Weight: 140 lbs., Height: 58″, BMI: 29.3.
Surgery:

- High Lateral Tension/Extended Abdominoplasty with associated liposuction to the abdomen, waist, and hips
- Total Removed Fat after Liposuction: 1300 ccs
- Excised Skin Weight: 6.0 lbs.

Post Op Photos: 8 weeks.

25.11 Fleur De Lis case 10

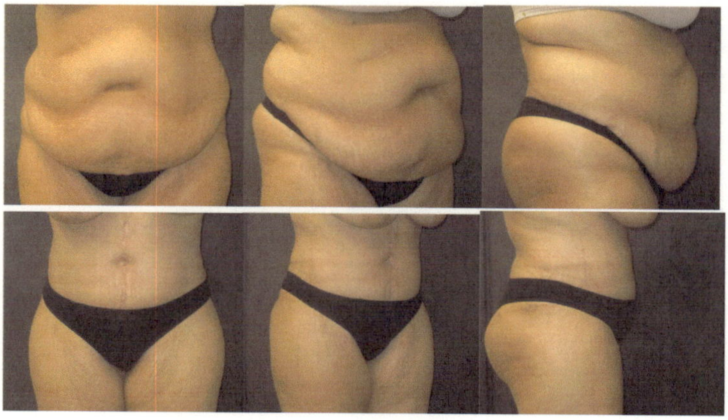

Pre Op: 49F, Weight: 230 lbs., Height: 66″, BMI: 37.1. Previous hx of emergent cholecystectomy with an abdominal incision.
Surgery:

- Fleur De Lis Abdominoplasty with associated liposuction to abdomen, waist, hips, mid back roll.
- Total Removed Fat after Liposuction: 4900 ccs
- Excised Skin Weight: 13 lbs.

Post Op Photos: 6 weeks.

25.12 Mini abdominoplasty case 11

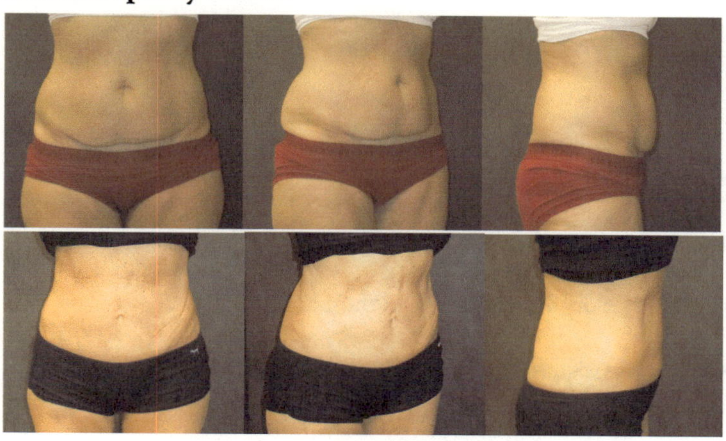

Pre Op: 58F, Weight: 131 lbs., Height: 64″, BMI: 22.5.
Surgery:

- Mini Abdominoplasty with associated liposuction to abdomen and waist.
- Total Removed Fat after Liposuction: 2200 cc
- Excised Skin Weight: 1.25 lbs.

Post Op Photos: 6 weeks.

Video materials

The video materials referenced in this chapter are available for download at the following link: https://bit.ly/49zzWnS

Author details

Andrew Sohn[1,2]* and Sebastian Gutierrez de Pineres[1,3]

1 Tulsa Surgical Arts Surgery Center, Oklahoma, USA

2 American Board of Cosmetic Surgery, United States

3 American Academy of Cosmetic Surgery, United States

*Address all correspondence to: sohndmd@gmail.com

References

[1] Barcelos F, Avelar L, Bordoni L, Barcelos R. Anatomical analysis of abdominoplasty. Revista Brasileira de Cirurgia Plástica. 2017;**32**(2). Available from: https://rbcp.org.br/details/1849/en-US/anatomical-analysis-of-abdominoplasty

[2] Nahai F, Nahai F. The Art of Aesthetic Surgery, Three Volume Set. 3rd ed. Thieme; 2020. pp. 2936-3025

[3] Nahai FR. Anatomic considerations in abdominoplasty. Clinics in Plastic Surgery. 2010;**37**(3):407-414. DOI: 10.1016/j.cps.2010.03.003

[4] Sivak W. Abdominoplasty. Plastic Surgery Key. 2020:60-62. Available from: https://plasticsurgerykey.com/abdominoplasty-6/ [Accessed: October 01, 2024]

[5] Nahai F, Brown RG, Vasconez LO. Blood supply to the abdominal wall as related to planning abdominal incisions. The American Surgeon. 1976;**42**(9):691-695

[6] Themes U. Anatomic considerations in abdominoplasty. Plastic Surgery Key. 2017:3. Available from: https://plasticsurgerykey.com/anatomic-considerations-in-abdominoplasty

[7] Rosenfield K, Lorne. High-tension abdominoplasty. Plastic Surgery Key. 2019. Available from: https://plasticsurgerykey.com/abdominoplasty-6/ [Accessed: October 02, 2024]

[8] Teitelbaum S. Demystifying high-lateral-tension abdominoplasty. Aesthetic Surgery Journal. 2006;**26**(3):325-329. DOI: 10.1016/j.asj.2006.03.006

[9] Bozola AR. Mini-abdominoplasty: Classification and treatment. Plastic Surgery Key. 2019:325-329. Available from: plasticsurgerykey.com/mini-abdominoplasty-classification-and-treatment [Accessed: October 02, 2024]

[10] Deos MF. Reverse abdominoplasty. Plastic Surgery Key. 2016. Available from: plasticsurgerykey.com/reverse-abdominoplasty-2/ [Accessed: October 02, 2024]

[11] Jaibaji M, Morton JD, Green AR. Dog ear: An overview of causes and treatment. Annals of the Royal College of Surgeons of England. 2001;**83**(2):136-138

[12] O'Kelly N, Nguyễn K, Gibstein A, Bradley J, Tanna N, Matarasso A. Standards and trends in lipoabdominoplasty. Plastic and Reconstructive Surgery. 2020;**8**:e3144. DOI: 10.1097/GOX.0000000000003144

[13] Marxen T, Shauly O, Goel P, Tsan T, Faria R, Gould DJ. The utility of lymphatic massage in cosmetic procedures. Aesthet Surg J Open Forum. 2023;**5**:ojad023. DOI: 10.1093/asjof/ojad023

[14] Hunstad JP. Abdominoplasty. Plastic Surgery Key. 2018. Available from: plasticsurgerykey.com/abdominoplasty-3/ [Accessed: October 02, 2024]

[15] Srivastava S, Patil A, Prakash C, Kumari H. Comparison of intralesional triamcinolone acetonide, 5-fluorouracil, and their combination in treatment of keloids. World Journal of Plastic Surgery. 2018;7(2):212-219

Chapter 14

High Definition Liposculpting

Pasquale G. Tolomeo and Manik S. Bedi

Abstract

High-definition liposculpting is an advanced body contouring technique designed to create a sculpted, athletic physique by selectively targeting fat layers and accentuating muscle definition. The advent of technologies like VASER (Vibration Amplification of Sound Energy at Resonance) and Renuvion (a helium plasma and radiofrequency device) has revolutionized this procedure, allowing for precise sculpting and improved definition of the body's contours. Ideal candidates are those seeking a more defined and athletic appearance with an emphasis on muscle visibility and skin tightening. The results yield a more esthetically pleasing silhouette. For optimal outcomes, patients must adhere to proper garment protocols and post-surgical lymphatic massages. Recovery is comparable to traditional liposuction but with the benefit of more dramatic, long-lasting results.

Keywords: high-definition liposuction, HiDef Lipo, Vaser, Renuvion, body sculpting, liposculpting

1. Introduction

A cosmetic surgeon performing high-definition liposculpting must possess both an artistic eye and a deep understanding of muscle anatomy to create a beautifully sculpted body. The artistic element comes into play when shaping the body's contours, as the surgeon must envision the final esthetic outcome, considering how light and shadow will enhance muscle definition. A thorough knowledge of the underlying muscles is crucial to ensure that fat removal highlights the natural curves and lines of the body, emphasizing a toned, athletic appearance [1]. By carefully blending artistry with anatomical precision, the surgeon can achieve a harmonious, balanced physique that looks natural and enhances the patient's overall proportions.

Traditional liposuction techniques have evolved from basic fat removal to more sophisticated contouring procedures aimed at revealing and enhancing the underlying musculature [2]. High-definition liposuction takes body sculpting to the next level, offering patients the possibility of achieving chiseled, athletic bodies. It focuses on strategic fat removal and redistribution to define specific muscle groups such as the abdomen, chest, arms, back, legs, and glutes.

In High-Definition Liposuction, the interplay of light, shadow, contour, and form is fundamental in achieving a sculpted, athletic look. Light and shadow naturally accentuate the body's peaks and valleys, so the surgeon strategically removes fat to enhance these contrasts, creating the appearance of a more defined muscle structure. By carefully shaping the body's contours, the surgeon highlights natural lines, ensuring a smooth, harmonious flow across areas such as the abdomen, chest, and arms. The precise removal of fat emphasizes the underlying muscle forms, allowing the body's inherent structure to become more prominent. This meticulous attention to how light interacts with the body's curves results in a physique that is not only physically toned but also visually striking, with muscles clearly defined and enhanced.

An essential principle in high-definition liposuction (HDL) is the use of positive and negative spaces to create balance and definition. Positive space refers to areas where muscle bulk or prominence is desired, such as the abdomen, chest, or arms, which are accentuated by removing fat around them, making the muscles stand out more distinctly. Negative space, by contrast, involves selectively removing fat to create depth and separation between muscle groups, enhancing the visual contrast between defined muscles and the surrounding tissue. By balancing these spaces, the surgeon can achieve a dynamic, three-dimensional appearance that results in an athletic, esthetically refined physique. Through the careful manipulation of positive and negative spaces, the body appears naturally contoured, with enhanced muscle visibility and a more appealing, well-proportioned form [2].

The success of HDL relies not just on the surgeon's skill but also on the use of advanced technologies. VASER liposuction provides more control over fat removal, while Renuvion delivers skin-tightening effects that complement fat reduction by addressing skin laxity.

2. High-definition liposculpting

2.1 VASER liposuction

VASER (vibration amplification of sound energy at resonance) liposuction, also known as ultrasound-assisted lipoplasty, uses ultrasound waves to emulsify fat cells, making fat extraction easier during traditional liposuction. The vibration emitted from the cannula breaks down the bonds between fat cells while preserving the surrounding blood vessels, nerves, and connective tissue [3]. This technique enables highly precise fat emulsification, particularly in fibrotic areas such as the male chest and back, where fat tends to be more resistant. VASER allows for targeted fat removal across various layers of the body, giving surgeons the ability to sculpt and accentuate the natural muscle contours for a more refined and defined appearance. Beyond fat emulsification, VASER also promotes skin retraction due to its thermal effects on the dermis, leading to improved skin tightening. Additionally, the technique minimizes blood loss, contributing to a safer and more efficient procedure with smoother recovery [4].

VASER affects adipose tissue through three primary mechanisms: cavitation, mechanical disruption, and thermal energy. Cavitation occurs when ultrasound vibrations in the tumescent tissue create bubbles that expand and eventually burst, causing fat cells to detach from the surrounding fibrous network. Mechanical disruption happens as the tip of the cannula physically contacts and dislodges adipocytes, facilitating their removal. The thermal effect arises when the cannula remains in prolonged contact with fat cells, generating heat that can potentially burn the tissue if not properly controlled [3, 5].

The use of VASER in high-definition liposuction offers numerous advantages. It can be applied to various areas of the body, including the neck, arms, chest, abdomen, back, thighs, flanks, and calves. VASER enables precise removal of superficial fat layers, enhancing natural-looking muscle contours with greater definition. Its selective fat disruption minimizes trauma to surrounding tissues, leading to reduced swelling, bruising, and a faster recovery process. Additionally, the emulsified fat obtained through VASER liposuction is of higher quality, as it undergoes less trauma compared to traditional liposuction methods, which improves its viability for autologous fat transfer procedures [6].

2.2 Renuvion

Renuvion is a device that has greatly changed the game of HDL. Renuvion combines helium plasma with radiofrequency to create a dual-modality approach for skin retraction. The effects of the energy are delivered to the surrounding tissue via two methods: direct contact with the helium plasma and the flow of radiofrequency through the plasma to the tissue.

The flow of energy is through the path of least resistance. When applied to the subdermal plane, Renuvion targets the fibro-septal network (FSN) as opposed to other devices that focus on the dermis [7]. More than 80% of adipocytes are found in the FSN. Targeting these cells potentially has the most effect on soft tissue contraction, which may lead to a volume loss of up to 45% [7, 8]. As the device is advanced along the plane, radiofrequency energy travels through the tissue proximal to the device, creating new paths of distribution leading to a 360-degree soft tissue treatment [7, 9]. The dispersion of energy allows for adequate soft tissue heating while minimizing the depth of thermal spread.

The final results typically become visible around 6 to 9 months post-surgery, once the processes of neocollagenesis and healing are complete. During this time, the body undergoes collagen production and tissue remodeling, which help tighten the skin and refine the contours. As swelling subsides and the skin retracts, the full effects of the procedure, including muscle definition and improved body contours, are revealed.

Combining VASER and Renuvion enhances fat removal precision while addressing skin laxity, resulting in smoother contours and more defined muscle highlights. VASER's emulsification of fat allows for controlled removal, while Renuvion tightens the skin to create a natural, toned appearance. Together, they enable three-dimensional body sculpting, accentuating natural musculature in areas like the abdomen, flanks, and arms for an athletic physique. This combination also offers customizable treatments, allowing for tailored results based on the patient's anatomy and goals, from non-invasive skin tightening to precise fat removal for high-definition contours.

3. Pre-operative planning

The pre-operative consultation is a pivotal step in the high-definition liposculpting process, often shaping the patient's entire experience and setting the foundation for a successful outcome. Given that many patients consult with multiple surgeons before making a decision, it is essential to make a strong, positive impression. The primary goals of the consultation are to thoroughly understand the patient's esthetic goals, gather detailed medical history, conduct a comprehensive physical examination, and provide a clear diagnosis. Surgeons also explain the recommended procedures, along with their potential risks and benefits. Additionally, this meeting offers a critical opportunity to manage the patient's expectations, helping them understand their condition and the various treatment options available. By ensuring that patients are well informed and have realistic expectations, the consultation plays a key role in preparing them for the procedure and enhancing overall satisfaction with the results.

3.1 Patient evaluation

A thorough pre-operative evaluation is crucial to ensuring the success and safety of any surgical procedure. The process begins by reviewing the patient's medical history and chief complaint, which should be described in the patient's own words to gain a clear understanding of their concerns and expectations. Open-ended questions are particularly effective for helping patients express their goals and worries. The evaluation also includes a detailed review of any medical conditions, current medications (including dosages and frequencies), allergies, and a complete surgical history including previous cosmetic procedures. Social factors, such as the use of tobacco or nicotine products, are vital to assess, as they can impair vascular health and negatively affect wound healing. Additionally, understanding the patient's occupation is essential, as it can influence post-operative restrictions and recovery plans.

The ideal candidate for HDL using VASER and Renuvion is an individual in good physical health who is near their ideal body weight. This procedure is best suited for individuals seeking enhanced muscle definition. Additionally, candidates with mild to moderate skin laxity can benefit from the skin-tightening effects provided by Renuvion, which works synergistically with VASER. Those patients who have unrealistic expectations are not candidates for HDL.

3.2 Patient examination

At this stage, the patient's overall body shape and appearance are carefully evaluated. Ideal candidates for HDL are individuals with localized fat deposits resistant to diet and exercise, coupled with well-developed underlying muscle anatomy. Patients with a body mass index under 30 are generally considered optimal candidates for this procedure. The assessment also includes screening for any skeletal abnormalities that could become more noticeable after fat removal, ensuring the results remain esthetically balanced.

The skin is then evaluated for scars, stretch marks (striae), and laxity. A pinch test is conducted to determine both the amount of fat available for resection and the degree of skin elasticity. Special attention is given to the abdomen, where any protrusion might indicate rectus diastasis or excessive intra-abdominal fat. In such cases, liposuction alone may not suffice to achieve a flat abdomen, and additional procedures may be required. Scars along the body are also assessed to identify any potential complications during or after the surgery, ensuring a smooth operative process and recovery.

3.3 Patient discussion

Both the patient and the surgeon must acknowledge that the human body is inherently asymmetric, and achieving perfect symmetry is rarely possible. It is the surgeon's responsibility to align the patient's desires with realistic, medically sound outcomes, ensuring that expectations are balanced with what can be safely achieved.

During the consultation, patients are encouraged to actively communicate their concerns and desired results. An informed patient, who understands the indications for specific procedures as well as the limitations and potential complications, is better prepared for the surgical journey. This open dialog fosters a strong surgeon-patient relationship, ensuring both parties are aligned in their goals, which contributes to a satisfying and realistic esthetic outcome.

3.4 Surgical preparation

Before surgery, patients must attend a pre-operative appointment to review the proposed treatment plan and consent forms including all associated risks and benefits. During this time, pre- and post-operative instructions are thoroughly discussed, such as stopping the intake of foods, supplements, and medications that may increase the risk of intra-operative bleeding, starting 2 weeks before surgery. Patients are advised to quit smoking at least 4 weeks before surgery and continue avoiding it for 3 months after to promote healing. Additionally, discontinuing birth control or hormone therapy 2 weeks before and after surgery helps reduce the risk of blood clots.

The appointment also covers the post-operative care plan, including the proposed schedule for manual lymphatic drainage and the proper use of compression garments, both of which are essential for optimal recovery and shaping results. Pre-operative photos are taken for documentation and comparison to assess the progression of results post-surgery. This thorough pre-operative preparation ensures the patient is well-informed and positioned for the best possible surgical outcome.

4. Pre-operative markings for male high-definition liposuction

Pre-surgical markings are essential for achieving optimal results in HDL. These markings guide the surgeon in highlighting the natural musculature while removing excess fat to create a sculpted, athletic look. On the day of surgery, the patient is marked in an upright position to ensure that natural body alignment is accurately reflected. Markings for male and female patients vary due to differing esthetic goals. Typically, men seek a sharper, more defined appearance, while women prefer softer contours.

The process begins with a thorough evaluation and palpation of the underlying musculature, which forms the foundation for the procedure. This initial assessment ensures that markings are precisely placed to enhance the natural muscle contours. Below is a step-by-step guide to the pre-operative markings for male HDL, focusing on the abdomen, chest, back, and arms.

4.1 Abdomen

The main goal of abdominal HDL is to enhance the appearance of the rectus abdominis and oblique muscles to create a defined, athletic core (**Figure 1**).

4.1.1 Anatomical landmarks

i. Linea alba: vertical line from the xiphoid process of the sternum to the pubis.

ii. Semilunar lines: lateral borders of the rectus abdominis muscle that separate from the external obliques.

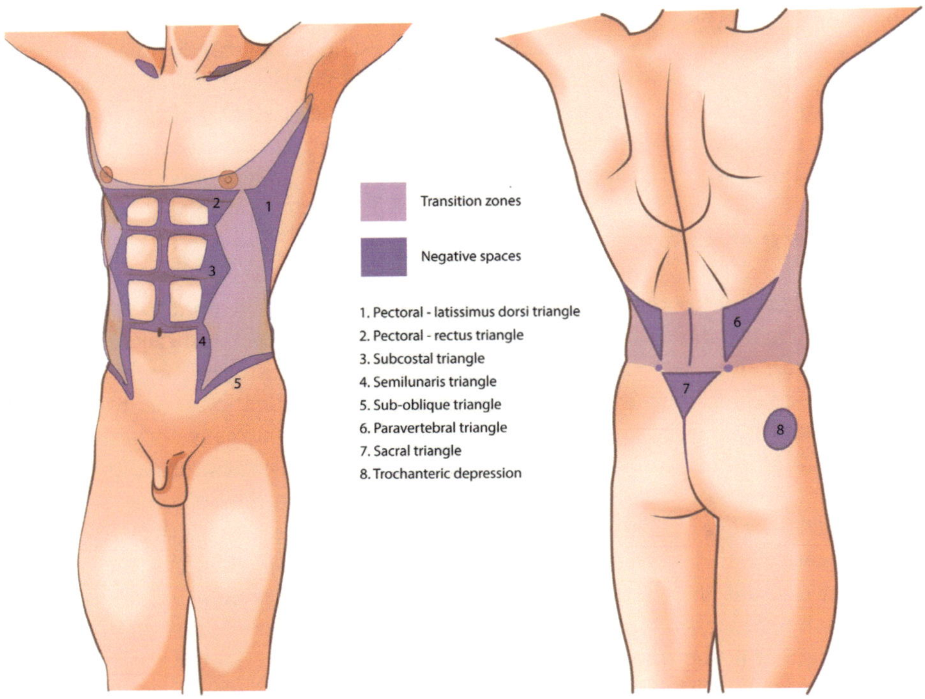

Figure 1.
Negative and transition zones for the male abdomen/Torso/back HDL [2]. Dark purple- negative space, light purple- deep fat extraction.

iii. Bellies of the rectus abdominis muscle: muscular intersections that form the six-pack look.

iv. Anterior superior iliac spine (ASIS): starting points for the V-line along the lower abdomen; enhances the lower abdominal contour and tapers the waist.

v. Inguinal ligament: runs from the ASIS to the pubic tubercle and defines the lower border of the V-line.

4.1.2 Surgical markings

a. The costal margins are marked bilaterally as the patient inhales deeply; this will mark out the cartilaginous thoracic arch.

b. Identify and mark the xiphoid process and the anterior superior iliac spines.

c. Mark the linea alba along the midline from the xiphoid process to the supraumbical area; no vertical mark is made below the umbilicus along the midline.

d. Mark the lateral border of the rectus abdominis; have the patient contract to assess the position of each belly of the rectus muscle and mark the intra-belly grooves.

e. Identify the transverse and oblique muscles bilaterally.

f. Mark the V-line by drawing from the ASIS down to the pubic area.

g. Mark the oblique lines following the natural slope of the external obliques, extending from the lateral ribcage down toward the ASIS.

4.1.3 Negative spaces: These areas form the shadows of the superficial anatomy

a. Sub-oblique triangle – region between the external obliques and transverse muscles

b. Subcostal triangle – region below the rib cage

c. Supraumbilical area following the midline

d. The region between the transverse inscriptions of the rectus muscle

e. Pectoral- rectus triangle- region between the supero-lateral border of the rectus abdominis and lower border of the pectoralis major

f. Pectoral- latissimus dorsi triangle- region between the lateral border of the pectoralis major and anterior border of the latissimus dorsi

4.2 Chest

For male HDL of the chest, the goal is to enhance the pectoral muscles, creating a firm, masculine contour while reducing fat deposits that may cause gynecomastia (excess breast tissue) (**Figure 2**).

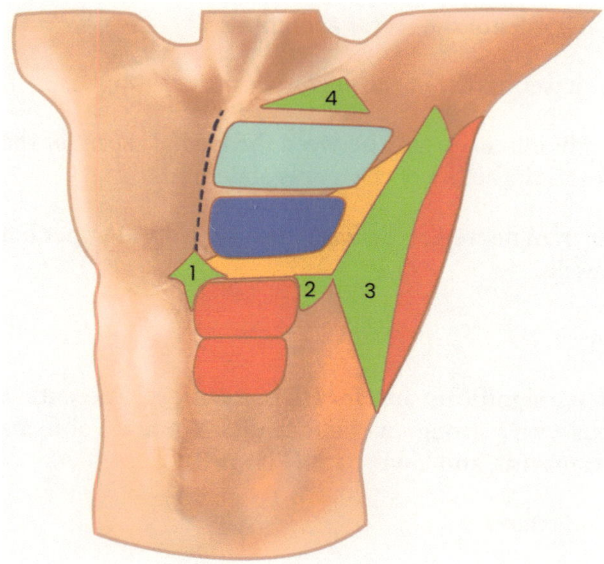

Figure 2.
Surgical landmarks and negative zones for the male chest HDL [2]. 1. Interpectoral rhomboid, 2. Subpectoral triangle, 3. Pectoralis-latissimus dorsi triangle, 4. Subclavicular triangle, orange-pectoral region for deep fat extraction, green- negative zone.

4.2.1 Anatomical landmarks

a. Sternal midline: vertical line in the center of the chest.

b. Inferior pectoral border: inferior edge of the pectoralis major muscle.

c. Lateral pectoral margin: outer edge of the pectoralis muscle that abuts the deltoid and anterior axillary fold.

d. Clavicular line: superior aspect of the pectoralis muscle along the clavicle.

4.2.2 Surgical markings

a. Mark a vertical line along the sternal midline.

b. Mark the inferior border of the pectoralis muscle, extending from the sternal border to the axilla.

c. Mark the lateral margin of the pectoralis muscle as it extends into the deltoid and axilla.

d. Mark the clavicular border of the pectoralis muscle to define the upper definition.

4.2.3 Negative spaces

a. Pectoralis-latissimus dorsi triangle- region between the anterior border of the latissimus dorsi and the lateral border of the pectorals major

b. Inferior pectoral triangle- region between the inferior border of the pectoralis and the lateral border of the rectus abdominis

c. Pectoral line- lower border of the pectoralis major

d. Interpectoral rhomboid- region between the medial aspect of the inferior pectoralis muscles and the bellies of the rectus abdominis

e. Subclavicular triangle- region between the clavicle and upper border of the pectoralis muscle.

4.3 Back/torso

The male back is a significant area for HDL, focusing on accentuating the V-shape that is synonymous with a strong, masculine build. The areas of focus include the latissimus dorsi, trapezius, and lower back (**Figure 3**).

4.3.1 Anatomical landmarks

a. Spinous processes: midline of the spine

b. Inferior scapular border: lower edge of the scapula; assists with marking the latissimus dorsi

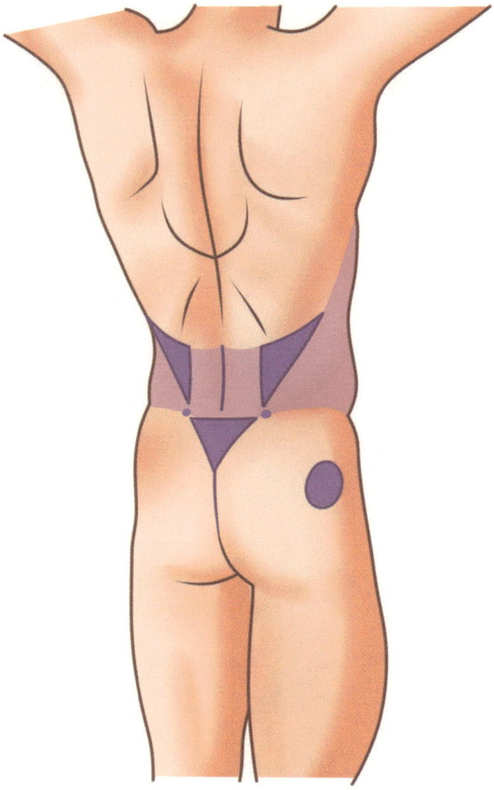

Figure 3.
Negative and transition zones for the male back HDL [2]. Light purple- fat extraction, dark purple- negative zone.

c. Posterior axillary fold: marks the lateral extent of the latissimus dorsi

d. Iliac crest: upper border of the pelvis

4.3.2 Surgical markings

a. Mark the spinous process along the midline to assist with symmetrical fat removal.

b. Mark the lateral border of the latissimus dorsi muscles bilaterally; the upper border begins at the inferior scapular border and extends down toward the axillary fold. The inferior portion of the muscle extends down toward the iliac crest.

c. Outline the bony borders of the scapulae.

d. Mark the lower back, following the natural V-shape created by the tapering of the latissimus dorsi to the iliac crest.

4.4 Arms

Defining the arms through HDL involves enhancing the contours of the deltoids, biceps, and triceps to create a strong, athletic look (**Figure 4**).

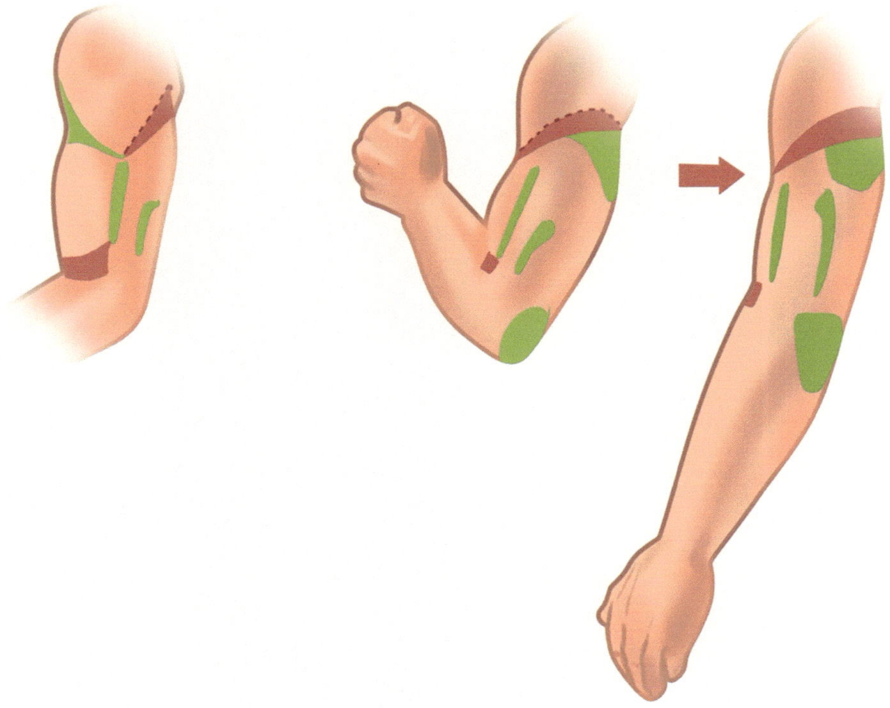

Figure 4.
Dynamic and negative zones for the male arm HDL [2]. Red zone- dynamic muscle movement, green zone- negative zone. Negative zone- bicipital groove, tricipital tendon and posterior triceps.

4.4.1 Anatomical landmarks

a. Deltoid insertion: tapering of the deltoid muscle into the upper arm.

b. Biceps groove separation between the bicep and triceps muscles.

c. Lateral and long heads of the triceps: major muscle group forming the posterior arm.

4.4.2 Surgical markings

a. Mark the borders of the deltoid muscle, extending from the acromion process to the insertion into the upper arm.

b. Mark the separation between the bicep and triceps muscles.

c. Mark the lateral and long heads of the triceps along the posterior aspect of the arm.

5. Pre-operative markings for female high-definition liposuction

Pre-operative markings are a critical step in high-definition liposuction for women. These markings guide the surgeon in sculpting the body to enhance feminine contours while reducing excess fat. Women typically seek a softer, more contoured appearance compared to the sharp, etched lines preferred by men. Markings for the torso, abdomen, chest, back, hips, breasts, and arms must reflect the patient's anatomical structure and esthetic goals, emphasizing natural curves and smooth transitions between regions.

The process starts with a comprehensive evaluation and palpation of the underlying musculature, which serves as the blueprint for the procedure. This critical assessment allows for precise placement of pre-operative markings, ensuring that natural muscle contours are highlighted and enhanced. What follows is a detailed, step-by-step guide to the pre-operative markings for female high-definition liposuction, focusing on the abdomen, breasts, hip, back, and arms.

5.1 Abdomen/torso

The primary goal for the female torso and abdomen in HDL is to sculpt a lean, toned core while maintaining a natural, soft, and feminine appearance (**Figure 5**). The objective is to create a narrower waist and subtly define the abdominal muscles, without over-emphasizing muscle definition.

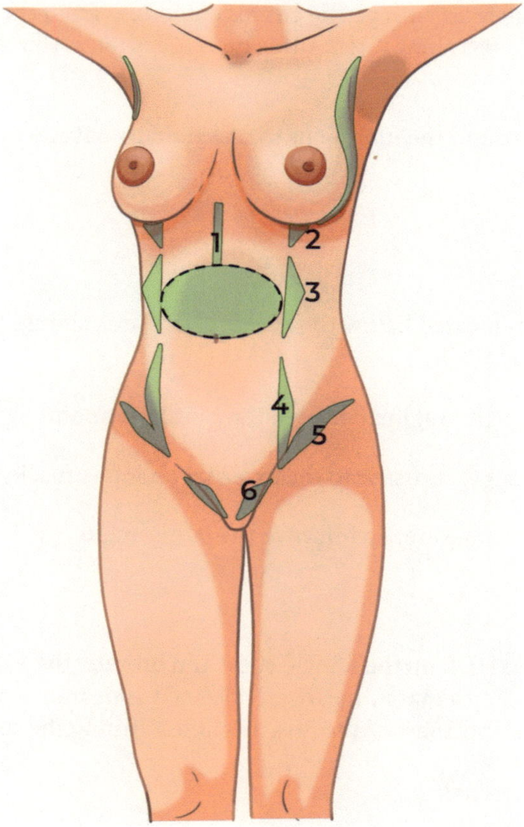

Figure 5.
Negative zones for the female abdomen HDL [2]. 1. Midline, 2. Submammary triangle, 3. Subcostal triangle, 4. Semilunaris triangle, 5. Sub-oblique triangle, 6. Pubis triangle.

5.1.1 Anatomical landmarks

a. Linea alba: central vertical line extending from the xiphoid process to the pubis.

b. Semilunar lines: lateral borders of the rectus abdominis, separating it from the obliques.

c. Umbilicus: natural center of the abdomen, around which markings should harmonize.

d. Anterior superior iliac spines (ASIS): landmarks for marking the lower abdomen and waist.

5.1.2 Surgical markings

a. Mark the linea alba from the xiphoid process to the pubic area.

b. Mark the lateral borders of the rectus abdominis, tapering these lines into the ASIS.

c. Draw curving lines from the lateral ribcage down toward the ASIS to emphasize the hourglass shape.

d. Mark the oblique lines with gentle curves extending from the lateral ribcage toward the iliac crest. In women, these lines are often softer and less pronounced than in men.

e. Mark the area around the umbilicus to maintain its natural position.

5.1.3 Negative spaces

a. Midline space.

b. Subcostal space- located below the rib cage, this area should be highlighted to enhance the waist.

c. Semilunaris triangle- region between the semilunaris and inguinal ligament.

d. Sub-oblique triangle- inferior to the external oblique muscle.

e. Pubic triangle- wedge area to improve the pubic angle.

5.2 Breast

When performing HDL on the female chest and breasts, the goal is to enhance natural curves while avoiding a masculine, overly defined appearance. Care must be taken to preserve the natural softness of the breasts while defining the surrounding contours.

5.2.1 Anatomical landmarks

a. Midline: vertical line that bisects the chest.

b. Inframammary fold: inferior boundary of the breast.

c. Lateral breast margin: lateral edge of the breast.

d. Clavicle: superior boundary of the chest.

5.2.2 Surgical markings

a. Mark a vertical line down the center of the chest.

b. Mark the inframammary fold to ensure that fat removal does not disrupt the natural shape and position of the breasts.

c. Outline the lateral breast margin where it blends into the chest and axilla to avoid removing fat that could flatten the upper chest.

d. Mark the clavicle to maintain the upper chest contour, especially in cases where fat removal near the clavicle is required to create a smoother transition to the shoulders.

5.2.3 Negative spaces

a. Sub-clavicular Triangle- space between the clavicle and the upper breast area, which should be left intact for a natural slope.

b. Inframammary Triangle- area beneath the breast should retain volume to ensure a natural, curved breast contour.

5.3 Back

For female patients, the back should be contoured to enhance the natural curves and accentuate the waistline. Pre-operative markings ensure that excess fat is removed from the upper and mid-back, creating a smooth, feminine silhouette.

5.3.1 Anatomical landmarks

a. Spinous processes: midline of the spine, serving as the central axis for symmetry.

b. Inferior scapular borders: lower edges of the scapulae, important for marking the lateral extents of the upper back.

c. Posterior axillary fold: lateral edge where the back blends into the arms and latissimus dorsi.

d. Iliac crest: upper boundary of the pelvis and lower back.

5.3.2 Surgical markings

a. Mark the spinous process along the midline from the cervical to the lumbar spine for symmetrical fat removal.

b. Mark the lateral borders from the inferior scapular edge down toward the iliac crest.

c. Mark the scapulae to maintain natural muscle contours and avoid over-resection.

d. Mark the natural curve of the lower back, enhancing the feminine hourglass shape by tapering toward the waistline.

5.3.3 Negative spaces

a. Thoracic triangle: area below the scapula and above the waistline that enhances the V-shape of the back.

b. Lower lumbar triangle: region between the spine and the iliac crest, which, when accentuated, enhances the waist-to-hip ratio.

5.4 Hips and buttocks

One of the most important areas for female HDL is the hips and buttocks, where the goal is to create a curvaceous and lifted appearance (**Figures 6** and 7). The pre-operative markings focus on accentuating volume in the buttocks while contouring the hips to create an hourglass silhouette.

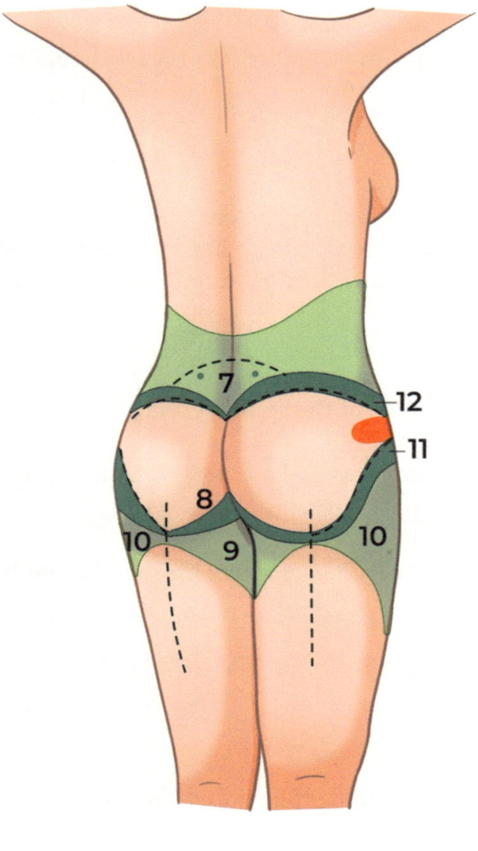

Figure 6.
Negative and transition zones for the female back and gluteal region HDL [2]. 7. Sacral triangle, 8. Internal gluteal angle, 9. Inner thigh triangle, 10. Outer thigh zone, 11. Lateral inferior gluteal Transition zone, 12. Lateral superior gluteal Transition zone.

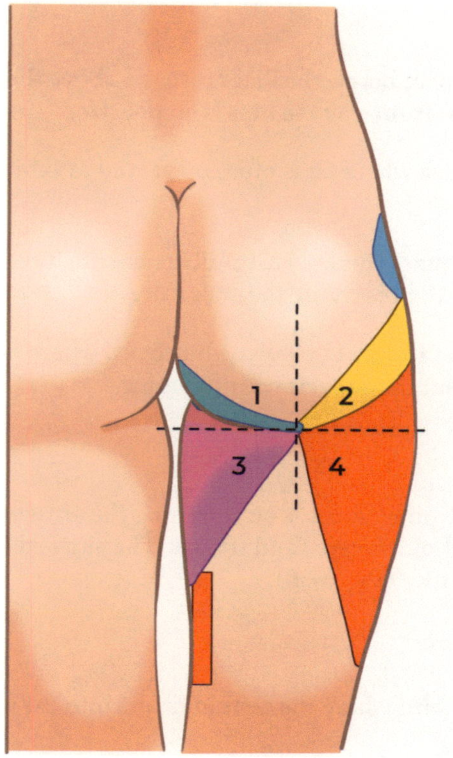

Figure 7.
Zones for the female inferior gluteal region HDL [2]. 1. Lower internal gluteal, 2. Lower external gluteal, 3. Inner thigh, 4. Outer thigh, 5. Blue arrow- zone of adhesion. Liposuction may be performed in these regions to accentuate the gluteal region. Liposuction is to be avoided along the middle inner thigh (blue arrow).

5.4.1 Anatomical landmarks

a. Iliac crest: upper boundary of the hips.

b. Greater trochanter: upper lateral edge of the femur, marking the widest point of the hips.

c. Gluteal fold: natural crease at the inferior border of the buttocks.

5.4.2 Surgical markings

a. Mark the natural inward curve of the waist and the outward curve of the hips, emphasizing the hourglass figure.

b. Outline the buttocks, ensuring the central and upper regions retain volume while lower fat is reduced to create a lifted appearance.

c. Mark the natural gluteal fold to ensure the area remains smooth and defined, avoiding an over-reduced or flattened look.

d. Mark the lateral edges of the hips to sculpt them in a way that maintains fullness and creates a smooth transition between the buttocks and thighs.

5.4.3 Negative spaces

a. Lateral hip curve: space below the iliac crest and above the greater trochanter, where the transition from waist to hips is emphasized.

b. Posterior hip dip: area where fat is often preserved to avoid flattening the hips and buttocks.

c. Lateral hip hollow: mark this area carefully to ensure it remains smooth, without excessive fat removal, preserving the curvature of the hips.

d. Sub-gluteal triangle: area just below the buttocks, where fat removal should be minimized to prevent the appearance of sagging.

5.5 Arms

HDL of the arms in women focuses on slimming the arms while enhancing the natural curves of the deltoid, biceps, and triceps. The aim is to create a toned but not overly muscular appearance (**Figure 8**).

5.5.1 Anatomical landmarks

a. Deltoid insertion: point where the deltoid tapers into the upper arm.

b. Biceps-triceps groove: natural separation between the biceps and triceps muscles.

c. Medial arm border: inner aspect of the arm, which should remain soft and smooth.

5.5.2 Surgical markings

a. Mark the deltoid muscle from the acromion to its insertion into the upper arm, preserving the natural curve of the shoulder.

b. Mark the groove separating these muscle groups to enhance arm definition.

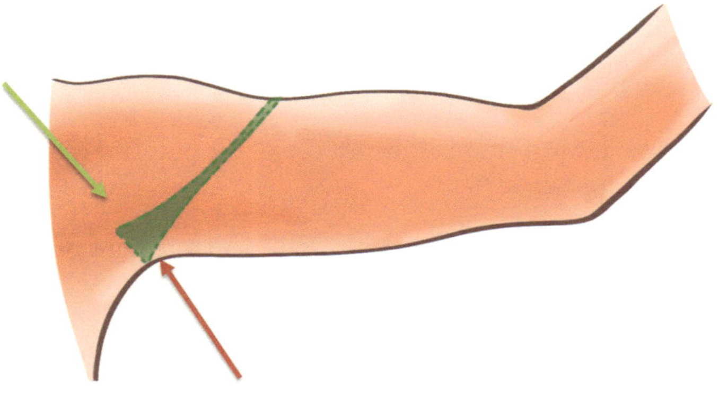

Figure 8.
Zones for the female arm HDL [2]. The negative zone is a curved triangle located between the posterior axillary crease (red arrow) and the insertion of the deltoid (green arrow).

c. Avoid marking the medial arm for aggressive fat removal, as this area should maintain a smooth, soft contour.

5.5.3 Negative spaces

a. Deltoid triangle: space around the deltoid muscle that enhances shoulder curvature.

b. Posterior triceps groove: space behind the triceps that, when subtly accentuated, helps define arm tone without creating an overly muscular look.

6. Surgical procedure

6.1 Tumescent anesthesia

Tumescent anesthesia is crucial for high-definition liposuction, enhancing both the safety and effectiveness of the procedure while significantly reducing discomfort for the patient. This technique utilizes a solution containing lidocaine, which provides localized pain control, and epinephrine, combined with tranexamic acid, to reduce bleeding and minimize post-operative bruising [10].

In addition to controlling pain and reducing bleeding, tumescent fluid plays a vital role in fat removal. By causing the fat cells to swell and become firm, it makes the fat easier to extract with less trauma to surrounding tissues. This gentler extraction process allows for greater precision in contouring and reduces the risk of damage to nerves, blood vessels, and connective tissue.

Overall, tumescent anesthesia significantly decreases trauma to surrounding tissues, minimizes blood loss, and accelerates the healing process. Patients benefit from a faster recovery, with less post-operative pain, swelling, and bruising, making the procedure more efficient and enhancing overall patient outcomes.

The author utilizes a tumescent anesthesia solution composed of 1000 cc of Lactated Ringer's, 1 mg of epinephrine, 250 mg of tranexamic acid, and 20 cc of 1% lidocaine. The generally accepted maximum safe dosage of lidocaine for tumescent anesthesia is 35 to 55 mg per kilogram of body weight, providing effective pain control while maintaining patient safety [11]. Additionally, the author follows a 1:1 ratio of tumescent anesthesia to the planned amount of fat removal; using a 1:1 ratio will decrease the excess stretch of the FSN which may lead to increase skin laxity.

Infiltration of the tumescent anesthesia is performed via surgical planned incisions. Hidden entry points are paramount to the HDL technique. The surgical area is first infiltrated with tumescent anesthesia along the deep layer, followed by infiltration into the superficial layer. This approach ensures that the anesthesia stays concentrated in the superficial layer, keeping it adequately hydrated throughout the procedure. Maintaining moisture in the superficial layer is essential during the emulsification stage as it facilitates more efficient fat breakdown and removal while also minimizing trauma to the surrounding tissues and promoting smoother contouring results.

6.2 Emulsification with Vaser

The emulsification process begins with the use of VASER technology along the superficial fat layer. The surgeon employs a 3-ring probe to initiate this process, with the VASER power setting adjusted based on the quality of the fat and the fibrous connective tissue. The author starts at 70% power in pulsed mode to minimize the risk of excessive heat damage to the skin. The VASER probe is used until the treated area feels smooth and free of resistance, indicating proper emulsification.

Next, the deep fat layer is treated with careful attention to keeping the probe superficial to the muscle to prevent any unintended damage to the underlying muscle tissue. This technique also ensures complete emulsification of the deep fat layer.

Once all the planned treatment areas have been addressed and both the superficial and deep layers feel smooth with minimal resistance, aspiration of the emulsified fat is performed, effectively removing the loosened fat and completing the contouring process.

6.3 Aspiration of fat

The author approaches the body from a bottom-to-top sequence. The author employs a 4-mm cannula to assist with the deep fat extraction. During liposuction, it is important for the surgeon to use one's non-dominant hand to always identify and locate the cannula tip to ensure proper positioning.

The goal of deep fat layer aspiration is to achieve a flap thickness of 0.5-1 cm. While aspirating the fat, the surgeon should minimize damaging the subdermal plexus by utilizing a cannula with openings that face away from the dermis and skin.

Once adequate fat has been aspirated from the deep layer, attention is turned to the superficial layer. The author employs a 3-mm cannula to begin this process. The aim of superficial liposuction is to develop the framing of the HDL. Along the previous marked lines, the skin is pinched, and aggressive liposuction is performed. The main areas to be treated are the surgical lines and negative spaces. While performing superficial liposuction, the surgeon must follow the natural contour of the muscle and bony framework to avoid achieving a "fake" look. Upon completion of the superficial fat aspiration, one can appreciate the proper depressions and convex contours.

The author approaches the body using a bottom-to-top sequence, beginning with deep fat extraction using a 4-mm cannula. Throughout the liposuction process, it is essential for the surgeon to use their non-dominant hand to continuously locate and identify the tip of the cannula, ensuring proper positioning and minimizing the risk of inadvertent damage.

The goal of deep fat layer aspiration is to achieve a flap thickness of approximately 0.5 to 1 cm. During fat aspiration, the surgeon must take care to avoid damaging the subdermal plexus by using a cannula with openings that face away from the dermis and skin, preserving the integrity of the overlying tissue.

Once sufficient fat has been aspirated from the deep layer, the focus shifts to the superficial layer. For this phase, the author utilizes a 3- and 3.5-mm cannula to begin sculpting and refining the contours. The objective of superficial liposuction is to frame the high-definition liposuction results, following the previously marked lines. The skin is pinched and targeted, and aggressive liposuction is performed along the surgical lines and in the negative spaces to enhance muscle definition and body contours.

When performing superficial liposuction, the surgeon must follow the natural contours of the muscles and bony framework to achieve an authentic, sculpted look, avoiding an unnatural or "fake" appearance. Upon completion of the superficial fat aspiration, the desired depressions and convex contours become visible, highlighting the refined and well-proportioned body silhouette.

Surgeons are strongly advised to avoid excessive subdermal liposuction, as this can significantly increase the risk of complications. Over-aggressive fat removal in this area can lead to a higher likelihood of seromas, contour irregularities, and damage to the subdermal plexus. Such damage compromises blood supply and tissue integrity, which can result in poor healing, increased scarring, and uneven skin contours. Maintaining a conservative approach in the subdermal layer is essential to preserving the overall health of the skin and achieving smooth, esthetically pleasing results.

6.4 Renuvion therapy

Upon completion of liposuction, it is crucial for the surgeon to ensure that no surface irregularities remain. Any noticeable skin inconsistencies, aside from the intentionally planned depressions, are addressed by the author using a 4-mm cannula in an off-suction mode. This technique is employed to blend and smooth the treated areas, ensuring a natural and even contour.

Following this, Renuvion therapy is applied to the FSN to further enhance skin tightening. The author utilizes a precise approach, performing three anterograde and retrograde passes over each treated area, with the device set to 75% power and a flow rate of 1.5 L/min. Each pass is spaced 1 cm apart to ensure uniform coverage and optimal tightening of both the superficial and deeper layers of the fibrous tissue. This controlled application provides consistent results, improving skin firmness and enhancing the overall esthetic outcome.

The combination of meticulous liposuction techniques and advanced skin tightening with Renuvion therapy offers a comprehensive approach to body contouring. By carefully addressing skin irregularities and applying plasma energy to stimulate tissue contraction, this method allows surgeons to achieve smooth, natural contours with enhanced skin tightening. Proper attention to technique ensures minimal complications, optimal esthetic results, and a quicker recovery, ultimately improving patient satisfaction.

7. Post-operative care

While the success of the surgery depends heavily on the surgeon's skill, post-operative care plays an equally crucial role in ensuring optimal results, minimizing complications, and promoting a smooth recovery.

7.1 Compression garments

One of the most critical components of post-operative care following high-definition liposuction is the use of compression garments. These garments apply consistent external pressure to the treated areas, offering several key benefits that enhance recovery and overall results:

1. *Reduction of swelling*: Compression garments help manage post-surgical swelling by applying evenly distributed pressure, which reduces fluid accumulation and promotes quicker resolution of edema.

2. *Skin retraction*: The applied pressure encourages the skin to adhere properly to the underlying tissue, facilitating smooth retraction and preventing sagging or irregularities in the skin.

3. *Improved circulation*: Controlled pressure from the garments enhances blood circulation, minimizing bruising and accelerating the body's natural healing processes.

4. *Support and comfort*: Compression garments provide essential support to the treated areas, reducing post-operative discomfort, and lowering the risk of complications such as seroma formation (fluid pockets). This support helps patients feel more comfortable and secure during their recovery.

Patients are instructed to wear compression garments according to their surgeon's recommendations, with the author advising the following schedule: wear the **faja** (compression garment) for 23 hours a day during the first month, followed by 12 hours a day during the second and third months. For optimal results, it is essential that the compression garment fits properly. It should be snug, providing firm support, but not overly tight. Excessive compression can compromise blood flow, potentially leading to tissue ischemia, while insufficient compression may delay healing and hinder skin retraction.

Maintaining proper hygiene, both in the garment and the skin, is crucial to preventing infections. Patients should be instructed to clean the garment regularly and ensure that the skin remains clean and dry under the garment.

To enhance post-operative compression, foam pads can be placed under the garment. Foam dressings help distribute compressive forces evenly, improving skin stabilization and contouring [12]. Patients should be advised to ensure that the skin is smooth and flat when applying the foam and garment to prevent any folds or creases in the skin, which can result in unwanted pressure marks or irregular healing.

7.2 Manual lymphatic drainage

Manual lymphatic drainage (MLD) is a specialized massage technique designed to stimulate the lymphatic system, reduce swelling, and promote healing after high-definition liposuction (HDL). By facilitating the movement of lymphatic fluid, MLD helps drain excess fluid and metabolic waste that has accumulated in the treated areas, significantly reducing post-surgical swelling. This drainage process also assists in the clearance of blood from surgical sites, which helps diminish bruising [13–15].

Two major benefits of MLD are the prevention of fibrosis and relief from pain. By continuously draining fluid from the tissues, MLD helps prevent the development of fibrosis (hardening of tissue) and supports the regeneration of healthy tissue. Additionally, the removal of fluid reduces tension on the skin, alleviating discomfort and minimizing post-operative pain [13–15].

The author recommends beginning MLD the day after surgery, with a schedule of two to three sessions per week during the first month, followed by one to two sessions per week during the second month. It is important to note that MLD is not the same as a deep tissue massage. It involves light, rhythmic movements designed to gently propel lymphatic fluid toward the lymph nodes, ensuring optimal drainage and promoting recovery without applying intense pressure to the treated areas.

7.3 Physical activity

Post-operative activity plays a crucial role in ensuring a rapid and successful recovery following high-definition liposuction. Patients are instructed to avoid heavy lifting and strenuous activities for the first 2 weeks after surgery to minimize stress on healing tissues. However, early ambulation is strongly encouraged, as walking immediately after surgery helps improve blood circulation, reducing the risk of blood clots (deep vein thrombosis) and promoting the healthy functioning of the lymphatic system, which aids in reducing swelling and fluid retention [16, 17].

After 2 weeks, patients can gradually resume light physical activity, including walking, slow jogging, and body weight exercises. At the 4-week mark, and if healing is progressing appropriately, patients are cleared for low-impact activities such as treadmill walking, cycling, and light weightlifting. By 6 weeks, most patients are cleared for all physical activities, assuming they have recovered without complications [16–18].

It is important for patients to listen to their bodies throughout the recovery process. Since each individual heals differently, patients should avoid activities that cause pain or discomfort and should wait until they are more fully recovered before resuming those activities. Additionally, as physical activity increases, so may fluid buildup in the treated areas. To manage this, the continued use of compression garments and manual lymphatic drainage (MLD) is recommended to reduce fluid accumulation and support proper healing.

7.4 Incision management

The author opts to avoid the placement of drains following high-definition liposuction (HDL). Instead, patients are instructed to maintain the patency of the liposuction incisions by using a Q-tip soaked in hydrogen peroxide or polysporin. This approach may help reduce the risk of surgical site infections by keeping the small incisions clean and preventing the buildup of bacteria. Additionally, keeping the sites open helps facilitate fluid drainage, reducing the risk of seroma formation [19, 20].

Patients are advised to open the liposuction sites three times a day for the first 2 weeks after surgery. This regular maintenance not only ensures the continued drainage of excess fluid but also helps prevent the early closure of the incision sites, which can lead to fluid accumulation and other complications. By following these guidelines, patients can effectively reduce the risk of seroma formation and promote proper healing [19, 20].

8. Results

See **Figures 9–17**.

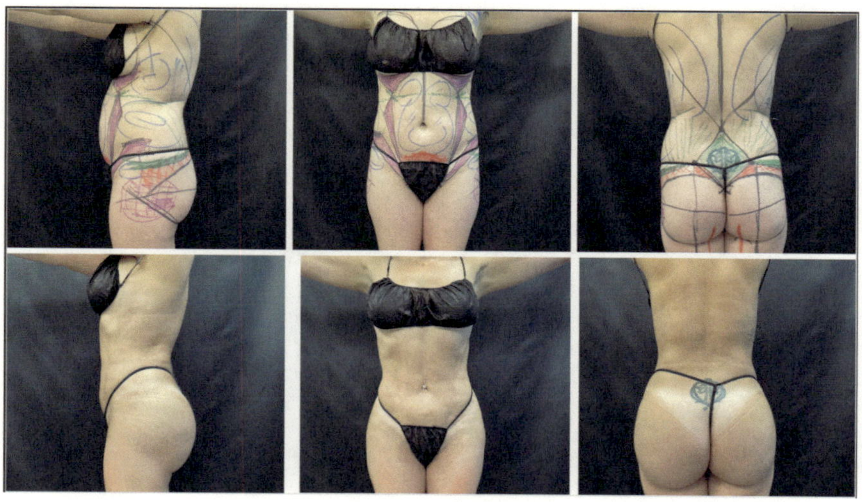

Figure 9.
Soft high-definition liposuction. Patient underwent a HDL 360 with gluteal fat transfer. Patient is 6 months post-surgery.

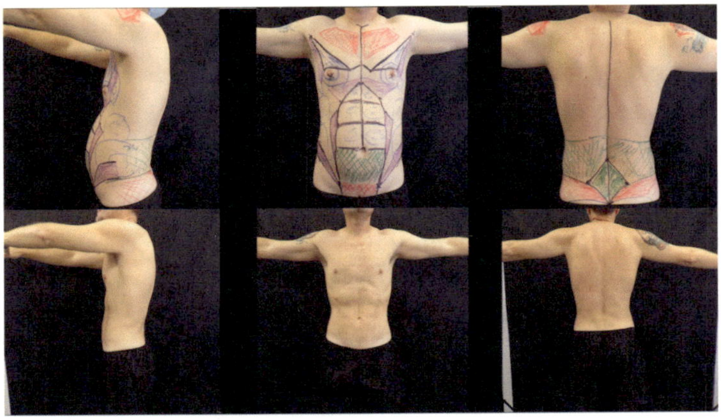

Figure 10.
Athletic high-definition liposuction. Patient underwent a HDL 360 with chest liposuction. Patient is 6 months post-surgery.

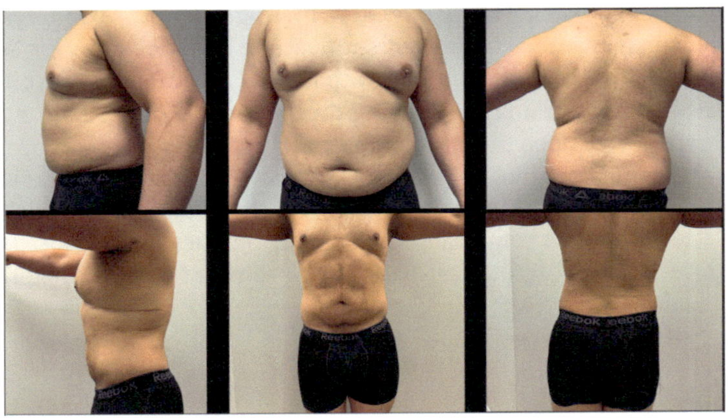

Figure 11.
Athletic high-definition liposuction. Patient underwent a HDL 360 with chest liposuction. Patient is 3 months post-surgery.

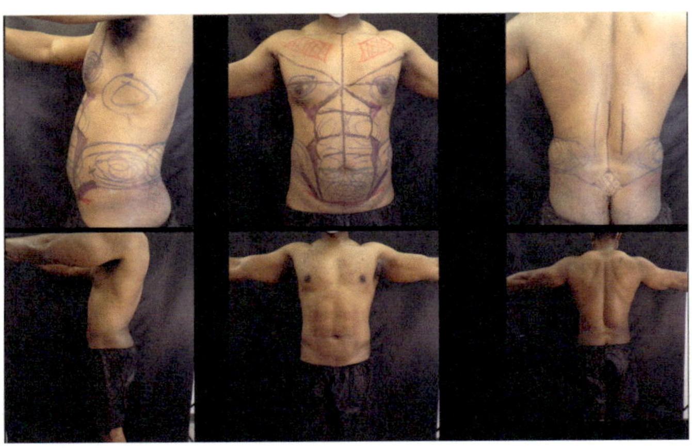

Figure 12.
Athletic high-definition liposuction. Patient underwent a HDL 360 with chest liposuction. Patient is 6 months post-surgery.

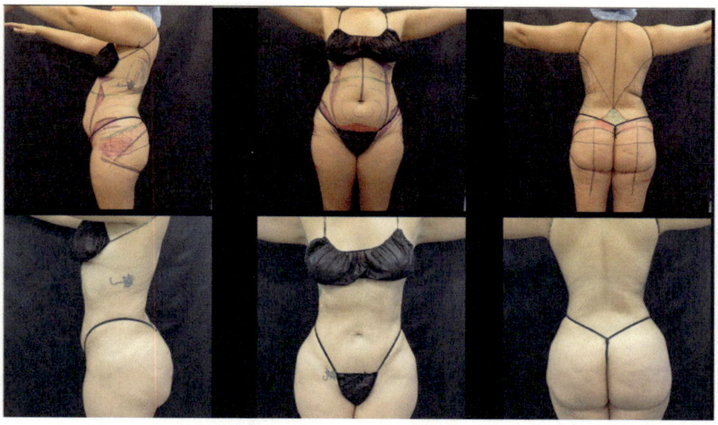

Figure 13.
Soft high-definition liposuction. Patient underwent a HDL 360 with gluteal fat transfer. Patient is 6 months post-surgery.

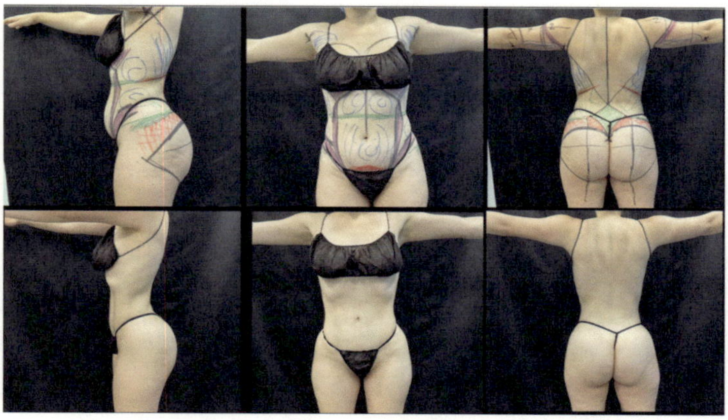

Figure 14.
Soft high-definition liposuction. Patient underwent a HDL 360. Patient is 9 months post-surgery.

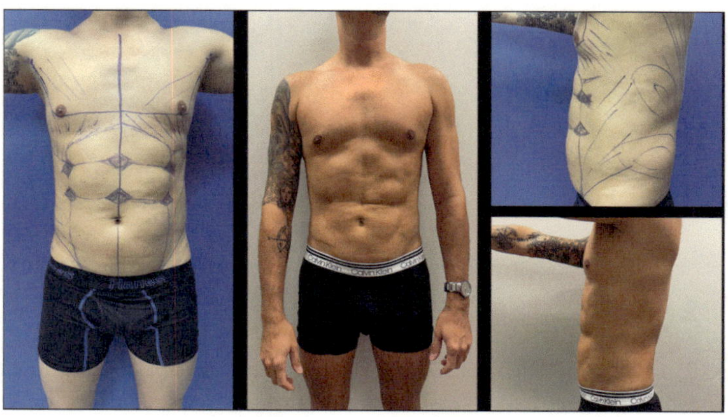

Figure 15.
Athletic high-definition liposuction. Patient underwent a HDL 360 with chest liposuction. Patient is 1-year post-surgery.

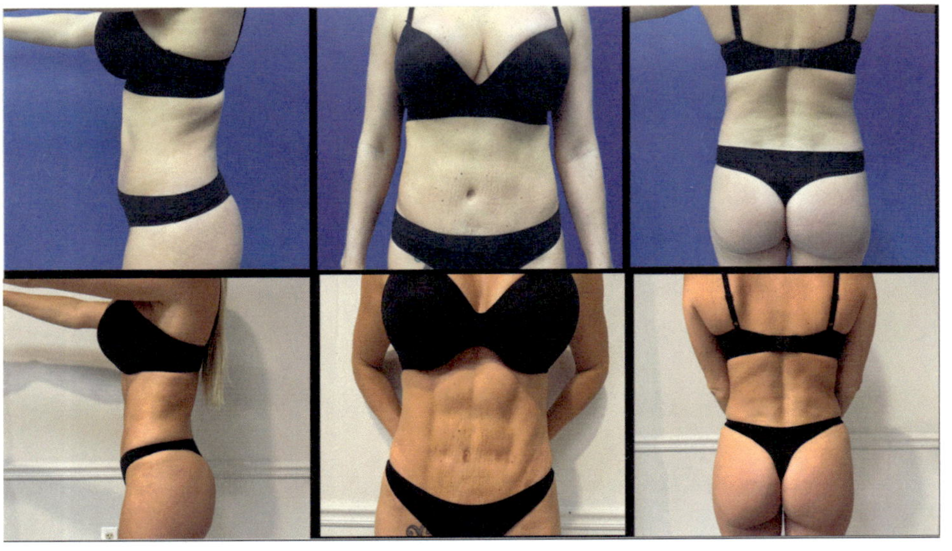

Figure 16.
Athletic high-definition liposuction. Patient underwent a HDL 360. Patient is 1-year post-surgery.

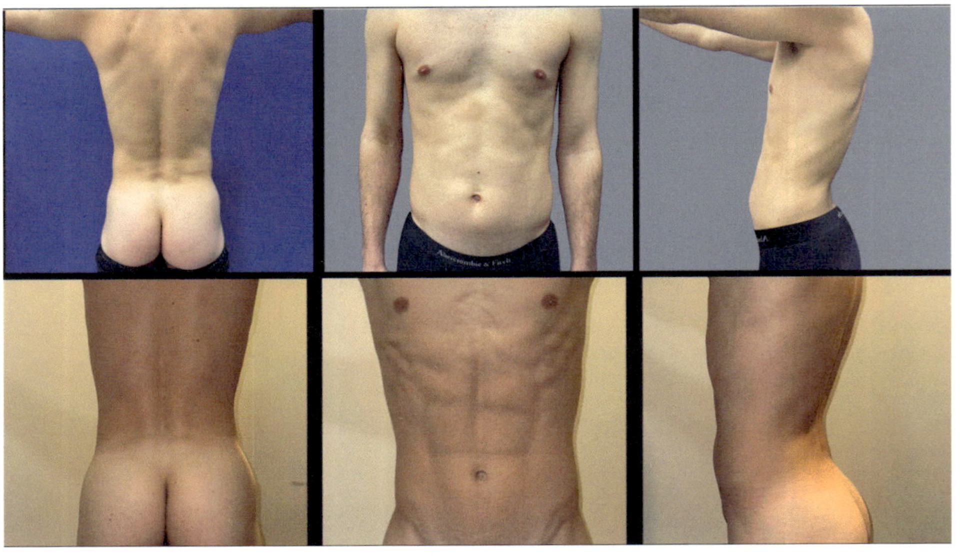

Figure 17.
Athletic high-definition liposuction. Patient underwent a HDL 360 with gluteal fat transfer. Patient is 1-year post-surgery.

9. Conclusion

High-definition liposuction (HDL) is a refined body sculpting technique that combines artistry with anatomical precision, enabling the creation of well-defined, athletic physiques. Achieving optimal results, however, extends beyond the surgery itself; it requires careful post-operative management to enhance the sculpted contours and ensure a smooth recovery.

Post-operative care following HDL is multifaceted, with key elements including the use of compression garments, manual lymphatic drainage (MLD), and a structured return to physical activity. Compression garments help manage swelling, improve skin retraction, and provide support during recovery, while MLD facilitates fluid drainage, reduces the risk of fibrosis, and alleviates post-surgical discomfort. Early ambulation and the gradual introduction of physical activity further promote healing by improving circulation and enhancing lymphatic function. Additionally, proper incision management is crucial for preventing complications such as infection and seroma formation.

The combination of advanced surgical techniques like VASER and Renuvion, along with meticulous post-operative care, allows for the creation of esthetically pleasing, natural contours with minimal complications. By following these carefully outlined post-operative protocols, patients can achieve superior results, a faster recovery, and long-lasting satisfaction with their high-definition liposuction outcomes.

Disclosure statement

The authors have nothing to disclose.

Author details

Pasquale G. Tolomeo[1]* and Manik S. Bedi[2]

1 Tolomeo Cosmetic Surgery, Fall River, MA, United States

2 Tampa Surgical Arts, Odessa, FL, United States

*Address all correspondence to: doctortolomeo@gmail.com

References

[1] Simblet S, Davis J. Anatomy for the Artist. New York: DK Publishing; 2001

[2] Hoyos AE, Prendergast PM. High Definition Body Sculpting: Art and Advanced Lipoplasty Techniques. Berlin, Heidelberg: Springer Berlin/Heidelberg; 2014

[3] Cimino WW. The physics of soft tissue fragmentation using ultrasonic frequency vibration of metal probes. Clinics in Plastic Surgery. 1999;**26**(3):447-461

[4] Nagy MW, Vanek PF Jr. A multicenter, prospective, randomized, single-blind, controlled clinical trial comparing VASER-assisted lipoplasty and suction-assisted lipoplasty. Plastic and Reconstructive Surgery. 2012;**129**(4):681e-689e. DOI: 10.1097/PRS.0b013e3182442274

[5] Cimino WW. Ultrasound-assisted lipoplasty: Basic physics, tissue interactions, and related results/complications. In: Prendergast P, Shiffman M, editors. Aesthetic Medicine. Berlin, Heidelberg: Springer; 2012. pp. 343-352. DOI: 10.1007/978-3-642-20113-4_40

[6] Di Giuseppe, A., Cimino, W.W., Giovagnoli, F. (2023). Ultrasound-assisted liposuction (UAL) with VASER technology in body contouring. In: Di Giuseppe, A., Bassetto, F., Nahai, F., Fat Transfer in Plastic Surgery (pp. 187-203). Springer, Cham. doi:10.1007/978-3-031-10881-5_13

[7] Zamora J, Roman S. Subcutaneous neck skin tightening. In: Advances in Cosmetic Surgery. New York: Elsevier; 2019. pp. 89-95

[8] Duncan DI. Nonexcisional tissue tightening: Creating skin surface area reduction during abdominal liposuction by adding radiofrequency heating. Aesthetic Surgery Journal. 2013;**33**(8):1154-1166

[9] Duncan DI. Helium plasma-driven radiofrequency in body contouring. In: The Art of Body Contouring. London, UK: IntechOpen Open Access; 2019. Available from: https://www.intechopen.com/books/the-art-of-body-contouring/helium-plasma-driven-radiofrequency-in-body-contouring

[10] Bayter-Marín JE, Hoyos A, Cárdenas-Camarena L, Peña-Pinzón W, Bayter-Torres AF, Díaz-Díaz CA, et al. Effectiveness of tranexamic acid in the postoperative period in body contour surgery: Randomized clinical trial. Plastic & Reconstructive Surgery - Global Open. 2023;**11**(11):e5403. DOI: 10.1097/GOX.0000000000005403

[11] Klein JA, Jeske DR. Estimated maximal safe dosages of tumescent lidocaine. Anesthesia and Analgesia. 2016;**122**(5):1350-1359. DOI: 10.1213/ANE.0000000000001119

[12] Schlesinger SL, Kaczynski AJ. Use of Reston foam in liposuction. Aesthetic Plastic Surgery. 1993;**17**(1):49-51. DOI: 10.1007/BF00455049

[13] Marxen T, Shauly O, Goel P, Tsan T, Faria R, Gould DJ. The utility of lymphatic massage in cosmetic procedures. Aesthetic Surgery Journal Open Forum. 2023;**5**:ojad023. DOI: 10.1093/asjof/ojad023

[14] Voss S, Wollina U. Postoperative manual lymphatic drainage after

cosmetic surgery. Journal of Cosmetic Dermatology. 2011;**10**(2):96-102

[15] Zerini I, Mori M, Sadigh PL, Fanoni D. Manual lymphatic drainage in aesthetic surgery: When and why it is effective. Plastic and Reconstructive Surgery. 2017;**140**(1):70-76

[16] Taylor MJ, Wilks D. Postoperative ambulation and recovery after cosmetic surgery: A review. British Journal of Surgery. 2005;**92**(9):1099-1103

[17] Shermak MA. Timing of physical activity after body contouring procedures. Plastic and Reconstructive Surgery. 2005;**116**(5):1423-1429

[18] Rohrich RJ, Pessa JE, Kenkel JM. Safety of post-liposuction exercise: A prospective study of low-impact versus high-impact exercise. Aesthetic Surgery Journal. 2000;**20**(4):303-308

[19] Chen R, Heller L. Management of seromas in body contouring surgery. Aesthetic Plastic Surgery. 2019;**43**(6):1577-1582

[20] Rohrich RJ, Pessa JE. Avoiding complications in liposuction: A comprehensive review. Plastic and Reconstructive Surgery. 2011;**127**(3):1226-1233

Chapter 15

Systematization Performing Multiple Body Contouring Procedures in One Stage after Massive Weight Loss with Minimal Complication Rate

Carlos del Pino-Roxo, Alicia Sigler-Moreno, María M. Cabrera-Cifuentes, Ana C. Weck Roxo and Víctor M. Whizar-Lugo

Abstract

Massive weight loss (MWL) results in excess, elastic and full of striae skin. The excess tissue in the arms, thighs, lower abdomen and breast ptosis causes difficult ambulation and sexual activity as well as psychological problems, including depression. This is a retrospective study analyzing the results of 1,435 massive weight loss patients who underwent multiple body contour procedures (at least 3) in less than 6 hours by the senior author and his team during the last 23 years of practice in public and private settings in Rio de Janeiro, Brazil. The preoperative markings and description of the surgical procedure techniques (lower body lift, fleur-de-lis pattern, breast lift, thoracoplasty, brachioplasty and thigh lift) are discussed. Postoperative management, including the lack of use of anticoagulation, using early ambulation and intraoperative measures for preventing DVT and PE is described. Mean operating time was 5.7 hours and average time to start ambulation, 4 hours. Seroma rate in lower body lift was 30–35%, lymphocele in brachioplasty less than 10% and skin suffering areas only 3–4%. No infections or necrosis has been documented. Low or no risk of severe complications such as PE, DVT or large blood loss was found.

Keywords: massive weight loss, body contouring after massive weight loss, markings for surgical body contouring procedures, complications after body contouring procedures, systematization for low or no risk during body contouring multiple procedures

1. Introduction

Morbid obesity has become a public health problem in many countries. The prevalence of obesity is estimated to be 603.7 million worldwide. The annual medical spending reported by Hua et al. is $1429 (42%) higher than that of people on normal weight; comorbidities and higher weights increased the gap of spending [1]. Bariatric surgery has become an effective and safe method for treating obesity with heavy weight loss as well as stable postoperative results. Approximately 252,000 obese patients undergo bariatric surgery per year in the United States. The most common procedures are sleeve gastrectomy and Roux-en-Y gastric bypass, gastric bypass, and gastric banding. These data vary from country to country [1, 2]. Massive weight loss (MWL) is defined as 50% or greater loss of excess weight. The effects of this massive weight loss are not as great as a patient would expect it to be, inevitably resulting in excess skin, which tends to be inelastic and full of striae. The face, breasts and buttocks deflate and there are rolls in the upper and mid-back; the mid and lower abdomen as well as the pubic area develop pannus. There is excess tissue in the arms, thighs, lower abdomen, as well as breast ptosis [2]. All these changes, besides the unaesthetic appearance, result in musculoskeletal pain, rashes, infection -intertrigo-, which may be, in many cases, refractory to conventional therapy. Patients also have difficulties in ambulation and sexual activity, and present psychological problems, including depression [2, 3].

Bariatric surgery has been demonstrated to improve medical conditions, as well as suicide rates, self-harm and substance use disorders in previously obese patients [4]. Furthermore, it has been published that post-bariatric surgery allows patients to reach a sustained quality of life improvement, and it also helps them to have better long-term weight control after both bariatric and post-bariatric surgery [2].

When the patient has had successful results with massive weight loss either by modifying eating habits or through bariatric surgery, there is a big possibility for a plastic surgeon to be involved in further plans to improve the patient's body contour by removing large amounts of skin and fat. Weight loss and body contouring surgery will boost the patient's self-esteem and confidence to wear more appealing clothes and to perform activities in public, improving their social relationships. Another important fact to consider, is that removing all the extra skin after massive weight loss, improves the hygiene of these patients in the crease areas of their bodies and subsequently avoids bad odor and skin infections such as the ones produced by fungus. There has been consensus on when to perform the body contouring procedures: the ideal patient's conditions are related to BMI, nutritional and psychological status, lab work results and general health issues. Cabbabe and colleagues describe that good candidates for bariatric plastic surgery are those who had bariatric surgery 1 year prior with stable weight for at least 3–6 months; the best candidates are those with BMI less than 30, have few or no medical conditions, do not smoke and have reasonable expectations [2]. The plastic surgeons make the decision on which surgical procedures should be performed on a first stage and which ones on a second and even on a third stage based on the knowledge that surgical time over 6 hours may involve blood loss that may require transfusions, general health decompensations, main complications that may be life threatening such as deep vein thrombosis (DVT) and pulmonary embolism (PE) and wound complications. It was previously published by the senior author that the variable of operating time was the primary factor influencing increase in plasma concentrations of stress markers, and therefore, of potential complications [5].

The main goal of this chapter is to show how multiple body contouring surgical procedures can be performed in one stage with minimal risk to the massive weight loss patient if the systematization proposed by the senior author is followed step by step, to avoid the main complications of blood loss, deep venous thrombosis (DVT), pulmonary embolism (PE) and other health problems such as hypothermia, wound complications, or poor postoperative healing due to an extended surgical time over 6 hours.

2. Method

We retrospectively analyzed 1435 massive weight loss patients (mean weight loss of 30 kg), who underwent multiple body contouring surgical procedures (at least 3) in a period of less than 6 hours by the senior author and his team during the last 23 years of practice. All surgeries were performed under general anesthesia in public or private hospital settings in Rio de Janeiro. The preoperative requirements for the patients to be considered as ideal candidates to undergo the proposed systematization plan were: normal physical and psychological health, this included patients whose comorbidities such as high blood pressure and diabetes mellitus were under control, adequate nutritional status which was proven by normal blood albumin levels; normal complete blood cell count (CBC), normal complete metabolic panel (CMP) as well as normal prothrombin time with INR (PT/INR) and partial thromboplastin time (PTT). A cardiovascular assessment based on a physical exam, electrocardiogram and lab work by a cardiologist, or an internist was performed in all patients. A urinalysis was done in all cases prior to surgery and, if any urinary tract infection was detected, it was treated. If a patient was found to have anemia, intravenous iron was administered every 3 days until achieving normal values.

3. Preoperative markings

Preoperative marking is vital in the surgical plan of these patients and must be carried out meticulously. Preoperative photographs and videos were obtained, trying to have the same positions, lights and shadows and taken in the same room to be able to compare objectively with postoperative ones. It is highly recommended to have plenty of time to plan where the incisions will be located in order to have the resulting scars in areas of the body where they will be easily hidden under clothes, undergarments and even beach clothing. The resulting scars ideally should be symmetrical, of excellent quality (not hypertrophic or keloid) and placed on areas that respect the esthetic units of the abdomen, torso, chest, arms and thighs.

The skin markings should be done 1 day before the surgery by the responsible surgeon who has had contact with the patient since the first office visit, who has evaluated and accepted the surgical case and has elaborated the plan in conjunction with the patient's desires, always in an orthostatic position. The surgeon uses a conventional marker in the beginning and, once the markings are checked and confirmed to be correct, they are re-marked with an indelible marker so that the markings on the skin will not disappear after the patient gets a shower the day of the surgery and after the body surface is scrubbed in the operating room (view https://youtu.be/aHzQC1iPsMs for full-body markings -lower body lift, breast lift and brachioplasty).

3.1 Lower body lift

The surgical procedure will have the goal of lifting the mons pubis or reversing the buried penis appearance. The most inferior point is on the midline, pulling with 2 fingers (maximum 6 cm at the end of the surgery), simulating the tension that the abdominal flap will do, above the base of the penis or above the vulvar commissure, under tension. The upper limit is marked in the umbilical area. On the lateral side, the pinch test is done; inferiorly, it begins at the quadriceps insertion. This is then transferred to the contralateral side, in a perfectly symmetric way. The points are then connected. The senior surgeon usually marks a more conservative line, and a more ambitious one; during the surgical procedure he decides which one of these will be taken into account, and this will change towards the most ambitious as the surgeon gets more experienced. Laterally, to do the markings that will connect the anterior and posterior aspects of the lower torso, one should imagine where the bikini or underwear will be, and using the pinch test, do the markings that will remove the extra skin and also lift the lateral aspect of the thigh.

On the posterior aspect, the inferior point in the midline is marked on the most superior part of the intergluteal crease, and then a mark is done around half a centimeter above it. Then the pinch test is done asking the patient to bend over before determining the superior point (this avoids dehiscence when the patient bends over postoperatively). Laterally to this point, using the pinch test, the markings are done where the effect of pinching lifts the buttocks in a more anatomical position and the skin sagging on them is pulled up giving a more natural appearance to the lower part of the buttocks. The lines are connected, and the marking is finished. In men, we recommend not to do an arched and pronounced line in the posterior aspect, because it will give a feminine appearance that is not wished by most, if not all men. On the other hand, in women, the final pattern looks like a butterfly shape that will lift the gluteal area and the resulting scar will have a curvilinear shape (the more laterally this butterfly shape opens, the more the lifting of the gluteal area will take place as well as for the lateral area of the thighs).

It is recommended to confirm the symmetry of the markings by taking the xiphoid process as a hallmark and measure the distance to the lateral points on both sides, on the upper, and lower lines, on the anterior and lateral aspects. On the posterior aspect, this can be done as well by measuring the different distances and confirming them to be equal (**Figure 1**).

For the Fleur de Lis pattern, to decide the lowest lateral point, it has to reach the midline marking on the mons pubis. The pinch test is performed all the way from the lower marking on the mons pubis to the xiphoid process (**Figure 2**) (view https://youtu.be/P4tsNl77B24 for lower body lift markings).

3.2 Breast lift

The smaller breast is always marked and operated on first. The first marking for a breast lift is found by the Pitanguy's maneuver to locate the ideal placement of the nipple. This is transferred from the smaller breast to the larger breast. Two centimeters above this marking is where a diagonal line will be drawn towards the medial and lateral breast and will have to measure 9 cm, 4 cm for the diameter of the areola and

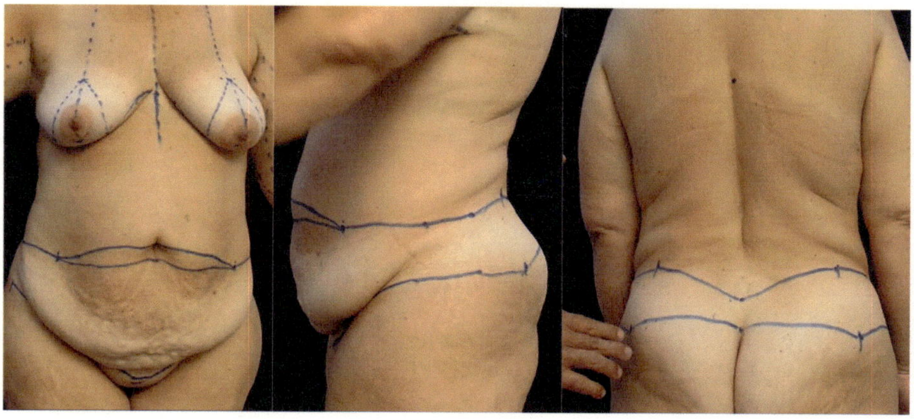

Figure 1.
Lower body lift markings.

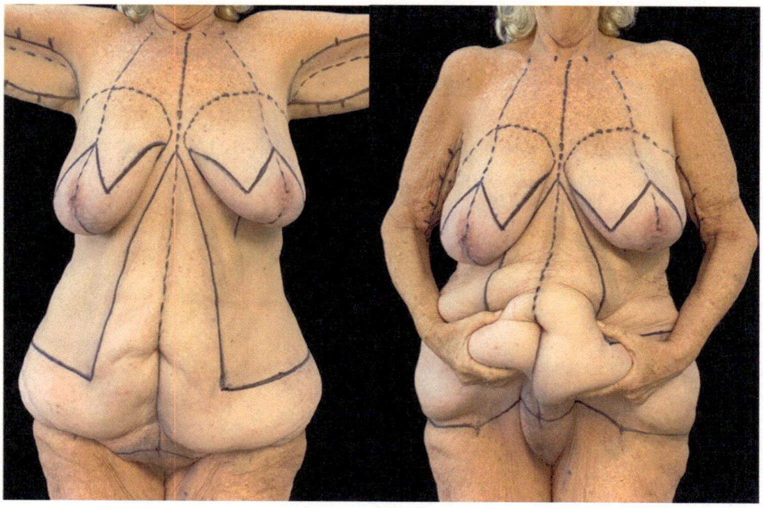

Figure 2.
Fleur de Lis pattern markings.

5 cm for the resultant vertical scar of the lift. To determine how oblique these two lines should be drawn, the surgeon should push with one hand the area below the areola inwards in order to approximate with the other hand the remaining area that corresponds to the pillars and gently approximate them with the breast crease that is already marked, The confluence point of the pillars with the crease on the meridian of the breast should be at 9–11 cm laterally from the midline, depending on how narrow or wide the patient's chest is (**Figure 3**).

3.3 Thoracoplasty

The scar on the back will follow the bra-line, and, as it is done simultaneously with the lower body lift, the pinch is verified at the same time for the thoracoplasty and the lower body lift, so there is no skin missing at the time of closure. The posterior scar

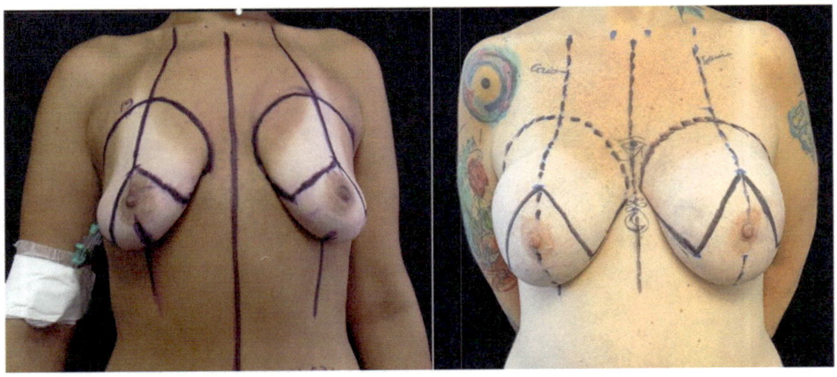

Figure 3.
Breast lift markings.

connects with the anterior aspect following the inframammary fold (**Figure 4**) (view https://youtu.be/51xkHl5tHjY for thoracoplasty markings).

3.4 Brachioplasty

A pinch test is performed involving the anteroinferior skin and tissue of the arm, drawing the site of the scar all along the bicipital groove and when it reaches the axilla, the patient is asked to lift the arm and a natural line is drawn on the skin showing where the marking should continue into the thorax if a thoracoplasty is planned with the arm lift and a breast lift (**Figure 5**).

3.5 Thigh lift

The markings of this procedure vary from men to women. It is important to remember that any resection of tissue on the skin where the groin area meets the

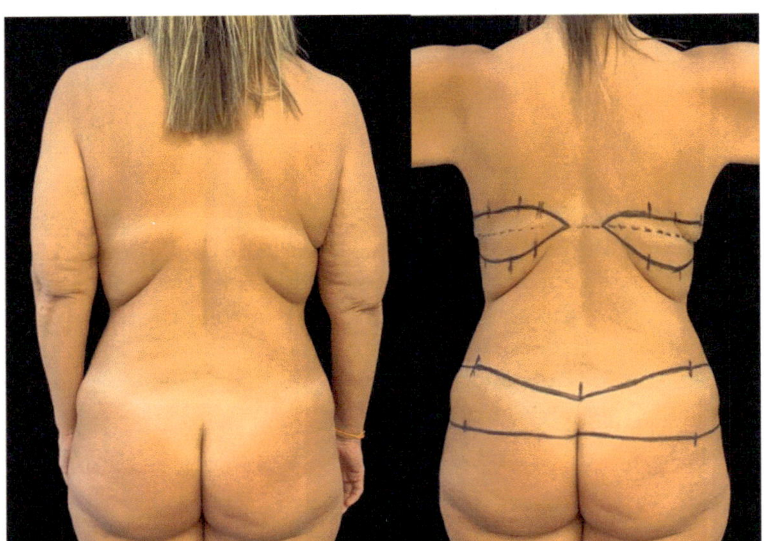

Figure 4.
Thoracoplasty markings.

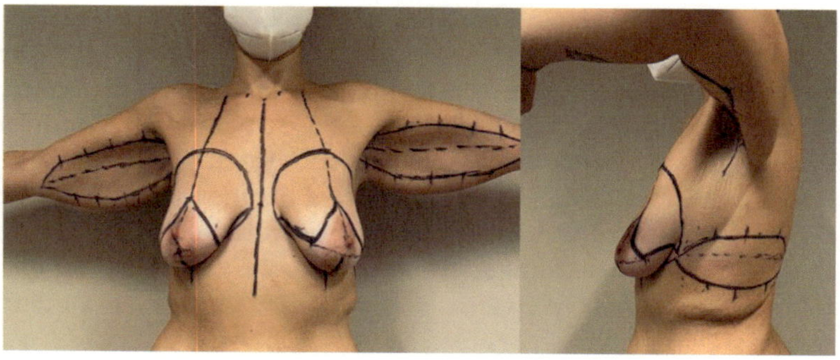

Figure 5.
Brachioplasty markings.

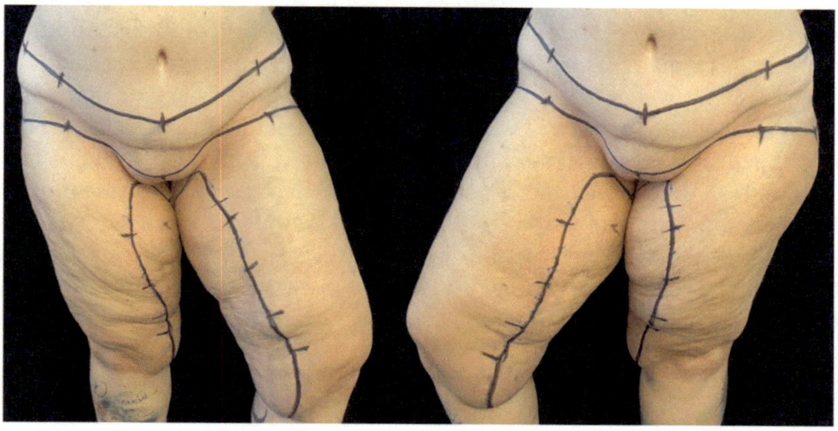

Figure 6.
Thigh lift markings.

thigh, will produce a scar that gravity and the lower tissues will pull downwards. The result will be a visible scar below the underwear or bathing suit and in women the labia majora will suffer distortion of their anatomy and could represent local disturbances in the vulvar region. That is why it is not recommended to make incisions in this area. In women, the recommendation is to hide the scar vertically on the medial aspect of the thigh, the amount of skin and fat to be resected is based on the pinch test and is done with an elliptical pattern. For the thigh lift on men, it is preferable a diagonal elliptical pattern that follows the sartorius muscle direction and the amount of skin to be resected is calculated with the pinch test (**Figure 6**).

4. Surgical procedures

No use of tranexamic acid or any fibrinolysis neutralizer is needed. Prior to the skin incision, a cefadroxil dose is administered to the patient. Patients who have intertrigo within the skin folds get a preoperative IV dose of fluconazole. All patients get intermittent compression stockings during surgery. During the whole procedure, electrocautery is used at 45 in coagulation mode. Before the skin is incised, the vertical lines drawn within the marking lines, are tattooed using the back of the knife and methylene blue; this assures that during the closure, both flaps are sutured at the exact point where they should meet. This technique involves no infiltration of the tissues, there are two reasons for this: it is not necessary because there is no undermining of the tissues, and its use would interfere with the action of the cautery as the main tool of dissection. It should be emphasized that no liposuction is performed during these combinations of surgical procedures to avoid seromas or altered blood supply to the wounds. As the leading surgeon finishes the dissection, performs skin removal and repositioning of the tissues, he moves on to the next area and the assisting surgeon/s start the closure of the area.

4.1 Fleur de Lis

The skin is incised superficially with a cold knife and further dissection is taken with electrocautery, in a perpendicular manner -not beveling or undermining- all the way down to the fascia (**Figure 7**). The umbilicus is excised as the dissection is done. For the neoumbilicus, a 2×10 cm flap is designed in the lateral aspects that will be de-epithelized as needed, once the dissection and skin resection are completed; this has previously been similarly described by Mendes et al. [6]. A conservative plicature is performed with 0 Vicryl™ with cross stitching. The flap reserved for the umbilicus is trimmed to an adequate size in the right position -it should be small rather than large because it widens with the healing and scarring process-. The umbilicus is fastened to the fascia once the plicature is done with two stitches at 12 and 6 o'clock. The wound is closed in two layers, the first involving Scarpa's fascia and the second involving the subcutaneous tissue.

4.2 Lower body lift

The procedure starts with the patient in a prone position, once the dissection and resection are done, the closure in two layers takes place with prior placement of a

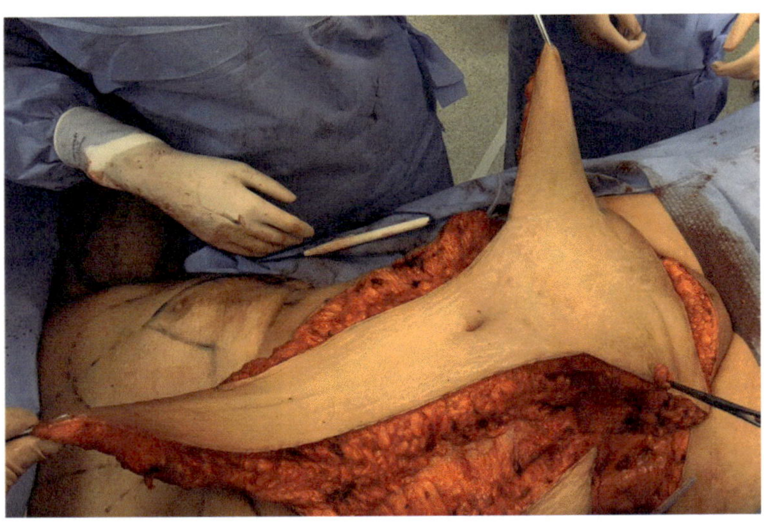

Figure 7.
Transoperative Fleur de Lis dissection.

drain that will go anteriorly and come out on the left side (**Figure 8a** and **b**). Then, the patient is turned on the table in a supine position. The anterior skin is incised with a cold knife and further dissection is taken with electrocautery, in a perpendicular manner -not beveling or undermining- all the way down to the fascia. The upper abdomen flap is undermined in a tunnel fashion preserving the abdominal perforators as recommended by Saldanha [7, 8], in an attempt to ensure the flap's viability. The patient's umbilicus base is preserved and a conservative plicature of the abdominal rectal muscles is performed with a 0 absorbable suture (**Figure 9**). The umbilicus is secured to the fascia once the plicature is done with two stitches at 12 and 6 o'clock. The skin on the abdominal flap is pulled down and a "Y" incision is done where the base of the umbilicus is located to suture their edges together to form the new belly button. The distance between the umbilicus and the abdominal wound should be 10–12 cm depending on the height of the patient. The extra skin and fat in the flap are excised. The wound is closed in two layers, the first involving Scarpa's fascia and the second involving the skin and then Prineo™ tape and cyanoacrylate glue are applied to all the wounds.

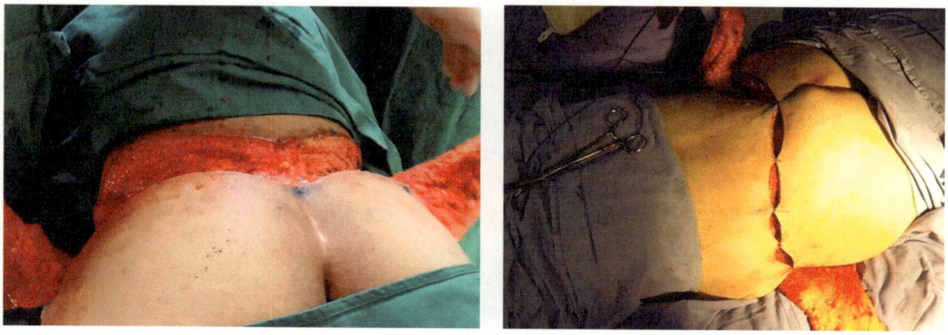

(a) (b)

Figure 8.
(a and b) partial dissection and partial closure.

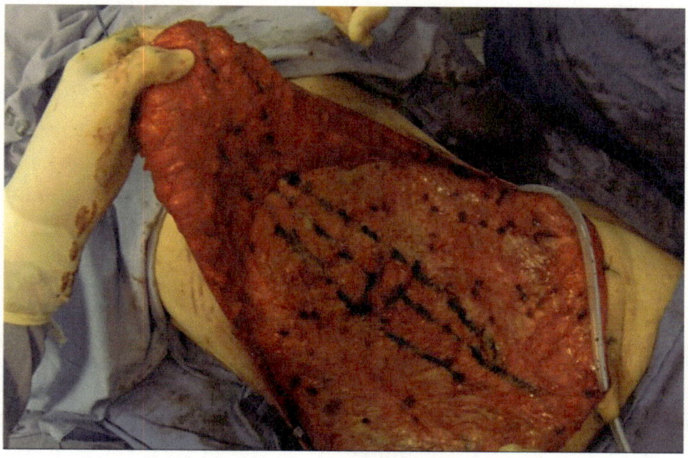

Figure 9.
Conservative recuts plicature.

4.3 Breast lift

For the breast lift in a massive weight loss patient, high profile round silicone gel breast implants, not beyond 280 ml in volume, are preferred, and placed in a subglandular pocket through a 5 cm incision on the crease marking. The upper limit of the pocket dissection is decided by pushing the breast tissue upwards to find the superior limit of the breast footprint. After a careful hemostasis, the pocket is closed with 2-0 Vicryl™ sutures. Then, the incisions are made on the markings already placed for the rest of the breast and around the areola (4 cm diameter) and a de-epithelization of the skin inside all these markings is done. The whole lower pole of the breasts is removed including breast tissue, fat and skin and closure is done with 3-0 nylon™ and 3-0 PDS™ in two layers.

4.4 Thoracoplasty

This procedure has to be planned depending on where the extra tissues have to be resected and the thorax contour corrected. In women, the areas of concern are below the axillary area and the upper back rolls. If the area below the axillary area is the problem, then a "J" pattern should be followed after finding the ideal markings with a pinch test. These markings should come from the axilla when the patient is extending superiorly the arms and be traced to join the sub mammary crease marking. When the excess of skin depends mostly on the upper back rolls, a horizontal line on the back where the resulting scar is desired should be traced with the marker and be placed where the brassiere will be covering it. The amount of skin and fat that will be removed will be determined by the pinch test on each side. In men, the markings have to be placed laterally on the chest and vertically, where the resulting scars can be covered by the arms in a resting position. Likewise, the excess of skin and fat to be removed should be based on the pinch test. Suturing is also based in doing it in two deep layers including the Scarpa fascia and the subdermal layer with 3-0 nylon™ and 3-0 PDS™.

4.5 Brachioplasty

Marking the skin should be done with the patient extending the arms laterally and tracing a line that will be the resulting scar on the bicipital groove or crease. With the pinch test the excess of skin is marked to trace the edges of an ellipse. The skin is incised with a cold knife through the subcutaneous tissue. On the distal third of the arm -around 5–6 cm from the most distal point near to the elbow, the dissection is superficial to preserve the lymphatic structures. Once that critical area is completed superficially, the rest of the dissection is taken all the way down to the fascia -this dissection is safe as all the critical structures are beyond the fascia-. Hemostasis is carried out with electrocautery and the wound is sutured in two layers with 3-0 nylon™ for the deeper layer and 3-0 PDS™ for the subdermal suture.

4.6 Thigh lift

The incisions and dissection should be made as already described for the lower body lift with the help of an electrocautery. After the skin and subcutaneous tissue are resected, the wounds are sutured in two layers as described for the brachioplasty after careful hemostasis with the electrocautery.

5. Systematizing the procedure

The systematization proposed to perform all possible combinations of these body contouring surgeries in less than 6 hours is based on the lead surgeon being the one marking the patient, performing the incisions and having all the other members in the surgical team intervene in different steps of the procedures such as removing the extra skin and fat and suturing the different layers of all the areas of the body being treated. This is the way it has been standardized:

a. The patient is on a prone position and the lead surgeon performs the incisions on superficial skin, then, the lead surgeon and the surgeon assisting on this phase will remove the half of the posterior flap on each side without undermining the remaining flaps which will be sutured (superior flap with inferior flap) together with the technique already described. A closed drain system will be applied for this area and the tube will exit the body through the mons pubis.

b. The patient is turned into a supine position and the excess of skin and fat located inside the markings for an abdominoplasty or a Fleur de Lis pattern is removed. The dissection of the flap to be removed goes from the lateral tissue of the flap to the medial one and the umbilical stalk is the one to be cut at the base once the surgeon has determined there are no hernias and it is safe to do so. If a hernia is encountered at any location of the abdomen, it should be reduced and treated

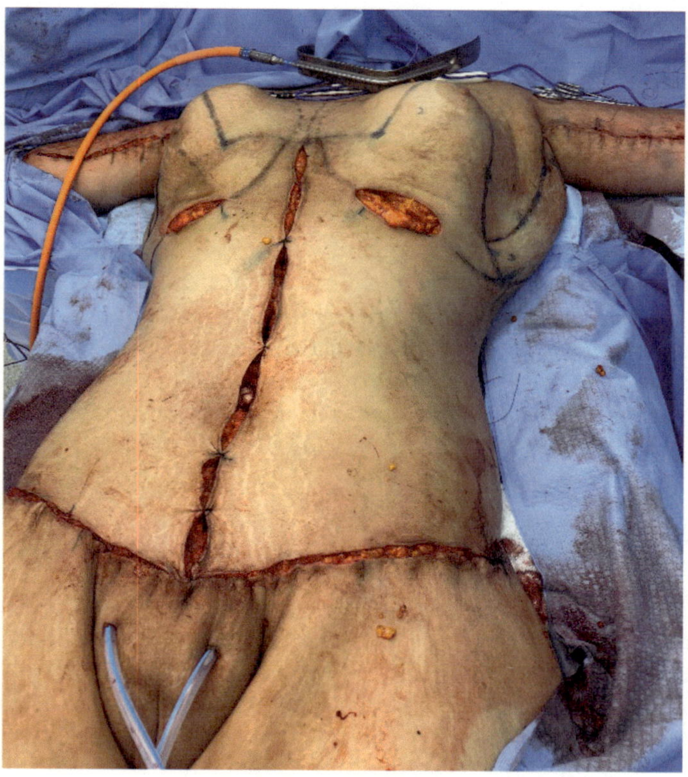

Figure 10.
Partial closure of abdominal and arms wounds, prior to mastopexy, with breast implants in place.

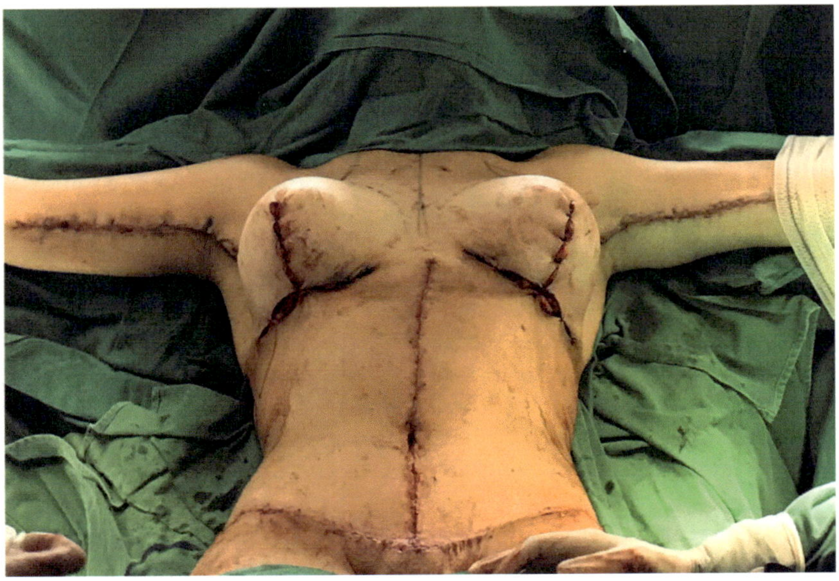

Figure 11.
Partial closure of abdomen, arms and breasts.

with a herniorrhaphy. The rectus abdomini plicature is then performed by the assistant surgeon, careful hemostasis must be done and the abdominal flap is pulled down to close the wound horizontally and vertically in case of the Fleur de Lis abdominoplasty is needed. The umbilicus is reconstructed in the "Y" shape method that has already been described. A closed drain system is left for the abdominal area and its tube is brought outside through the mons pubis. While this is being done, the lead surgeon starts the mastopexy as described before with the help of another plastic surgeon. When the implants have been placed and the extra skin and lower pole of both breasts have been removed, then the lead moves on to performing the brachioplasty with the lateral thoracoplasty if needed. The sutures for the arms and thoracoplasty are performed by the other assistants and the lead surgeon moves on to performing the thigh lift on both sides, leaving the sutures on one side to the surgeon that has already finished the abdominal wall treatment and the lead surgeon suturing the other thigh wound. If a bra-line thoracoplasty is performed, this should be done when the patient is in the prone position at the beginning of the surgery (**Figures 10** and **11**).

6. Postoperative management

After all the wounds are closed in two layers, cyanoacrylate glue and mesh tape (Prineo™) are applied to the wounds, then the patient is draped on kinesiotape which has been found to lower the postoperative swelling, ecchymoses and pain, and avoids seroma formation. The wound areas are left without the taping so that they can be closely checked for dehiscence or signs of infection (**Figure 12**).

As commented before, there is no need for the patient to be put in any anticoagulant medication postoperatively. If the patient had a urinary catheter put in place, as requested by the anesthesiologist, it comes out right after the surgery is finished. For

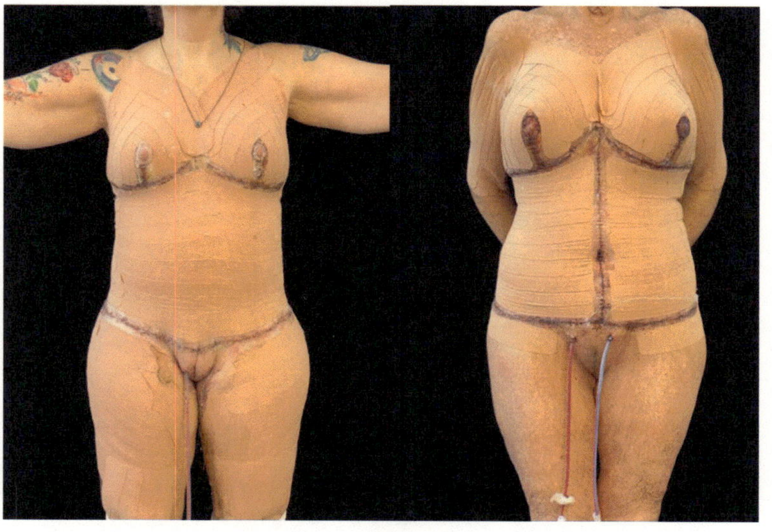

Figure 12.
Postoperative management.

outpatient pain management, ketorolac is administered orally; all patients are asked to take cefadroxil (azithromycin if allergic) for 7 days after the surgery. Patient exits the operating room to a recovery room and then transferred to the room to stay overnight under monitoring. The patient is encouraged to eat a healthy diet based on fiber and water -for a fast and healthy wound healing and recovery- avoiding anything that can cause allergy (seafood) and avoiding the use of laxative medication to prevent bacterial translocation to happen. The patient starts ambulation within 4 hours (late cases even within 2 hours) after the procedure and is discharged after evaluation the next day. Compression garments are ordered to be worn during 1 month for the areas treated. Drain tubes are removed within 7 days postoperatively or when the drain amount is below 30 ml per day.

After 1 week post op, the patient starts visiting the physical therapist, who changes the kinesiotapes and starts lymphatic massages, which are applied once a week for 3 to 4 weeks. Patients are encouraged to walk and do as many activities as possible, even going out to buy new clothes.

7. Results

The combinations of procedures performed are as follows: Lower body lift with or without Fleur de Lis pattern plus breast lift, with or without implants and thoracoplasty if needed, in 100% of the procedures; 50 to 60% may have a brachioplasty and/or thigh lift associated.

The mean time for these combinations of procedures performed was 5.7 hours and the average time to start ambulation is 4 hours. All patients are discharged after 1 day of hospital stay. No patients needed blood transfusion nor transfer to an Intensive Care Unit. None of them had DVT or PE either.

It is important to note that the psychological status of all patients improves amazingly, several patients got pregnant after surgery as their sexual health changed; they also got to wear clothes they never thought they would be able to

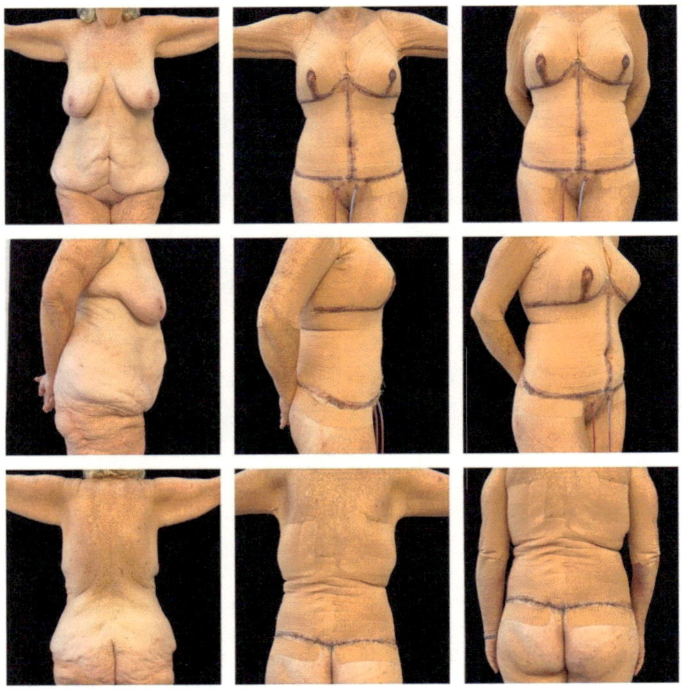

Figure 13.
72 year old female patient, ex-volleyball athlete, who lost 86 Kg after gastric sleeve 10 years before the procedure. The weight before surgery was 104 Kg, with a BMI of 30.6 and 27.05 after the surgery. The tissue removed in the procedure weighed 10.3 Kg. Surgery time was 4 hours and 56 minutes. She started deambulation 3 hours after surgery, did not require blood transfusion and was discharged after 24 hours.

wear, and got involved in many activities they had stopped joining due to the excessive weight. We show the example of a 72-year-old female patient, ex-volleyball athlete, who lost 86 Kg after gastric sleeve 10 years before the procedure. The weight before surgery was 104 Kg, with a BMI of 30.6 and 27.05 after the surgery. The tissue removed in the procedure weighed 10.3 Kg. Surgery time was 4 hours and 56 minutes. She started ambulation 3 hours after surgery, did not require blood transfusion and was discharged after 24 hours (**Figure 13**). A 62-year-old male patient who lost 150 Kg after bariatric surgery 20 years before the body contour procedure. The weight before surgery was 98 Kg, with a BMI of 39.36 and 33.44 right after the surgery. The tissue removed in the procedure weighed 14.5 Kg. The surgery time was 4 hours and 30 minutes. He started ambulation 4 hours after surgery, did not require blood transfusion, and was discharged 24 hours after the procedure (**Figure 14**).

8. Complications

In terms of postoperative complications, its incidence has lowered since the beginning of the senior author's practice, 23 years ago. Seromas have been found only in the lower body lift. No seromas in brachioplasty, thoracoplasty, mammoplasty or thigh lift. Currently, the seroma rate in lower body lift is 30–35%, the mean volume drained is 150–200 ml, with the largest having approximately 800 ml. Seromas are

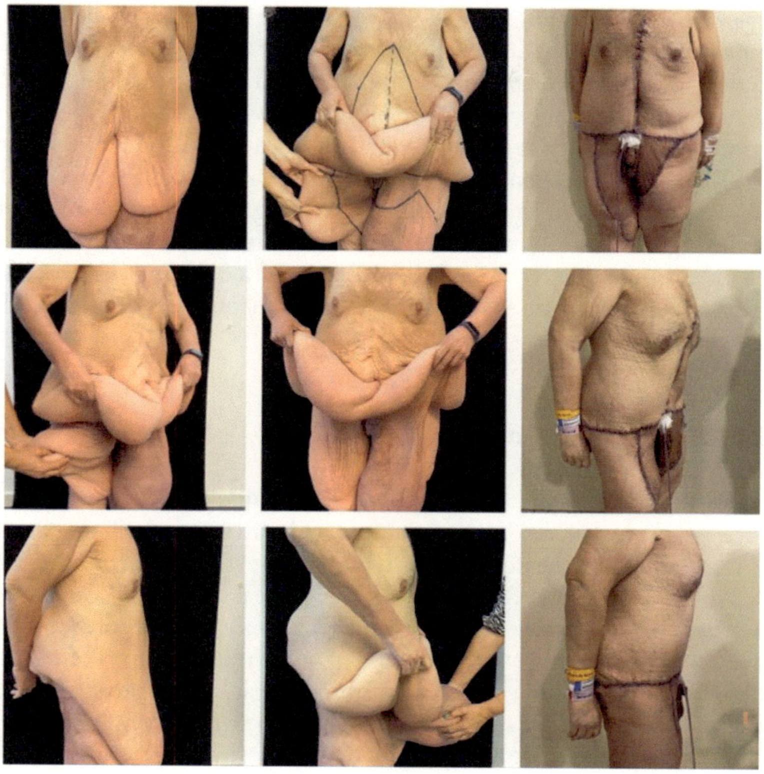

Figure 14.
62 year old male patient who lost 150 Kg after bariatric surgery 20 years before the body contour procedure. The weight before surgery was 98 Kg, with a BMI of 39.36 and 33.44 right after the surgery. The tissue removed in the procedure weighed 14.5 Kg. Surgery time was 4 hours and 30 minutes. He started ambulation 4 hours after surgery, did not require blood transfusion, and was discharged 24 hours after the procedure.

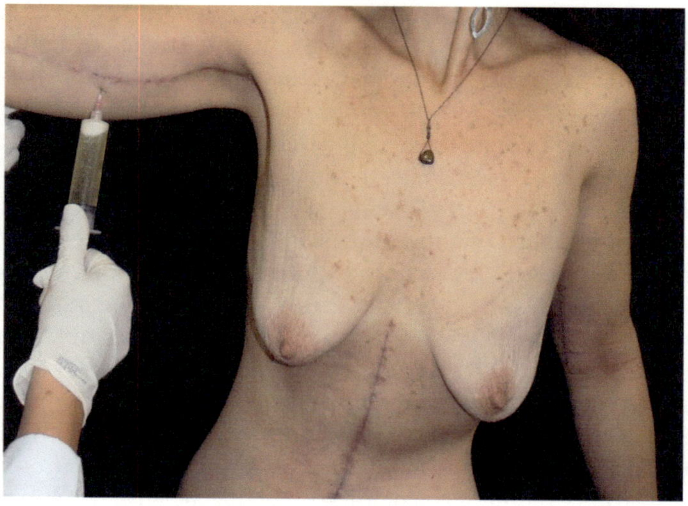

Figure 15.
Lymphocele drainage in office.

drained twice a week until they resolve, which usually takes 4–6 weeks. Lymphoceles in brachioplasty are less than 10%; they are drained at the surgeon's office (nearly 5 ml of clear liquid is drained on each session), resolving in 2 to 3 weeks (**Figure 15**).

There have been some minor skin suffering areas which are no bigger than 4–5 cm; in the beginning of the practice its incidence was close to 10%, currently the rates are close to 3–4%. The management is always conservative, and this usually happens more in the lateral aspects of the abdominoplasty, thighs and coccyx (the bending of the patient during the marking of the patient has lowered dehiscence in this portion to zero). No infections or necrosis have been documented during the procedures.

No patient in this series has required blood transfusions, nor DVT or PE has occurred.

9. Anesthesia considerations

Morbid obesity induces metabolic and physical changes that are not fully corrected after massive weight loss. One of these changes is the airway, which must be meticulously evaluated and have the necessary devices for the management of difficult intubation. Anemia is another frequent factor in these patients; although it is possible to take them to surgery with mild anemia, it is preferable to correct this deficit promptly; oral or parenteral iron, oral folic acid, and frequent doses of erythropoietin are indicated. Other comorbid conditions are also crucial factors to consider; type 2 diabetes mellitus, insulin resistance, sarcopenia, chronic kidney failure, obstructive sleep apnea, oxygen desaturation, altered thyroid function, etcetera; aspects that are not always corrected after massive weight loss.

Medical tourism continues to grow exponentially, especially in plastic and obesity surgery. Tourist patients represent an additional challenge; pathologies typical of their race, their country of origin, acute changes secondary to prolonged travel, languages and customs different from the place where they will be operated on, stress, fatigue, anxiety, and other aspects that must be meticulously assessed by the medical team [9].

Anesthesia in this group of patients has special challenges, so it is desirable, although not essential, for the anesthesiologist to have experience in this field. The pre-anesthetic evaluation must be anticipated, not only to get to know each patient, but also to establish empathy and have enough time to request the opinion of other specialists and to be able to correct existing deficits when possible. Although some plastic surgery centers use regional anesthesia [10], it is more common to use general anesthesia, which may or may not be balanced with opioids, alpha2 agonists, ketamine, and/or regional anesthetic techniques. In pre-anesthetic medication, a pharmacological scheme that includes anxiolytics, amnesia, pre-emptive analgesics, and antiemetic's is recommended. Sublingual doses of lorazepam 1–2 mg, oral melatonin 10 mg, oral etoricoxib 90 to 120 mg, iv keratin 50 mg, iv magnesium sulfate 2 gr, and 8 mg of ondansetron are strongly recommended. Discontinuation of semaglutide-based medications should be considered prior to general anesthesia due to gastrointestinal side effects including delayed gastric emptying [11]. Anesthetic induction with propofol and a fast-acting neuromuscular relaxant such as rocuronium facilitate orotracheal intubation. Maintenance of anesthesia may be with desflurane or sevoflurane, with or without opioids. The use of neuromuscular relaxants eases mechanical ventilation, which should be volume controlled, recommending physiological PEEP, FiO2 0.5% with a mixture of air and oxygen.

The physiological changes caused by obesity change the response to some drugs, so it is mandatory to know the unique characteristics of the administered agents in order to provide safe anesthetic care. The variability in the tissue content of these patients justifies a different, personalized approach [12].

10. Discussion

Capla et al. suggest that prior evaluation includes standard medical and surgical history, as well as aspects of weight loss history (total weight loss, length of stable weight, type of weight loss surgery, etc). The safe cutoff accepted is BMI of 30 or less, stable weight for at least 3 months, ideally 6 months. Medical conditions that did not resolve with massive weight loss should be properly addressed prior to surgery [3]. Our criteria for eligibility for the procedures were mentioned above. Cabbabe and colleagues consider a patient candidate for post bariatric surgery 1 year after weight loss surgery and stable weight for 3–6 months. They operate on BMI's 25–35, with poor candidates being with BMI 35 or greater, active smokers, poor overall medical condition, on anticoagulants and unrealistic expectations [2, 3].

The study by Marchica and colleagues describes a series of modifiable and non-modifiable predictors for complications in abdominoplasty in massive weight loss patients; factors such as preoperative obesity and body mass index, active smoking, preoperative anemia, use of fibrin glue or quilting sutures were considered modifiable and factors as advanced age, diabetes mellitus, and surgical mode of weight loss were considered non-modifiable predictive factors for complications. A study by Bayter-Marin and colleagues including 409 patients to compare the use or not of blood management measures (iron and erythropoietin administration, use of normovolemic hemodilution, temperature maintenance) among patients undergoing body contouring surgeries, they found that hemoglobin value 24 and 72 hours after surgery was significantly higher in the intervention group; they also found an association between lower hemoglobin levels at 24 and 72 hours and longer time in the prone position [13]. We have described the results of the senior author's study describing that the surgery time less than 6 hours is predictive of complications [13, 14]. The senior author has found that, unlike what is suggested, the electrocautery does not cause skin necrosis or dehiscence complications; we recommend its use on a regular basis for all the dissection, for it allows a bloodless and faster procedure. No transfusions were performed in any patients.

The Dermabond™ Prineo™ Skin Closure System combines 2-Octyl cyanoacrylate with a self-adhering mesh for safe and reliable skin closure. It forms a watertight barrier over the incision, and it has been suggested that it forms a microbial barrier as well as providing an even distribution of tension across the incision. Although complications such as rash and allergic contact dermatitis have been described with its use, it is very convenient for skin closure without any of these, and its use is important to lower wound dehiscence and infection rates as well as lowering operating time by using it. Its use in these procedures started in 2007 [15].

Regarding skin suffering areas, these are thought to be due to the poor nutritional state of patients; in the beginning of the practice its incidence was close to 10% (now being 3–4%), by that time, the tension of the flaps, low protein levels, type of sutures used and layered closure may have played a role in dehiscence rate seen. The absence of wound infections or dehiscence nowadays, is most likely to be due to the particularity of not practicing undermining, not so many layers being sutured, and a good nutritional status of the patients.

Kinesiotaping has been recently added to the postoperative management of these patients. It is an elastic tape with longitudinal interwoven elastic fibers and acrylic glue with an elasticity of 130–140% that influences the skin and subcutaneous layers. Among the mechanisms of action to control edema, are that the pre-tension lifts the skin, improving lymphatic flow and directing it to pathways that suffer less congestion and providing a massage-effect during active movement. We have found that its use, which we started in 2020, added to the previously applied lymphatic massage, reduces postoperative edema and improves patient's recovery [16].

11. Conclusions

During 23 years of experience, 1435 procedures have been performed, with a complication rate of 12%. The most common complications have been seroma, lymphocele and small skin suffering areas. These complications were more prevalent in the first years of practice, and have been lowered as the technique and perioperative management practices have been improved. By reviewing the cases performed, the lower body lifting technique improves and even corrects the urinary incontinence in some patients, possibly because the urethral angle is repositioned.

Among the benefits of this systematized approach, we include: lower costs (hospital stay, medication, postoperative complications), one surgical stage opposed to 2 or 3 stages depending on the case (which involves more hospital admissions, anesthesia associated problems, more disability time and recovery periods), low/no risk of severe complications such as PE, DVT or large blood loss.

This is a reproducible technique, once the markings are correctly and accurately done, any plastic surgeon can perform each procedure and get it done with the same ideal results. If the markings are appreciated and respected, the scars will be put within the transition lines of the different esthetic units of the body. If the systematization proposed here is followed by other teams, then the time lapse for the combination of the procedures mentioned above will be as low as 6 hours or less, with diminished health risks and avoiding the use of anticoagulant medications.

The next step is to evaluate and report the patient's-reported outcomes, to correlate them with complication rates and surgeon-reported outcomes, for a more objective analysis.

Conflicts of interest

The authors declare that they have no conflicts of interest to disclose.

Author details

Carlos del Pino-Roxo[1], Alicia Sigler-Moreno[2]*, María M. Cabrera-Cifuentes[3], Ana C. Weck Roxo[4] and Víctor M. Whizar-Lugo[5]

1 Facultad de Medicina de Vassouras, Rio de Janeiro, Brazil

2 Hospital Ángeles, Tijuana, México

3 Hospital General Dr. Manuel Gea González, México City, México

4 Hospital Pedro Ernesto – UERJ, Servico de Cirugía Plástica Universidade do Estado do Rio de Janeiro, Brazil

5 Lotus MedGroup, Tijuana, México

*Address all correspondence to: aliciasiglerplasticsurgeon@gmail.com

References

[1] Hua Y, Lou YX, Li C, Sun JY, Sun W, Kong XQ. Clinical outcomes of bariatric surgery – Updated evidence. Obesity Research & Clinical Practice. 2022;**16**(1):1-9. DOI: 10.1016/j.orcp.2021.11.004

[2] Cabbabe SW. Plastic surgery after massive weight loss. Missouri Medicine. 2016;**113**(3):202-206. DOI: 10.1016/j.cps.2018.08.002

[3] Capla J, Shikowitz-Behr L. Patient evaluation and surgical staging. Clinics in Plastic Surgery. 2019;**46**(1):9-14. DOI: 10.1016/j.cps.2018.08.002

[4] Gastón-Panthaki A, Serrano A, Virani N, Sylvestre J, Crisafulli BF, Becker CB. Food insecurity, weight-based discrimination, weight self-stigma, and mental health in post-bariatric surgery patients. Body Image. 2023;**45**:46-53. DOI: 10.1016/j.bodyim.2023.01.009

[5] Roxo AC, Del Pino RC, Marques RG, Rodrigues NCP, Carneiro DV, et al. Endocrine-metabolic response in patients undergoing multiple body contouring surgeries after massive weight loss. Aesthetic Surgery Journal. 2019;**39**(7):756-764. DOI: 10.1093/asj/sjy195

[6] Mendes FH, Donnabella A, Fagotti Moreira AR. Fleur-de-lis abdominoplasty and neo-umbilicus. Clinics in Plastic Surgery. 2019;**46**(1):49-60. DOI: 10.1016/j.cps.2018.08.007

[7] Ribeiro O, de Souza EB, Novaes W, Pazetti CE, Lopes EM, et al. Lipoabdominoplasty with selective and safe undermining. Aesthetic Plastic Srugery Journal. 2003;**27**:322-327. DOI: 10.1007/s00266-003-3016-z

[8] Ribeiro O, de Souza E, Novaes W, Lucon R, Magalhaes F, et al. Lipoabdominoplasty without undermining. Aesthetic Surgery Journal. 2001;**21**(6):418-526. DOI: 10.1067/maj.2001.121243

[9] Whizar-Lugo V, Flores-Carrillo JC, Campos-León J, Parra-Beltrán P, Azamar-Llamas D. Perioperative care of tourist-patients. Journal of Anesthesia & Critical Care Open Access. 2015;**3**(6):00119. DOI: 10.15406/jaccoa.2015.03.00116

[10] Whizar LV, Cardenas MC. Anesthesia for plastic surgery procedures. Chapter 1. In: Anesthesia topics for plastic and reconstructive surgery. Ed. Whizar-Lugo V. Intechopen. London 2019. Whizar-Lugo VM, Cisneros- corral R, Reyes-Aveleyra M, Campos-León J, Domínguez J. Anesthesia for plastic surgery procedures in previously morbidly obese patients. Anest México. 2009;**21**(3):186-193

[11] Fezza R, Rains B, Fezza T, Fezza JP. Emerging anesthesia risks with semaglutide. Plastic and Reconstructive Surgery. Global Open. 2023;**11**(11):e5427. DOI: 10.1097/GOX.0000000000005427

[12] Willis S, Bordelon GJ, Rana MV. Perioperative pharmacologic considerations in obesity. Anesthesiology Clinics. 2017;**35**(2):247-257. DOI: 10.1016/j.anclin.2017.01.010

[13] Bayter-Marin JE, Cárdenas-Camarena L, Peña WE, Durán H, Ramos-Gallardo G, et al. Patient blood management strategies to avoid transfusions in body contouring operations: Controlled clinical trial. Plastic and Reconstructive Surgery. 2021;**147**(2):355-363. DOI: 10.1097/PRS.0000000000007524

[14] Marchica P, Costa AL, Brambullo T, Marini M, Masciopinto G, et al. Retrospective analysis of predictive factors for complications in abdominoplasty in massive weight loss patients. Aesthetic Plastic Surgery. 2023;**47**(4):1447-1458. DOI: 10.1007/s00266-022-03235-5

[15] Parvizi D, Friedl H, Schintler MV, Rappl T, Laback C, et al. Use of 2-octyl cyanoacrylate together with a self-adhering mesh (Dermabond™ Prineo™) for skin closure following abdominoplasty: An open, prospective, controlled, randomized, clinical study. Aesthetic Plastic Surgery. 2013;**37**(3):529-537. DOI: 10.1007/s00266-013-0123-3

[16] Hörmann J, Vach W, Jakob M, Seghers S, Saxer F. Kinesiotaping for postoperative oedema – What is the evidence? A systematic review. BMC Sports Science, Medicine and Rehabilitation. 2020;**12**:14. DOI: 10.1186/s13102-020-00162-3

Section 3

Enhancing Healing in Cosmetic Surgery

Chapter 16

Enhancing Postoperative Healing with Hyperbaric Oxygen Therapy: Applications in Plastic Surgery Procedures

David Borg, Kristian Bugeja and Kurt Lee Chircop

Abstract

This chapter examines the application of Hyperbaric Oxygen Therapy (HBOT) in cosmetic surgery, focusing on its efficacy in enhancing wound healing and improving postoperative outcomes. Through a review of scientific principles and clinical data, the chapter outlines the mechanism of action of HBOT, which involves increasing tissue oxygenation to support critical healing processes, such as angiogenesis, collagen synthesis, and fibroblast activation. Clinical applications are discussed through case studies and research findings that highlight reduced recovery times and lower complication rates. The chapter also addresses potential risks and economic considerations associated with HBOT, alongside emerging research and technological advancements that may expand its use in cosmetic surgery. The overall assessment is that HBOT represents a valuable yet underutilized modality in cosmetic surgical recovery.

Keywords: Hyperbaric Oxygen Therapy, cosmetic surgery, wound healing, postoperative recovery, clinical applications of HBOT

1. Introduction

1.1 Objective

The primary aim of this chapter is to delineate the relevance and efficacy of Hyperbaric Oxygen Therapy (HBOT) within the realm of cosmetic surgery, particularly focusing on its role in enhancing wound healing. As cosmetic procedures continue to surge in popularity globally, the need for advanced therapeutic techniques to optimize healing and reduce recovery time is paramount [1]. HBOT presents a significant opportunity in this regard, offering accelerated wound healing and potentially superior outcomes in terms of both function and esthetics [1].

1.2 Background

Hyperbaric Oxygen Therapy, which involves the administration of 100% oxygen at elevated atmospheric pressures, has historically been utilized for a broad spectrum of medical conditions, including decompression sickness, chronic nonhealing wounds, and acute carbon monoxide poisoning. Its application has expanded into the domain of cosmetic surgery, where precise and effective wound healing is crucial for successful outcomes [2]. This therapy leverages the physiological benefits of increased oxygen availability to enhance tissue repair and angiogenesis, processes critical to effective postsurgical recovery [3]. Figures of Hyperbaric Oxygen Therapy chambers are shown in **Figures 1–3** below.

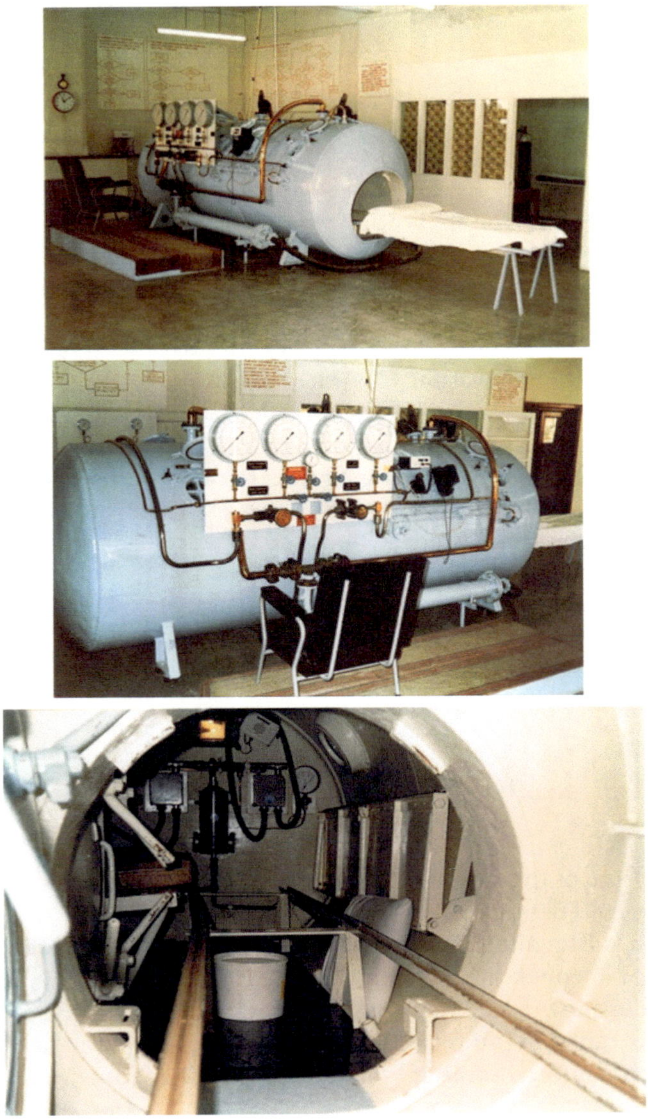

Figure 1.
Photos of the first Hyperbaric Unit at Kalafrana, Malta, and Europe. Pictures courtesy of Hyperbaric Unit staff [4].

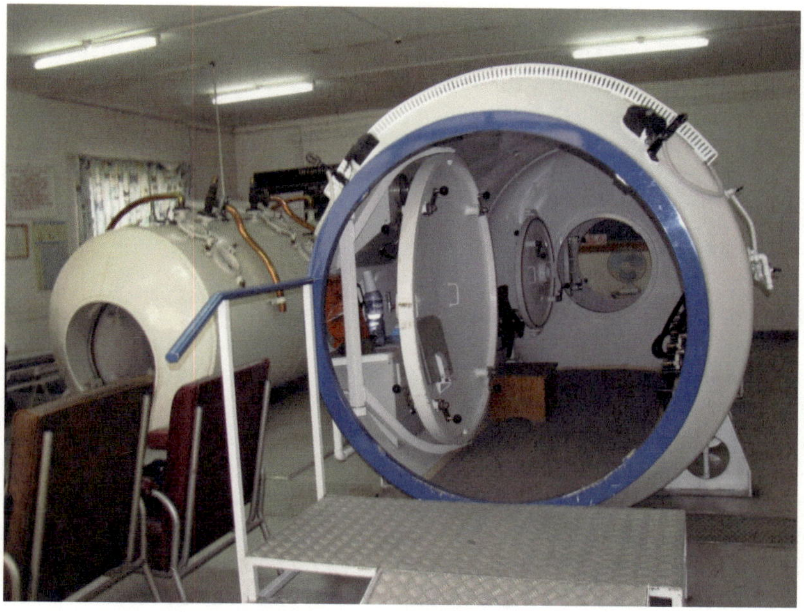

Figure 2.
Photos of the old-World War 2 era Japanese recompression chamber and the Italian recompression chamber obtained in 1994 at the former St. Luke's Hospital Hyperbaric Unit, Malta, and Europe. Pictures courtesy of Hyperbaric Unit staff [4].

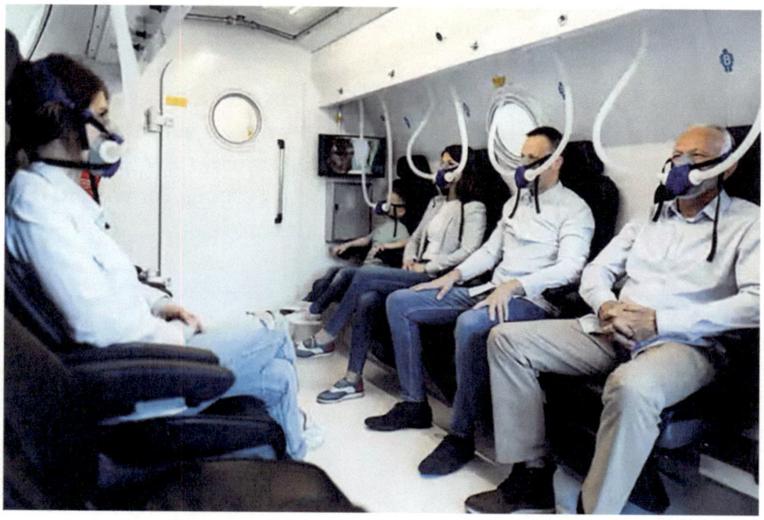

Figure 3.
Modern Hyperbaric Oxygen Therapy chamber with four patients and a qualified hyperbaric nurse [5].

1.3 Scope

This chapter will explore the integration of HBOT into cosmetic surgical procedures, highlighting its mechanisms of action and the empirical evidence supporting its use. It will address various cosmetic surgeries that can benefit from HBOT, supported by data from recent studies and clinical trials. Additionally, the discussion will extend to the limitations and potential risks associated with HBOT, providing a comprehensive overview that balances the therapy's advantages against its constraints and challenges. This approach aims to furnish practitioners and researchers with a nuanced understanding of HBOT's role in cosmetic surgical recovery, backed by current scientific and clinical evidence.

2. Theoretical foundations

2.1 Mechanism of action

Hyperbaric Oxygen Therapy (HBOT) operates on the principle of increasing atmospheric pressure to enhance the solubility of oxygen in the blood, which allows for higher levels of oxygen to be delivered to tissues [6]. This is represented in **Figure 4** below. Under normal atmospheric conditions, oxygen transportation is primarily hemoglobin-bound in the red blood cells. However, as represented in **Figure 5**, under hyperbaric conditions, oxygen dissolves directly into the plasma, cerebrospinal fluid, and other body fluids, substantially increasing tissue oxygenation without being reliant on hemoglobin. This elevated oxygen level under pressure saturates the tissue, promoting mitochondrial respiration and energy production, which are essential for cellular repair and regeneration processes [9].

2.2 Biological impact

The biological responses to HBOT are multifaceted and crucial for effective wound healing:

1. *Angiogenesis*: HBOT stimulates the release of growth factors such as vascular endothelial growth factor (VEGF) and stimulates the formation of new blood vessels. This process is vital for supplying sufficient blood flow to regenerating areas, improving oxygen and nutrient delivery which is crucial for wound healing.

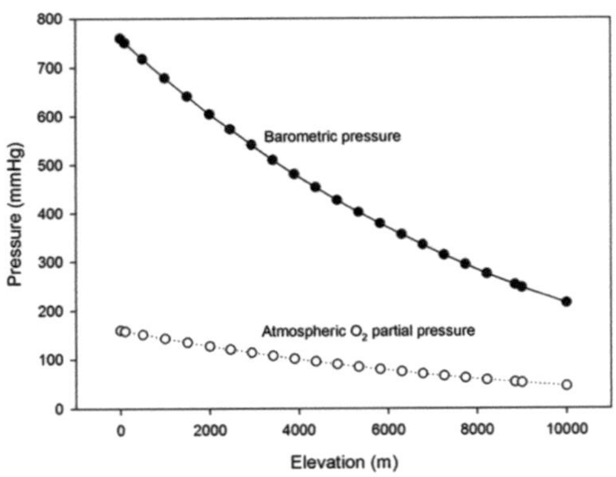

Figure 4.
Relationship between elevation and Barometric Pressure (filled circles) and Atmospheric Partial Pressure of Oxygen (hollow circles). Calculations were based on the standard atmosphere [7].

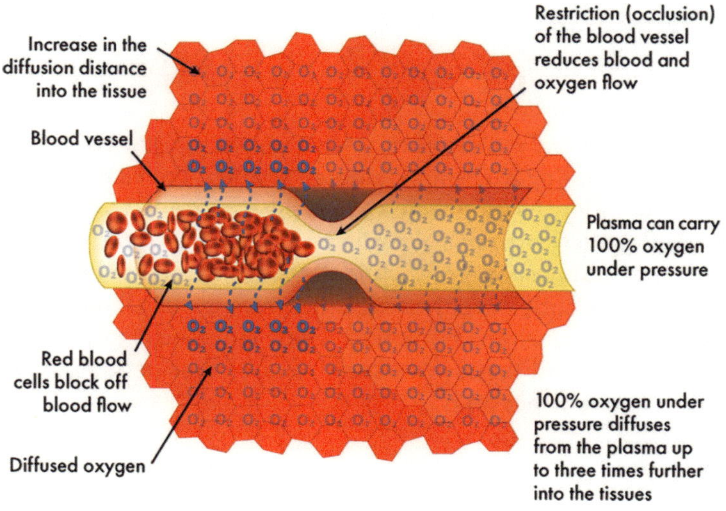

Figure 5.
Figure representing the direct transfer of oxygen to plasma and surrounding tissue because of increased diffusion, a direct result of hyperbaric oxygen [8].

2. *Fibroblast activation*: Fibroblasts play a critical role in the wound healing process by secreting collagen and other extracellular matrix components. Exposure to high oxygen levels enhances fibroblast proliferation and differentiation, thereby accelerating the maturation of the extracellular matrix and enhancing wound strength and durability.

3. *Collagen synthesis*: Collagen is the main structural protein in the extracellular space in the various connective tissues in the body. Increased oxygen levels boost the hydroxylation of proline and lysine, two amino acids necessary for the stable formation of collagen molecules. Enhanced collagen synthesis under HBOT conditions leads to more robust and resilient tissue repair.

4. *Reduction of inflammation*: HBOT has been shown to reduce local and systemic inflammation by decreasing pro-inflammatory cytokines and enhancing the activity of anti-inflammatory mediators. This reduction in inflammation can decrease swelling and pain, further aiding the healing process.

5. *Bacterial oxidative killing*: The high levels of oxygen delivered during HBOT are toxic to certain anaerobic bacteria and enhance the oxidative killing capacity of leukocytes. This is particularly beneficial in wound healing, as it reduces the risk of infection, a common complication in surgical interventions.

By understanding these mechanisms and biological impacts, practitioners can more effectively utilize HBOT in cosmetic surgery to enhance outcomes and reduce recovery times. This scientific foundation not only supports the clinical application of HBOT but also guides further research into optimizing protocols for specific types of cosmetic procedures [10].

3. Clinical applications in cosmetic surgery

3.1 Case studies

Several clinical trials and case studies have demonstrated the efficacy of HBOT in enhancing wound healing in cosmetic surgery settings. For example, a controlled study published in the Journal of Plastic and Reconstructive Surgery compared postoperative healing in two groups of patients undergoing facelifts: one group received HBOT pre- and post-surgery, while the control group did not. The HBOT group exhibited significantly faster healing times, reduced swelling, and fewer complications, such as hematoma formation. These outcomes suggest that HBOT can be a valuable adjunct to traditional postoperative care in cosmetic surgery, enhancing patient outcomes and satisfaction [11].

3.2 Procedure types

HBOT has been found beneficial across a variety of cosmetic procedures, including:

- *Facelifts (Rhytidectomy)*: Enhances recovery by reducing swelling and bruising, leading to a quicker return to normal activities.

- *Breast augmentations*: Supports healing by promoting vascularization, which is crucial for the survival of fat grafts and reduction of capsular contracture.

- *Skin grafts and flaps*: Increases the success rate of grafts and flaps by improving oxygenation and reducing ischemic complications.

These examples highlight the versatility of HBOT in cosmetic surgery, catering to a range of procedures that require enhanced tissue repair and healing [1]. **Figures 6–8** are examples of the latter.

3.3 Treatment protocols

Typical HBOT protocols for wound healing in cosmetic surgery involve sessions lasting approximately 90–120 minutes, with patients receiving 100% oxygen at pressures between 1.5 and 2.5 atmospheres absolute (ATA). The frequency of treatments

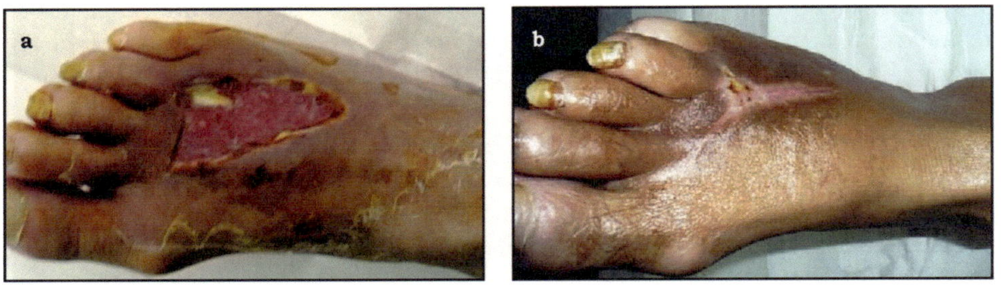

Figure 6.
Foot ulcer before (a) and after (b) hyperbaric treatment [12].

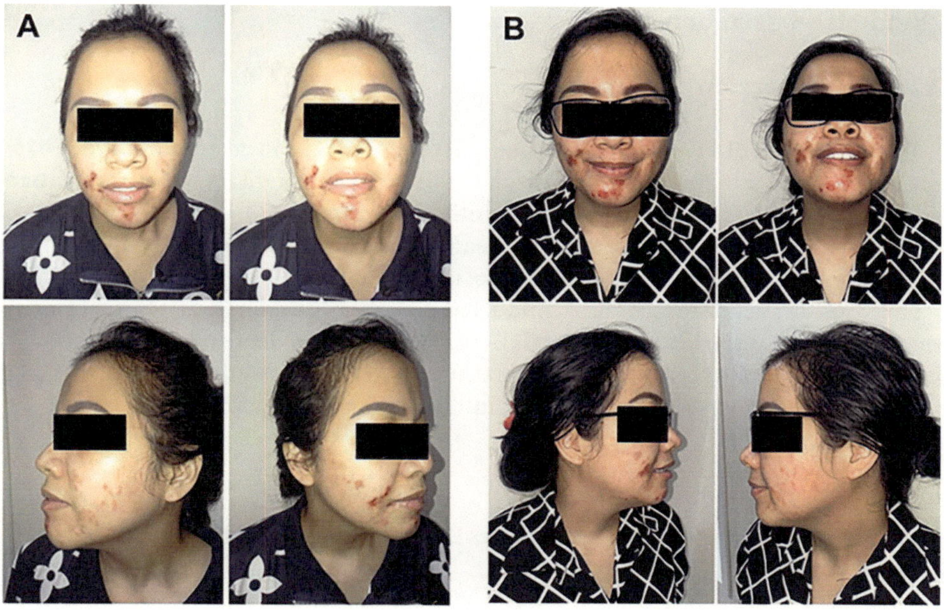

Figure 7.
Post thread lift allergy leading to facial excoriations. (A) Multiple wounds on the nasolabial folds and jawlines before HBOT. (B) Inflammation resided and wounds turned bright red as vascularization improved after 1 month of HBOT [13].

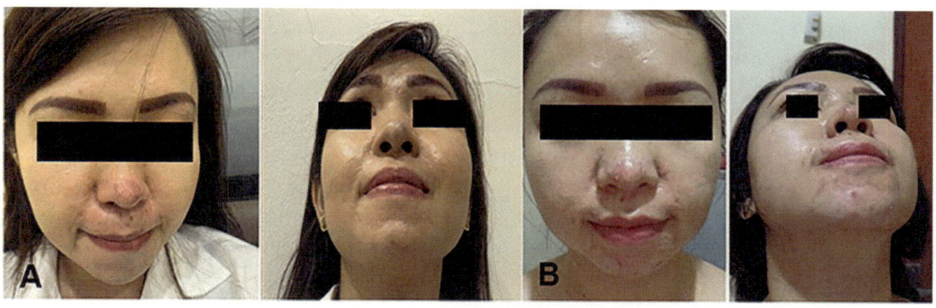

Figure 8.
Post-filler vascular occlusion of the nasal tip. (A) Erythema and blanching of the nasal tip before HBOT. (B) Excoriations turned bright red as vascularization began to improve after 1 month of HBOT [13].

can vary depending on the specific needs of the procedure and patient conditions, but commonly, a total of 5–10 sessions are recommended for optimal results [14]. For instance, in the case of facelifts, HBOT may be administered daily for the first few day's post-surgery to maximize the reduction in swelling and bruising. Treatment protocols should always be tailored by medical professionals based on individual patient assessments and the specific type of surgery performed [10].

The integration of HBOT into cosmetic surgical practices offers a promising tool for improving outcomes. Its use is supported by scientific evidence demonstrating its benefits in speeding up the healing process, reducing the risk of complications, and enhancing the overall success of cosmetic procedures. As HBOT becomes more recognized in this field, its protocols continue to be refined, providing valuable insights for practitioners aiming to achieve the best possible patient outcomes [14].

4. Evidence-based benefits

4.1 Research overview

The utilization of Hyperbaric Oxygen Therapy (HBOT) in cosmetic surgery has been substantiated by numerous research studies that highlight its benefits in enhancing wound healing. These studies consistently show that HBOT increases oxygen delivery to surgical sites, accelerates the healing process, and reduces the incidence of complications such as infections and necrosis.

For example, a landmark study conducted on patients undergoing rhinoplasty demonstrated that those treated with HBOT showed a 35% decrease in healing time compared to the control group. The study attributed this improvement to the enhanced oxygenation and reduced inflammatory response facilitated by HBOT.

4.2 Statistical data

Statistical evidence further underscores the efficacy and safety of HBOT in cosmetic surgery:

- *Infection rates*: Research indicates that HBOT can reduce postsurgical infection rates significantly. A meta-analysis of over 3000 cosmetic surgery patients revealed that the infection rate in the HBOT group was only 2%, compared to 10% in the non-HBOT group [14].

- *Healing times*: A systematic review focused on breast reconstruction surgeries found that patients receiving HBOT had a 40% reduction in healing times, with improved scar quality and reduced incidence of revision surgery [15].

- *Complication rates*: Data from a multicenter study involving facelift surgeries showed a reduction in complication rates from 15% in the control group to 5% in the HBOT group. Common complications such as hematoma and seroma were notably less frequent among patients treated with HBOT [14].

5. Challenges and limitations

5.1 Risks and complications

While Hyperbaric Oxygen Therapy (HBOT) is generally considered safe, it does carry potential risks and complications, particularly when used in the high-risk environment of postoperative care in cosmetic surgery. Common risks associated with HBOT include:

- *Barotrauma*: Due to changes in air pressure, patients can experience ear pain or more severe injuries such as a ruptured eardrum.

- *Oxygen toxicity*: If administered improperly, the high levels of oxygen can lead to oxygen toxicity, affecting the central nervous system and pulmonary systems.

- *Claustrophobia*: The enclosed space of the hyperbaric chamber can induce feelings of claustrophobia in some patients.
- *Fire hazard*: Due to the high levels of oxygen used in HBOT chambers, there is an increased risk of fire if safety protocols are not meticulously followed.

5.2 Limitations in research

Despite the growing body of evidence supporting HBOT in cosmetic surgery, there remain significant gaps in the current research:

- *Lack of standardization*: There is considerable variability in the HBOT protocols used in studies, including differences in pressure levels, duration, and frequency of sessions. This lack of standardization makes it difficult to compare results across studies or establish optimal treatment guidelines.
- *Small sample sizes*: Many studies have relatively small sample sizes, limiting the generalizability of their findings.
- *Long-term effects*: The long-term effects of HBOT on cosmetic surgery outcomes are not well-documented, with most studies focusing on short-term results.

5.3 Cost-effectiveness

Incorporating HBOT into cosmetic surgical practices also presents economic considerations:

- *Initial investment*: The cost of acquiring and maintaining hyperbaric equipment is substantial. Additionally, the operational costs—including staffing, training, and safety compliance—can be significant.
- *Insurance and reimbursement issues*: In many regions, HBOT is not routinely covered by insurance for cosmetic procedures, potentially placing a financial burden on patients and limiting the accessibility of this treatment.
- *Cost vs. benefit*: While HBOT can reduce the time to recovery and decrease the incidence of complications, these benefits must be weighed against the high costs of the therapy. Economic analyzes are needed to determine whether the improved outcomes justify the additional expenses [16].

In conclusion, while HBOT offers promising benefits for enhancing wound healing in cosmetic surgery, it is crucial for practitioners to consider the associated risks, research limitations, and economic implications. Future research should aim to address these gaps, particularly through large-scale, randomized controlled trials, to better define the role of HBOT in cosmetic surgery and establish clear, evidence-based guidelines for its use.

6. Future directions

6.1 Emerging research

The field of Hyperbaric Oxygen Therapy (HBOT) in cosmetic surgery is ripe with potential for new research avenues that could further elucidate and expand its applications. Current research efforts are focusing on:

- *Extended applications*: New studies are examining the effectiveness of HBOT in less common cosmetic procedures, such as body contouring and nonsurgical facial rejuvenation techniques. These studies aim to establish broader, evidence-based applications for HBOT in cosmetic surgery.

- *Optimal treatment protocols*: Ongoing clinical trials are aimed at determining the most effective treatment protocols for HBOT, including the optimal number of sessions, duration of treatment, and specific pressures to be used for different types of cosmetic surgeries.

- *Patient-specific outcomes*: Researchers are also focusing on how individual differences, such as age, health status, and smoking habits, affect the outcomes of HBOT in cosmetic surgery. This could lead to more personalized treatment plans.

6.2 Technological advancements

Technological innovations continue to enhance the safety, efficiency, and applicability of HBOT:

- *Portable hyperbaric chambers*: Advances in technology have led to the development of portable hyperbaric chambers, which could be used in outpatient settings, making HBOT more accessible to patients.

- *Real-time monitoring systems*: Integration of real-time monitoring systems within HBOT setups can enhance patient safety by providing continuous feedback on patient vitals and the internal environment of the chamber. This can help prevent complications such as oxygen toxicity.

- *Automated pressure adjustment technologies*: New technologies that automate the adjustment of pressure levels based on real-time physiological responses are being developed. These systems aim to optimize the therapeutic effects of HBOT while minimizing risks.

7. Summary and conclusions

7.1 Recapitulation

This chapter has explored the integration of Hyperbaric Oxygen Therapy (HBOT) into cosmetic surgery, examining its scientific underpinnings, clinical applications, and the body of evidence supporting its efficacy and safety. The key points include:

- *Mechanism of action*: HBOT enhances the oxygenation of tissues, which supports various physiological processes crucial for wound healing, including angiogenesis, fibroblast activation, and collagen synthesis.

- *Clinical applications*: HBOT has been effectively applied in a range of cosmetic surgeries, including facelifts, breast augmentations, and skin grafts, demonstrating significant benefits in reducing recovery times and improving overall surgical outcomes.

- *Evidence-based benefits*: Research and statistical data have shown that HBOT can reduce infection rates, speed up healing processes, and lower the incidence of complications, making it a valuable adjunct in cosmetic surgical care.

- *Challenges and limitations*: Despite its benefits, HBOT comes with risks such as barotrauma and oxygen toxicity, and there are economic and practical considerations that can limit its application.

- *Future directions*: Emerging research and technological advancements are likely to enhance the effectiveness, safety, and accessibility of HBOT in cosmetic surgery.

7.2 Final thoughts

Looking ahead, the future of HBOT in cosmetic surgery appears promising. Continued research and technological development are crucial for overcoming current limitations and expanding its use. It is recommended that:

- *Standardized protocols*: The development and adoption of standardized treatment protocols based on robust clinical evidence will be essential for optimizing treatment outcomes and ensuring patient safety.

- *Personalized treatment plans*: Further studies should focus on how individual patient factors affect HBOT outcomes, which can lead to more personalized, effective treatment approaches.

- *Cost-effectiveness analysis*: Comprehensive economic evaluations are needed to better understand the cost-benefit ratio of HBOT in various cosmetic procedures, which will help in making informed decisions about its broader adoption.

In conclusion, HBOT holds significant potential to transform postoperative care in cosmetic surgery. By continuing to build on the current foundation of scientific research and by leveraging new technologies, practitioners can enhance the therapeutic benefits of HBOT, ultimately leading to better patient care and satisfaction in the field of cosmetic surgery.

Acknowledgements

The authors acknowledge the use of Grammarly for the language polishing of this chapter.

Author details

David Borg*, Kristian Bugeja and Kurt Lee Chircop
Department of Surgery, Mater Dei Hospital, Malta

*Address all correspondence to: davidborgdavid@outlook.com

References

[1] Simman R, Bach K. Role of hyperbaric oxygen therapy in cosmetic and reconstructive surgery in ischemic soft tissue wounds: A case series. Eplasty. 2022;**22**:e61. DOI: 10.1097/PRS.0000000000003416

[2] Winocour J, Gupta V, Ramirez JR, Shack RB, Grotting JC, Higdon KK. Abdominoplasty: Risk factors, complication rates, and safety of combined procedures. Plastic and Reconstructive Surgery. 2015;**136**(5):597e-606e. DOI: 10.1097/PRS.0000000000001700

[3] Francis A, Baynosa RC. Hyperbaric oxygen therapy for the compromised graft or flap. Plastic and Reconstructive Surgery. 2017;**139**(2):395-402. DOI: 10.1097/PRS.0000000000003103

[4] A Shallow Dive into the Hyperbaric Unit [Internet]. Malta: divinginfo.mt; 2023. Available from: https://www.divinginfo.mt/a-shallow-dive-into-the-hyperbaric-unit/ [Accessed: August 26, 2024]

[5] Shabir O. Alzheimer's disease: Hyperbaric oxygen proposed as treatment in new study. The Conversation. 2021;**1**:1. Available from: http://theconversation.com/alzheimers-disease-hyperbaric-oxygen-proposed-as-treatment-in-new-study-167818 [Accessed: August 26, 2024]

[6] Feldmeier JJ, Hopf HW, Warriner RA, Fife CE, Gesell LB, Bennett M. UHMS position statement: Topical oxygen for chronic wounds. Undersea & Hyperbaric Medicine. 2005;**32**(3):157-168. DOI: 10.15462/uhm.2005.32.3.157

[7] Ortiz-Prado E, Dunn JF, Vasconez J, Castillo D, Viscor G. Partial pressure of oxygen in the human body: A general review. American Journal of Blood Research. 2019;**9**(1):1-14

[8] HyOx - Hyperbaric Oxygen Therapy Clinic [Internet]. What Are the Benefits of Hyperbaric Oxygen Therapy? The HyOx Team Explains. Available from: https://www.hyox.com/what-are-the-benefits-of-hyperbaric-oxygen-therapy [Accessed: August 26, 2024]

[9] Kindwall EP, Gottlieb LJ, Larson DL. Hyperbaric oxygen therapy in plastic surgery: A review article. Plastic and Reconstructive Surgery. 1991;**88**(5):898-906. DOI: 10.1097/00006534-199111000-00023

[10] Neel OF, Mousa AH, Al-Terkawi RA, Bakr MM, Mortada H. Assessing the efficacy of hyperbaric oxygen therapy on facelift outcomes: A case–control study comparing outcomes in patients with and without hyperbaric oxygen therapy. Aesthetic Surgery Journal Open Forum. 2023;**5**:ojad065

[11] Parnis J, Magrin AMF, Hassan H. The role, safety, and efficacy of hyperbaric oxygen therapy in aesthetic practice: An evidence-based review. Aesthetic Plastic Surgery. 2023;**47**(1):110-117. DOI: 10.1007/s00266-023-01641-4

[12] Cimen KM. Wound healing and hyperbaric oxygen treatment. Journal of Wound Care. 2008;**17**(9):406-412. Available from: Semantic Scholar

[13] Oley MH, Oley MC, Mawu FO, Aling DMR, Faruk M. Hyperbaric oxygen therapy in aesthetic procedures. Clinical, Cosmetic and Investigational Dermatology. 2021;**14**:1257-1264. DOI: 10.2147/CCID.S321111

[14] Oley MH, Oley MC, Mawu FO, Aling DMR, Faruk M. Hyperbaric oxygen therapy in managing minimally invasive aesthetic procedure complications: A report of three cases. Clinical, Cosmetic and Investigational Dermatology. 2022;**15**:63-68. DOI: 10.2147/CCID.S344408

[15] Bassetto F, Bosco G, Brambullo T, Kohlscheen E, Tussardi IT, Vindigni V, et al. Hyperbaric oxygen therapy in plastic surgery practice: Case series and literature overview. Plastic and Reconstructive Surgery. 2020;**145**(4):817e-825e. DOI: 10.1097/PRS.0000000000006607

[16] Zhou D, Fu D, Yan L, Xie L. The role of hyperbaric oxygen therapy in the treatment of surgical site infections: A narrative review. Medicina (Kaunas, Lithuania). 2023;**59**(4):762

Chapter 17

Perspective Chapter: Lymphatic Therapy and Post-Operative Care – The Science of a Seamless Recovery

Brandy Fenwick

Abstract

This chapter explores the history of manual lymphatic drainage (MLD) and its importance. Complete decongestive therapy (CDT), which utilizes both MLD and skilled wrapping techniques or garment compression for patients living with lymphedema and lipedema, or basic MLD for autoimmune disorders or general selfcare, has been historically utilized. Interestingly, the beauty of the lymphatic system and its function has come to the forefront of more recent conversation as it relates to pre/post-operative care. This profound technique has evolved through the hands-on experience and science-based findings of post-operative specialists internationally. This revolutionary concept of lymphatic work or "therapy" (MLD technique) as a foundational tool of complete post-operative care has truly optimized patient outcomes. These specialists, armed with staged treatment techniques, play a vital role in ensuring ideal results for patients who have experienced body altering procedures. Facilitating esthetically pleasing results based on each patient's unique procedure and needs is the primary goal. Despite meticulous surgical planning and care, post-operative complications can still arise. There are multiple facets to the recovery process. Therefore, having the right post-operative care facilitated by surgeons, surgical staff, and post-operative specialists is essential.

Keywords: manual lymphatic drainage, lymphatic therapy and post-operative care, stages of healing, lymphangiogenesis, compression

1. Introduction

The art of body altering procedures has been around for centuries. However, in 1990, the volume grew tenfold. Surgeons became more innovative in their approach as new techniques and technologies surfaced. The utilization of tumescent (meaning swollen and firm) introduced by Dr. Klein in 1985 allowed efficiency and efficacy of surgeries, reducing blood loss and decreasing the sympathetic response of the body during trauma while under either local or general anesthesia [1]. Adversely, this new process introduced an exponential amount of fluid within the extracellular matrix (ECM).

Within the cosmetic and plastic surgery industry, there was a paradigm shift around 2018, posing the concept of incorporating MLD as potentially helpful for cosmetic surgery patients [2]. In late 2019, receiving "lymphatic massages" after a cosmetic procedure, was becoming a trend. Surgeons were beginning to encourage this treatment. However, this technique seen across social media platforms was and is not lymphatic drainage, lymphatic massage, or lymphatic therapy. Rather, it is post-surgical drainage, literally manually "milking" the patient's torso to rid them of interstitial post-surgical fluids. This technique is beneficial when performed gently rather than with oils and aggressive strokes. Aftercare should not induce additional pain or trauma to the patient or their tissues.

This misinformation became a segway for certified providers to originally implement MLD as a foundational tool along with post-operative care. This application of MLD has gradually morphed into a more applicable title of lymphatic therapy. The additional post-operative components include educating patients on the recovery process, drain management, compression guidance, incisional care, scar work, umbilicus training, hygiene, taking measurements and photos to document patient progress, selfcare instruction, incorporating mobility and neuromuscular re-education, encouraging proper nutrition, establishing home programs, and providing emotional support within our scope of practice.

As the number of patients undergoing cosmetic procedures continues to increase, there is a need for adjunctive therapies that promote patient recovery which is paramount to improve post-operative outcomes and enhance patient's satisfaction. The Esthetic Society reported in 2022 that with 11,078 reviews of patient satisfaction across various platforms, esthetic appearance was the strongest predictor of rating across all procedures. Buccal fat removal (98.8%) and abdominoplasty (98.1%) had the highest satisfaction, and Brazilian butt lift had the lowest (88.2%). Additional significant contributors included staff interaction, bedside manner, health outcomes, complications, and post-operative care [3].

Although in its infancy, post-operative specialists are gaining traction as an intricate part of the surgical experience. In the past 5 years post-operative care has revolutionized the final outcomes of body altering procedures. Through the author experience, it has been expressed by surgeons that a patient at their 6-week follow-up may present as looking 6 months post-op. This may not always be the case. However, the science is there, and the critical thinking involved with creating a seamless recovery is a beautiful thing to see come to fruition.

2. History of complete decongestive therapy (CDT)

The original method of MLD was developed by Dr. Emil Voder and his wife, Estrid Voder, in the 1930s. Dedicating their studies to the lymphatic system and the techniques involved with intuition and practical treatments. The practice of MLD was first introduced in North America in 1972 and is taught in countries all around the world [4]. The utilization of compression and exercise came in the 1950s when Dr. Keith Stillwell published results for treating lymphedema post-mastectomy with massage, compression, and exercise. This later evolved in the 1980s when Professor Michael Foeldi combined both Vodder's and Stillwell's approaches and revolutionized what is now known as Complete Decongestive Therapy (CDT) [5–7].

DOI: http://dx.doi.org/10.5772/intechopen.1008360

3. Anatomy and mechanisms of the lymphatic system (LS)

The lymphatic system is nothing short of remarkable as it works silently in the background, parallel with the circulatory system. It is supportive of the immune system and aids in homeostasis. When it comes to surgery and the recovery process it plays a crucial role.

3.1 Anatomy

The lymphatic system (LS) is an open system. At the capillary loops in the dermis, the initial lymph capillaries (ILC) effectively retrieve approximately 20% of the interstitial fluids (IF), comprised of 96% water, and the remaining 4% being plasma proteins, debris, bacteria, long chain fatty acids, and other cells too large to be picked up by the circulatory system at the capillary loops located in the corium papilla. Once the IF is within the LS, it is considered lymphatic fluid (LF). As illustrated in both **Figures 1** and **2**, there is a sequence of events that occur to filter this fluid prior to reintroducing it to the circulatory system. Throughout this process, the LF is being transported via the superficial and deep

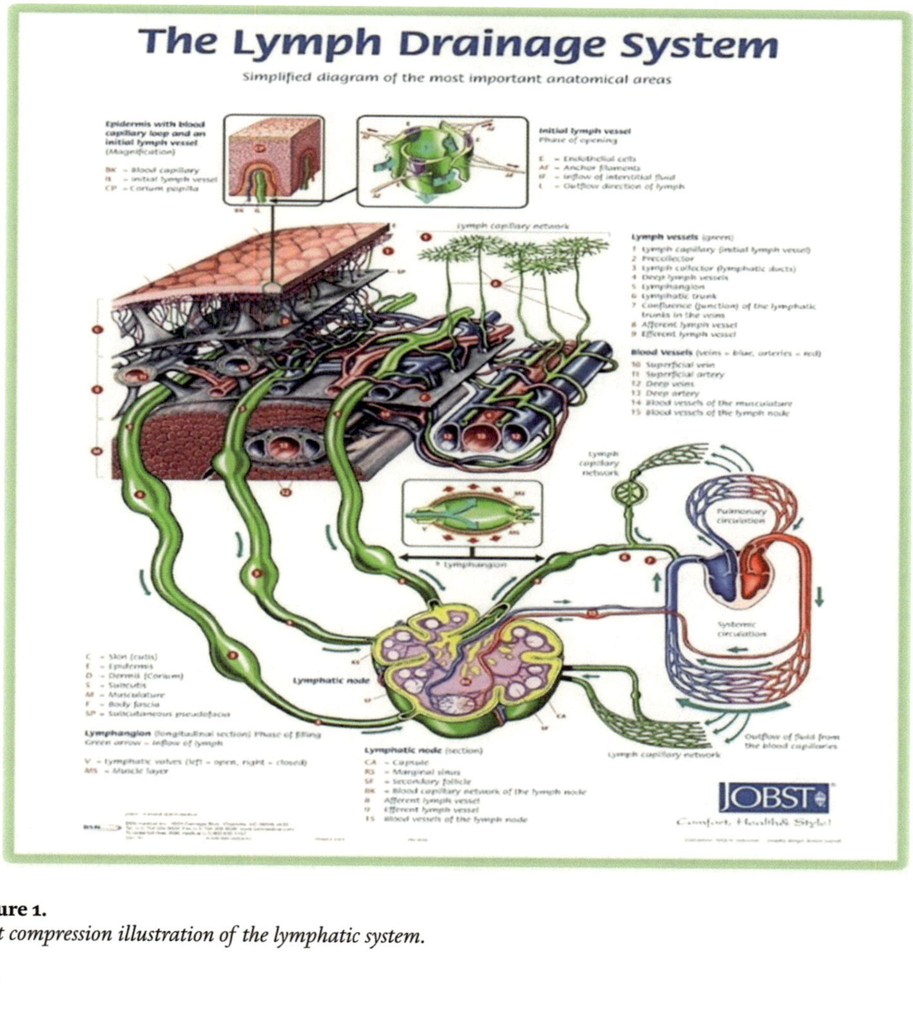

Figure 1.
Jobst compression illustration of the lymphatic system.

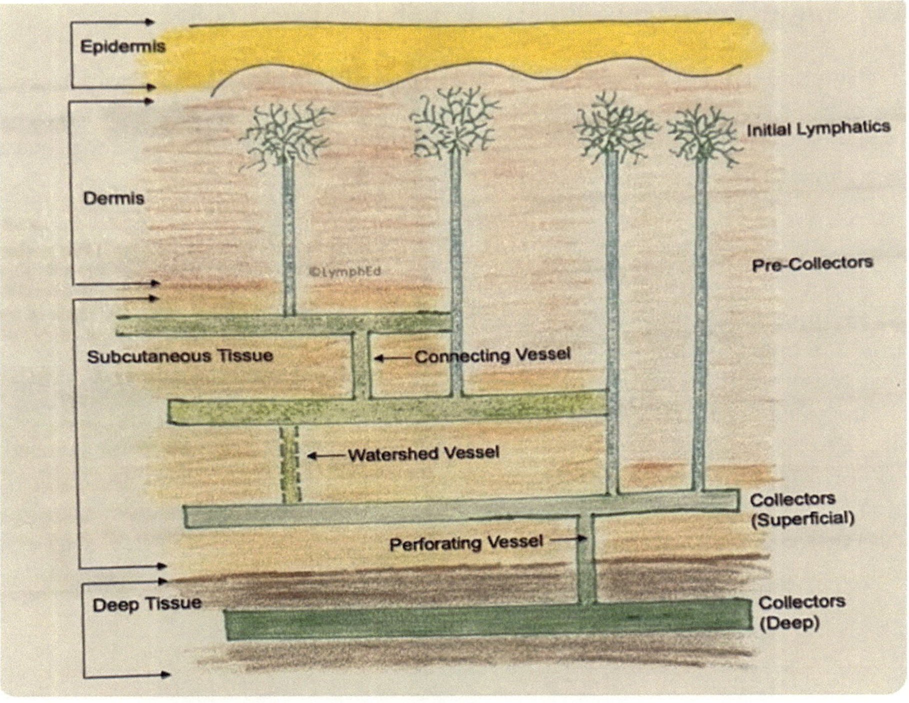

Detailed Drawing of tissue dissection and presentation of the lymphatic vessel system from superficial to deep.

Figure 2.
DiCecco, Shelly. Lymphatic system: Vessels, lymphed manual. 2021 [6].

LS and filtered through 300-900 lymphnodes throughout the body. This movement is then carried onward to the lymphatic trunk (the largest lymph vessel) stationed behind the diaphragm. The lymphatic trunk manages the cyclic process of bilateral lower quadrants and the upper left quadrant of the trunk and extremities, the upper right quadrant is effectively managed by the right lymphatic duct. Then LF is transported from the lymphatic ducts to bilateral venous angles (supraclavicular fossa). Progressing to provide nutrients to vital organs and cells, provide any immune response, and finally the residual being expressed from the body through urination. This directional system can be compromised and become insufficient either dynamically or mechanically. A body altering procedure elicits a high-volume dynamic insufficiency, ultimately returning to normal function (**Figures 1–3**) [5–7].

The body is segmented into quadrants: four quadrants of the trunk, four of the face, and 2 of the breasts (25% sternal and 75% axillary). These established quadrants are separated by vessel blockades called watersheds. In the process of managing a post-surgical patient, there are multiple anastomoses that allow for redirecting LF during the dynamic insufficiency stage. The inguinal to/from

- ➢ NO CENTRAL PUMP
- ➢ Dynamic insufficiency: Healthy system is overwhelmed due to trauma
- ➢ one-way "directional", open system, the initial lymph vessels can pick up interstitial fluid at any point. It then converts to lymph, is transported and processed through the lymph nodes, and then drains at the venous angles into the blood stream.
- ➢ It's interstitial fluid until it turns into lymphatic fluid once it's in the lymphatic system
- ➢ Superficial and deep system:

-superficial initiates in epidermis at the capillary loop (corium papilla) – dermis (corium)

-deep transitions via (perpendicular)perforating precollectors the to (parallel) collectors located in muscle/fascia/joints. Ex: Sternocostal joints, Intercostal muscles, pubis symphysis

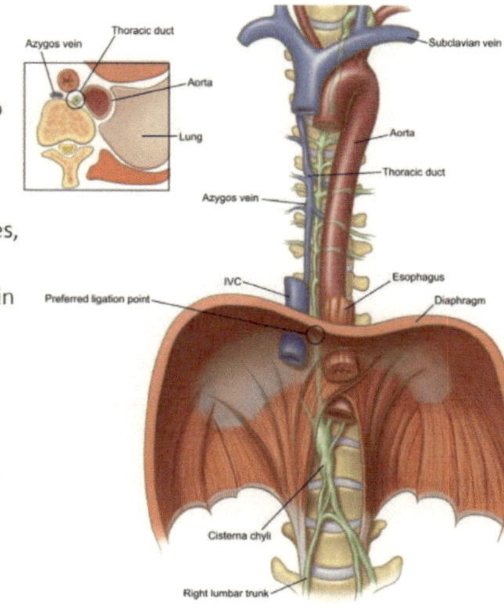

Figure 3.
Summary of lymphatic anatomy and its functional mechanisms.

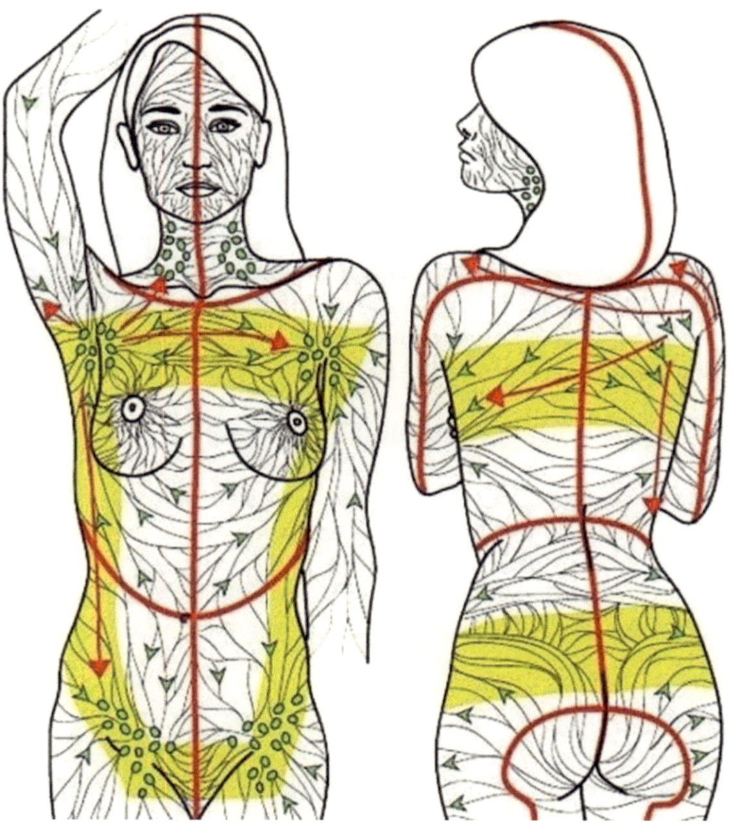

Figure 4.
Illustration of watersheds (RED), major lymph node bundles (GREEN), and anastomosis (YELLOW).

axillary anastomosis is a primary mechanism for redirecting during the recovery process (**Figures 2** and **4**).

3.2 Lymphatic load and diffusion distance

The transport capacity (TC) of the LS is 10x greater than the lymphatic load (LL) in normal conditions. However, with a high-volume dynamic insufficiency such as *trauma induced from surgery*, the lymphatic vessels have been damaged, severed, or compromised thus effecting their function. With the influx of fluids introduced to the body both by external forces such as the injecting of tumescent and the natural inflammatory response, the LL will then exceed the transport capacity of the LS. When this occurs, the diffusion distance in skin-to-body relation increases and impedes the metabolic and healing processes. Therefore, a mechanism to facilitate reducing the diffusion distance is crucial for returning the body to homeostasis [5–7].

3.3 Lymphangiomotoricity

Lymphangiomotoricity is the speed at which the angions of the LS contract. Typically, the LS pumps at 10–12 pulses per minute (ppm) with a maximum of 60 ppm. With a sluggish or insufficient system due to trauma, lack of movement, and anesthesia, a therapist will in effect work to mimic the LS with a slight increase to approximately 20–30 ppm to "trick" the system and progress toward homeostasis [5–7].

4. Non-surgical to post-surgical

Putting the LS anatomy and mechanisms into perspective once the "normal system" is impacted by an invasive cosmetic procedure is strategic. The fundamental knowledge of the LS, the impact of surgery, proper awareness of body system responses, residual effects of surgery, and how to bridge the surgery to recovery gaps, are the greatest puzzle pieces of putting together a seamless recovery.

4.1 Dynamic insufficiency VS mechanical insufficiency

The body takes on physiological responses, a massive increase of interstitial fluids, and patients wake in a fight or flight sympathetic state. A body altering procedure is a high-volume dynamic insufficiency. However, it has the potential to evolve into a mechanical insufficiency if an excessive number of lymphatic passageways, superficial or deep, are damaged, or scar tissue impedes lymphatic flow. This can ultimately compromise the LS permanently.

4.2 Lymphatic therapy (LT)

With the growing popularity of post-operative care, there have been small roadblocks due to misinformation or misinterpretation. Through this author's communication, patients have voiced fear of having "lymphatic massages" because of the word massage as it relates to the kneading of the skin. Others are fearful of being squeezed or having skin pulled on too harshly and unnecessarily to manually drain fluids, as seen in social media. Therefore, the post-op specialists currently in the industry are progressing toward the utilization of verbiage such as "lymphatic therapy," a distinct transformation from MLD to a more medically based, critical thinking technique of post-op care. Application of LT facilitates the beginning of a healing journey. The body is overloaded with tumescent, which includes lidocaine, a lipophilic substance that is easily sequestered in the fat and remains for several days, contributing to an already damaged and sluggish LS post-operatively. The superficial LS has endured a significant amount of damage, now having severed or traumatized lymphatic vessels, cauterized lymph nodes or potentially removal of lymph nodes [8].

LT continues to incorporate the Voder Method, utilizing both vertical and horizontal skin stretch strokes to move toward proper regional lymph bundles. These mentioned strokes are then modified in accordance with the palpation of the tissues and recognition of the stage of healing an individual is in. Thus, the reason hands-on palpation is crucial and truly supersedes machine use in the first 5–6 weeks of post-operative care. Famous osteopathic physician Viola Fryman said: "Palpation cannot be learned by reading or listening; it can only be learned by palpation" [9]. According to the Academy of Lymphatic Studies (ACOLS) the amount of pressure applied may vary from 5 to 10 g per cm^2, with the typical hand 10 cm x10 cm = 500 g–1000 g.This combined with Dr. Guimberteau's (the founder of Kinesio Tape) Pressure 60 g – 130 g force (no more than the weight of a cell phone) to engage epidermis/dermis gives parameters necessary for engaging in LT and post-operative care (**Figure 5**) [7, 10].

4.3 Stages of healing

The four stages of healing are major components of understanding a treatment protocol post-surgically. As displayed in **Figure 6**, there is a vast amount of overlapping within the recovery process. Individuals recover at varying speeds depending on preoperative status. Regardless, all have a core healing process in effect. The four stages of healing are observable and palpable guides in the morphology of the tissue matrix. Ultimately a director of transforming each treatment session accordingly.

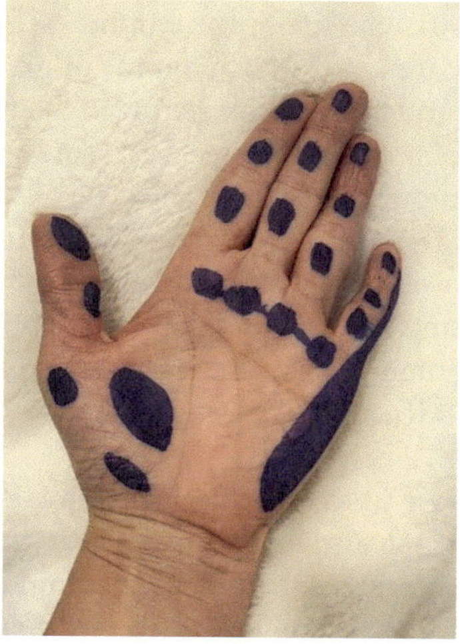

Figure 5.
Symbolizes points of contact when palpating and when providing lymphatic skin stretch strokes; hand application will vary, but markers indicate all contacting surfaces.

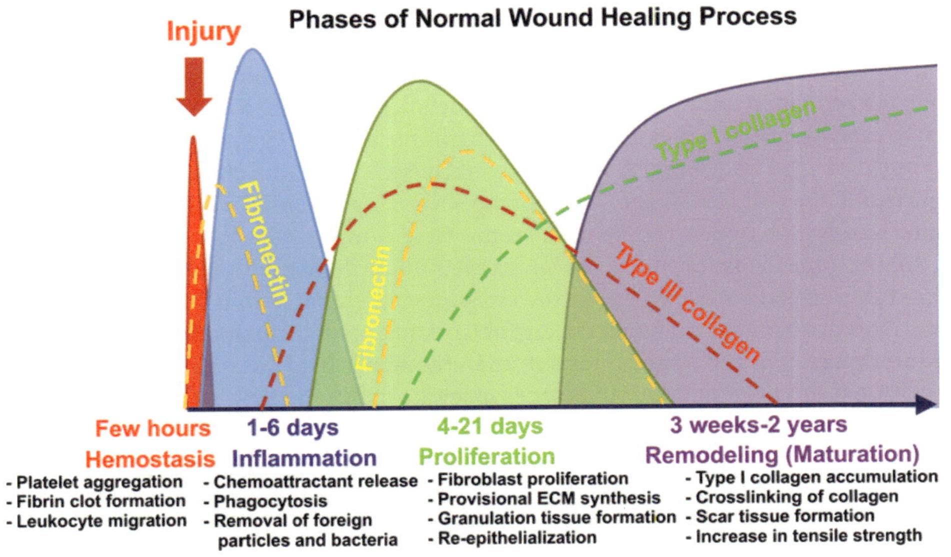

Figure 6.
Graphical presentation of the four stages of healing.

i. Stage 1: Bleeding stage is when initial and overlaps more noticeably for 1–6 days after a cosmetic procedure. The body's reaction to trauma is to establish homeostasis rapidly, with platelets adhering to the sub-endothelial wall and the first fibrin strands begin to adhere within about 60 seconds [10]. Now imagine this occurring with a mass influx of tumescent. This influx of fluids impedes the fibrin attachment, thus creating a post-surgical sensation, which is described as velcro pulling apart and tissues filling with "hot lava."

ii. Stage 2: Inflammatory stage is now when the injured vessels leak transudate (made of water, salt, and protein), causing localized swelling. Inflammation both controls bleeding and prevents infection. The fluid engorgement allows healing and repair cells to move to the site of the wound [11]. Patients undergoing a body altering procedure are impacted by a "wound" of greater surface area. The damaged cells, pathogens, and bacteria are removed from the wound area and white blood cells, growth factors, nutrients, and enzymes create the swelling, heat, pain and redness commonly seen. With the influx of transudate plus tumescent the body takes on a larger diffusion distance. Inflammation is a natural part of the wound healing process and is only problematic if prolonged or excessive. Therefore, implementing lymphatic therapies post-op day, one initiates the process of lymphatic homeostasis, which aids in reducing the expanded (greater than normal trauma) diffusion distance.

iii. Stage 3: The proliferative phase of wound healing is the rebuilding of new tissue made up of collagen and extracellular matrix. In the proliferative phase, the surgical tissues contract as new tissues are laid down. This is an important stage for lymphangiogenesis, angiogenesis, and neurogenesis. These network vessels are now reconstructed so that the granulation tissue can be healthy and receive sufficient oxygen, nutrients, and information. Myofibroblasts cause the wound to contract by gripping the edges of surgical incisions and surface tissues after liposuction and pulling them together or attempting to draw the tissues closer to the body's fibroseptal network using a mechanism like that of smooth muscle cells. This stage is also important to understand for any dehiscence that may occur post-surgically. It tactilely presents the firmness of the tissues impacted by the cosmetic procedure. When collagen is laid down, it is disorganized [11]. Treatment from week 2 and thereafter is required to help reduce the presence of indurated tissues, facilitate the next stage of healing and minimize risks of irreversible fibrosis (**Figure 7**).

iv. Stage 4: The remodeling/maturation stage of wound and post-surgical healing is when collagen is remodeled from type III to type I. The cells used to repair tissues in phase 3 are no longer needed, thus removed by apoptosis, or programmed cell death. Collagen is now aligned along tension lines, and water is reabsorbed so the collagen fibers can lie closer together and cross-link. Cross-linking of collagen reduces scar thickness and makes the skin area of the wound stronger. Generally, remodeling begins about 21 days after an injury and can continue for a year or more. Even with cross-linking, healed wound areas continue to be weaker than uninjured skin, generally only 80% of the tensile strength of unwounded skin [11]. Manual sculpting is a perfect touch at this stage of healing. It's the opportune time for patients to focus highly on "snatching" their waist, if this is the desire for their recovery journey. The stages of healing can be a fragile process, and it requires knowledge and understanding of each stage both in wound healing and tissue morphology to progress a patient through their recovery (**Figure 8**).

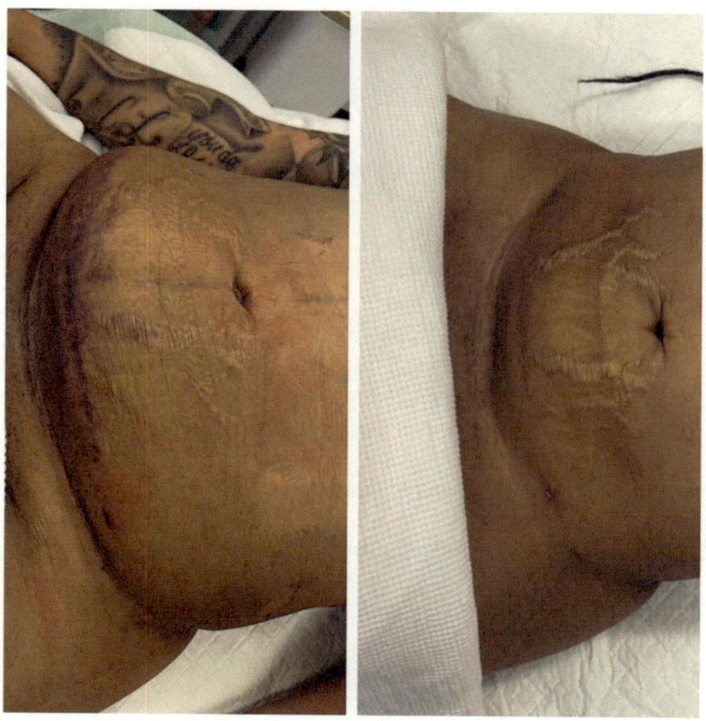

Figure 7.
Stage 3, significant induration of the lower abdomen before and after four sessions and proper garment wear.

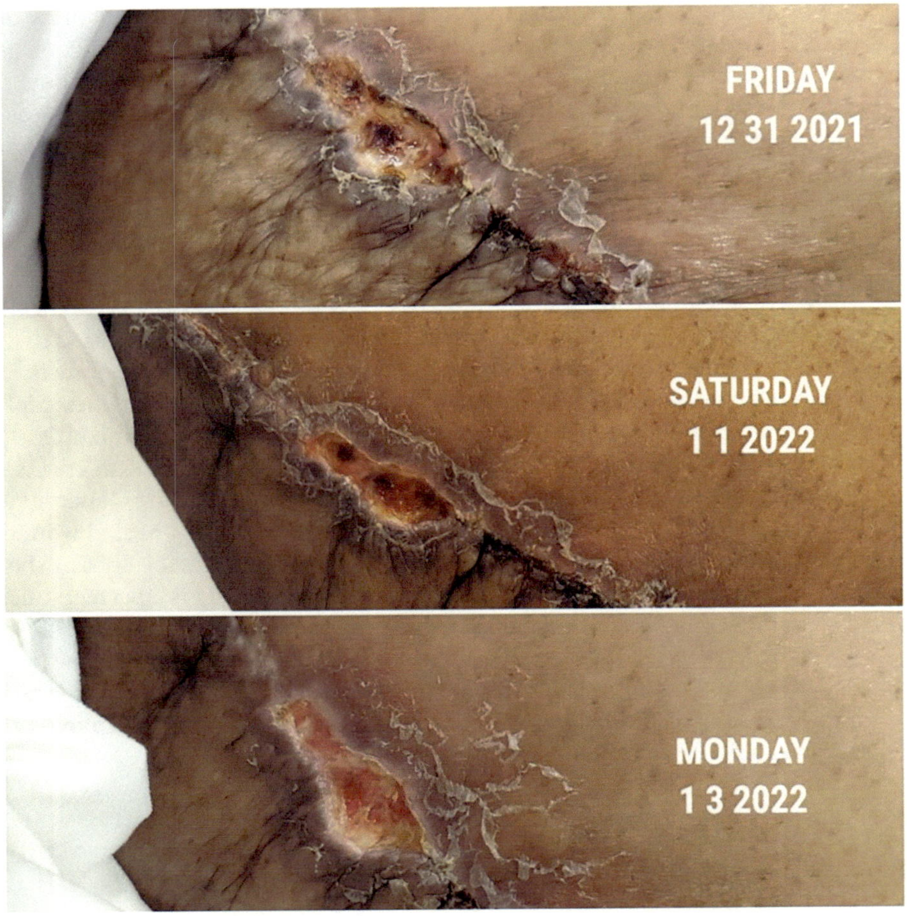

Figure 8.
Inner thigh lift dehiscence 4-day progression in healing.

4.4 The significance of day 1 treatment

There is significant value in day 1 post-operative treatment. This is the beginning of an import process. In **Figure 9**, this 1-day post-op patient has had multi-procedure surgery; educating and assessing her are highly beneficial to her first week of recovery. A post-op specialist has several things to provide and carry out in this session:

i. Establish patient trust in care received

ii. Assess skin through palpation and observation

iii. Give patient the understanding that it is "ok to touch yourself"

iv. Check drain (if applicable) for proper function

v. Educate patient on selfcare and things to expect the first week of recovery

vi. Determine treatment plan of frequency and duration

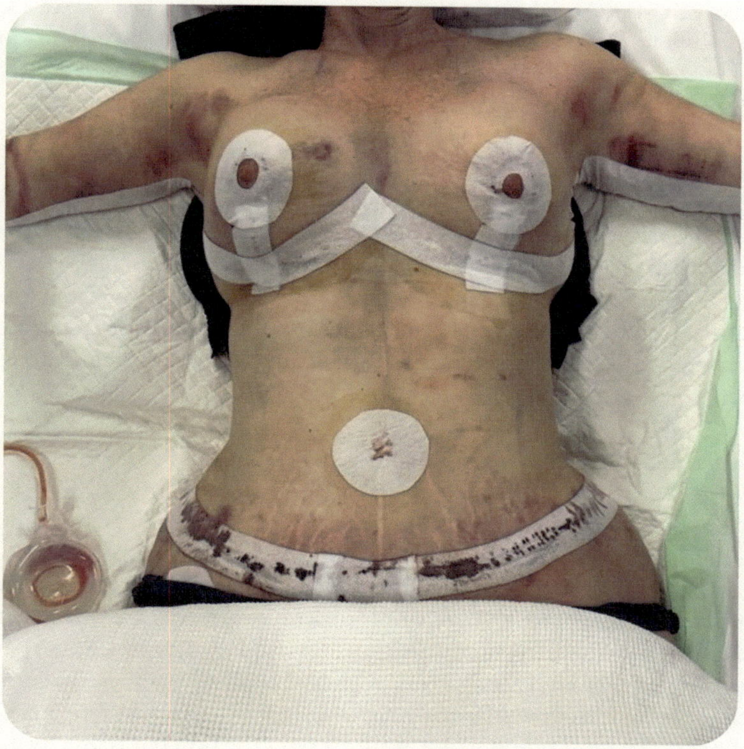

Day 1 Post-op: Brachioplasty, extended breast lift, breast reduction, breast augmentation, tummy tuck with abdominoplasty

Figure 9.
Picture of day 1 post-op multiple procedure case.

From a medical standpoint, the post-op specialist assesses and provides:

i. An analgesic (parasympathetic) effect.

ii. Controlled modification of the skin stretch stroke of lymphatic therapy.

iii. Monitor for infection or skin reactions.

iv. Observing the patient for negative physiological effects that may need medical attention.

v. Skin assessment of all bruising and any discoloration indicative of decreased blood flow to and incision site.

vi. Communicate any findings to surgical staff or surgeon.

5. Lymphatic therapy in tandem with all post-operative care

As previously mentioned, LT is not to be mistaken for massage. It is skin stretch stroking of the superficial tissues and intermittent slightly deeper work pumping perpendicularly to the deeper lymphatics *via* joints, muscles, and fascia. Not a soul application for post-operative care but the key component throughout the patient's journey. The treatment protocol will gradually shift, the use of LT decreases but it is always a part of the treatment. As the shift in treatment evolves, several distinct processes should occur.

5.1 Palpation for any tissue anomalies

Palpation is the key to understanding the body's progressive needs in treatments. There is potential for small absences, or unexpected occurrences as shown in **Figure 10**. The use of a cellulite release procedure followed by a Brazilian butt lift (BBL) resulted in channels of loose liquefied fat. Finding this anomaly in a timely manner allowed the patient to communicate with her surgeon to keep abreast of the issue and care for as needed.

5.2 Skin assessment for seromas, hematomas and allergic reactions

The prevention of seromas, hematomas, and allergic reactions is first and foremost in the immediate aftermath of surgery. The presence of a seroma is palpable as a "waterbed" if superficial enough. However, at times they may be deep or in an unexpected area such as the mons pubis. Observation and palpation are a must in after care to find these pockets of fluid and to listen to the patients explanation of what they may feel. Some patients will report pain and feeling bulgy, others do not even realize they have these 10 cc–500 cc or greater pockets present. Hematomas are more challenging to find if there is not a discoloration of the skin. There is a fluid like sensation under the skin but is less "waterbed" like and more gelatinous in palpation. Allergic reactions can be very traumatizing to the patient considering they are in post-surgical pain and now they are itching nonstop (**Figure 11**), this can be mitigated with over the counter products but may ultimately require surgeon intervention for use steroids etc

5.3 Improving active range of motion (AROM) and functional mobility

It is natural to guard when in pain. After patient's initial surgical instructed range restrictions such as tummy tuck or a breast augmentation, it is imperative

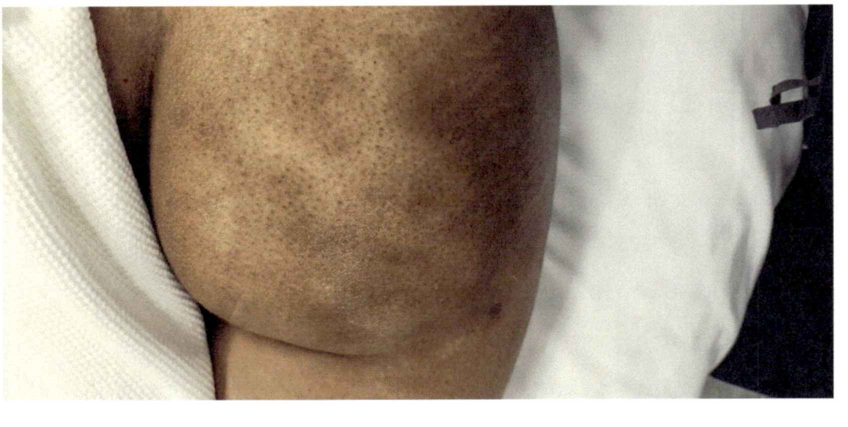

Figure 10.
Effects of BBL and cellulite release performed at the same time. These fat grafted channels (lighter skin areas) are palpable anomalies and are filled with liquefied fat that did not take.

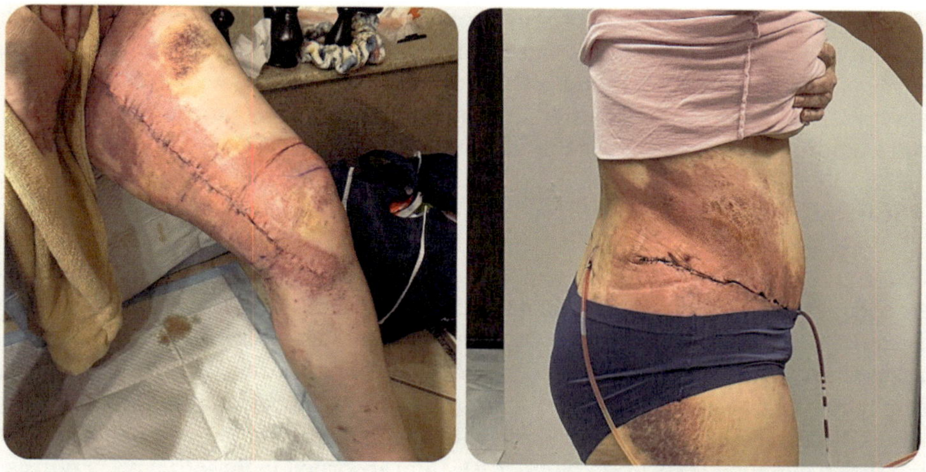

A. Hypersensitivity to surgical skin adhesive

B. Reaction to a combination of adhesives and white surgical binder and "other".

Figure 11.
A. After 3 surgeries and some closure technique, the patient's body reacted to surgical skin adhesive. The surgical skin adhesive migrated into the incisions and continued to create a systemic reaction for several months. B. Patient had an initial unknown reaction. It was later determined she reacted to the elastic binder and adhesives.

to incorporate small diagonal, postural, or extremity movements to begin slowly returning back to normal activities of daily living. There are exceptions; for example, if additional anchor sutures for a tummy tuck were placed, a patient should remain flexed at 45 degrees for a few days or weeks longer per specific surgeon's protocol. In the case of a breast augmentation with added mesh or securing pocket sutures, the protocol may be to not reach over the head and not lie on the side for several weeks.

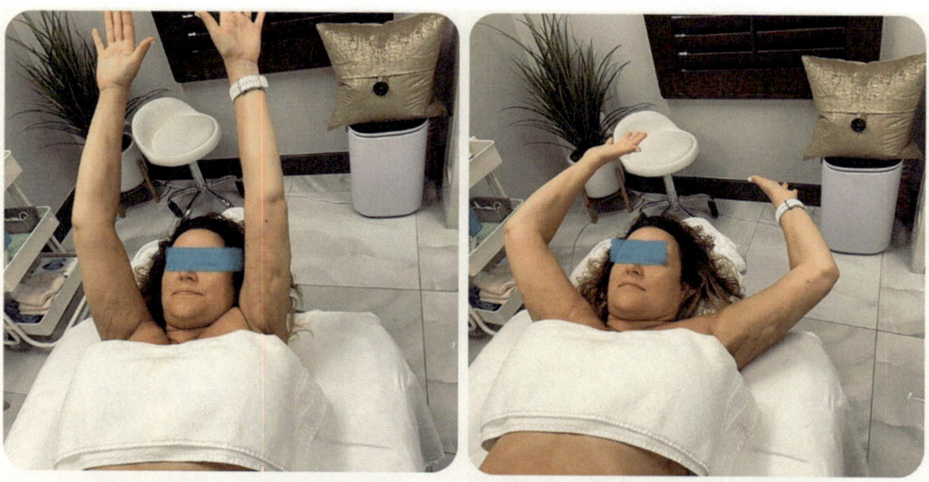

A. Arm liposuction 3 weeks post-op. Limited AROM to include shoulder flexion and shoulder abduction. Vertical adhesions in bilateral axilla, and significant induration of surgical site and surrounding tissues detected.

B. 60-minute session. incorporating lymphatic therapy, manual soft tissue work to indurated tissues, and PROM stretching throughout entire session. Patient reports tremendous progress in her ADLs due to increased AROM.

Figure 12.
A. Patient is very limited due to stage 3–4 induration and natural holding patterns (guarding). B. 1 hour later, the patient has quality improvement in her AROM for normal activities of daily living.

With no surgical restrictions after arm liposuction, **Figure 12** displays limited upper extremity AROM. This was hindering the patient's work and caused axillary discomfort. This treatment session reduced these issues and improved her work day. Postural awareness is of extreme importance and can be highly problematic if not addressed from a holding pattern and mechanical standpoint (**Figure 13**).

5.4 Scar and adhesion work

Scar and adhesion work is instrumental in the laying down of the scaffolding of the new collogen. Although early scar massage is advised against in wound care literature, it is advisable through observation and practical application to apply modified LT strokes across covered incisions from any body altering procedure. This aids in stimulating lymphangiogenesis and improving the patterning of the underlying scar tissue. In week 4, actual scar work begins along with any incisions to aid in releasing adhesion and 30-day dissolvable sutures (Monocryl), fully absorbed in 90–120 days (**Figures 14** and **15**) [12]. Paying close attention to patients showing a history of Keloids, as this will require more frequent monitoring and care to reduce excessive scar production. Optimizing scar appearance spans from the preoperative period to scar maturation.

After extensive scar/incisional work in the first 5–6 weeks, it is truly beneficial to implement silicon scar tape during the day and scar repair creams or gels at night, thus allowing the skin to aerate. From multiple applications, this author

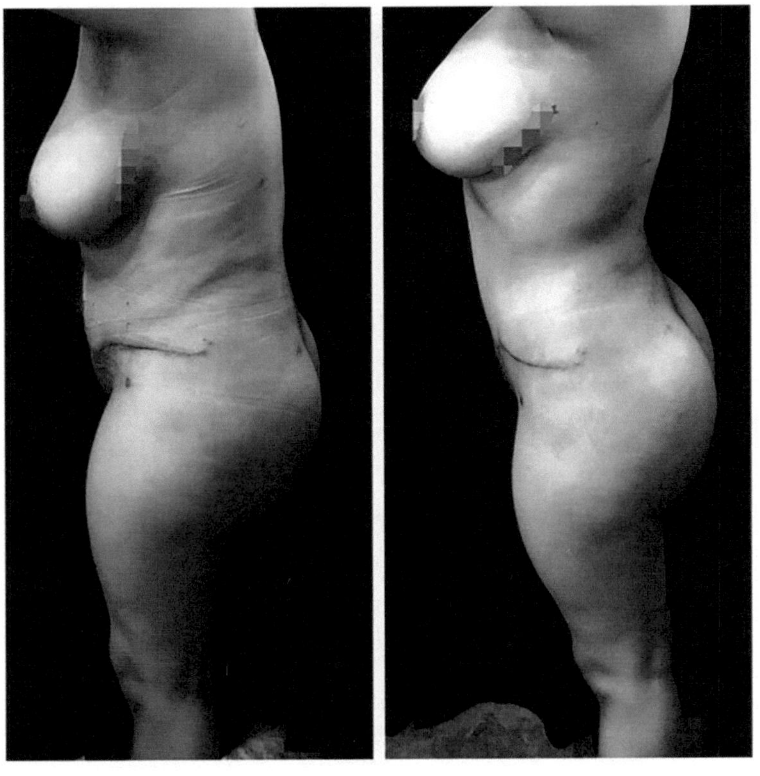

Figure 13.
Beginning at 4 weeks (first visit) to weeks, postural correction evolved with lymphatic therapy and manual tissue mobilization. Progression.

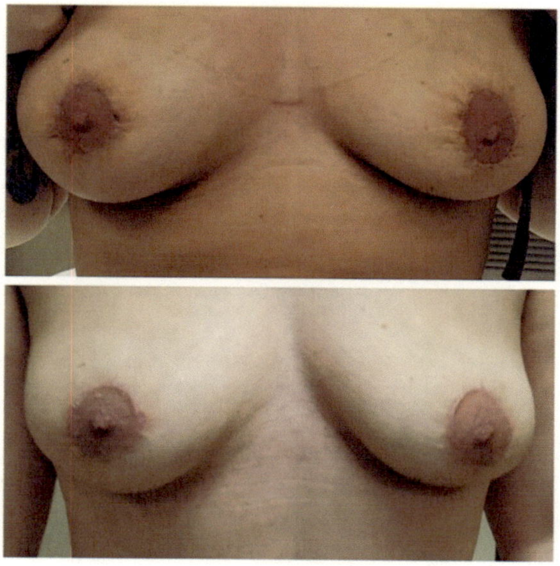

Figure 14.
Top. Nipple reduction 5 weeks post-op. She began post-operative care in her 5th week of recovery with no scar release work. Bottom. After 2 sessions the areolas relaxed from manual scar massage, Monocryl suture releasing and mild adhesion releasing, the incision smooth for a more natural outcome.

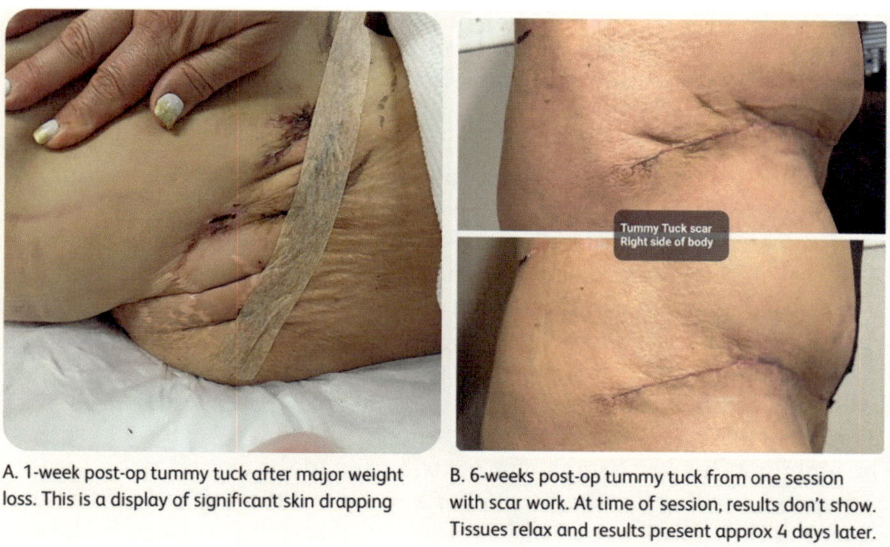

Figure 15.
A. This draping of tissue is necessary after major weight loss followed by a tummy tuck to ensure approximation of incisional tissues. B. With scar work beginning 1–6 days after surgery and continuing on in week 4 to incorporate scar massage, Monocryl suture release, and adhesion release, the drape scar that began can become more cosmetically pleasing.

has found that the use of thicker post-surgical silicone strips presents a more effective micro-level scar massage throughout the day with active movement. The suggested guidelines for post-op patients (**Table 1**) give a baseline standard for optimal outcomes [13, 14].

Scar treatments noninvasive guideline		
Product	**When to initiate treatment**	**Duration of treatment**
Paper tape	POD 7	≥ 6 wk.
Scar gels/creams	Wk. 6 or once scabbing has resolved	3–6 mo. alternating with use of Silicone sheets
Silicone gel sheets	Wk. 6	3–6 mo. 12/ hours, alternating with scar gels/creams
Scar massage	3 wk.	≥ 6 wk.

Table 1.
Table of suggested effective guidelines in the use of silicone scar tapes and scar repair creams or gels.

Scar work helps reduce compensatory strategies due to adhesions developing from patients holding patterns and guarding mechanisms. As Jan Trewartha (2016) states, "the aim is to re-integrate the scar tissue into the three-dimensional fashion matrix or fashion septal network by directly changing the tissue tension and enabling the system to recognize itself. Therapies can change the appearance of scars and the way in which they influence the surrounding tissues thus leading to the client having more freedom mobility and improved sensory function" (p. 18) [15].

Additional adhesion work will become palpable in week 3–4. The treatment required may be a simple as stretching to add to the curvature of the vertical adhesion and contour the waist line. However, it can be as complex as manually releasing (popping) to improve posture, mobility, and decrease and discomfort ensued from this occurrence. It is imperative that the post-op therapist can palpate the differences in regular adhesions and hi-def ab etching. Hi-def sculpting, ab etching, soft sculpting, all have the same intention, to create a canal for fibrotic tissues to laydown and create a natural looking abdomenal physique. This intentional scarring must not be confused with vertical adhesions or indurated tissues by the post-op specialist or patient. If they are not trained properly in manual work, they could potentially be ruined or have a less defined definition than intended by the surgeon (**Figure 16**).

5.5 Reducing risks of umbilical stenosis

The umbilicus is a key component contributing to the overall esthetics of the abdomen following liposuction 360 or any style of tummy tuck. This can be introduced at the time of surgery after closure. An earplug is placed in the umbilicus for approximately 1 to 2 weeks and then removed and replaced for several weeks thereafter [16]. There are certainly surgeon preferences on the process with umbilicus training. Some surgeons choose to defer this to the patient or post-op specialist in which **Figure 17** depicts the process for a post-operative session (**Figure 17**). Of researched articles, Dr. Milind Kachare [16] found "Most of the articles indicated that a smaller umbilicus was found to be aesthetically pleasing, but a numerical range of values were not specified" [17]. Therefore, helping optimize the presentation of the patient navel and training them how to carry over this routine care until no longer needed is a quality adjunct treatment during the post-operative session progression.

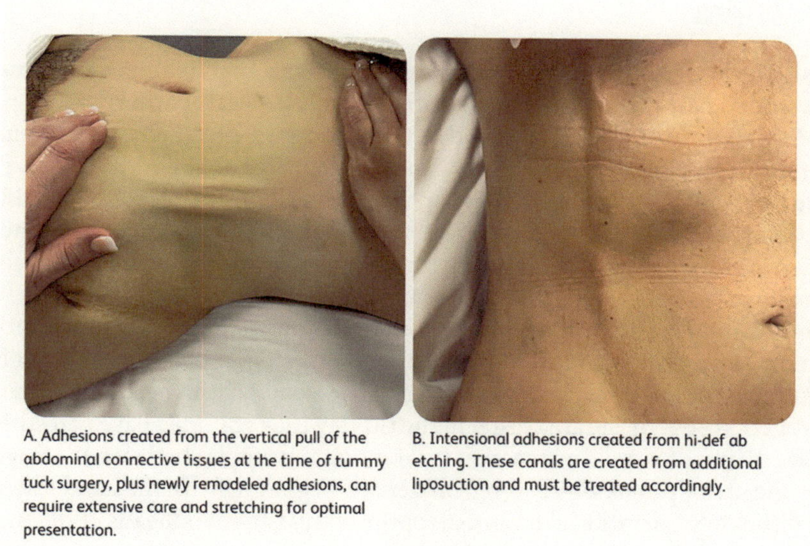

Figure 16.
A. Natural body adhesions B. Intential scarring/adhesions for hi-def abs along semilunaris.

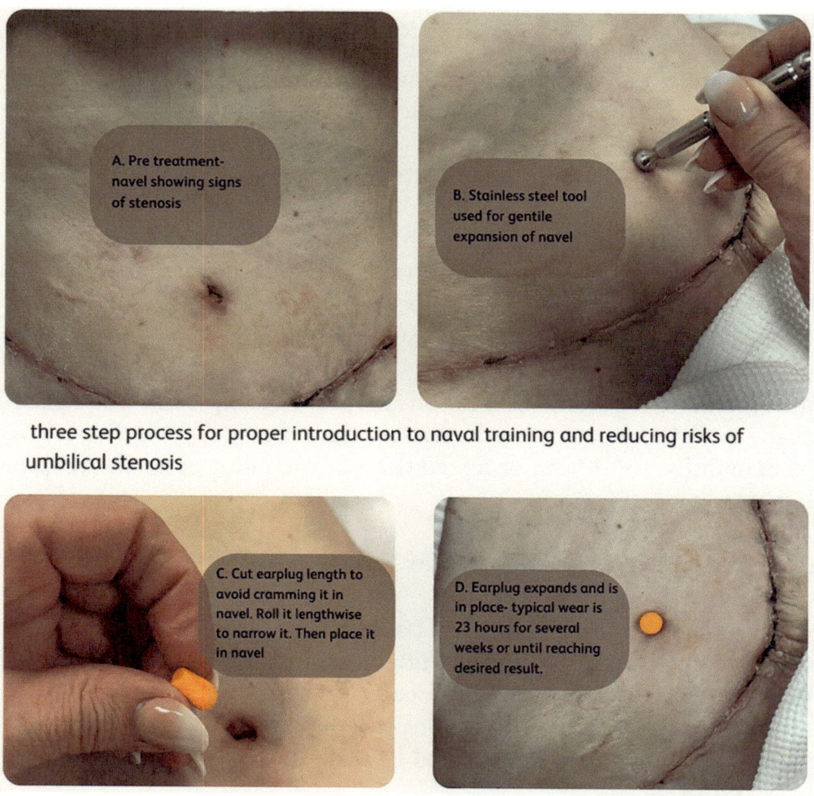

Figure 17.
A. Umbilicus in its narrowed state post-surgical B. Use of tool to manually do scar work and lightly stretch the navel. C. Shortening an ear plug to prevent cramming it in the umbilicus D. Utilizing the expanded and shortened ear plug as a soft dynamic stretch to the umbilicus to reduce umbilical stenosis.

5.6 Desensitizing

During the healing process, the body has natural internal itching, can be numb for an extended period, can be hypersensitive, and have neuropathic pain, or paresthesia. Mechanotransduction is defined as the process by which physical stimulation is converted intracellularly into various types of electrical or chemical signals [15], when the tissue matrix encompasses peripheral nerve endings/receptors [17, 18]. These specialized nerve endings may take up to 6 weeks or longer to regenerate and be responsive to stimuli. Until healing is complete, the above-mentioned occurrence of odd sensations or lack thereof may be normal for the patient.

Desensitization is a manual technique used in treatment and taught to the patient. For example, with a breast lift, reduction, or augmentation, the nipples may not have any sensation or lack symmetrical sensations, the torso may be hypersensitive to touch after liposuction 360, or the area distal to the tummy tuck scar may have paresthesia. For the nipples, there is a simple instruction for rotating the nipples between the fingers. For the body, the use of progressively rough materials, beginning with the hand, then wash rag, and ultimately tolerating a dry brush for the body is another means of desensitizing.

6. The optimal post-operative care knowledge

With post-op care, there are many things to take into consideration. When taking in the patient's information on medical history it is a helpful guide for care. Patients having comorbidities like diabetes, lipedema, or connective tissue disorders and may require adjustments to the treatment protocol.

6.1 Treatment metamorphosis and milestones

Regardless of comorbidities or not, each patient is an individual in their recovery process. The foundation of recovery "norms" is to be expected. However, it is safe to say that approaching each new case with a fresh template leads to quality care. Treatment is dictated by the patient's healing speed which will relay over to that individualized treatment metamorphosis.

From this authors repeated observation and personal experience, the patient will typically experience positive milestones in their recovery typically at 4 weeks, 4 months, 6 months, and 1 year, provided there are no unexpected interruptions in the healing process.

6.2 Emotional support *being equipped with the knowledge to educate*

Patients become hyper-aware of their body after a body altering procedure. They will observe asymmetries in the breast, buttocks, and body after a procedure. This is a normal occurrence due to our body not caring about symmetry while healing. Additionally, several aspects of a cosmetic procedure may involve "shape shifting" for 6 to 12 months as shown in **Figures 18** and **19** as it relates to the breast and buttocks (**Figures 18** and **19**).

Structural anomalies may give a distorted appearance of the results of a breast, tummy, or buttocks procedure regardless of if the patient knows they have a possible leg length discrepancy or scoliosis (**Figure 20**) or not; the realization of these impacting results can be emotional.

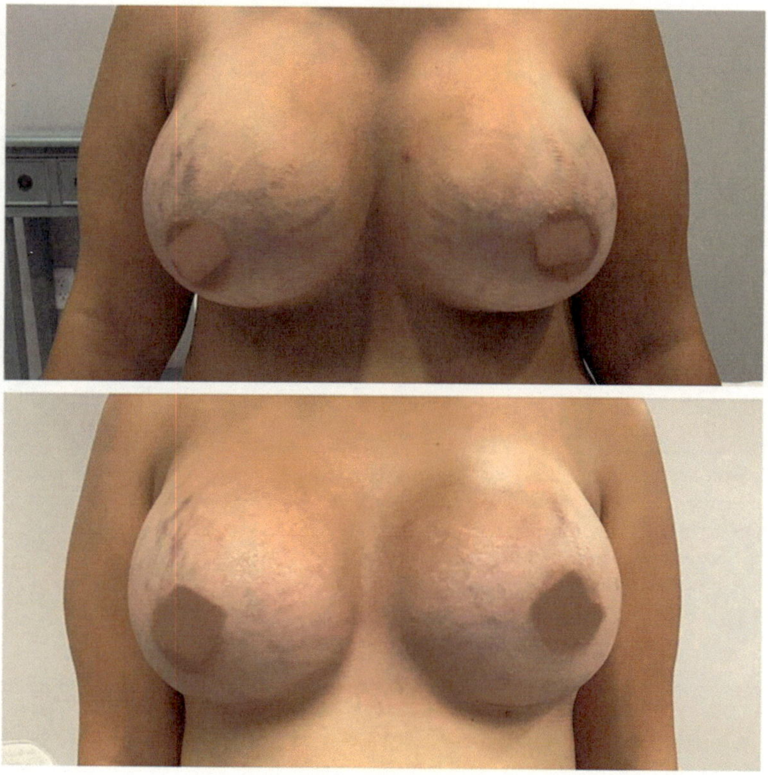

Figure 18.
Manual work weekly for 6 weeks along with patient training for pocket manipulation in the shape shifting process.

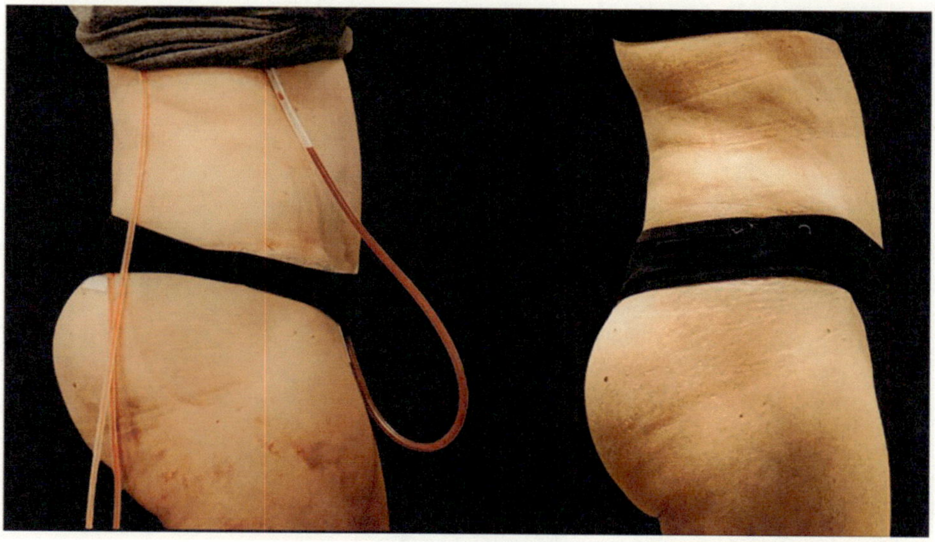

Figure 19.
At 4 weeks there is a dropping process after a BBL. The firm injected fat cells, and angry tissues begin to relax and soften, this begins the "fluffing" process. However, some patients fear they have lost their butt at this milestone and require education on the recovery process.

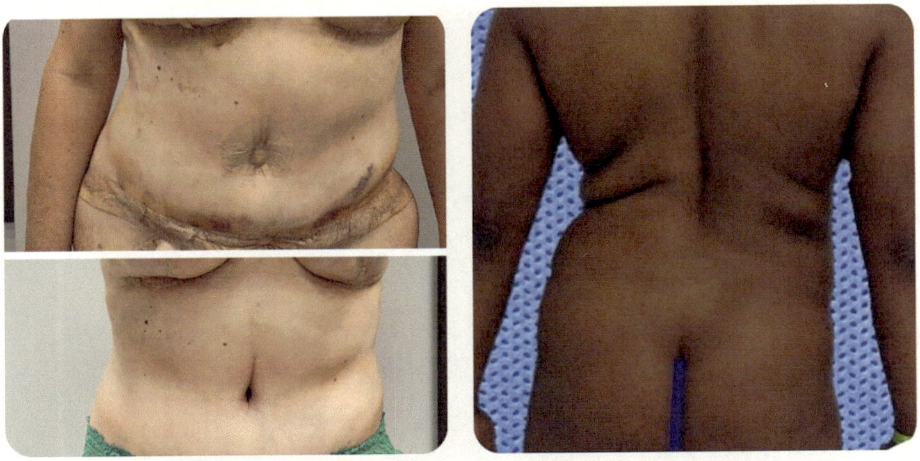

Figure 20.
A. Scoliosis was recognized after major weight loss and a tummy tuck. B. Scoliosis possible altering the outcome of a BBL.

The breast will go through possible shape shifting. However, when a patient begins to encounter a capsular contracture, this can be another emotional barrier to recovery. A patient may have a history of body dysmorphic disorder (DDD). Their body is something they have chosen to invest in and when things do not meet their expectations, they may begin to or already struggle with body image. The first several weeks of recovery can be an emotional roller coaster (**Figure 21**).

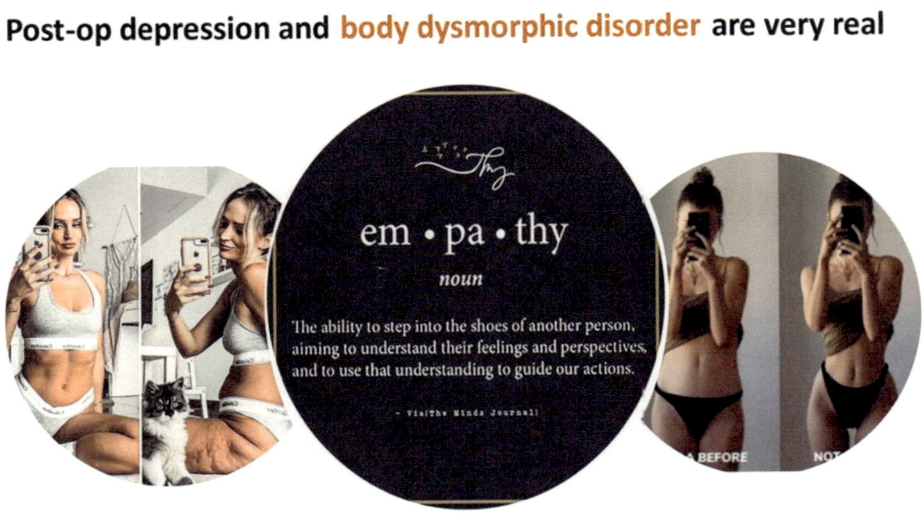

Figure 21.
Body dysmorphic disorder is not in our scope of practice to resolve. However, it is something a post-op specialist must be aware of to guide the patient through some education to ease their worries.

DOI: http://dx.doi.org/10.5772/intechopen.1008360

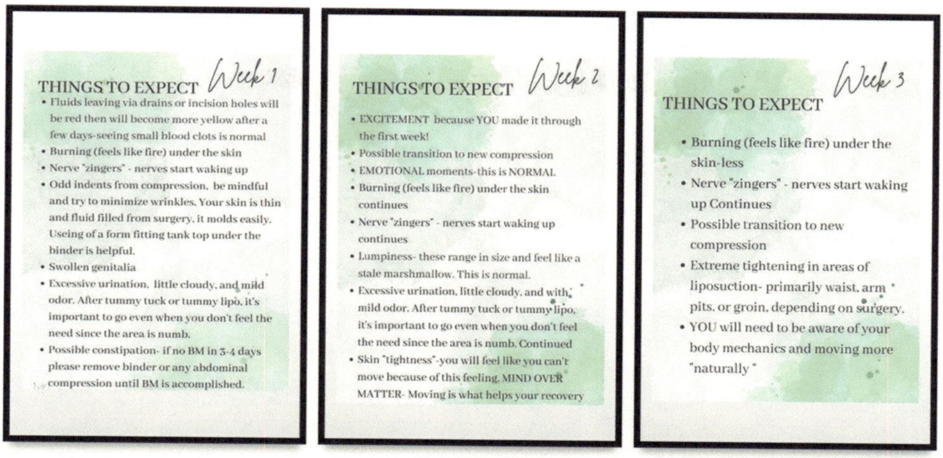

Figure 22.
A weekly list of possible things to expect post-surgically.

6.3 Patients' concerns - Normal or complication

Patients should be educated on things to expect (**Figure 22**).

i. Burning or sensation of hot lava inside of the tissues as a result of liposuction

ii. Electrical bolts or zingers as nerves begin responding

iii. Swollen genitalia after torso liposuction or tummy tuck

iv. Asymmetries and shape shifting of area recovering due to swelling and normal healing processes.

7. Patient home programs

For a year or more, recovery ensues, during this time the patient must become self-sufficient. With the proper therapist on board, they will be given home programs and have a means of communication for continued guidance. Post up care consists of multiple facets, tandem with patient's education and selfcare. The goal toward optimizing outcomes is to empower our patients. Giving them selfcare home programs makes them a part of the recovery team. Below are great examples of home programs (**Figures 23** and **24**).

8. Compression garments and recovery accessories

Not all compression garments are created equal, nor do they have standardized sizing. Compression is a necessary and beneficial component of aftercare. However, knowledge is key. Misinformation on social media can make this process with a patient somewhat difficult. The social media and patient goal may be to "get snatched," but this does not require a patient to squeeze their body unnecessarily into

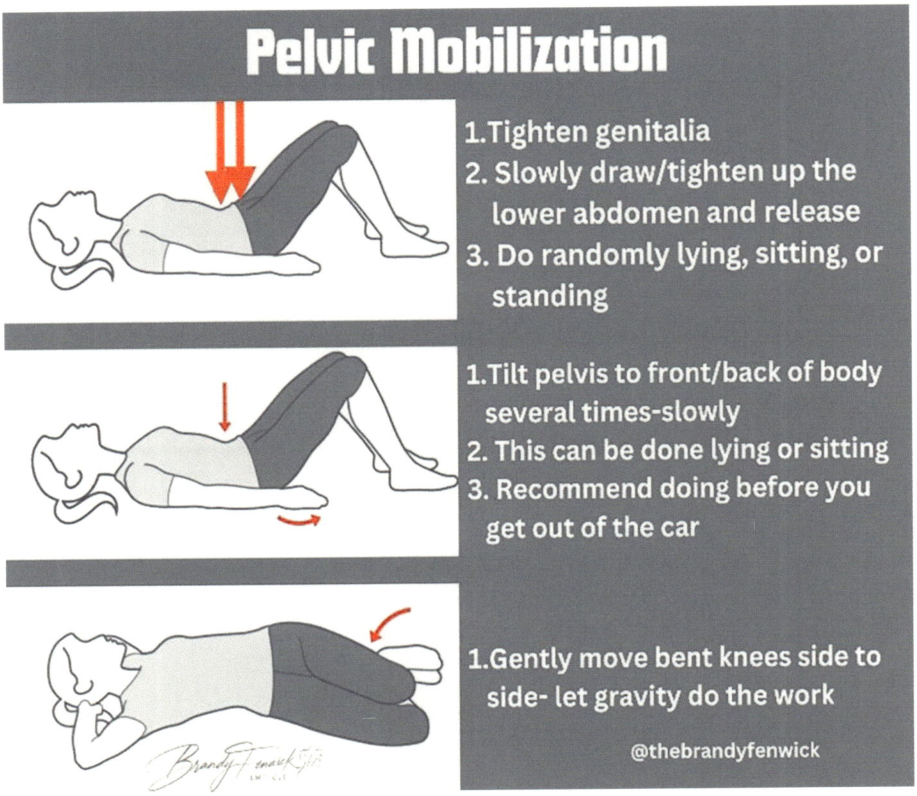

Figure 23.
At 2 weeks post-op liposuction or ant style of tummy tuck with abdominoplasty benefits from neuromuscular re-education and pelvic mobility.

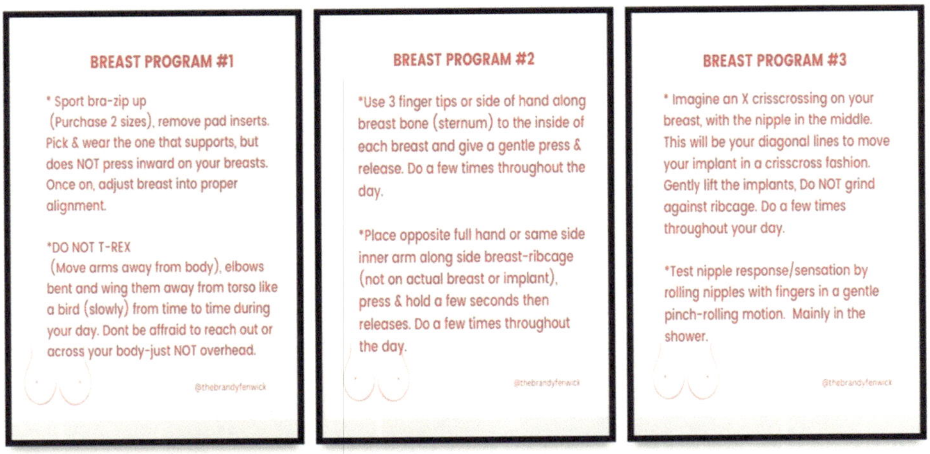

Figure 24.
Properly sequenced to give out at weeks 1, 2, and possibly weeks 3–5, depending on recovery. This breast program helps reduce the risks of capsular contracture.

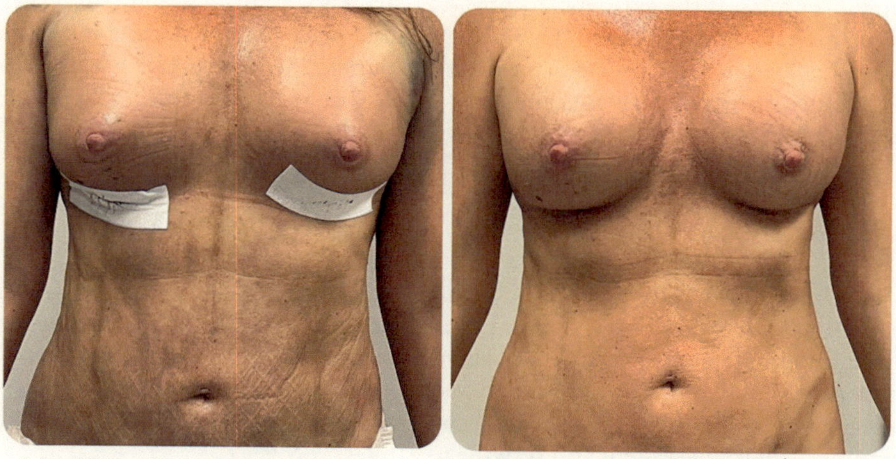

A. Day 1 Post-op Breast Augmentation

B. Week 8 post-op Transformation. Utilized 1 x weekly Lymphatic Therapy and Post-Op care to include home program and sequential garment wear.

Figure 25.
Breast augmentation, 8-week results.

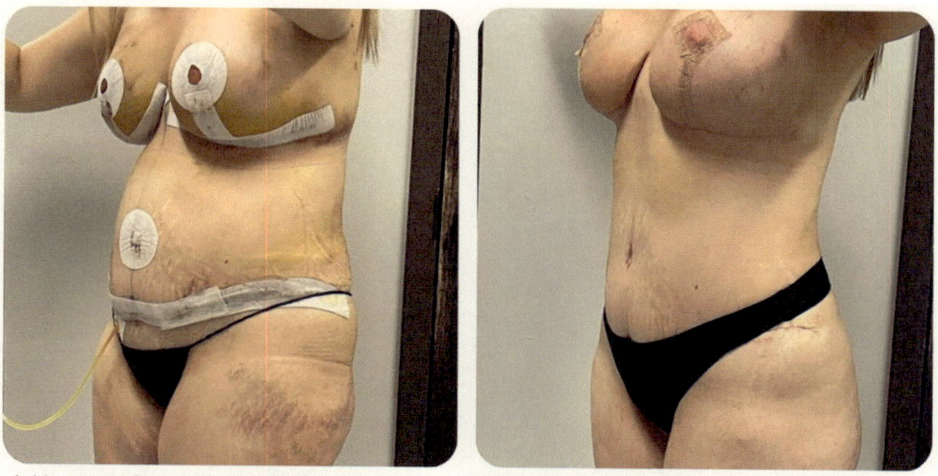

A. Mommy make over: Breast lift, breast augmentation, and tummy tuck with abdominoplasty

B. Same patient 8 weeks post-op

Figure 26.
Mommy makeover Breast lift, breast augmentation, and tummy tuck with abdominoplasty 8-week results.

excessively tight garments or fajas along with added accessories. Compression should be a firm hug, roughly 30–40 mmHg. The initial priority is to reduce the diffusion distance while allowing the natural healing, quality circulation, and intestinal peristalsis. Later as the stages of recovery progress, then the compression may progress and intensify. This is typically known as stage 1, stage 2, and stage 3 of post-surgical garments or fajas. If the garment fits properly, there is very little need for accessories such as lipofoam and ab boards. There is a time and place for add-ins and it is helpful to have the guidance of a post-op specialist. No patient is cookie cutter in the fitting and shaping process of garments and accessories. Our goal as a surgical and post-operative team is optimizing outcomes like the results in **Figures 25** and **26**.

9. Conclusion

MLD has evolved into a newfound practice of lymphatic therapy and post-operative care in the body altering esthetics industry. Critical thinking, understanding the science, and implementing proper treatment strategies help empower the patient. Ultimately the collaboration between the patient, surgeon, staff, and a post-op specialist will facilitate the quality outcomes desired by all involved. We are here to help protect their investment and provide a seamless recovery.

Disclosure Statement

The Author has nothing to disclose.

Author details

Brandy Fenwick
Tulsa Surgical Arts, Tulsa, OK, USA

*Address all correspondence to: postop@lacurvamethod.com

References

[1] Kleinlipo. Tumescent Liposuction [Internet]. 2019. Available from: https://kleinlipo.com/tumescent-liposuction/ [Accessed: September 29, 2024]

[2] Marxen T, Shauly O, Goel P, Tsan T, Faria R, Gould D. The utility of lymphatic massage in cosmetic procedures [Internet]. Aesthetic Surgery Journal Open Forum. 2023;5:ojad023. DOI: 10.1093/asjof/ojad023

[3] The aesthetic society. The positive patient experience: A comprehensive analysis of plastic surgery Online Reviews [Internet]. 2022. Available from: https://pubmed.ncbi.nlm.nih.gov/35417545/ [Accessed: September 25, 2024]

[4] Dr. Vodder School International. Manual Lymph Drainage History (MLD) [Internet]. 2024. Available from: https://vodderschool.com/manual_lymph_drainage_history [Accessed: September 28, 2024]

[5] Null M, Arbor T, Agarwal M. Anatomy, Lymphatic System. [Internet]. Available from: https://www.ncbi.nlm.nih.gov/books/NBK513247/ [Accessed: October 5, 2024]

[6] DiCecco S. Lymphed Preparation Course for CLT-LANA. Course Manual. Atlanta GA: LymphEd; 2021

[7] Academy of Lymphatic Studies. Complete Decongestive Therapy. Course Manual. Sebastian Florida; 2004

[8] Vascular Endothelial Growth Factor Signaling in Development and Disease [Internet]2018. DOI: 10.1242/dev.151019 [Accessed: September 28, 2024]

[9] The Essence of Palpation: How Do you Feel? [Internet]. 2008. Available from: https://leonchaitow.com/2008/06/14/the-essence-of-palpation-how-do-you-feel-2/ [Accessed: October 10, 2024]

[10] Lavigne T. Sensory Approach to Massage Therapy. Course Manual. Quebec Canada; 2018

[11] Woundsource. The Four Stages of Wound Healing [Internet]. 2016. Available from: https://www.woundsource.com/blog/four-stages-wound-healing [Accessed: September 25, 2024]

[12] Understanding Monocryl Sutures: Advantages, Uses, and Techniques in Surgical Practice. [Internet]. 2024. Available from: https://medicogrp.com/monocryl-suture/ [Accessed: October 15, 2024]

[13] Lee E. Updates on Postsurgical Scar Management [Internet]. 2016. Available from: https://www.ncbi.nlm.nih.gov/pmc/articles/PMC4961501/ [Accessed: September 25, 2024]

[14] Woundsource. Scar Management [Internet]. 2019. Available from: https://www.woundsource.com/patientcondition/scar-management#:~:text=Other%20clinical%20observations%20include%20continued.is%20restored%20by%20six%20weeks [Accessed: September 25, 2024]

[15] Avison J, Blyum L, Scarr G, Sharkly J. Scars, Adhesions and the Biotensegral Body Science, Assessment and Treatment. Boston MA, Pencaitland East Lothian, and London UK: Handspring Publishing; 2020. pp. 3-131

[16] Fell C, Kachare M, Moore A, Wilhelmi B. Does size really matter? A

DBT and Art for
Youth Suicide Prevention

of related interest

DBT-Informed Art Therapy in Practice
Skillful Means in Action
Edited by Susan M. Clark
ISBN 978 1 78775 208 5
eISBN 978 1 78775 209 2

DBT-Informed Art Therapy
Mindfulness, Cognitive Behavior Therapy, and the Creative Process
Edited by Susan M. Clark
ISBN 978 1 84905 733 2
eISBN 978 1 78450 103 7

Art Therapy with Transgender and Gender-Expansive Children and Teenagers
Kelly Darke and Shannon Miller
ISBN 978 1 78592 808 6
eISBN 978 1 78450 847 0

Art Activities for Children and Young People in Need
Helping Children to Develop Mindfulness, Spiritual Awareness and Self-Esteem
Diana Coholic
ISBN 978 1 84905 001 2
eISBN 978 0 85700 368 3

DBT and Art for Youth Suicide Prevention

When Art Saves Lives

Marney Schorr

Foreword by Rita M. Willey

Jessica Kingsley Publishers
London and Philadelphia

First published in Great Britain in 2022 by Jessica Kingsley Publishers
An imprint of Hodder & Stoughton Ltd
An Hachette Company

2

Disclaimer: The information contained in this book is not intended to replace the services of trained medical professionals or to be a substitute for medical advice. You are advised to consult a doctor on any matters relating to your health, and in particular on any matters that may require diagnosis or medical attention.

A CIP catalogue record for this title is available from the British Library and the Library of Congress

ISBN 978 1 78775 353 2
eISBN 978 1 78775 354 9

Printed and Bound in Great Britain by CPI Group

Jessica Kingsley Publishers' policy is to use papers that are natural, renewable, and recyclable products and made from wood grown in sustainable forests. The logging and manufacturing processes are expected to conform to the environmental regulations of the country of origin.

Jessica Kingsley Publishers
Carmelite House
50 Victoria Embankment
London EC4Y 0DZ

www.jkp.com

For my Dad
For cleaning up my spills
For being my rock
For believing in me when I couldn't believe in myself.

Contents

Part 3: DBT-Informed Art Therapy

Part 4: Other Risk Factors for Suicide: Trauma and Addiction

Part 5: Resources for Helping Professionals

List of Figures

There are additional images online that can be downloaded from https://library.jkp.com/redeem using the voucher code HGCYNEW

References to these images are marked with the symbol throughout the book.

Foreword

I have known Marney Schorr for nearly a decade in my capacity as both a primary care physician and a professional colleague. When I first met Marney, she was struggling, walking the tightrope of emotional and psychological distress. She felt as though she couldn't make it. Her soul was shattered with despair. Despite her recurring ups and downs, she did make it. She was able to overcome her obstacles by diving deep into her work in art therapy with young people who struggled much the same way she had. She plunged through and made it to the other side. Seeing her progress through the many stages brought on by hard and seemingly unendurable conditions has brought a light to the end of a long, dark tunnel.

When I learned Marney had met with our local healthcare system to design an arts-based suicide prevention program for young people, I was thrilled. Our small, rural county in Western Massachusetts is under-resourced to help teens and young adults at risk for suicide. As a healthcare professional, I have witnessed too many youth in the throes of what has become an epidemic—drug use, cyberbullying, rejection, depression, confusion of sexual and gender identity, and ultimately suicide. What Marney has created in only a few years has changed the way we can help our young residents in Berkshire County. Her program, Arts in Recovery for Youth (AIRY), has paved the way for adolescents and young adults to not only stay safe and recover from this epidemic, but to create full, meaningful lives. They have become empowered by artistic outlets for personal expression and through connecting with their peers in a healthy and hopeful way. AIRY has equipped them with the tools to survive, make meaningful contributions to society, and see bright futures ahead.

It did not take long for Marney to gain a widespread successful reputation as the go-to person in youth suicide prevention in the Berkshires. Her work has affected the lives of countless families and helping professionals throughout our community. I was not surprised by Marney's success, as I had always seen her strength, and the gifted and talented woman she is. I am in admiration of the way she has used her own personal experience to help others in crisis. Marney's own journey has been the catalyst for this life-changing program.

I am honored to write a foreword for this powerful and compassionate book about art therapy and suicide prevention with young people. In the book, Marney chronicles five years of inspired stories of the adolescents and young adults in the AIRY program while showcasing their beautiful artwork and describing the richness of their transformation. She thoroughly explains the details of the program, breaking down each component in a hands-on manner. She explores all of the research she has built upon from both the historical and contemporary canons of art therapy and suicide prevention literature. She posits that the keys to moving past youth suicidality involve learning skills with DBT-informed expressive arts therapy, increasing a sense of hope and belonging, and sharing the power of lived experience. Her book is both practical and evidence-based. It provides useful resources for parents, educators, mental health professionals, and the media, and a number of art therapy activities that youth have enjoyed in her art studio.

I feel blessed knowing Marney. I am delighted that I encouraged her to be all she can, knowing she had this deep, inspirational talent that others could learn and grow from. She continues to inspire me and I know her work will inspire others in a profound and personal way.

Rita M. Willey, DNP, FNP-BC, MBA, RN

Acknowledgments

I would like to thank all the individuals and organizations who have supported my work in youth suicide prevention and the growth of the Arts in Recovery for Youth (AIRY) program.

First and foremost, I am thankful to the 135 young people who have come through my studio door, shared their stories with me, and trusted me to help them. You have all inspired me and shown me the path toward hope. To my youth staff, Kiara, Rachael, and Jack—thank you for always having my back, for being willing to take direction and putting up with my endless handouts. Your strength has helped save so many lives. And to the many parents who have worked with me—with special thanks to Bonnie Bresett and Jeanne Kelly, we are all in this together.

I could not have persevered in this work without the support of my healthcare providers with whom I have developed long-term caring relationships. Thank you for holding space and supporting me through both my darkest times and triumphs: Holly, Antoinette, and Rita, you are remarkable women who have mentored and inspired me.

To my art therapy mentor, Ellen Joffe Halpern, I cannot express to you enough gratitude for allowing me to process my emotions with you each step of the way. Your kindness and compassion have kept me going and provided bricks for me to solidify the foundation of my work.

To my many colleagues that have supported my work, including my dear friend Peggy Morse—thank you for seeing my vision and for advocating for AIRY since day one. And to Stephanie Cohen, Kristen Vorisek, Joy Ruben, Jacqueline Pelzak, Lauren Muller, Megan Cooper, Leo Mazzeo, Tammara Leminen, Misa Chappell, Caroline Kelley, Myk Daigle, Joanie Ciolfi, Kathy Gideon, Karen Jacobs, Claudia Shuster, Craig Rand, Judith Fitzgerald, Frances King, Annemarie Jones, Jess Sweeney,

Katie Haig, Mary McGuiness, Allison Bayles, Nina Kryzak, Katy Holt, Em Reim Efrach, Cate Wolff, and Christina Marks. Thank you from the bottom of my heart.

In this small rural community, there have been so many organizations that have supported and collaborated with AIRY. Special thanks to the Berkshire Coalition for Suicide Prevention, Berkshire Taconic Community Foundation, the Barr Foundation, Berkshire United Way and Covid relief partners, the Local Massachusetts Cultural Councils in the Northern Berkshires (Pittsfield, Lenox, Great Barrington, Stockbridge, and West Stockbridge), The Golub Foundation/Price Chopper, Berkshire Bank, Annamaria College, the MA Department of Public Health, the MA Coalition for Suicide Prevention, Senator Adam Hinds, State Representative Tricia-Farley Bouvier, the Northern Berkshire United Way, Barrington Stage Company, Berkshire Theatre Group and the Colonial Theatre, CommonFolk, the Whitney Center for the Arts, 18 Degrees, Berkshire Health Systems, the Youth Zero Suicide Prevention Program, Berkshire Pulse, Brien Center, Bushnell-Sage Library, Clinical Support Options, Colonial Theatre, Counseling Center of the Berkshires, Extra Special Teas, Roots Teen Center, the Northern Berkshires Youth Coalition, *The Berkshire Eagle*, *The Berkshire Edge*, Mass Appeal, Channel 22 News, Unitarian Universalist Church, NUarts Studios and Gallery, and private donors in the community. Thank you all for believing in our vision.

Introduction

From the person to the profession—my story

This is my art studio. It is my safe place. It's where the magic of art therapy happens. It's a private space and a shared space. Hundreds of people have made art here and have left their mark on the tables.

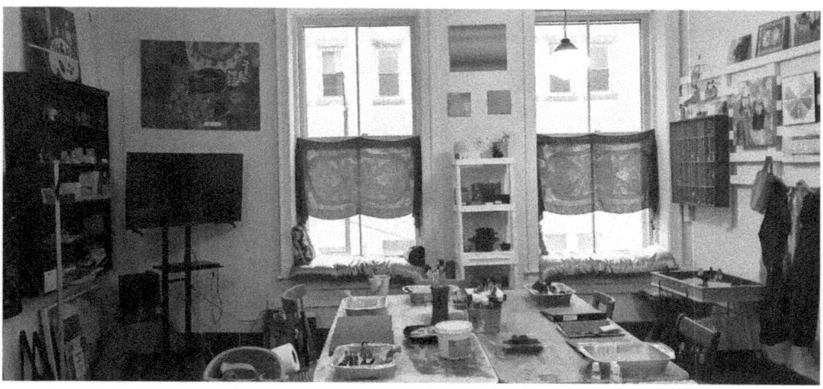

Figure 0.1 Art studio

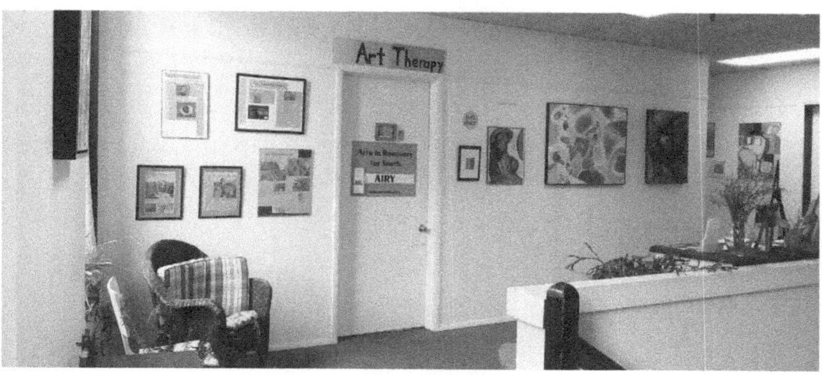

Figure 0.2 Art studio

I have been an artist for as long as I can remember. My first memories of art were my mother's paintings. In the living room she had used oils to portray a beautiful Spanish dancer at a bullfight. The canvas was decorated in a gold ornate frame that to me was like a museum masterpiece. I was completely captivated by the woman in the picture, her thick and luscious dark hair, her romantic red and white dress, her pure and passionate expression, her ruby red lips. I could not believe that someone in my family could paint such an enduring work of art. I find it ironic that to this day, my mother has never called herself an artist, she just was.

From a young age, my artistic instinct was heavily influenced by my mother's creativity. Growing up, art materials were scarce and she was resourceful. She taught me how to develop my own materials from household items and I learned to keep my eye out for them. She introduced me to the craftsmanship of the arts with things like calligraphy, sewing, garden design, stone sculpture, and production of decorative items to sell at craft fairs. She let me strum her acoustic guitar and exposed me to the Beatles, folk and traditional Irish music, as well as 50s dances like the Lindy.

It was easy for me to construct my own world of the arts and this world became my own private safe haven. I held it dear to my heart and took it seriously. As a child, I spent hours in my room designing my own board games, fan clubs, newsletters, poetry books, doll clothes, purses, and, of course, drawings. Since dance and music were also very popular in my home, and with money being tight, I spent my free time enveloped in art, music, and dance. I learned to tap dance, pirouette, do the Irish jig and 70s dances like the hustle. I sang and tried my hand at playing the spoons, harmonica, piano, bongos, and hand drums.

The arts were most definitely my therapy. As thankful as I am to have grown up with so much creative expression, it wasn't just for pleasure. It was how I coped. In hindsight, my own suicidal thoughts began as early as ten years old. I wrote a poem about wanting to be dead and drew clouds and a rainstorm. I was sad. I had the feeling that I was dead inside and wanted to just be gone. I had an instinctual sense that I lived with mental illness in my day-to-day life. After decades of processing it all, I have come to view my childhood and adolescence through the lens of trauma and adversity. Financial hardship, unemployment, loss, alcoholism, and violence were among the environmental factors around me contributing to my suicidal thoughts.

We were an Irish Catholic family of six, and we all attended Catholic school. There were no arts in my school curriculum, but nevertheless, I remained faithful to creative practices. Perhaps because of this, I never seemed to fit in. Bullying began early and followed me into my teen years. Moreover, I was quite a sensitive and eccentric child, desperately wanting to express the pain I felt in an outward fashion. Feeling that my voice was suppressed often resulted in dramatic and provocative behavior.

In my grammar school years, my father lost his job and my family moved from New York to Tennessee. We became isolated in a small rural town amongst farm animals and a completely different culture. I was able to use nature to self-soothe, running through open fields with nothing around but the sun and the wind. I helped my mother bake pies, tended to a variety of animals, and found solace in creating miniature worlds of pretend play.

When we moved back to New York, my grandmother died. The tone of the house was maudlin for a long time. My parents fought and my siblings and I tried to adapt.

When I was 11 years old, I went through further traumatic experiences within my family. Back then, there were very few resources for therapy, let alone dialogue about feelings. Seeking treatment for mental health issues was unpopular and often shameful. The words "mental illness" were never spoken. We lived in secrecy and silence. But I could express myself in drawing, painting, and poetry. I carried a sketchbook with me most of the time and had started drawing from observation. Sometimes my words and images were dark, but they served as a container for my experiences.

My first major onset of depression at age 12 prevented me from getting out of bed or leaving the house for over three months. I remember being terrified of the school bullies, lacking friends or any type of community connection. I learned I could stuff all those fears into a state of tired numbness, and usually stay in bed. I stopped making art or writing poetry or playing with my siblings. I isolated myself further and even deeper feelings of shame were reinforced.

When I didn't show up for school for three months, the courts intervened. I was ordered to mandated therapy with an agency social worker. I attended the sessions but didn't know how to vocalize what I was feeling other than in my art. I was resistant, I lied, and stayed angry for self-protection. In some strange way, the art-making and the destructive behaviors kept me from killing myself. I learned I could project those feelings outward and became a high-risk teenager. I got involved with alcohol and drugs, self-injury, and dating older boys to feel secure. I sold some of my art in exchange for drugs. I got high and drew more pictures and wrote more poems.

Daily life as an adolescent felt like navigating a minefield. Rather than talking about it, my siblings and I began to go our separate ways. Our motto was "every man for himself." Outside of the house, I attached myself to an older boy who played guitar in a rock band. Attending music gigs at local dive bars prompted me to channel my art into promoting the band. I drew flyers and album covers and explored photography of the band in my father's darkroom.

Major depressive episodes continued into my adulthood. To cope with my feelings, I published student art and poetry magazines, attended music events, and took long walks across campus. In my second year of college, I was repeatedly flooded with feeling suicidal. I remember driving my car home from college, wishing I could drive straight off a bridge, but at the same time, trying to just get home, to just stay steady. I don't know if I wanted to die or to just not live this life. The buildup of my psychological pain had just burst and I was truly powerless. Being suicidal was a complete mystery. We didn't talk about it and it was sinful. Despite my good grades, I had to drop out of college because, simply put, I couldn't cope. There were so many essential life skills that I lacked. But I did continue making art and I did stay alive.

After that, I stayed in therapy for nearly a decade. Not once did we talk about suicide.

I had returned to school to study visual art, gotten married, and was working full time as a paralegal, when I had my first psychiatric hospitalization. After eight years of sobriety, I felt myself in the midst of a nervous breakdown with the fear of my marriage ending. During that hospitalization, I learned what I was experiencing was a manic episode. Right away, it made sense. I had become inexplicably over-productive without appetite or need for sleep. I found myself taking risks in several areas of my life that were uncharacteristic for me. My mind and speech operated faster, and my creative ideas felt so fantastic it was like I had special powers. But I was also in the heart of a hurricane, where the urge to die by suicide completely consumed me. I tried hard to hide it, both from myself and from my loved ones. Inevitably it came crashing down and I no longer trusted myself to stay alive.

On the first day, I regretted my decision to sign myself in for treatment, because I quickly experienced the feeling of being trapped, knowing I was in "lockdown" on a psychiatric unit. It drove me into a state of panic and I had to be sedated. By the second day, my husband had delivered my art supplies and so that is what I did, make art to survive. It was during that hospital stay that I met two female staff in white lab coats who called themselves art therapists. It was their job to help people through the medium of art. This interested me right away, and although I first applied for my master's in fine art, I subsequently changed my mind to pursue art therapy as a career.

Five years after that first hospitalization, I thought I had recovered. I had no intention of killing myself when I awoke in my apartment that June day, though deep emotional pain had its grip on me—I was grieving a divorce, a job change, a geographic relocation, and the death of my cat of 15 years. My table was piled with books on existentialism and a few of yesterday's beer bottles. I was questioning the point of life. Mine lacked meaning and purpose after a broken marriage and not bearing children as I had planned. I couldn't see a new path. I was spinning my wheels and going nowhere. Close family and friends had drifted. I did not know how isolated I had become.

I never viewed myself as someone who would kill herself. In fact, I feared going to Hell with my religious upbringing. But I've come to learn that ideas about morality don't actually help solve the suicide problem. Becoming suicidal doesn't discriminate. White middle-aged males have the highest rate of death by suicide, but it runs wide across the spectrum from wealthy CEOs to homeless veterans, from working mothers to teens on social media devices, all feeling disconnected and alone.

In many ways, I thought I was fine and just in a state of transition. I tried to intellectualize everything but it wasn't working. Something that afternoon just snapped in me when the man I was dating gave me his reasons for our breakup. What I heard in my head was that I wasn't worthy of something normal, I was a failure, and I'd never fit in the world the way I wished I could. The dark voice of depression took over and I just had no more fight in me. I convinced myself that my family was better off without me and another needy phone call. Besides, I couldn't muster the words to ask for help. Hope was gone.

When I came to the next day, I was honestly shocked that I was still here. I wasn't sure if I wanted to be alive, but I was. I felt numb, confused, and shamed by the people around me. Someone had called the police when I emailed my suicide note. I was pretty sure I should have died and had no idea what to do next. It was all very strange and surreal and demoralizing. But somehow in that hospital gown locked away for a week I managed to put one foot in front of the other and found a room down the hall where I could make art. And that was what I did because that was what I knew.

That day was one of three suicide attempts, six psychiatric hospitalizations, and following that, the fourth of nine day-treatment programs. It took nearly 30 medications before I found the right ones and was properly treated for bipolar disorder. It has been an exhausting uphill trek to get where I am now. I am grateful for the discovery of dialectical behavior therapy in those treatment programs, which has shown me how to recover in an immensely practical way. I am grateful for a diagnosis I understand and the willingness to remain committed to my treatment. I eventually earned my master's in art therapy and began my own journey of using art to help others.

It took a while after leaving my job in Brooklyn and moving to the Berkshires before I discovered a way of life that suited my recovery. After decades of sacrificing my kitchen and living room to have an art studio, I finally opened a community accessible art space and an office in a small rural city known for its down-to-earth art scene. My two studios are among 18 others that form an artist's cooperative known as NUarts Studios and Gallery. We are art and expressive movement therapists, painters, sculptors, mixed media artists, jewelry makers, musicians, videographers, and writers, occupying the entire second floor of an old brick building downtown.

I am completely at home in my office and studio like I have never felt before. The studio is filled with a lifetime of art-making and the paint marks of over a hundred youth who have passed through. The tall windows pull in light from the north and the west, and their sills are lined with creative projects—clay figures, wire trees, painted rocks, homemade storybooks, and sand gardens—and plants and a sound machine. The rough wood floors are often covered in paint spills and glitter. The teens have painted my office in our program colors—spring green and white—and posters of our community events are pinned to the wall. A bright pink shag rug filled with pillows is coveted as a self-soothing sitting spot by all.

I am a suicide attempt survivor. I am also an artist, art therapist, educator, staff supervisor, presenter, and, now, an author. I have chosen to share my personal experiences in this book with the hope of offering a unique perspective—how my personal and professional growth led to my work in youth suicide prevention, and in developing the Arts in Recovery for Youth program. This I consider to be my life's work. So often do we not get to hear the personal stories of the therapists who create these safe havens for people in our communities, what we have learned and endured on our journeys to serving society, and what motivates us to do this work. It is my wish to reinforce the impact and value of sharing lived experience in finding solutions to the problem of youth suicide.

PART 1

Art Therapy and Youth Suicide Prevention

Chapter 1

The Development of Arts in Recovery for Youth

In an instant, the idea was born. It was a crisp autumn day in the heart of the Berkshires when I attended the local meeting for school adjustment counselors and other helping professionals who gathered to share resources in the auditorium. I was trying to spread the word about a new art therapy group for youth that we called the CIA—Culture, Identity, and Art. The group was fueled by my work with a 20-year-old intern from Springfield College and her desire to make a difference using art as a form of social action. We had been practicing guerilla art throughout the city—secretly leaving messages of hope in books at the public library, taping artwork on the bathroom walls of fast-food restaurants, placing traveling art on park benches, and writing thoughtful questions in sidewalk chalk on pedestrian crossings. We were hoping to recruit more underserved youth who needed a safe space to connect, make art, and ignite their own subculture in the city.

Following the meeting I was approached by an administrator of a new hospital program for youth suicide prevention. The hospital-based program had been spearheaded by the Department of Public Health as part of a national initiative to curb the dramatic rise of youth suicide. The administrator was excited about my work and asked me if I would be interested in doing an arts-based group for youth suicide attempt survivors with a focus on peer support. I remember the conversation quite vividly. I looked up at her sincere light blue eyes and paused. That was the moment, the very moment, that was about to change my life. So boldly, I said to her, "I am a suicide attempt survivor." And again there was a pause as she looked at me with great intent. She was pleased to hear it. It was a strange feeling. Suddenly, my recovering from a suicide attempt was a preferred job qualification. Our culture was changing. The value of lived experience was evident.

It took about five seconds for me to say yes. I didn't have to think about it, I just knew deep in my soul that this would be a life-changing journey personally and professionally. I had witnessed the power of art therapy to help all kinds of situations from depression, anxiety, and trauma to developmental disabilities, addiction, and recovery from cancer. Immediately my brain awakened. What if we, as a community, could create a safe space for youth to have their struggles heard and held, to challenge myth and stigma, to attack suicidality on the front lines with art? Why not use art therapy to prevent youth suicide? There was work to do and I wanted to do it. And so the mission began, fired by passion, sweat, and perseverance, guided by the force of a small community who cared more deeply than I could have imagined.

What transpired was an entirely grant funded program for youth suicide prevention through the arts. When I pitched the idea to the local coalition for suicide prevention that November, a unanimous vote gave us the green light to begin with a modest budget. After the first 12 weeks, our pilot group showed to be an astounding success. The phone began to ring with referrals from therapists of youth struggling with suicidal thoughts, from the hospitals where youth were being discharged after a suicide attempt, and from youth themselves who hadn't told anyone about feeling suicidal but had heard about the program from a friend. Soon after, I asked for more support and the community responded. We received additional funding from area cultural councils and helping organizations. We tripled in size within six months.

While some may have said don't put the cart before the horse, I didn't blink. I dove in with my heart and my mind and it all just fell into place. Those kinds of moments are rare in life, where another door opens with every step taken. I believed in what was happening and found it was simultaneously healing me. Creating and directing Arts in Recovery for Youth had become a new reason for living. There was no turning back.

Within four years we had served over a hundred youth. They were all safe and showing improvement. Teens and young adults with histories of multiple suicide attempts were in complete remission. Suicidal thoughts were decreased. A network of young people were regularly helping each other to recover, based on a foundation of non-judgmental acceptance, safe talk, healthy boundaries, and the expressive arts. Word reached the State Coalition for Suicide Prevention, the Massachusetts Statehouse, and the Senator, who presented us with an award for leadership in suicide prevention. We were invited to speak at the Annual Massachusetts State Suicide Prevention Conference. We were in the news and on tv. And then I took home the Top 25 Award for the Most Influential, Creative, and Dedicated People of the Berkshires.

What had happened? One day I was just doing what I do. And someone asked for my help. I thought back to the last day I had tried to end my life, to the horrific feelings of shame afterward, to the damage that had been done in my life, and the building, brick by brick, back to wellness. I could not have conceived that I would be writing this book. And when I thank the universe for keeping me alive, I like to imagine this is why.

When I began my research in suicide prevention, I had a felt sense of understanding specific to suicide attempt survivors. Not only could I cognitively process theory and practice, and creatively apply it, but I could also embody it from my own experiences. I could intuitively feel how it worked, and this was a gift. At times, I was faced with my own suicidal thoughts and applied what I was teaching others to my personal recovery. It reassured me. With my history, I realized that if I could do it, so could they.

When battling my own depression, I was able to express to the youth in the program what was happening with me and how I was coping. My 30-plus years of working toward recovery is a factor in the mentorship aspect of our work. My shared lived experience is authentic yet safe. There is a light at the end of the tunnel for all of us and they understand that we are in it together.

Arts in Recovery for Youth (AIRY™) is a unique hybrid program for adolescents and young adults who are at risk for suicide or who have survived a suicide attempt. It combines art therapy, dialectical behavior therapy (DBT), best practices in suicide prevention, and recovery-oriented peer support in an art studio setting. The premise of the program is that suicidality can be lessened and managed through creative expression, skill development, and sharing and valuing lived experience.

In group art therapy, suicidal urges are decreased through creative adaptation of DBT skills and in developing reparative bonds that form a new kind of social connectedness amongst peers. Expressive arts therapies offer a variety of learning styles to accommodate all growing young people. Peer support functions as a framework for building shared narratives of survival and recovery. From the depths of adverse experiences and the lens of the expressive arts, youth discover personal meaning, strengths, and talents, and learn they can make a difference.

AIRY was created by listening to the voices of caring and devoted community members in the rural towns of Western Massachusetts. We looked at what issues the contemporary young person was facing that were contributing to suicide, and how we could help. We met with parents of suicidal youth, survivors of suicide loss, clinicians, adolescents and young adults, behavioral healthcare agencies, youth organizations, our local Suicide Prevention Coalition, the administrators of hospital-based intervention programs for suicidality, the Department of Public Health, and the Senator's office. We also collaborated with area artists and art organizations that are prominent in the Berkshires, and who have a strong helping hand in the community. Collaboration was key in the formation and rapid growth of the AIRY program.

Our development was a direct response to the tragedy of youth suicide in our neighborhoods. We are a rural community with a population of approximately 126,000, with the largest number of people in the city of Pittsfield, centrally located in the County. There are benefits and disadvantages to living in a rural community. There is a lack of resources that are only found in a big city. There are fewer choices and less diversity. But on the other hand, anonymity is rare. People know each other and there is a short degree of separation from community members. Word spreads quickly. Residents band together to make change. I believe that the environment of the Berkshires played a crucial role in the success of Arts in Recovery for Youth. And for this I am very grateful.

Having served over a hundred youth between the ages of 13 and 26 in the last four years, we have measured an average reduction of suicidality by 77 percent within 8 to 12 weeks, 86 percent within six months, and 95 percent within one year (see outcomes data in Chapter 22). Graduates of the program report feeling safe, loved, and wanted; making great strides in personal goals for the future; a sense of belonging and connectedness; and the knowledge of what to do if they or someone they know is feeling suicidal.

The Arts in Recovery for Youth program has implemented a number of strategies developed from research in suicidology and the peer recovery movement, as well as best practices in suicide prevention and art therapy, and the adoption of skills from DBT.

Solutions to feeling suicidal depend on learning new life skills. These skills can be learned organically through the expressive arts. Art therapy is both serious and fun, expressive and contained, structured and spontaneous. The art studio itself is a unique, experiential world, and often a different encounter than youth are accustomed to. I meet young people who have never picked up a paintbrush, sensed a piece of clay in their hands, or been given permission to tear out images from art magazines. The fascination and exploration of art materials is a new, exciting expedition all of its own. Since the skills are taught in an art studio setting, the clinical atmosphere and its barriers are removed.

To provide a summary of how the arts work in therapy for youth who are feeling suicidal is a large task, which will be explored in depth in this book. While initially there was a bit of trial and error, our program has deepened and expanded at a rapid pace as young people contributed their insights about what works for them. I have sought constant feedback from both youth and their parents to make sure I am not asking too much of them. What I have discovered is that teens and young adults want to be challenged, and that attentively inviting them to examine their thinking and behavior gives them a sense of confidence and power. It is a beautiful thing to witness how they each have the capacity to become their own healers.

In this book, I have also included the stories and testimonials of members of our community who have helped keep the AIRY program alive and growing. Below are testimonials from youth, parents, and area artists who share their experience about the program.

A testimonial from a young adult who graduated AIRY

I was first introduced to AIRY when I was a sophomore in high school. I had a friend who had recently come out of hospital from a crisis and they were referred to the AIRY program as a new outlet to help them out. I was asked by them to come along and provide support because they had no clue what AIRY was or what they'd really be walking into. I've had a wonderful relationship with that friend for years but what I really have to be grateful to them for is introducing me, even if by accident, to one of the best programs I've ever experienced.

Since about the age of 12 or 13 I've struggled with depressive symptoms and I remained in a state of public denial for years about it, only telling my closest of friends and one of my brothers details of how I felt; to everyone else I was happy, energetic, and animated. Every day in my early teen years I would get home from school and collapse, my energy would drain, my focus would soften, and it was open season for terrible thoughts and depressive behaviors to take hold. It was as if I took a mask off and hung it on my bedroom door when I'd get home. Without that mask I was freed from the feeling that I had to be happy, which left me more sad and broken-hearted than ever.

Not even my own mother, who I loved more than anyone else, was aware of my constant inner dialogues and how low I had begun to sink in those years. Marney's studio just across town from me was the first place I was ever able to take off my mask with several other people around, not just other people but strangers, a small group of folks that above any difference of background or lens, I could relate to because of the experience we shared with depression and suicidal ideation. It didn't even take long, maybe two or three weeks in a row at the studio alongside my friend, before I felt comfortable showing what I believed were my true colors. I was able to openly discuss where my depression had led me and how I too was struggling with managing dark and turbulent thoughts that derailed my life.

In other programs that I had been a part of in school and within my community, I would spend months at a time getting to know people and working with groups that at a glance would seem similar to AIRY, but I could never open up in the way that I wished I'd been able to. The tone and deep level of discussions in AIRY were unlike anything I'd experienced before. Through the process of making art (for which I had no confidence in myself) I was able to open up gateways of conversation and interpersonal understanding that I wouldn't have thought possible. I figured out how to combat my mental health issues.

I was shocked at the reception I received when I took the time in groups to talk openly about my day-to-day experiences and my feelings. I fully believed that any attempt to explain myself and discuss my depression would be met with pity and pseudo-inspirational chatter to convince me to simply try again the next day. I thought my true colors would show the group a hopeless loser with no fighting chance to get back to the kind of happiness he felt as a child but everyone at the table saw more than what I did. They told me I was insightful, well spoken, empathetic, earnest, and (after a while when I started to crack jokes) pretty funny to boot. I would go home on Wednesday nights after a group at the studio, look in the mirror, and see what they could see. After a very long and painful period in my life I could look in the mirror and smile.

AIRY members have a process to go through when they join, with the referral, intakes, consent forms, therapist communication, and all that to make sure that a member of the group is well equipped to use the group to full effect. I skipped all those steps my first day, thanks to my just popping in on a session mid-season with the excuse "I want to support a friend of mine, can I start showing up here?" Marney could see that I was having a positive effect on my friend's time with AIRY. But when I told her that I wanted to stay for a while I was met with those consent forms and intake meetings, that all seemed fair to me, and so I signed on properly without thinking of the horrible side effect that would come with it—I had to tell my mother about my depression.

My denial was still in full effect and my mom did not know what I often had felt for the past three years. When my mom pulled around the corner of North Street to drop me off, I asked her to come up with me to see the studio. How I had the courage to ask I may never fully know, and she agreed. It took maybe ten minutes after I asked her to come up when Marney broke the news about how much this group deals with depression, anxiety, mental illness, and suicide. Those were words that a parent never wants to associate with their kid.

It took another five minutes for Marney to pull out a consent form and hand it to my mother. She read it through. She asked me why she would have to mark a box stating that she was aware of her child's struggles with depression and suicidal thoughts. She was truly scared and she wanted to hear from me that this is what I wanted. We walked into the hallway together and had the most awkward and heart-breaking conversation I've ever been a part of. Honestly it took a lot out of the both of us, but it opened up a dialogue between me and my parents that I had never been able to start before.

My mom started to research depression in teens and young adults, and talked with Marney and myself after group every single week. She stood by me at every chance she could to help me to understand and overcome that dark, dangerous cloud spinning around in my dome. A gift like that is completely invaluable. My relationship with my mom has changed for the better and it will never go back to how it was when I felt alone in a fight against my own feelings.

I continued with AIRY for two years before graduating from the Step-Up program that Marney led, the whole while writing poetry, painting, attending events and conferences, and learning from people like me what they would go through and how they would cope. Those years were amazing for getting me to a place where I could put on less and less of a facade at home and in school. Over time I became more comfortable in my day-to-day life, and I discovered more of what made me who I am.

Where am I after graduating from AIRY? I could discuss here any of my opportunities or achievements, my dreams and goals for the future, or the kind of person I've become as I near 19 years old with high school behind me. But I want to make it much more simple than that. I am alive. I have a lot to improve on, a lot to strive for, and so much support surrounding me. For that I am thankful. But above all, I am alive. Whether I would be without AIRY is really impossible to know. I am more than glad to be in the timeline where I joined and can confirm that I wake up every day.

My discovery of the program, falling head over heels for it, breaking the ice wide open with my family, and using AIRY to get better and become more of myself for as long as I was able to stick with it, has all changed my perspective on the value of my own life and my individuality. It has allowed me to feel like I'm a small part of a much larger family, one that I never have to stop being a part of. I am immensely grateful for all Marney and AIRY have given me.

A testimonial from an AIRY intern

I came to AIRY as an intern with interest in learning about art therapy, and I gained knowledge in AIRY of therapeutic methods. I was a college student at MCLA (Massachusetts College of Liberal Arts) and was navigating through the choices of wanting to be an art therapist or an art educator. When I found AIRY, it was my beginning step in this field. It turned out to be the best decision of my life because AIRY deeply moved me.

I have gained skills and knowledge while interning with AIRY. It allowed me to learn the language of art therapy and its techniques. The skills helped me personally and to see how they benefit the lives of many people. I learned about mindfulness, regulating emotion, self-care, and peer support.

My most favorite thing that I created in AIRY was an abstract painting I did. The painting was structured around an emotional regulation exercise. The task was to identify an emotion that we were consistently feeling all week and then figure out what the opposite of that emotion was. Then, we would demonstrate the two emotions in whatever way we envisioned or felt it to be or look like. And the reason that I enjoyed it the most is because it redirected my thinking and emotion to a positive outcome, and helped to evolve my mindset.

One of my most memorable moments in AIRY was the very first day when I was introduced to AIRY, Marney, and the kids that we were working with together. AIRY is a safe space that allows you to be who you are and develop into a stronger individual.

A testimonial from a parent

The AIRY suicide prevention program is rapidly gaining repute as a "go to source" for counseling, skills, teen camaraderie, support, guidance, and a healthy avenue for teens to feel connected to others like themselves who are dealing with suicidal ideation and other mental health issues. Art therapy provides therapy without pressure, without a clinical environment in which many youth do not feel comfortable, therapy without seeming like therapy—Marney provides a tremendously fabulous blend of counseling and art and healing and teaching the kids to listen to themselves, and to listen to others—really listen—not like your common gatherings with teens—not social media—not online—but face to face—in a calm, supportive, and creative atmosphere.

Without the AIRY program we can assure you that our own son was in direct and acute danger of potential death by suicide. My husband and I were not qualified to recognize the distress signals that he was presenting—but Marney was—she stressed the importance of seeking immediate inpatient treatment when it was necessary—and he got treatment—but we strongly believe that the reason our son was able to successfully pull himself up and out of his despair was because Marney had provided him with essential tools that he was able to draw from and utilize during and after his treatment. Had he gone to treatment without having met Marney first, without having had that time to work with her and learn from her and get those tools, we are not certain the outcome would have been as successful. Marney saved his life. Of that we have no doubt. The AIRY program saved his life.

We shudder to think of what will happen to the many youth out there if the AIRY program is discontinued. Currently Marney is working to grow the program in order to accommodate more youth as the word spreads that this program works—to be able to reach out and ask for help without being looked upon as a problem—without stigma—and with the love and support that is necessary to survive. AIRY is truly a valuable resource in the Berkshires—and hopefully eventually beyond the Berkshires.

A testimonial from a parent

The Arts in Recovery for Youth (AIRY) suicide prevention program in the Berkshires is unlike any other program available to youth at risk of suicide. AIRY offers expressive arts, counseling in a safe space, peer support, a sense of hope and belonging, coping skills, and an outlet to discharge suicidal thoughts and emotions.

The first clinician my daughter ever encountered completely dismissed her suicidal thoughts, making her feel even worse. Marney has always validated my daughter's feelings and has been the one consistent support person we could count on for the past four years.

AIRY uses the expressive arts to help youth who are suicidal and in a way that breaks the stigma of receiving mental health services. My daughter is not one to open up and talk about her feelings in a clinical setting, and Marney's approach not only made her think, but also allowed her to heal. In fact, Marney has had such an impact on my daughter's life that she is now enrolled in college pursuing a degree in psychology and art and plans on attending graduate school to become an art therapist.

Without the AIRY program, I feel that my own daughter would not be here today. Marney has helped my daughter in more ways than one can imagine. She has given her hope, supported her, boosted her self-esteem, inspired her to fulfill her dreams, and given her the necessary skills to recognize the danger signs and act upon them immediately. My daughter has gone through the 16-week program as a young teen, currently participates in a Step-Up group, and has become a skills counselor, while also serving as an intern. This program literally saved her life, and for that I am forever grateful.

Without the AIRY program, my daughter and many other suicidal youth who are in dire need of support will be in danger.

A support letter from Berkshire Theatre Group

I am the Administrative Director of Education for Berkshire Theatre Group. I have worked with Marney Schorr for the past two years in planning our community awareness event for youth suicide prevention during Valentine's week, called Love Yourself—a collaboration between Arts in Recovery for Youth (AIRY) and Berkshire Theatre Group at the Colonial Theatre in Pittsfield. We share a mission with AIRY, increasing access to the arts for underserved populations in our county and creating opportunities for creative youth development.

Since 2018, I have worked hands on with Marney and the many youth who are served in the AIRY program. I have heard the stories of young people, as they emerge from a place of high risk for suicide to a place of resilience and transformation. This winter, seven of these teens and young adults stepped up to do the planning of our event, collaborating with six local professional artists and performers in the community such as the Berkshire Theatre Group Youth Chorus and the Dancers of the Berkshires. The event was an outstanding success and AIRY received an Official Citation from State Representative Tricia Farley Bouvier who came to the event to support this very important program.

Simply put, AIRY uses the arts to save lives. Youth move into leadership roles, not only enhancing their skills in suicide prevention and the arts but making a significant contribution to society and culture.

Allison Rachele Bayles, Berkshire Theatre Group

A support letter from the Pittsfield Cultural Council

The Pittsfield Cultural Council, of which I am Secretary, has supported the work of Marney Schorr, the Founder/Director of AIRY for the last three grant cycles. Through her arts-based suicide prevention program she has relentlessly and successfully worked to save the lives of over 90 teens and young adults at risk for suicide.

Since 2017, AIRY has served 18 towns in Berkshire County and the surrounding area. The program directly addresses the public health problem of youth suicide. Sadly, this demographic area has the highest rate of suicide in the state of Massachusetts.

When AIRY began its arts programming for families of youth facing suicidal tendencies, the Pittsfield Cultural Council approved a grant at the highest allowable amount. With the success of the first year and the growth of AIRY, we continued to approve grants at the highest allowable amount.

Ms. Schorr has collaborated with established cultural organizations in Berkshire County and has organized and promoted a variety of shows, art exhibitions, poetry readings, and music in which her clients were participants. These cultural programs helped to move her clients from introverted and seriously depressed/anxious states to improved self-esteem, improved social skills, the ability to handle social situations they could not have done previously, and so much more. Furthermore, through these collaborative efforts there has been a high level of community engagement in the arts as all have been free and open to the public which has led to increased access to the arts for under-served populations. AIRY has saved many lives. The benefits of AIRY have been unprecedented in serving the teens and young adults in Berkshire County.

Berkshire County benefits from this program in many ways. Not only does it teach youth suicide prevention, but it also provides creative avenues for self-expression where youth learn the skills they need to thrive as emerging young adults. Several youth who have attended the program have moved forward into leadership roles and are now making significant contributions to society.

Through AIRY's collaborative design, the Pittsfield Cultural Council has proudly assisted in effecting change for the young adults who attend the program and many other youth. The work this program does is so very significant. It is my hope that AIRY can become a sustainable resource for young people and their families, and to continue the important work it is doing in Western Massachusetts.

Karen Jacobs, Pittsfield Cultural Council

In the chapters ahead, we will look at the origins and development of art therapy with suicidal individuals and go deeper into how art therapy benefits adolescent development and youth suicidality. Best practices for suicide prevention and safety planning are explained, as well as current theory in suicidology, the lived experience model, and what it means to be a survivor. In later chapters, we will examine dialectical behavior therapy for use in art therapy and the ingredients of a youth art therapy group for suicide prevention. I will discuss the effects of the global pandemic on the AIRY program and how to help youth cope with collective trauma. Factors that contribute to suicidality such as addiction are also examined more closely. Finally, chapters in self-care for helping professionals and art therapy directives for youth suicide prevention are included as well as several appendices with further resources and information.

Chapter 2

Origins of Art Therapy with Suicidal Individuals

I have found over the years that not many people know about art therapy. It is a highly specialized field. During the years in which I studied art therapy in graduate school, I learned a vault of knowledge that I didn't know existed. I became utterly fascinated by its history and development which is by no means simplistic. The discovery of art therapy ignited a fire within me that continues to burn bright. I believe it will be useful to the reader to provide an overview of the origins of art therapy and how it was applied with suicidal individuals, beginning with an evolutionary perspective.

Evolutionary perspectives of art

Using art to help youth who may be feeling suicidal is not actually a new idea. While the term "art therapy" first arose in 1942, the practice of using art as a means to stay alive is inherent in our ancestry. Since the beginning of time, art-making has been used in civilizations with a variety of implications for survival. This suggests art-making has an evolutionary basis for our species.

Steven Pinker (1997) investigated the biological roots of the significance of art and the idea that "evolution created psychology" (p.210). We have an aesthetic inheritance that promotes our adaptation as a species. Pinker suggests that art-making arises from the inborn tendencies of our ancestors. They needed to hone their perceptual abilities to survive and to communicate knowledge of survival in symbolic form.

We can look as far back as cave art in examining the roots of art therapy. John Pfeiffer (1982) explored prehistoric cave art in the Upper Paleolithic or Stone Age. He suggests that art-making was used to indoctrinate the young, to enhance memory, and to transfer knowledge for survival in the group.

Contemporary researchers expand upon this idea, indicating that cave art was essential in communication. For example, linguist Shigeru Miyagawa studied the timelines of cave art in France, Spain, Indonesia, and Southern Africa, estimated to be between 40,000 and 120,000 years old (Miyagawa, Lesure, and Nóbrega 2018). He observed that acoustics were a principal reason for the placement of drawings within caves, located in deeper, harder-to-access areas. The convergence of sound and drawing in the caves creates a "cross-modality information transfer" of auditory information and visual art which characterizes human language (p.1).

According to Alland (1977), the ancient origins of art-making may be a by-product of evolutionary mammalian behavior. Art-making was a form of play and exploratory behavior, verbal communication, and a capacity for perceptual discrimination. It prepared the young for adult life and for navigating the environment. It played a crucial role in the formation and continuance of social groups necessary to survival of the species.

Ellen Dissanayake (1995) describes art as a universal behavioral propensity of the human species—a part of our biological heritage. She explains that art arose from the evolutionary desire to make important things special. It was also used as a protective mechanism to detect threat in the environment. More than aesthetic, art was used in daily life for passing on cultural values. Art served as a form of bonding and ritual crucial to survival. Art allowed people to participate in behaviors such as singing, dancing, storytelling, body painting, and decoration of possessions.

In addition to works found on walls within caves, and art forms used in daily life, historians look to the portable sculptural artifacts of the Upper Paleolithic period to tell us more about the evolution of art-making. One of the oldest known works of art is the Venus of Willendorf (25,000 BCE), sculpted from oolitic limestone, one of three figurines unearthed at Paleolithic archeological sites at Willendorf in Austria.

In 1908, Josef Szombathy, an Austro-Hungarian archeologist, discovered the Venus of Willendorf during excavation by the Natural History

Museum of Vienna, outside the small Austrian village near the Town of Krems, at just under 4½ inches high. According to Zygmont (n.d.), the object's small scale signified a remarkable allocation of time and effort, and was deliberate for the purpose of carrying during nomadic travels in search of food. The sculpture, which retains traces of a red-ochre pigment, is noted to be a representation of the reproductive and child rearing aspects of a woman, whose function is related to fertility (Witcombe 2013).

Such artifacts hold great symbolism for communities. Even in the earliest times, art expressed aspects of human nature such as pain and suffering. In a fascinating book by Ron Brown, *Art of Suicide*, the earliest known image of "self-killing" is identified. The death of Ajax by sword is represented on a small Corinthian seal dated c. 700 BCE. This image of suicide is seen to be both male and heroic, and enmeshed with mythology. This and other images provide information about evolving cultural attitudes toward suicide since the dawn of civilization.

For instance, although there was no word for suicide in the languages of Greek antiquity, images from this time portray that "to die by one's hands was not wrong in itself, but good reason was required" (Brown 2004, p.22). On the other hand, Brown opines that the lack of images of suicide in pre-Christian and pagan times may reflect that the visual representation of suicide was actually taboo. From the early Christian era to the 15th century, images of suicide appear as a product of diabolical despair, linked to sin and the supernatural. Most imagery from this period reflects suicide related to religious discourse.

How suicide is imagined in visual terms is also the subject of the book *Suicide and the Creative Arts*, by Steven Stack and David Lester. They set forth the idea that the visual arts can offer insights into the nature and causes of suicide, including social and cultural predictors. Historical art as early as Sophocles' plays from 2500 years ago suggested motives for suicide that include "trauma or grief over the death of a significant other, shame over deviant behavior, reunion fantasies, blocked anger and suicide to escape suffering" (2009, p.8). In another example—the frequently painted narrative of the Queen of Egypt—Cleopatra's self-inflicted death in 30 BCE from a poisonous snake bite is seen as a heroic suicide to escape capture by the Romans.

It is important to note that art has not just portrayed suicidality or functioned as a means for survival. It has also offered direct practical applications to suicide prevention. Stack and Lester note that "artistic work itself has been thought of as a life-saving behavior for some suicidal artists" (2009, p.1). Studying 646 artist suicides, they provide case studies to increase understanding about the high incidences of suicide and mental disorders among artists. They suggest such suicide rates may be in part due to the insecure nature of artistic work as an occupation dependent on clients. This is not to be misunderstood. Art and the art-making process itself are not a cause of suicide. Expressing oneself through art often provides relief from feeling suicidal. However, it has sometimes been the case that the *perceptions* of artists—as to whether their art product meets social approval—can contribute to low feelings of self-esteem that many artists struggle with. Worrying about how society receives their art could trigger social aspects of suicidality for some artists, such as feeling alienated or like an outsider.

Art historian Fred Cutter examined how cultural attitudes of suicide are reflected in art in his book *Art and the Wish to Die*. He argued that art has more of an effect on public attitudes about suicide than do scientific works. Changing public opinion about artistic images to include anti-suicide messages can support efforts in suicide prevention (1983, p.x).

In *Art as Therapy* (de Botton and Armstrong 2013), philosopher Alain de Botton outlines seven core psychological functions of art that can be helpful in suicide prevention. He suggests that art helps us feel less alone in our suffering. Art provides a form of hope. Art is about remembering and self-understanding.

Studying the evolution of artistic images through recorded documents of history shows us the multiple advantages of art in life—from how art-making evolved into language, ritual, and even a mechanism for survival to driving cultural attitudes about suicide and conveying the psychological forces of human suffering. It is a fascinating expedition to trace the timeline of the function of art in becoming the therapeutic practice that it is today. We now turn to exploring later movements in art history alongside the development of psychoanalysis to further reveal early contributions to the field of art therapy and its application with suicidal individuals.

Romanticism, psychoanalysis, and emotional expression in the arts

Romanticism was a movement in Western history that occurred from the late 18th to the early 19th century. It was seen as a rebellion against the Age of Enlightenment and all its scientific advances. The movement spurred the development of both psychology and psychiatry. This was especially true in Germany where the idea of the unconscious transpired. It is also where verbal psychotherapy or "talk therapy" began (MacGregor 1989). These developments changed the way we view the human psyche. The cause of mental disturbance, as revealed later in the 19th century by Sigmund Freud, Carl Jung, and others, was no longer evil possession, but a conflict of the mind. This is where art therapy had some of its first underpinnings.

The art of the Romantic period was radical. It depicted, for the first time, pure emotional expression. Artists came to believe that the strongest emotions to be expressed in art came from "the dark side of the mind" (MacGregor 1989). The best artists came to be viewed as mad geniuses who were often rejected by society.

In light of the new Romantic art, doctors took an interest in what was called the "art of the insane." This study evolved into using art for diagnostic measures and as a therapeutic tool (MacGregor 1989). As a means of cataloguing patient art, doctors began to group and classify artworks by disorders. Paul-Max Simon, a French psychiatrist, published studies of the drawings of the mentally ill as early as 1876, followed by Cesare Lomboso in 1887. In 1901, French psychiatrist Reja classified artwork of patients into subtypes. The first drawing tests for psychiatric use were developed by Fritz Mohr in 1906. Walter Morganthaler studied and wrote about the artwork of his patient Adolph Wölfli in 1921.

The 1922 publication of Viennese psychiatrist and art historian Hans Prinzhorn is most widely cited by scholars today as the seminal work classifying the art of psychiatric patients. *Artistry of the Mentally Ill* studied the formal qualities of art present in the work of Prinzhorn's patients with schizophrenia. Prinzhorn recognized art as a mode for aesthetic and communicative potential. He discovered that art was a creative means for self-healing (Rubin 1986).

In this work Prinzhorn discusses the psychic functions of major characteristics in the art of his patients. He explores aspects of art such as the expressive urge and the urge to play. He catalogued the many aspects and functions of art he observed in his patients:

- intuition and fantasy
- the decorative roots of art
- art's relation to the animal kingdom
- form, arrangement, rhythm, and order
- visual perception
- the need to imitate
- the eidetic image
- symbolic significance
- extraction of meaning.

Prinzhorn found that the "productive forces" of untrained artists with mental illness, and especially those with schizophrenia, may have been born out of their mental illness. He also found that specific components in their art were related to the symptoms of schizophrenia. These included the arrangement of formal elements and a tendency toward repetition and ordering. He found patients with schizophrenia showed "an uninhibited stream of invention" (1922, p.266). Art for them was connected to an incapacity to adapt to reality.

Prinzhorn's work was novel, inventive, and groundbreaking. He opened the first real door to art therapy that would be explored for decades to come.

> With the aid of the pictures we found new insights into the psychic life of patients...which may through a critical evaluation of analogical phenomena, offer us insights into and solutions to many problems in psychopathology...pictorial creative power is present in every person... this primeval process which incorporates the subconscious components in almost pure form. (Prinzhorn 1922, pp.273–274)

As doctors like Hans Prinzhorn and Emil Kraepelin wrote textbooks about mental illness, the use of patient art for psychiatric research became more legitimized. They looked at patients who were supported in making art in asylums. One example is Wilhelm van Kaulbach, who is known for his depictions of mental hospitals as early as 1835. He experienced a catharsis in making his drawings. Art for him "was undertaken with the goal of helping him to recover from his depression...as a means of salvation from mental illness" (MacGregor 1989, p.22).

Another example of a patient artist in the nineteenth century is Charles Meryon, who was provided with a studio and supplies while living at an asylum in Charenton in 1855. He had been diagnosed with "delirious melancholia" (MacGregor 1989, p.84). His symptoms included paranoia and isolation. Meryon's architectural drawings have become well known and were published in a catalogue, *Charles Meryon: Prints and Drawings* (Burke 1974).

The recognition of the "art of the insane" coincided with the emergence of psychiatry and neurology. At the same time a growing number of exhibitions of Romantic art were held. Francisco Goya was a Romantic artist who depicted the art of the insane in his paintings such as *Corral de locos* (1794) and *The Madhouse* (1812–1819).

The progression of historical art movements that depicted the art of the insane moved from Romanticism to Expressionism and later to Art Brut. The Expressionists drew their inspiration from the primordial nature of children's art and the art of other cultures, especially Oceanic and African. Their search for the primitive led them to the discovery of the art of the insane. This became evident in their style.

The Expressionist period in art was significant for another influential psychiatrist and art historian, Ernst Kris. Like Prinzhorn, Kris studied the art of his patients from both a psychoanalytic and historical point of view. He noticed that his patients returned to a primitive, childlike mental state in order to work through the confines of their illness. He termed this process "regression in the service of the ego." "The essence of his thesis is the regulation of the ego and the individual's ability to bind, neutralize and channel energy toward creative work" (Robbins and Sibley 1976, p.29).

Kris theorized that during art-making there existed a paradoxical space in the human psyche where a patient could remain intact while suffering from symptoms of a psychiatric illness. This he called the "conflict-free sphere" (Kris 1952).

An example of Kris's theories can be seen in the work of Expressionist artist and patient Ernst Ludwig Kirchner. Around 1905, Kirchner joined a subgroup of Expressionism in Dresden, known as Die Brücke ("the bridge"). Many of the Die Brücke artists addressed the human condition at a time when Germany was involved in two world wars. They explored themes of suffering, sorrow, and passion. They often elicited political overtones that responded to Hitler's banning of their art as "degenerate" in Nazi Germany. Sadly this was one of the harrowing events that led to Kirchner's suicide in 1938 (Arnason 1998).

Kirchner suffered a nervous breakdown while serving in the First World War and subsequently lived in a sanatorium for two years. "He experienced severe delusions of persecution and physical symptoms that were probably the result of hysterical paralysis, and at times, was so dangerously suicidal as to necessitate constant supervision" (MacGregor 1989, p.226).

Kirchner had stated that he used his work to keep himself alive. In his regression he found enough strength to survive his psychoses, demonstrating Kris's notion of a conflict-free sphere.

Studying the works of "insane" artists led to an unprecedented common ground amid doctor and patient. A new triad of relationships grew that is at the heart of art therapy—that between patient, doctor, and art (MacGregor 1989). Psychiatrists discovered that art materials could offer patients a means to experience organization of the mind and to measure reality testing. Psychoanalysts used art to develop assessments for their patients, such as the Rorschach in 1921, the Thematic Apperception Test in the 1930s, and the Holtzman inkblot test.

Even Freud used artwork in his case studies such as a drawing by the father of Little Hans, the first case of child analysis, in 1905. Freud also made use of patient art in the case of the Wolf Man in 1918. He described how his patient made a drawing of his dream.

Freud's concept of the "id" describes the rawest material of the psyche. The id is analogous to the content and methods of achieving Romantic art. Like the id, this art is pure, expressive, and uninhibited. It represents the fulfillment of wish fantasy that is a major tenet of psychoanalysis.

While these developments moved forward in psychiatry and art history, veterans of the world wars were introduced to art for its therapeutic qualities. In 1942, war painter Adrian Hill coined the term "art therapy" in his book *Art Versus Illness*. Hill had served with the Honourable Artillery Company during the First World War and was commissioned by the Imperial War Museum to record the conflict on the Western Front in drawings. He went on to work with veterans in the Second World War to treat mental disorders using art.

During the Second World War, group therapy and art therapy began being integrated into rehabilitation movements for traumatized war veterans. Psychiatrist Karl Menninger established the Menninger Foundation in 1941 and founded the Winter Veterans Administration Hospital in Topeka, Kansas, which offered art therapy as part of their psychiatric services to returning Second World War veterans. Menninger asked artist Mary Huntoon to organize one of the first art therapy studios in the United States.

Clearly the progression of the roots of art therapy spans centuries—from art as a means of survival and ornamentation in human evolution, to historical periods representing the art of the insane; from a means of emotional release for patients in asylums, to its use as an aid in psychiatry and with veterans returning from war, and to yet another field that influenced its development, that of art education, explored in the next chapter.

References

Alland, A. Jr. (1977) *The Artistic Animal: An Inquiry into the Biological Roots of Art.* New York: Anchor Books.
Arnason, H.H. (1998) *History of Modern Art* (4th edn). New York: Harry N. Abrams.
Brown, R. (2004) *Art of Suicide.* London: Reaktion Books.
Burke, J.D. (1974) *Charles Meryon: Prints and Drawings.* Toledo, OH: Toledo Museum of Art.
Cutter, F. (1983) *Art and the Wish to Die.* Chicago: Nelson/Hall.
de Botton, A. and Armstrong, J. (2013) *Art as Therapy.* New York: Phaidon Press.
Dissanayake, E. (1995) *Homo Aestheticus: Where Art Comes from and Why.* Seattle, WA: University of Washington Press.
Hill, A. (1942) *Art Versus Illness.* London: Allen and Unwin.
Kris, E. (1952) *Psychoanalytic Explorations in Art.* Madison, CT: International Universities Press.
MacGregor, J.M. (1989) *The Discovery of the Art of the Insane.* Princeton, NJ: Princeton University Press.
Miyagawa, S., Lesure, C., and Nóbrega, V.A. (2018) Cross-modality information transfer: A hypothesis about the relationship among prehistoric cave paintings, symbolic thinking, and the emergence of language. *Frontiers in Psychology 9*, 115.
Pfeiffer, J.E. (1982) *The Creative Explosion: An Inquiry into the Origins of Art and Religion.* New York: Harper and Row.
Pinker, S. (1997) *How the Mind Works.* New York: W.W. Norton.
Prinzhorn, H. (1922) *Artistry of the Mentally Ill.* New York: Springer-Verlag.
Robbins, A. and Sibley, L.B. (1976) *Creative Art Therapy.* New York: Brunner Mazel.

Rubin, J.A. (1986) From psychopathology to psychotherapy through art expression: A focus on Hans Prinzhorn and others. *Art Therapy* 3, 1, 27–33.
Stack, S. and Lester, D. (2009) *Suicide and the Creative Arts*. New York: Nova Science Publishers.
Witcombe, C.L.C.E. (2013) *Venus of Willendorf*. Apple Books.
Zygmont, B.J. (n.d.) Venus of Willendorf. Khan Academy. Retrieved from www.khanacademy.org/humanities/prehistoric-art/paleolithic-art/a/venus-of-willendorf on November 8, 2019.

Chapter 3

The Influence of Art Education

The roots of art therapy are unique—a hybrid ranging from evolution and art history to the development of both psychiatry and art education. We will now take a look at where art education began and how art educators became pioneers in the field of art therapy. The marriage of art education with psychoanalysis shows us another fascinating avenue into this specialized field.

As early as 1792, Benjamin Franklin advocated for art education in his book *Proposed Hints for an Academy*. Developments around the world over the next century explored the use of art in education in a myriad of ways, opening the door to its many uses to help youth (Whitford 1923).

The first documented book for teaching art in the United States happened in 1825 with William Bentley Fowle's *An Introduction to Linear Drawing*. Over a decade later another significant development occurred. Fredreich Frobel opened the first kindergarten in Germany in 1837. Kindergarten was a radically new educational method and philosophy using games, play, songs, stories, and crafts to stimulate imagination and develop physical and motor skills.

These and other moments in the timeline of art education were catalysts of what was to become the Progressive Education Movement in the 1880s (Reese 2001). This was a period that began to move away from the Euro-American tradition of classical preparation for the university dependent on social class, toward an opportunity for all. Scholars like John Dewey argued that the purpose of learning was to allow children to grow mentally, physically, and socially while becoming creative critical thinkers. According to Dewey, education was a social and interactive process that should reflect all areas of development of humans in society, including art. In 1883 the National Education Association designated a Department of Art to promote art education in the classroom.

Shortly after, Franz Cižek began the Child Art Movement in Vienna (Malvern 1995). He held exhibitions of paintings and woodcuts by his students in Great Britain to raise money for his Juvenile Art Class. Such exhibitions of child art, along with the child art movement, promoted the idea of the "child as artist" and supported the free "natural" art-making of children as opposed to the traditional regimented school art of the time. In this new tradition, Alfred Stieglitz opened an exhibition in 1912 of children's art at his New York 291 gallery. Stieglitz saw children's artwork as displaying "universal humanity" through its genuine, expressive, and free qualities.

At the same time, Italian educator Maria Montessori developed the Montessori method that included reasoning, imagination, and creativity in the classroom. Rudolf Steiner began the first schools of Waldorf education which holistically integrated practical, artistic, social, and academic experiences. Through hands-on activities, Steiner focused on developing artistic expression, social capacities, critical reasoning, and empathic understanding.

In 1924, Margaret Mathias wrote one of the first well-known books on art education, *The Beginnings of Art in the Public Schools*. American educator Ruth Faison Shaw is credited with introducing finger painting as an art education medium. She developed her techniques in Rome, Italy, before patenting a safe non-toxic paint in 1931. After developing her expressive medium for children, Shaw devoted her attention to the therapeutic benefits of finger painting. At the request of Karl Menninger, Shaw taught at the Southard School at the Menninger Foundation in Topeka. Later she served as a consultant to the Department of Psychiatry at Memorial Hospital at the University of North Carolina at Chapel Hill.

Following the Great Depression, the Federal Art Project (FAP) was created to provide work relief for artists in various media—painters, sculptors, muralists, and graphic artists—with various levels of experience. The program sought to bring art and artists into the everyday life of communities in art centers, exhibitions, and classes (Library of Congress 2015).

The arts brought hope following such a sad time in history. The FAP was just one of several government-sponsored art programs of the period. Others included the Public Works of Art Project (PWAP) (1933–1934), the Department of the Treasury's Section of Painting and Sculpture (1934–1942), and the Treasury Relief Art Project (TRAP) (1935–1938).

A marker moment in the intersection between art education and art therapy was Viktor Lowenfeld's book *Creative and Mental Growth* in 1947. It was to become the single most influential textbook in art education. Lowenfeld classified children's development into artistic stages. Art therapists continue to use these stages as a guide in their work with youth. For example, toddlers aged two to four exhibit development through what is called the Scribbling stage. This stage marks the first development of a child to visualize in pictures. The next stage is the Preschematic stage where children four to six years old begin to create circular images with lines that suggest a human or animal figure. They also explore the emotional aspects of color. From seven to nine years old, children enter the Schematic stage and progress toward spatial relationships, often drawing pictures of their family and their environment. From 9 to 11 is the stage of Dawning Realism where children develop perspective and show their own point of view. Finally, from 11 to 13 is the Pseudo Realistic stage which conveys more subjective experiences in art.

In the 1950s two seminal art educators turned their focus to using art therapeutically. Margaret Naumburg and Edith Kramer began using art therapy in school settings and then later in psychiatric settings (Vick 2003; Rubin 2010). These two women are often viewed as the art therapy pioneers responsible for the development of the two schools of thought about art therapy, commonly known as "art as therapy" and "art psychotherapy."

Both introduced the therapeutic use of art in schools to help children with behavioral problems. While no formal training had yet been established in art therapy, Naumburg and Kramer, along with a handful of other individuals, began to define the discipline in art therapy literature.

Edith Kramer (1916–2014) was a social realist painter, art educator, and psychotherapist from Vienna. While studying in Prague, she taught art to the children of political refugees. During the Second World War she took refuge herself in America, working in New York City first as a machinist in a tool and die shop. She also taught sculpture at a progressive school. Eventually she was hired as an art therapist at the

Wiltwyck School for Boys, a residential treatment facility for children with behavioral and emotional needs. Later she worked at Jacobi Hospital in their child psychiatric ward.

Kramer adapted concepts from Freud's personality theory to explain the art therapy process. Art therapy was "conceived of primarily as a means of supporting the ego, fostering the development of a sense of identity, and promoting maturation in general" (Kramer 1987). Kramer termed this process "art as therapy." She particularly focused on the role that the Freudian defense mechanism of "sublimation" had in art-making. Through sublimation, a patient's negative and destructive emotions and urges could be transformed into a socially acceptable and constructive visual product. Making art in itself was thereby therapeutic. In 1971 Kramer published her notable work in *Art as Therapy with Children.*

As presented in the theory of Ernst Kris, Kramer saw that in every creative act, temporary regression is a necessary phase. Regression may lead to the uncovering of unconscious material. During regression the client often feels inspired and heightened creatively. Regression may also lead to direct acting out, in which case the art therapist may intervene to help the client maintain a sense of control. Kramer would assist the client in what she called "third hand intervention."

Margaret Naumburg (1890–1983) also recognized the unconscious processes in the creation of art (Naumburg 1966). She was an American psychologist, educator, and artist, who opened the Walden School in 1951 in New York City. She also worked at NY State Psychiatric Institute with adults and children, where she published a series of case studies using art for assessment and diagnosis. Naumburg developed the approach of "dynamically oriented art therapy" where art promoted "the release of spontaneous imagery" through symbolic content and free association (Rubin 2010, p.145).

With roots in psychoanalysis, Naumburg focused on the "transference" inherent in the relationship between therapist and the client who makes art. Transference involves a client projecting feelings onto the therapist as a part of the therapeutic process. It is an ingredient in repairing childhood wounds. "The client's art productions were viewed as symbolic communication of unconscious material in a direct, uncensored, concrete form" (Vick 2003, p.9).

Naumburg opined that her patients were able to express forbidden impulses through images. This expression helped them to gain detachment from their conflict. Art allowed them to see and verbalize problems with more objectivity. Like Kramer, Naumburg believed the art-making process could help strengthen the ego, gradually reducing dependence on the therapist.

In Naumburg's "art psychotherapy," the emphasis is placed upon the *process* of creating the expression and eliciting the client's interpretation verbally. In contrast, Kramer's "art as therapy" places emphasis on the end *product.* Process versus product is an ongoing debate in art therapy. Simply put and at the risk of overgeneralizing for the reader, the therapeutic process can have different focuses in art therapy. For Naumburg, the focus was on talking about the art and the creative process. For Kramer, the focus was the act of creating itself.

In later decades and because of the work of these pioneers, art therapy became increasingly legitimized as its own profession. By the 1960s art therapy broadened with the advent of performance art, interactive curricula, and encounter movements originating in California. By 1969, the American Art Therapy Association was formed and in 1973 produced its professional journal *Art Psychotherapy.* Along with an increasing number of publications in art therapy, the professional identity of the art therapist evolved into its present-day applications as a human services profession.

There are numerous perspectives and windows into the world of art therapy. Diane Waller touches upon these perspectives, suggesting that art therapy involves learning, emotions, and communication (Waller 1993).

I believe it is important to emphasize the contribution of art educators to the field of art therapy. In the last 50 years, advances in art therapy led to its becoming a mental health profession, but sadly it has been separated from some of its roots in the classroom. What is so brilliant about art therapy is its intersection with so many fields. This core aspect of the origins of art therapy should not be lost in the field's effort to gain legitimacy and approval by insurance companies.

For this and other reasons, I work with schools to help them have more access to art therapy methods and practices that can be employed in classrooms and offices with school counselors. It is one of my goals to acknowledge that school staff are also on the frontlines working with some students who may become suicidal. We need to build a bridge to schools to help save young lives. If schools are equipped with best trauma-informed practices and more creative ways to teach coping skills, we can, simply put, save more lives. This has become more important than ever as the suicide rate climbs in response to trauma such as the global pandemic.

Another important aspect of building this bridge is acknowledging the complex relationship between suicidality and adolescent development. Suicidality often compromises young people's ability to learn and to acquire social skills that are primarily developed in the learning environment. It is a catch-22 because risk factors for suicide may happen at school and yet intervention usually happens outside of school.

Art therapists can not only be employed by schools but can help train school staff. They can teach educators to implement what are often simple, evidence-based strategies that can be used directly in the classroom. I have received nothing but positive feedback from teachers about this. They are witness to a significant change in the learning environment when they can spend just five minutes at the beginning of class utilizing expressive arts therapy methods.

If we can work past the red tape of the separate professions and learn from the past, art therapists and educators can harmoniously work together to help solve the youth suicide problem. Let us not let other agendas interfere with our uniting to save young lives.

Art therapy began with so many roads. Whether it was Neanderthals in caves, patient artists in psychiatric institutions, historical art movements, veterans recovering from war, or with psychoanalysts and art educators, one thing is clear. Art therapy began with making art and has been shown to be beneficial in working with suicidal youth.

References

Kramer, E. (1971) *Art as Therapy with Children*. New York: Schocken Books.

Kramer, E. (1987) Sublimation and Art Therapy. In J.A. Rubin (ed.) *Approaches to Art Therapy*. New York: Brunner/Mazel.

Library of Congress (2015) New Deal programs: Selected Library of Congress resources. Federal Art Project. Retrieved from www.loc.gov/rr/program/bib/newdeal/fap.html on October 17, 2021.

Lowenfeld, V. (1947) *Creative and Mental Growth*. Toronto, ON: The Macmillan Company.

Malvern, S.B. (1995) Inventing "child art": Franz Cizek and modernism. *The British Journal of Aesthetics 35*, 3, 262–272.

Naumburg, M. (1966) *Dynamically-Oriented Art Therapy.* New York: Grune & Stratton.
Reese, W.J. (2001) The origins of progressive education. *History of Education Quarterly 41*, 1, 1–24.
Rubin, J. (2010) *Introduction to Art Therapy: Sources and Resources.* New York: Routledge.
Vick, R.M. (2003) A Brief History of Art Therapy. In C. Malchiodi (ed.) *Handbook of Art Therapy.* New York: Guilford Press.
Waller, D. (1993) *Group Interactive Art Therapy.* London: Routledge.
Whitford, W.G. (1923) Brief history of art education in the United States. *The Elementary School Journal 24*, 2, 109–115.

Chapter 4

Art Therapy and Suicide Prevention

THE LITERATURE

Last year I was given this poem to share with my readers. It was written by an adolescent in the program and is called *Curtain Claustrophobia*:

If I choose to close my eyes please call me by my name,
The hypocrite who fell back first onto a bed where
it was easiest to hide the shame.

My luxury of isolated energy,
trapped in a shallow box,
fostering and festering the mold
creeping through the hardwood floors.

Flooring the flooding and pressuring
support beams of a bedpost,
hidden beneath covers and curtains
wrapping up your problems like a gift on Christmas day
and leaving them at your feet, always found yet never
willing to stay.

If I choose to close my eyes please call me by my name,
The hypocrite who fell back first into a bed where
it was easiest to hide the shame.

Don't defend me,
I've a thousand thoughts, plans, and promises
to do that for me.

While literature directly addressing art therapy and suicide prevention is scarce, this author found promising results from art therapists when working with suicidal individuals.

For example, in *Art Psychotherapy* Harriet Wadeson (1980) explores working at an inpatient hospital with 93 individuals hospitalized for psychotic depression, many of whom were suicidal. Twenty-four of her patients made pictures in art therapy associated with suicidal ideation. The pictures depicted apparent suicide messages, anger, depression, hopelessness, self-hate, and, at times, feelings of harmfulness to others. She states:

> Hopelessness is often the direct result of feelings of profound isolation. That most of the foregoing patients were able to express their suicidal feelings and know someone was listening was extremely helpful in undercutting the hopelessness and isolation. For many of the patients, the pictures and their comments about them were their most complete communication of suicidal feelings. In some instances picture-making probably replaced destructive ways of enacting these feelings and facilitated the patients' own exploration and understanding of their suicidal wishes. (p.96)

Wadeson concluded that art therapy served individuals who were suicidal in four ways. The first was that it provided ventilation or release of pent-up feelings, and helped to circumvent more destructive feelings. Second, art therapy was a form of communication in which patients were often more expressive in pictures than in other modes of expression. Third, the relationship with the art therapist provided contact that helped break isolation. Finally, art therapy as a form of therapeutic work helped them better understand and transcend their suicidal ideation.

Shirley Riley (1999) found that art expression "is a powerful condensation of the verbal narrative of suicidal intent into a visual statement" (p.122). She stressed the importance of taking seriously any talk of suicide. Therapists should recognize that for adolescents any crisis, such as a relationship conflict, separation from friends or family, pressures at home or school, and rejection from peers, calls for acting promptly with intervention.

Riley (2003) offers techniques for working through resistance with adolescents. She finds they often need to distance themselves. For example, instead of making direct eye contact, she suggests having them turn their focus toward looking at and discussing their art. "If the therapist enters the adolescent's worldview by offering art as a means of communication, there is a good possibility of creating some alternative visions for these despondent youth" (p.220).

To foster a greater sense of mastery, the art therapist could try asking them how they would handle a situation if they were in control and letting them decide the direction the art will take. Because suicidality is often fused with feelings of ambivalence, it can be helpful to offer opportunities to express this in the art. One example is "polarity drawings" that depict opposites or differing views. Finally, Riley advocates using art styles that are most familiar to teens, such as street art or graffiti.

Robbins and Sibley (1976) raise another point of view, that of the art therapist as a symbolic form of a primary maternal figure. The art therapist offers nurturing and can help build the world of the imagination. They suggest that when working with clients who are potentially suicidal, there may be a hunger for direction and mothering on a very basic pre-symbiotic level. In this way, the therapeutic relationship "contains all the trusting qualities of an early mother–child relationship where the basic mode of communication is one of a soft touch or perhaps a sweet sound" (p.31). The task of the art therapist is to meet the client where they are on the continuum of closeness and distance.

> The therapist aids separation and individuation by being with the patient and withstanding fits of rage, anxiety, and loss. Materials solidify this encounter by making minimal verbal demands on the patient. Techniques are introduced with an attitude of acceptance and understanding. An implicit statement is constantly made: "I am available, I am with you, I will listen but not take over." (p.63)

In other instances, where the client is consumed by feelings of helplessness, the art therapist uses materials to externalize conflicts and provide a means of alternative perspectives. Like Riley, Robbins and Sibley suggest that the art therapy process helps them develop a sense of mastery in a safe atmosphere.

In Chapter 2 of *Art Therapy Practice: Innovative Approaches with Diverse Populations*, Harriet Wadeson (2000) examines the work of several art therapists who worked with suicidal children and adolescents in brief treatment in psychiatric hospitalization. Ruth Evermann found that applying structure to art activities provided children with the boundaries needed to help them feel safe. Making art served to help calm them, improve eye contact, and provide a form of visual and spatial containment for strong urges and feelings.

Evermann is one among many art therapists who use their creativity to problem solve with young people within the limits of restrictive conditions. For example, when several of her suicidal patients refused to draw pictures of themselves, she brought in a mirror. Through the mirror, they were able to establish eye contact and conceptualize images of themselves. In another case, creating puppets helped an 11-year-old to change her feelings from those of urges of self-destruction to ones of pride. For her, art therapy provided "building blocks for [her] own imagery and symbol formation" at a time of crisis (Wadeson 2000, pp.54–58).

In describing the work of other art therapists, Wadeson refers to Laura Jacob who found that the art process helped her suicidal patients to reveal their issues more readily than did verbal therapy (Wadeson 2000, p.60). Robin Lee Garber worked with young people in a hospital creating large-scale scenery using the entire body (Wadeson 2000). This helped them to explore issues of mastery and body awareness, as well as to sublimate feelings of rage, tension, and anxiety. Painting large areas provided teens with a much-needed energy release.

Art therapist Michael Hanes (2008) worked with jail inmates at risk for suicide. While the suicide rate is three to nine times higher with inmates than in the general population, most inmates did not exhibit any warning signs. He developed a road drawing technique, as a simple and familiar task with universal significance. He found the road drawings could be used as a "therapeutic metaphor for a person's capacity to undergo reparation and change" (p.79). The idea of a "road of life" often parallels the client's life circumstances.

Hanes illustrated four case examples where roads drawn reflected suicidal ideation. One client drew a "Highway to Heaven" in which she viewed suicide as an escape from a troubled and traumatic past. Another client drew a road map where all paths led to a "Dead End." The drawing helped her disclose suicidal thoughts as a feeling of entrapment, with no way out. A third client drew roads depicting a "Wrong Way" sign. Subsequently, that client also drew a path to "Heaven" indicating a need for refuge and escape. The last client drew a crossroads with himself at the intersection. His path then tapered off into a "Dead End" which he described as a path of despair. The art therapist was able to open a discussion about the crossroads being a critical junction with the possibility of a path away from self-destruction.

Hanes's case studies illustrate the benefits of art therapy in helping individuals who are reluctant to verbally disclose their suicidality. It also demonstrates how art-making can be used to help a suicidal individual "self-assess his or her capacity for change, shift destructive patterns of thought and action, and instill hope and optimism for the future" (p.83).

Walsh and Minor-Schork (1997) conducted a study to explore the reactions of 17 hospitalized, suicidal adolescents to an "art future image intervention." The adolescents were asked to consider their futures while creating a future caricature of themselves. The authors explained that while the teens found the art directive to be both irritating and humorous, it proved to help them rekindle their dreams and establish a sense of control over their future.

Harden, Rosales, and Greenfield (2004) studied the effect of art therapy with suicidal adolescents in outpatient treatment. Their target goals were to repair poor self-esteem and identity confusion, provide a container for emotions, and a way to transition to making verbal connections. In their research, they found drawings by hospitalized suicidal adolescents commonly depicted themes of death, violence, isolation, hopelessness, helplessness, and feelings of failure. More particularly, adolescents were found to illustrate specific suicidal methods.

In one of their initial sessions, a 14-year-old suicidal female adolescent with a history of physical abuse was asked to draw a symbol representing herself. She drew a picture with the Star of David inside a cross, with a dagger piercing it. She described the cross and the star as representing hope and faith, and her desire to trust and confide in an adult. The dagger, on the other hand, represented death, destruction, and despair, and her assertion that "her life would never get better" (p.171). The symbol was seen by the art therapist to encapsulate the extremes of the client's life experiences thus far: hope versus violence and abuse.

In further art therapy sessions, they worked to identify the client's strengths and past successes and signs of hopefulness to affirm the possibility of change. One intervention involved drawing a "huge red wall" to depict her feelings of anger, sadness, and the desire to be protected. The concept of the wall was used in verbal processing in ensuing sessions, and the client was able to open up about her shameful feelings related to experiences of parental abuse.

Over the course of 48 outpatient art therapy sessions, the client eventually began drawing pictures of positive memories and age-appropriate adolescent themes. Her depression resolved and there was improvement in her interpersonal relationships. She said that she no longer felt suicidal.

The authors concluded that outpatient art therapy can open, in a more complete and compassionate way, access to the individual's inner world. When combined with verbal methods, it bridges the sense of isolation and alienation experienced by many adolescents. Most of the adolescents saw improvement after exploring themes central to the recovery of suicidality, including mistrust and despair, anger, and self-esteem.

In the next chapter, we will look at how art therapy contributes to adolescent development and learning, as well as some practical considerations for use with young people at risk for suicide.

References

Hanes, M. (2008) Signs of suicide: Using road drawings with inmates on suicide observation at a county jail. *Art Therapy: The Journal of the American Art Therapy Association 25*, 2, 78–84.

Harden, B., Rosales, A.B., and Greenfield, B. (2004) Outpatient art therapy with a suicidal adolescent female. *The Arts in Psychotherapy 31*, 165–180.

Riley, S. (1999) *Contemporary Art Therapy with Adolescents.* London: Jessica Kingsley Publishers.

Riley, S. (2003) Using Art Therapy to Address Adolescent Depression. In C. Malchiodi (ed.) *Handbook of Art Therapy.* New York: The Guilford Press.

Robbins, A. and Sibley, L.B. (1976) *Creative Art Therapy.* New York: Brunner Mazel.

Wadeson, H. (1980) *Art Psychotherapy.* New York: John Wiley & Sons.

Wadeson, H. (2000) *Art Therapy Practice: Innovative Approaches with Diverse Populations.* New York: John Wiley & Sons.

Walsh, S.M. and Minor-Schork, D. (1997) Suicidal adolescent perceptions after an art future image intervention. *Applied Nursing Research 10*, 1, 19–26.

Chapter 5

Art Therapy and Adolescent Development

When I met Colby, he presented as reluctant, introverted, and socially awkward. He had been bullied at school and did not like leaving home. He was quiet and shy and relied on his parents to speak for him. He was skeptical of me and of art therapy.

During intake, I learned quickly that Colby's inner world was filled with characters in comic books and video games. Accustomed to being isolated at home, he wasn't sure he "belonged" in a group setting and was even concerned that the nature of his suicidal thoughts did not merit enough qualification to attend. He looked around at the colorful paintings in the studio and quickly assured me he could only work in black and white pencil drawings of comic book characters. He set a boundary right away and needed acceptance.

Colby was questioning whether the world of his pencil drawings which safeguarded his identity would be at risk if he joined the group. He held onto them tightly for self-preservation in a sea of social confusion with peers, and a host of personal phobias that he struggled with in the external world. He explained that he had been developing this specific set of characters for several years. Together, his "war heroes" fought off a common enemy to protect the ones they loved.

On the one hand, the drawings held his identity and gave him a sense of safety and assurance. On the other hand, his insistence on only drawing his comic book characters kept him from trying new ways of relating to others and advancing his social skills. Considering this, I made him a deal. He could spend the first ten minutes of every session drawing comics provided he remained open to learning new skills through materials exploration and group discussion. If he tried other materials and didn't like them, he could continue to work solely on his characters in pencil. He found this option to be fair and agreed.

Within the coming months, Colby continued his pencil drawings as well as participating in the use of other materials such as clay, collage, and painting on canvas. He began to enjoy the experimentation and being afforded the chance to express himself in a variety of ways. He soon enjoyed being part of the group, sharing ideas and art materials, and gradually became open to discussing his thoughts and feelings amongst peers.

I eventually purchased a quality drawing paper book for the continued development of his characters that he used in group, school, and at home. He kept it close and talked about it in almost every session. At the same time, he started to allow his sense of humor to become apparent, and further connect to the group. After several months, I began putting colored pencils, gel pens, and dual-tipped brush markers in front of him. Group members suggested he try adding color to his comics, and he did.

While taking the risk of adding color to his protective world, Colby also started to challenge himself in other ways. Soon he was able to conquer many fears. He made new friends at school and began describing himself as the leader of his group. After a year in the program, we put together his own art show which depicted the evolution of his war hero characters from black and white to color, and from paper to canvas. He showcased hundreds of drawings for the public and was well received. At the same time, he graduated middle school and transitioned to high school with confidence and ease.

Group art therapy was transformative in Colby's ability to overcome phobias and his capacity to build and participate in peer relationships. He became comfortable and competent in social situations while maintaining a strong sense of personal identity. As his identity was accepted and nourished in group art therapy, he became less preoccupied with feeling socially awkward and fearful, and no longer experienced suicidal thoughts. This made space for him to focus on future goals and his role in society. He volunteered in a summer program making art with children and became an intern in the art studio. He is pursuing a vocational track in high school and making plans to explore a career in design.

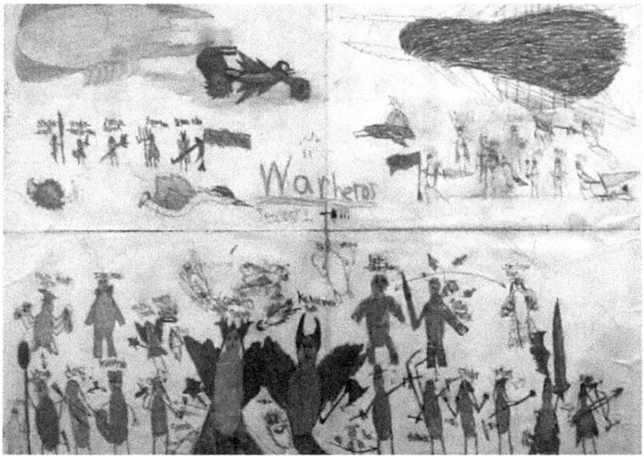

Figure 5.1 Case of Colby

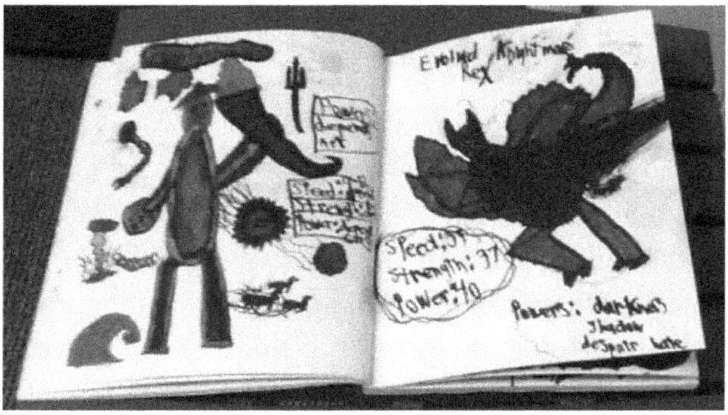

Figure 5.2 Case of Colby

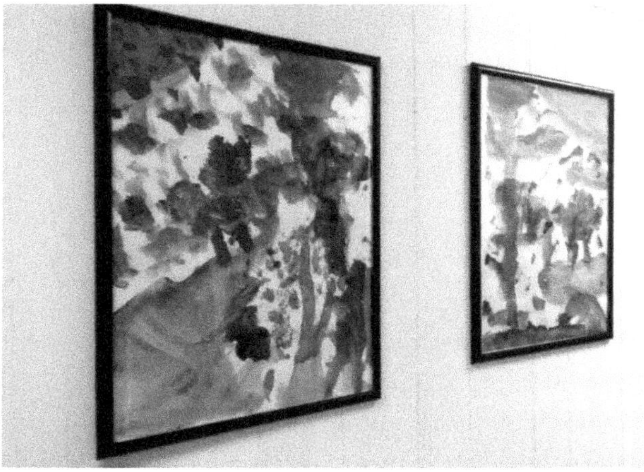

Figure 5.3 Case of Colby

Through visual, social, and emotional learning in the art therapy studio, Colby moved through tasks of adolescent development and psychological maturation supported by peers and the process of creative expression. He was able to conceptualize his life in a new way and socially integrate with others while securing his emerging identity. He and many others have been able to acquire a new skill set through the expressive arts which targeted and resolved feelings of suicidality.

Art therapy and adolescent development

The field of art therapy has become increasingly beneficial in the overall developmental processes of children, adolescents, and young adults. According to Riley (1999), the goal of art therapy with young people is to find ways that will assist them to compensate for the distress of the complexities of the 21st century. In the AIRY program, we examine their current external circumstances and discuss their concerns, stressors, and pressures. Rather than searching for pathology, each young person is viewed as a survivor navigating the rite of passage into adulthood. They are the guide, and the art therapist provides them with a safe place to express how they see themselves and their world.

Adolescent development has been defined by stages of growth. As adolescents seek to find their individual selves, societal pressures are mounting which influence their psychological process of maturation. In the last five years, I have learned a great deal about what is happening for our youth today. They are growing up in a digital age with guns, war, and the opioid epidemic. They are subject to ever-increasing isolation and fear, to disconnectedness, depression, anxiety, academic pressure, bullying, environmental trauma, and insecurities about the leadership of our country. They experience things that we as adults can barely manage. They are at risk for a variety of psychosocial difficulties from substance abuse, depression, and early sexual behaviors, to eating disorders, self-injury, and family conflicts (Holmbeck *et al.* 2006, referring to the American Psychological Association 2002). As a result, adolescents often lose trust in the adult world, and hence may put themselves in danger before seeking help from authority figures.

> Adolescence is a transitional developmental period between childhood and adulthood that is characterized by more biological, psychological

> and social role changes than any other stage of life except infancy. (Holmbeck *et al.* 2006, p.421)

Although the words adolescence and puberty may at first seem synonymous, they are not. Adolescence is a separate entity from puberty because there is a difference between physical growth and psychological maturation. Sexual drives, body changes, and cognitive potential progress at individual rates in each child. In implementing any kind of therapy, it is therefore important to evaluate the teen developmentally instead of chronologically and to take into account that no two young people are the same. A review of theories of adolescent development is included here to help us explore in more depth what it means to be an adolescent in the contemporary world and perhaps why so many youth are feeling suicidal.

Art therapists recognize that adolescents are moving through stages, such as Erik Erikson's fifth stage of development "identity versus role confusion." According to Erikson (1968), adolescence presents a psychosocial crisis where the psychological need for personal identity—exploring values, beliefs, goals—may conflict with the social need to define their role in society. His eight stages of development are a modification of Freud's psychosexual theory, in which people are motivated by the need to achieve competence in certain areas of their lives. At each stage there is a crisis or task that we need to resolve. Failure to master these tasks leads to feelings of inadequacy.

In Colby's case he needed to preserve his identity as a comic book artist and at the same time allow himself to become part of a social group. After a consistent period of time of bonding with peers while being open to learning new art forms in the studio, he was able to master this task and no longer felt suicidal.

In adolescence, Erikson asserts that the main task is developing a sense of self, a strong sense of identity in which youth are able to remain true to their beliefs and values in the face of adversity. Teenagers who struggle to adopt a positive role will likely struggle to "find" themselves as adults. While in search of an identity young people may present with confusion about a number of stressors in their day-to-day life, ones that we as adults struggle with after years of experience navigating society. Without the ability to visualize solutions, youth are faced with deep psychological pain and hopelessness, which can lead to feelings of suicidality.

Blos (1962, pp.12–14) suggests there are many categories of adolescent maturation including advances in types of thinking and use of judgment, as well as socialization and sexualized feelings. He also discusses the development of self-image, identity, and body image. Group art therapy is an ideal setting for young people to safely process the enormity of these tasks of adolescent development. The creative process of the individual allows for exploration of identity and an opportunity to build new kinds of relationships outside of the home and the pressures of the school setting.

Contemporary researchers in the field of adolescent development base their models on those presented by Holmbeck and Steinberg as well as Hill and Grotevant. The frameworks these authors have presented suggest that the developmental changes of adolescence have an impact on the outcome of adolescence by the interpersonal contexts in which adolescents develop (Holmbeck *et al.* 2006).

Strand's "developmental-constructivism" approach considers the social issues of the adolescent. He asserts that the tasks of adolescent development include "the emergence of the capacity for abstraction and self-reflection, the development of values, and participation in mutual relationships" (Strand 1997, p.330).

Rutter and Rutter (1993) believe that:

> Freudians, Piagetians, and Ericsonians seem to ignore the social life of children. Psychosexual and operational changes have given way to a focus on attachments, on the way relationships influence others, on the development of social understanding, and on the way children make inferences about another person's thoughts and beliefs. (In Riley 1999, p.32)

Vygotsky (1978) also argued that psychological processes have a social basis. He suggests that cognitive processes are influenced by social interactions, particularly verbal communication. "Some of the social cognitive developmental tasks that may influence progress in therapy include the development of social perspective taking and empathy skills, the role of affect in understanding people, attributional processes in social situations and prosocial behavior" (Holmbeck *et al.* 2006, p.433).

Steinberg (2005) suggests that adolescents undergo changes in social role definition in the interpersonal, political, economic, and legal areas. More specifically, there are changes in familial status as well as the ability to vote, work, drive, and marry. Preparing to leave home in later adolescence also serves to redefine one's social role. He asserts that adolescents often struggle to sort through the conflicting role expectations.

Identity formation is expressed in a variety of ways in the art therapy studio. Youth may "try on" identities or personas in stereotyped art from a number of contemporary cultural references, such as language, music, tv, games, fashion, artistic style, and representation of the ideals of their idols. Symbolically they can explore who they are becoming in a wide range of modalities, whether making a mask that imbues identity conflicts or developing a clay figure of a hidden part of themselves. Storytelling in the form of art therapy provides them with an open forum for how they may make future choices. They can safely relate to how characters express themselves along with the possible outcomes of their decisions.

Art therapists also take into consideration how adolescents develop cognitively. Piaget's stage theory (1977) has dominated this field of study. His stages of intellectual development appear to be related to brain growth, which is not fully developed until after adolescence. From the age of 12 onward, he termed the stage *formal operations*. Here, adolescents develop the ability to think about abstract concepts, logical thought, deductive reasoning, and systematic planning. Adolescents who are successful in this stage are able to think in greater terms of complexity and possibilities, and develop the ability to think realistically about the future (Holmbeck *et al.* 2006).

In the last few decades, we have been able to understand much more about adolescent development and art therapy through another science, that of the brain. Findings in neuroscience suggest that art therapy can assist in the brain's capacity to strengthen, renew, and, to a certain degree, rewire. The brain structurally adapts to the repeated practice of making art and consistently communicating with others through art forms (Hass-Cohen and Carr 2008). To discuss each process that takes place in the brain during group art therapy with youth is beyond the scope of this book; however, we can briefly review some details and important conclusions.

Adolescence is unique in that one's physical and mental self is in flux. It is a time of profound brain growth and change. Even the brain of a younger adolescent, when compared to an older adolescent, differs in anatomy, biochemistry, and physiology (Weinberger, Elvevag, and Giedd 2009). By the end of adolescence, the human brain will have formed over a hundred trillion neuronal networks.

A great advantage of art therapy with youth is being able to help guide and shape brain development affecting cognitive, emotional, and social function. As the brain continues to develop during adolescent and young adult years, the frontal lobes myelinate and reorganize, a process referred to as synaptic pruning (Hass-Cohen and Carr 2008). Brains of infants and children experience in their early years differing types of pruning, whereby the brain removes synapses that it no longer needs. The pruning that takes place in adolescence involves higher cognitive functions (such as inhibitory control and emotion regulation) responsible for the social–emotional turmoil characteristic of the teen years (Huttenlocher and Dabholkar 1997). This pruning process also affects factors such as cause-and-effect thinking, managing conflicting choices, and planning for the future.

Research into adolescent brain development has been conducted with brain imaging techniques and very precise hormonal probes, as well as new methods of observation and analysis (Weinberger *et al.* 2009). Specifically, the prefrontal cortex of the frontal lobes appears to be critical for decision making and impulse control, as well as initiating and inhibiting appropriate behavior, strategic thinking, organization, goal setting, empathy, and insight (Weinberger *et al.* 2009). Those parts of the brain related to higher order functions like learning and socialization appear to show the greatest changes in adolescence. Once adulthood is reached, such parts of the brain level off and become stable (Weinberger *et al.* 2009).

The frontal lobes are brain sites that enable adolescents to make sense of the floods of information constantly being gathered by their five senses, the experience of emotion, the passage of time, and working memory (Ackerman 2007). As greater insulation occurs in the frontal lobes, and as the cingulate gyrus matures, youth develop faster signaling required to meet the increasing demands on the adolescent's attention (Ackerman 2007). Several other brain structures increase in volume up to the age of 18. These include the amygdala, which aids in processing emotions; the hippocampus, which is crucial for the formation of memories; and the corpus callosum, where the brain translates the data from our five senses into mental perceptions and to the regions concerned with language (Ackerman 2007).

> A young person will have gained a new capacity for abstract thinking, the ability not only to dream but also to plan, and the consolidation of a

> core identity, which in turn opens the way for deeper love relationships and for enduring satisfaction in work, friendships, and many other areas of life. (Ackerman 2007, p.3)

According to Kaplan (2000), among the many benefits of art therapy, visual art expression can facilitate language development, self-esteem, problem solving, feelings of pleasure, and successful functioning. As experience with art increases, brain systems involved in language acquisition and motor skills increase. Manual dexterity and language go hand in hand (Kaplan referring to Calvin 1996).

Sylwester (1998) asserts that the arts provide training in skilled movement which impacts the neurotransmitter serotonin and influences levels of self-esteem. Harth's (1993) neural model of visual perception proposes that mental images activate the same neural pathways as from images from the external world. Therefore, art-making allows us to externalize images into reality for problem solving.

While using art therapy to learn how to regulate their emotions, young people's brains are relaying connectivity between the subcortical, limbic, and cortical aspects of the brain. The tactile and kinesthetic sensations in working with specific art materials activate the primary somatosensory cortex, which can help young people express, experience, and learn how to handle their feelings. At the same time, art therapy can facilitate integration or balancing of the right and left hemispheres of the brain necessary for achieving stable mental states (McNamee 2003).

Furthermore, the relationships that occur between the art therapist and the individual, as well as those between group members, can evoke a neurobiological process called empathic resonance (Gallese 2006). According to Siegel, this process involves mirror neurons, empathic imitation, and observation of another's actions. He uses the acronym FACES to describe how emotional resonance teaches young people to increase "flexible, adaptive, coherent, energized and stable states of mind (FACES)" (Siegel 2018).

Art therapy by nature focuses on non-verbal communication. This provides the advantage of accessing and regulating emotions through art rather than language. Art materials can serve to calm the somatic nervous system in a pleasurable way, and to provide a sense of mastery and control. Art-making can promote balance of the sympathetic and parasympathetic nervous systems (Hass-Cohen and Carr 2008).

Working in youth suicide prevention requires a thorough knowledge and understanding of how adolescents develop. Teaching skills in suicide prevention through the facilitation of art therapy involves understanding the process of how young people learn. This will be examined in the next chapter.

References

Ackerman, S.J. (2007) *The Adolescent Brain—The Dana Guide*. The Dana Foundation. Retrieved from www.dana.org on June 15, 2009.

Blos, P. (1962) *On Adolescence*. New York: The Free Press.

Erikson, E. (1968) *Identity: Youth in Crisis*. New York: W.W. Norton.

Gallese, V. (2006) Intentional attunement: A neurophysiological perspective on social cognition and its disruption in autism. *Brain Research. Cognitive Brain Research 1079*, 15–24.

Harth, E. (1993) *The Creative Loop: How the Brain Makes a Mind*. Reading, MA: Addison-Wesley.

Hass-Cohen, N. and Carr, R. (2008) *Art Therapy and Clinical Neuroscience*. London: Jessica Kingsley Publishers.

Holmbeck, G.H., O'Mahar, K., Abad, M., Colder, C., and Updegrove, A. (2006) Cognitive-Behavioral Therapy with Adolescents: Guides from Developmental Psychology. In P.C. Kendall (ed.) *Child and Adolescent Therapy: Cognitive-Behavioral Procedures*. New York: The Guilford Press.

Huttenlocher, P.R. and Dabholkar, A.S. (1997) Regional differences in synaptogenesis in human cerebral cortex. *The Journal of Comparative Neurology 387*, 2, 167–178.

Kaplan, F. (2000) *Art, Science and Art Therapy: Repainting the Picture*. London: Jessica Kingsley Publishers.

McNamee, C.M. (2003) Bilateral art: Facilitating systemic integration and balance. *The Arts in Psychotherapy 30*, 283–292.

Piaget, J. (1977) *The Essential Piaget*. New York: Basic Books.

Riley, S. (1999) *Contemporary Art Therapy with Adolescents*. London: Jessica Kingsley Publishers.

Rutter, M. and Rutter, M. (1993) *Developing Minds: Challenge and Continuity across the Life Span*. New York: Basic Books.

Siegel, D.J. (2006) An interpersonal neurobiology approach to psychotherapy: Awareness, mirror neurons, and neural plasticity in the development of well-being. *Psychiatric Annals 36*, 4, 248–256.

Siegel, D.J. (2018) Integration: A Central Process in the Journey to Thriving. *Science of the Mind*. Retrieved from https://www.garrisoninstitute.org/blog/integration-a-central-process-in-the-journey-to-thriving on January 6, 2022.

Steinberg, L. (2005) Cognitive and affective development in adolescence. *Trends in Cognitive Sciences 9*, 2, 69–74. Review.

Strand, P.S. (1997) Toward a developmentally informed narrative therapy. *Family Process 36*, 4, 325–340.

Sylwester, R. (1998) Art for the brain's sake. *Educational Leadership 56*, 3, 31–35.

Vygotsky, L.S. (1978) *Mind in Society*. Cambridge, MA: Harvard University Press.

Weinberger, D.R., Elevag, B., and Giedd, J.N. (2009) *The Adolescent Brain: A Work in Progress*. Washington, DC: The National Campaign to Prevent Teen Pregnancy.

Chapter 6

Art and Adolescent Learning Styles

When problem solving with suicidal youth, art therapists must consider the myriad of ways in which they learn. They are developing an increased capacity for abstract thinking while also forming their beliefs and values. To reduce or eliminate suicidal thinking, they need to learn new life skills. An art therapist assists how they process information with the space they create, with the materials they use, with facilitating group dynamics, and building a therapeutic relationship.

Many factors can influence a young person's preferred learning style. Social, cultural, and educational experiences influence perception, as does the growing cognitive structure of their brains. Growing up in the technological age is another factor. Adolescents and young adults are accustomed to enhanced visual images associated with various computer, phone, and television-based games and game systems (Gardner 2006). All of these advances have made visual images more pervasive and common.

For example, digital storytelling involves drawing a story on a computer screen with one's hands or a drawing tool. Creating scenes with facial expressions, body language, and other content has been used in art therapy as a way of learning about emotions, what healthy relationships look like, and identity formation.

For example, we created a digital story in the studio on tablets. In *The Story of Indigo Phoenix*, a group of youth come upon a mannequin in a dumpster. The character, Georgia, immediately identifies with "feeling like someone's prop, left behind." The group of characters, feeling like outsiders, work together to remake the mannequin. In doing so, they give it a relatable and acceptable identity in an adolescent world filled with social pressures.

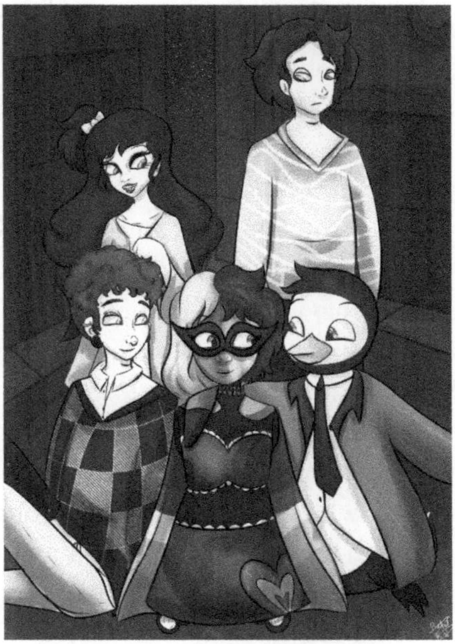

Figure 6.1 Indigo Phoenix

Visual learners, or spatial learners, process information through images. Researchers using brain-imaging technologies have been able to find out the key areas of the brain responsible for each learning style. For instance, the occipital lobes at the back of the brain manage the visual sense. Both the occipital and parietal lobes manage spatial orientation.

How young people perceive, interact with, and respond to art therapy calls for use of a variety of learning modalities in the studio, which may differ from traditional methods used in other environments. To build self-efficacy in groups of young people, they must have the opportunity to develop skills in a myriad of ways.

Walter Burke Barbe and colleagues (1979) proposed three learning modalities—a visualizing modality, an auditory modality, and a kinesthetic or tactile modality. Visual modalities include learning with pictures, shapes, sculpture, and painting; auditory modalities with listening, rhythms, tone, and chants; and kinesthetic modalities with gestures, body movements, object manipulation, and positioning. Barbe and colleagues reported that learning modality strengths can occur independently or in combination, they can change over time, and they become integrated with age. They also pointed out that modality *strengths* are different from *preferences*; a person's self-reported modality preference may not correspond to their empirically measured modality strength.

Richard Bandler and John Grinder (1979) developed neuro-linguistic programming in the 1970s, adding that social learning occurs through observing the behavior of others.

An example of relational or social learning in the art therapy studio involves working in pairs on a single canvas. This is an ideal way to practice hands on an emotional regulation skill called opposite action, which is a method of behavior used in dialectical behavior therapy, to reduce the intensity of one emotion by focusing on another. In the studio, one youth paints an intense emotion on the right side of the canvas while the other youth paints an action that is opposite to that emotion on the left side. In the middle of the canvas they work together to find a middle path by which they can get to the opposite emotion.

By working together in this way a language, sometimes non-verbal, is created about emotional experience. Each youth is required to respond to a peer in the art. Additionally, youth must navigate the physical space between, deciding spatial boundaries in the art and amongst themselves. In Figure 6.2, a clear boundary is drawn between the two artists.

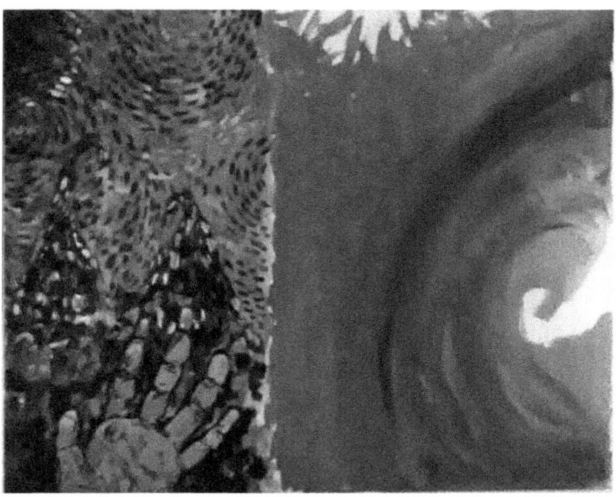

Figure 6.2 Opposite action painting

Later, the relationship between the artists differs—their space is closer, the content of one mirrors the other, and the process is more integrated.

David Kolb published his learning styles model in 1984 from which he developed his learning style inventory. Learners are described by their ability to look at things from different perspectives, whether they prefer to watch or do, work hands on, work in groups, apply logic and practicality or an experiential "gut" instinct approach, problem solve, prefer technical tasks, or interpersonal/social aspects of learning.

Some youth prefer to learn by observing the group. They are given the freedom to participate when they feel ready and no time sooner. Watching others gives them the time they need to be reflective of their observations.

The group created a 3 by 4 feet mural over the course of multiple art therapy sessions. While some artists preferred to watch and learn before developing their images, others took risks right away, claiming their place in the group space.

Anthony Gregorc and Kathleen Butler organized a model describing different learning styles rooted in the way individuals acquire and process information differently (see Butler and Gregorc 1988). This model posits that an individual's perceptual abilities (concrete and abstract, random or sequential) are the foundation of their learning strengths. Concrete perceptions involve registering information through the five senses, while abstract perceptions involve the understanding of ideas, qualities, and concepts which cannot be seen. In regard to the two ordering abilities, sequential ordering involves the organization of information in a linear, logical way, and random ordering involves the organization of information in chunks and in no specific order.

In Figures 6.3 and 6.4, adolescents processed information through mixed media art-making with shapes and words—through concrete perception, some in sequence, some in random order.

Felder and Silverman (1988) introduced learning styles in the following areas: preference in terms of type and mode of information perception (sensory or intuitive, visual or verbal), approaches to organizing and processing information (active or reflective), and the rate at which students progress towards understanding (sequential or global). The instrument associated with the model is known as the Index of Learning Survey (ILS) (see also NC State University n.d.).

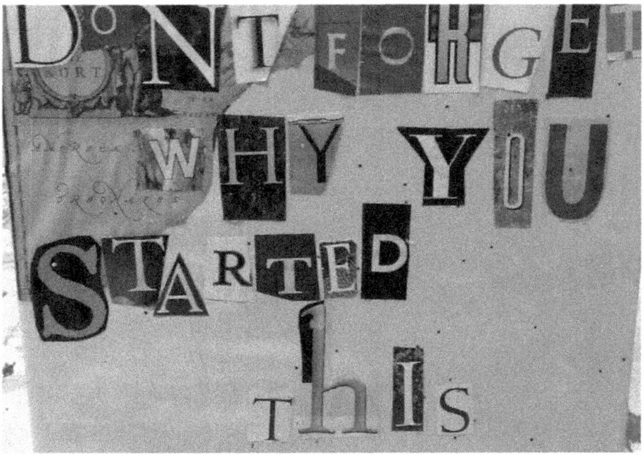
DONT FORGET
WHY YOU
STARTED
THIS

Figure 6.3 Shapes and words 1

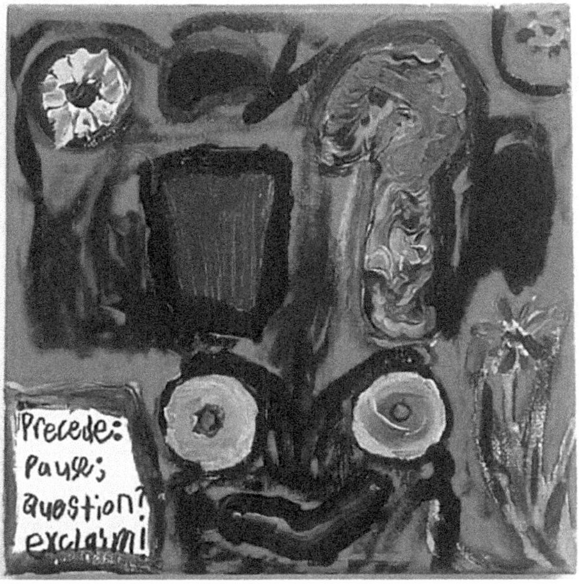
Precede:
Pause;
Question?
exclaim!

Figure 6.4 Shapes and words 2

In Figures 6.5 and 6.6, adolescents explored materials as they related to their sense of touch in a tactile manner—pouring, scraping, sliding, building, and mixing paint with sand and glue. The art therapy directive taught ways to use art materials to self-soothe during times of distress, calling upon sensory and intuitive information perception. This allowed free discharge of emotions from a felt sense rather than through thoughts, ideas, or concepts.

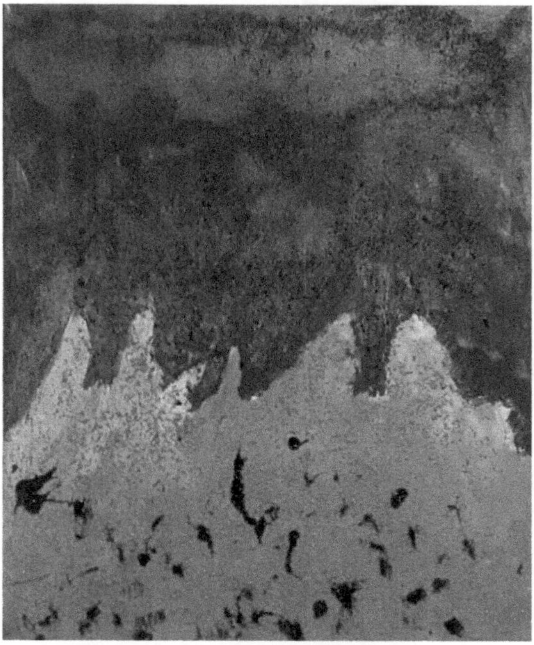

Figure 6.5 Tactile painting

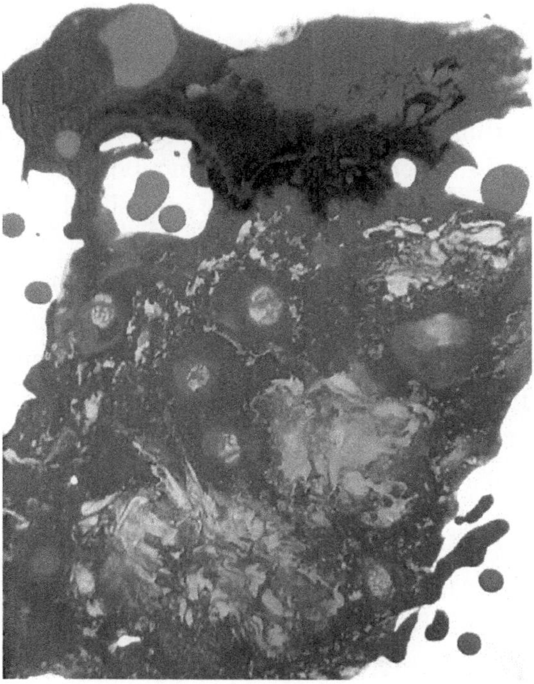

Figure 6.6 Pour painting

Physiologically, young people are attracted to sensory experiences found in the expressive arts. Through the exploration of art materials, they develop kinesthetic awareness and sensory integrated experience. This teaches the ability to regulate their bodies and soothe their emotions. Group members often make requests for creating sensory aids in the studio. Examples such as cloth bags of rice, homemade scented putty, glitter slime, modeling clay, painting their hands, and peeling dried glue from their arms have been instrumental in calming the parasympathetic nervous system, reducing anxiety, and quelling urges to self-harm. Music therapy and auditory experiences like Tibetan singing bowls, as well as olfactory aids such as essential oils, also help regulate the senses and support young people to learn through sensory modalities.

Howard Gardner's theory of multiple intelligences proposes eight types of intellectual abilities which may affect learning styles: verbal–linguistic (language), logical–mathematical (problem solving), visual–spatial (graphical information), musical intelligence (sound), naturalistic (types of plants, animals, and weather formations found in the natural world), bodily–kinesthetic, interpersonal (other people), and intrapersonal (self). Gardner believes that learning is fluid and complex, and it's important to avoid labeling students as one type of learner (1993).

In other artworks, youth explored intuitive color choices and rhythm in what Gardner might have called bodily–kinesthetic and visual–spatial methods of learning. The controlled yet fluid movement of the brush-strokes provided another way to regulate emotions. This art form differs from those where the need was to let go of control and focus on primary discharge.

For art therapy to be effective in resolving feelings of suicidality among teens and young adults, it is necessary to provide opportunities to explore these varieties of learning styles. The art therapist offers such experiences through a range of methods and materials in the studio. Preparing for and conducting the process of art therapy, as well as considerations about the art product when working with young people, are further explored in Chapter 7.

By familiarizing ourselves with adolescent development and learning styles, we are left with a sense of compassion for the struggles of young people. It often amazes me how they endure. In the midst of these changes, they can develop strong leadership skills in the art therapy studio. Their voices matter and they have a lot to say. I am witness to each of these youth transforming their pain and adversity into something beautiful and meaningful as they let us into their private worlds through art, word, music, dance, and film. Art therapy teaches them how to channel their emotions into works that we benefit from as a community, and that enhances our artistic culture. To take hold of their adversity and exercise willingness to stay alive through these difficult changes contributes greatly to our world.

References

Bandler, R. and Grinder, J. (1979) *Frogs into Princes: Neuro Linguistic Programming.* Boulder, CO: Real People Press.

Barbe, W.B., Swassing, R.H., and Milone, M.N. (1979) *Teaching through Modality Strengths: Concepts and Practices*. Columbus, OH: Zaner-Bloser.

Butler, K.A. and Gregorc, A.F. (1988) *It's All in Your Mind: A Student's Guide to Learning Style*. Columbia, CT: Learner's Dimension.

Felder, R.M. and Silverman, L.K. (1988) Learning and teaching styles in engineering education. *Journal of Engineering Education 78*, 7, 674–681.

Gardner, H.E. (1993) *Multiple Intelligences: The Theory and Practice*. New York: Basic Books.

Gardner, S.F. (2006) Preparing for the Nexters. *American Journal of Pharmaceutical Education 70*, 4, Article 87.

Kolb, D.A. (1984) *Experiential Learning: Experience as the Source of Learning and Development*, Vol. 1. Englewood Cliffs, NJ: Prentice-Hall.

NC State University (n.d.) Learning styles and Index of Learning Styles. Retrieved from www.engr.ncsu.edu/stem-resources/legacy-site/learning-styles on October 18, 2021.

Chapter 7

Preparation, Process, and Product in Art Therapy with Young People

Setting a space for healing

If we are to help young people, we must provide them with safe spaces to heal. Environment is a crucial ingredient in the process of art therapy. The sacred space that we have mindfully co-created in the studio holds feelings, memories, process, expression, and more. It responds to youth with safety, comfort, creativity, and mirroring.

The art studio setting feels comfortable to young people, perhaps because it is not an office, hospital, or a classroom. It is perceived as a place to play, discover, and try out new things. It conveys a certain freedom for self-exploration and disclosing innermost thoughts, emotions, and sensations. The space itself can be an entry point for transformation.

When considering a space for group art therapy with young people who feel suicidal, a secure setting with clear boundaries is necessary to do the work called for. It is important early on to establish what is theirs to engage with and what is not, including materials and the personal belongings of others.

It is also essential to establish group rules in and out of the setting. I find it is best to make this part of the group process in the first session. By allowing young people to determine what they find is appropriate and safe in group dynamics, as well as what their personal needs are regarding boundaries, sets up an atmosphere of trust. For example, some of our members have stated they do not like to be touched or crowded; consequently one of our group rules is no touching or hovering without permission. Another rule developed by the group is to respect the health and wellbeing of others by calling out sick. This arose when a member expressed his phobia of germs.

In the AIRY program, group members collaborated to come up with a "safe word" indicating when a member is feeling threatened—whether by something spoken, a physical gesture, or thematic content of discussion. The safe word is posted with clear visibility in the room, along with the other rules agreed upon. Some of these include respecting our "judgment free zone" by not gossiping or criticizing, and by practicing cultural and gender-informed sensitivity; respecting time for individual sharing without interruption or dominating conversation; and being mindful of volume and making sudden or jarring noises.

My personal rules in running a suicide prevention art therapy group include "no methods talk," that is, not sharing specific details about methods of self-harm or suicide plans or attempts, or graphic depictions of any kind of violence. I also maintain and lock up any "sharps" in the room and permission to use them responsibly is necessary. My biggest rule in working with adolescents and young adults is—without exception—safety. On day one, I explain my safety policy clearly and firmly. Youth know they can tell me anything in confidence, but if there is a safety concern, a parent or other trusted adult will be notified and included in a conversation about safety planning.

This sometimes involves having conversations with parents after group, and it is necessary to consider the space for this. It is important to protect the confidentiality of other members and their artwork before inviting parents into the studio, which involves careful consideration of covering or storing any art in progress.

In addition to the shared studio space in which boundaries have been defined and confidentiality preserved, youth may need an additional, private, and secure space in which they can take a break from group dynamics. This space is for being able to self-soothe, whether to manage anxiety, overstimulation, or other factors that arise in groups. Creating a separate holding environment for youth to regain their composure may be in the form of a quiet waiting area or hallway space with chairs and pillows, and ideally sensory aids, that is not open to the public. Without this secondary space designed for such circumstances, some youth can feel trapped in the group setting and become resistant to the process of art therapy.

Also, as technology has progressed, it is helpful for the art therapist to recognize the relationship some young people have formed with their phones. The phone and the ability to communicate with someone as needed may represent a secure object of attachment, especially when dealing with invalidating home environments. Being able to step outside to use their phone in times of distress may be restorative and help them return to the group with more ease and focus.

The issue of whether use of phones is acceptable during group art therapy is posed to the group on day one. We have had groups in which one member collects the phones to be kept in a special box or tray until the session is over. We have also had groups where phones are on the table. They are used during art-making to find images or to play music that the group votes on.

Ultimately, therapists need to feel secure about their ability to hold the group and its individual members. Trial and error often reveals how best to prepare for this.

Art therapists know well that materials play a very important role. They should be considered with the group ahead of time. Some members struggle with certain smells, sounds, or textures, with getting their hands dirty, or with allergies or sensitivities to specific materials. These are factors I ask about during each individual intake, along with any food allergies, special needs, or medical conditions. However, additional concerns may also arise during the group. Latex gloves have been provided as needed, and some materials are removed from the planned directive when necessary. Considering sensitivities to materials has included the smell of alcohol-based markers, the texture of different clays, images in magazines, and the sometimes regressive nature of paint or finger painting.

As previously noted, when choosing materials for group art therapy with adolescents and young adults, it is important to understand their developmental processes and learning styles. I have found that purchasing some high-quality materials (such as a set of Prismacolor or dual-tipped brush markers, Bristol, vellum, watercolor, or arches paper, academic-level acrylic paints, some professional grade brushes, and having digital options for storytelling) can help them feel empowered and less infantilized by adults. Youth are also taught how to properly clean and care for the materials, which make the materials feel more special.

Finally, the storage of artwork is a factor every art therapist must plan for and is explained in greater detail in the next section.

The art product: an agent for change

It is essential to the process of change and growth for young people that art therapists consider the life of the art product both within and outside of the studio. The art they make has great meaning and influence in their lives. These works become so much more than art-making. The creative process of each individual is a coping tool for living in the world.

The art product particularly plays an important role in the recovery of youth who are feeling suicidal. It is a safe way to try on new aspects of identity in relationship to self and others. The artwork defines ownership of self (it's mine to decide), boundaries and trust (I choose who to share it with), self-preservation (it's a tangible, forever, part of me), and empowerment (it can communicate to others on my behalf).

Youth have the power to choose what is to become of their expression (the art product), and when and with whom that expression may be received. Some choose to keep their artwork safely stored in the studio and beyond the reach of others as a transitory process. They may need their art to live somewhere else apart from them because it reflects something too intense to bring into their day-to-day lives at this stage of their development.

A thoughtful decision-making process occurs in finding a new home for their art. Each person is granted time and space to choose. They may bring it home and tuck it away. Or they may display it somewhere as a reminder—of something important they learned, of a relational connection to a person or persons in the group, or as a transitional object that helps them adjust to new situations.

The art is an alternative form of communication with an infinite life expectancy. In the concrete nature of the art product, thoughts and feelings are externalized and preserved. This creates objective distance necessary for the development of new thought processes. It also provides a record of progress and the potential for limitless self-discovery.

Choosing to revisit the image with others outside the studio can offer validation, acceptance, empowerment, new perspectives, and other ways to communicate. Sharing it with a chosen person when they are ready, youth can open conversations metaphorically. This can be safer and easier when direct confrontation in words is too difficult.

For example, in group art therapy, a 15-year-old created an expressive drawing to convey feelings of both anger and fear about her mother's ongoing physical illness. While normally she felt safest to leave her artwork in the studio, this day she chose to bring it home with the intention of sharing it with her family. She had struggled to communicate with words which her mother had perceived as her having a stubborn teenage attitude. Instead of openly declaring her feelings and risking "disappointing my family" and "being too emotional," she was able to explain what was happening in the picture to her mother in an objective way. (This picture is about being angry and scared; this is me; this is you.) The picture served as a bridge between expressing her emotions and maintaining a self-perception of being strong for her family. It opened a constructive dialogue at home in which she could share a specific view, a defined space, of her inner world.

These examples illustrate how the art product becomes a teaching tool for boundaries between self and other. Oftentimes, when words and emotions are the only available language, it is too much for the young person to bear. They fear their emotional lability, and their minds may become flooded, making it difficult to express themselves in the moment. They don't know where to start or stop. The original content can become deflected or dismissed when there are no boundaries for their expression. Talking about their art changes this.

The idea of the art product as an agent for change creates opportunities for youth to become empowered outside of the therapy setting by serving as a link to communication in other environments. For example, young people may choose to share their creative expressions with peers, in art shows, conferences, and other community events. Their art can make a statement, express beliefs and opinions about the world, or stand for something in an externalized and empowering way. Their art can reflect their belongingness to a group or set of values. This helps develop and strengthen an emerging identity.

The art products created in the studio often tell personal stories individually or collectivized as a group. Their stories can pass on a legacy that affects others, whether in the form of a single or group art show or other community event. The ripple effect of sharing their art can positively impact communities, serving to educate, break stigma, and raise awareness.

Art therapy as a language

Developmentally, adolescents and young adults have a strong desire to "make their mark" and to communicate in symbols and metaphors, a language of art (Riley 2001). Working hands on with art materials offers a complement to their digital world.

Let us return to Colby and his love of drawing comic book characters.

During one session, participants were asked to draw pictures of their families doing something—Kinetic Family Drawing (Burns and Kaufman 1987). Colby had lost a primary caregiver a few months earlier and had difficulty discussing his family when verbally prompted. However, when asked to draw, he became immediately motivated to express images of his family in the style of video game characters.

His picture involved a battle scene of various creatures trying to invade his home. His grandmother stood in the kitchen cooking dinner while warding off the invaders with her frying pan. He was able to communicate how he perceived her as a protective symbol of strength in the family and how all the family members were involved, together, in protecting the home (Figure 7.1).

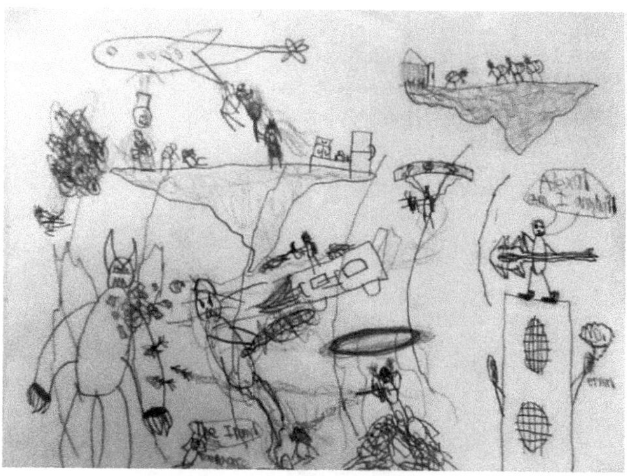

Figure 7.1 Family drawing

As previously mentioned, the development of characters is prevalent amongst young people and an open door for the efficacy of art therapy, such as those we have seen in Colby's comic book characters and the group's digital storytelling of Indigo Phoenix. As authors of their own stories, youth can choose how the story will end. From this concept, new fields of art therapy have emerged including digital art therapy, narrative therapy, and film and video therapy.

In expressing the developing identity, art therapy creates an alternative language, one that feels safe and non-confrontational. This process can break down barriers of resistance, increase receptivity to treatment, and offer material and insight about the young person that may go unexplored in other forms of treatment.

According to Riley, making images stimulates metaphorical conversation which enriches the possibility of communication (1999). Adolescents are comfortable talking through metaphor and they enjoy telling a narrative through allegory. Metaphor can be a way to circumvent disclosure yet still have a meaningful dialogue. Exploring a topic by relating it to the art reinforces the comfort of distance until a stronger alliance is formed. Even looking at the art rather than direct eye contact with the adolescent can provide greater comfort. Discussing alternative outcomes to the narrative of the art simultaneously can provide new perspectives to problem solving and a vision of hope and change. Changing the outcome to a story is easier for adolescents to translate than directly being asked to make behavior changes.

In this example, the image serves as a first step toward telling the story of a young person's "coming out." Figure 7.2 expresses gender identity in color, shape, and symbol.

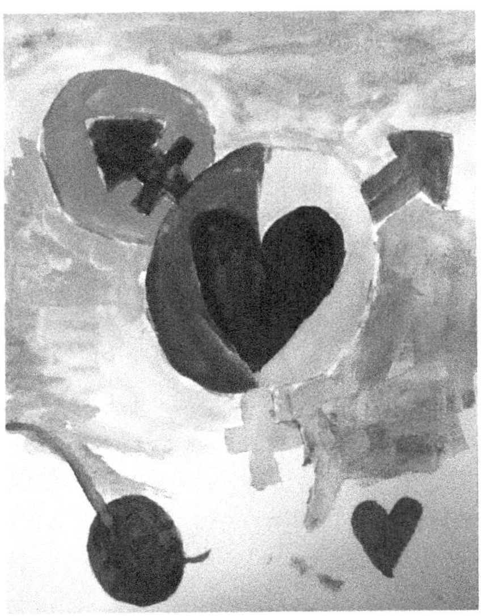

Figure 7.2 Gender identity painting

Working with adolescents and young adults in contemporary society means competency, information, and support for adolescents on the LGBTQIA+ (lesbian, gay, bisexual, transgender, queer, intersex, asexual, nonbinary) spectrum, who will share through their images meaningful experiences in exploring gender identity and emerging sexual orientation. Young people often enjoy teaching the adult what it's all about for them.

Riley (1999) also suggests that the alternative language of art therapy serves as a utilitarian approach to working in the real world with families and their adolescent children:

> Art therapy is a great way to get past the initial wall that surrounds the troubled teenager, and a fine therapeutic tool to encourage the story the youth would like to tell. Adolescents want to let others know how "screwed up" they find the world, but they do not trust enough to use words. They can more comfortably employ the silent form of communication through images. As long as they are not pressed to talk, paradoxically, they will. The art form is safe and under their control. (p.21)

Art therapy can help teens and young adults stay focused and provide a vehicle for communication, including feelings of suicidality. The skill of the art therapist is to engage the teenager's natural talent for creativity, where they are at developmentally, and through a learning style that suits them. From there, the art therapist helps them channel their creativity into therapy with a new language—one that is metaphorical and autobiographical at the same time. This can open doors to direct conversation with adults necessary to solve the problem of youth suicide.

Art therapy and therapeutic relationship

One of the most unique facets of art therapy is how it changes the structure of traditional therapy by presenting a therapeutic triad between client, therapist, and the art. In traditional therapy, the therapist and the client are the two elements fundamental to the process of change. In art therapy, a third element is introduced. The art itself forms a triangle of therapeutic activity.

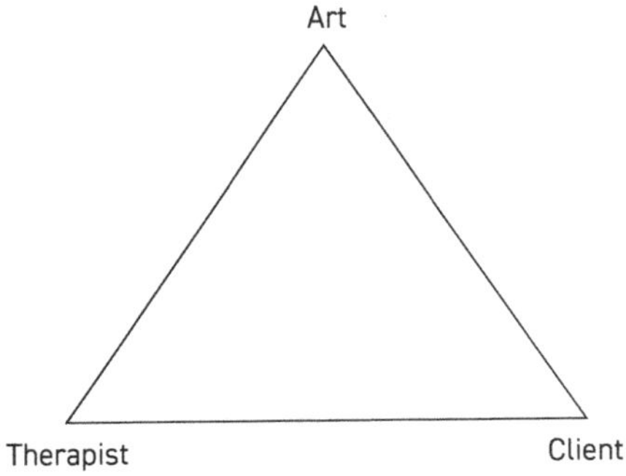

In group art therapy, another dynamic is presented. Peers bear witness and form relationships that are youth-driven and developmentally reparative. The art therapist plays a collaborative role. Through the group and the art product their voices are heard in a new way, giving them a sense of personal power.

Youth are less resistant to art therapy than conventional individual therapies that operate from an authority-based model. In a world run by adults, youth are often frustrated by needing consent or permission to make decisions that will affect their lives. Moreover, group art therapy is a pleasurable and fun experience that most youth do not associate with behavioral healthcare. For families, too, the expressive arts do not present the attached stigma surrounding many clinical treatments for mental health. Art therapy allows for a natural extension into developing a sense of community and breaking isolation through collective enjoyment of the arts.

In this chapter, we have looked at how art therapy can serve as an alternative language, an agent for change, and a way to form new kinds of relationships. We have also discussed how art therapy can impact the greater community, opening a nonjudgmental dialogue about suicide. Utilizing the expressive arts in group therapy is an effective tool for helping teens and young adults cope with the challenges of the contemporary world we live in.

Like me, they have learned through the AIRY program that their lived experience is valuable and can help save each other's lives. Every year they astound me and teach me about hope, possibility, and the power to overcome. I am so glad I am able to show up for them and be witness to their transformation—from surviving to thriving—to leading us in the fight against youth suicide.

References

Burns, R.C. and Kaufman, S.H. (1987) *Kinetic Family Drawings (K-F-D): An Introduction to Understanding Children through Kinetic Drawings*. New York: Brunner/Mazel.

Riley, S. (1999) *Contemporary Art Therapy with Adolescents*. London: Jessica Kingsley Publishers.

Riley, S. (2001) Art therapy with adolescents. *Western Journal of Medicine 175*, 1, 54–57.

PART 2

Youth Suicide

Chapter 8

Best Practices in Suicide Prevention

On August 12, 2014, I was informed by media that Robin Williams had died by suicide. Our nation was shocked since we as an audience were accustomed to his upbeat positivity and humor. He just always appeared happy, which logically stumped us because of preconceived notions that happy people don't kill themselves. For many people, it was unimaginable that he could take his own life. Many years later, we continue to read about it in social media and the press and feel its profound effect in our lives.

I remember personally experiencing passive suicidal thoughts in response to hearing this news. Without getting into specific details, I can say that having a suicide plan in the far recesses of my mind is something that has never gone away, despite my recovery. When I heard about Robin Williams's method of suicide, for some strange reason I thought about it as a possibility. It triggered ideas about my suicide plan, even though I had no intention of killing myself. Later, when I experienced episodes of depression, I recalled this again. It has been imprinted in my mind ever since.

I hope this personal example can illustrate the potential harm caused by media reports of suicide. It is important that we are able to acknowledge, destigmatize, and mourn deaths by suicide. However, since suicidality itself is traumatizing, learning best practices in suicide prevention in all facets of society is essential to helping solve the problem.

Unfortunately, suicide contagion and suicide clustering are real things. In a perfect world we could count on the media to report suicide in a way that does not influence contagion. It is helpful for anyone working in suicide prevention to share information with media about responsible reporting (see WHO 2008).

Suicide contagion

Suicide rates have increased when celebrity deaths reach mainstream media, such as the deaths of icons like Kurt Cobain and Robin Williams.

Between 1947 and 1968, David Phillips of San Diego University studied the effects of suicides just after a highly publicized suicide story (Williams 2001). The more widely engaged with the public the individual was the greater the increase in suicides, particularly in the geographic areas where the suicide occurred. A similar study by Brian Barraclough in the United Kingdom examined recorded suicides in the newspapers and an increase in suicide deaths that followed in the next few days (Williams 2001).

Phillips also studied the effects of attempted suicides and suicide deaths shown on soap operas during 1977 on US television. Even with fictional portrayals, the suicide rate increased in the later part of the week after being seen on tv. Arnold Schmidtke studied the number of railway suicides following a related fictional portrayal broadcast on television and reported that an extra 60 deaths by suicide occurred as a result of this fictional episode. In 1999, Keith Hawton saw the same effect, when suicides by poisoning increased by 17 percent just after a death by overdose on BBC's drama *Casualty*.

The debate about whether accounts of suicide in the media cause people to imitate them has a long history. For example, in 1774 with the publication of Goethe's *The Sorrows of Young Werther*, the author was accused of encouraging suicidal behavior when a young man ends his life by shooting himself in the head. Coroners all over Europe began to believe that the "Werther effect" sentimentalized suicide and contributed to a wave of imitative youth killing themselves in the name of love. Emile Durkheim agreed that "no other phenomenon is more readily contagious" (quoted in Williams 2001, p.128).

For this reason, it is imperative that those in the media take precautions when reporting suicides. Detailed descriptions of suicide methods should not be given, even in fictional portrayals, so that risk of suicides following such events can be reduced. Media should not make simplistic conclusions about why an individual has died by suicide, for it may falsely portray the complexity of the situation. The consequences of suicide and its effect on communities should not be minimized; however, they should also not be dwelt upon in a way that could increase feelings of victimization by those at risk. Additionally, the media should avoid extensive or unnecessary repeated coverage (see WHO 2008).

A more recent example of this are the youth suicides that followed the debut of the television show *13 Reasons Why* (Netflix). The show featured the suicide of the main character with a graphic depiction of the teenager's death. In the month following the show's debut in March 2017, there was a 28.9 percent increase in suicide among Americans between the ages of 10 and 17. The number of suicides was greater than that seen in any single month over the five-year period researchers examined (Bridge *et al.* 2020).

In recovery practices for suicide attempt survivors, a strengths-based focus can turn fearful news into a learning opportunity. Asking youth to share what they have learned, how they survived, and how they are overcoming adversity can lead to a fruitful conversation. It can reinforce that help is available and that others, by comparison, do not have to try to kill themselves to get that help. They can reach out before they act upon suicidal thoughts, and there will be people who will listen, care, and mobilize support. This may seem apparent, but it isn't. So many people that I encounter do not know what resources exist for suicide prevention. We as a society are responsible for sharing that information in our communities. Suicide prevention phone numbers should be as well known as dialing 911.

The public health problem of youth suicide

No continent is alone in this fight against youth suicide. It is now the leading cause of death for youth in Australia and the leading cause of death for 10–14-year-olds in Japan. Japan reports that among those between 15 and 39, suicide has been the dominant cause of death since 2012. (About half of those who killed themselves were in their 20s.) In England, the suicide rate has risen since 2013, particularly for 10–24-year-old females where the rate has increased significantly since 2012 to its highest level.

In the United States, suicide has become the second leading cause of death for people ages 10–34, the first being accidental deaths. Between

2007 and 2017, suicide deaths by youth ages 15–19 increased by 76 percent. Suicide rates for youth ages 10–14 increased by 56 percent, more than twice the homicide rate. And suicide rates for 20–24-year-olds increased by 36 percent. Despite some fluctuations in these rates, there remains a steadily increasing rise of suicide at record breaking highs.

In 2017, it is estimated that 47,000 people died by suicide in the United States. That number is equivalent to 128 suicide deaths per day, or five per hour. There are people dying to suicide as you read this.

What's more is that for every person who dies by suicide, more than 30 others attempt suicide. This number equals 1,410,000 suicide attempts in one year, or nearly 4000 per day, meaning that, on average, 166 people every hour of every day try to kill themselves in the United States.

Every suicide attempt and death affects countless other individuals. Family members, friends, co-workers, and others in the community all suffer the long-lasting consequences of suicidal behaviors. This ripple effect is destroying communities across the nation. We need to become competent in suicide prevention, learning how to talk about it, and how to help those who become suicidal.

At the Federal level, the 2012 *National Strategy for Suicide Prevention* was developed in a joint effort by the Office of the US Surgeon General and the National Action Alliance for Suicide Prevention. The US Department of Health and Human Services, Office of the Surgeon General, states:

> Reducing the number of suicides requires the engagement and commitment of people in many sectors in and outside of government, including public health, mental health, health care, the armed forces, business, entertainment, media, and education…the Surgeon General is drawing on suicide prevention experts across the nation to help make Americans aware of the heavy burden suicide imposes on our nation and to facilitate the prevention of suicide and related problems.

The four categories of goals in the National Strategy include:

1. creating supportive environments that promote healthy and empowered individuals, families, and communities

2. enhancing clinical and community preventive services

3. promoting the availability of timely treatment and support services
4. improving suicide prevention surveillance collection, research, and evaluation.

The National Strategy states that suicide prevention efforts should:

> Foster positive public dialogue, counter shame, prejudice, and silence; and build public support for suicide prevention...address the needs of vulnerable groups...and seek to eliminate disparities...promote changes in systems, policies, and environments that will support and facilitate the prevention of suicide and related problems...promote efforts to reduce access to lethal means among individuals with identified suicide risks; and apply the most up-to-date knowledge base for suicide prevention.

Despite the strategy implemented in 2012, the suicide rate has continued to rise.

Massachusetts and other states developed state and regional suicide prevention coalitions that advocate for increased funding for suicide prevention. The coalitions strive to save lives at the local level in communities through education, awareness, and prevention strategies.

Amongst the barriers to suicide prevention and help-seeking, the Massachusetts Strategic Plan for Suicide Prevention identified lack of understanding that suicide is a preventable public health problem and stigma.

Arts in Recovery for Youth (AIRY) addresses the lack of understanding through open and direct dialogue about suicide in every group session, and through awareness and education for parents, youth, and communities by means of handouts, check-ins, and parent involvement. The program functions to reduce the barrier of stigma with its focus on the lived experience/peer support model (as opposed to clinical models focused on mental disorders). This promotes new environments for change where old systems can be challenged in favor of what works now. We talk about our experiences with suicidality while emphasizing coping skills specific to suicidality.

Furthermore, by means of the expressive arts, the program has created a stigma-free, neutral format for learning suicide prevention, as well as for advocacy and community-building. Youth and their families, as well as our collaborators, have become proud of its success, and grateful to represent a program that breaks stigma. They happily engage with press in the news, tv, and radio, speak at conferences, and advocate locally and at the state level. Art shows bring the community together to take part in the resilience of youth in the program.

AIRY has collaborated with over a hundred artists and area organizations, increasing collaborations and partnerships in the community, which gives the program a significantly greater impact. Groups are held in the studio of an artist collective, increasing exposure and access to the arts. The program partners with a variety of types of guest artists, movement, yoga, and other expressive therapies, art centers and galleries, filmmakers, musicians, dance and theatre groups, and nature and animal-based organizations, as well as its local suicide prevention coalition. Through such collaborations and its community events, AIRY fosters positive public dialogue, counters shame, prejudice, and silence, and builds public support for suicide prevention.

Another area identified in the state strategy that AIRY includes in its programming is open participation and input from its members and their families. Youth and their parents are involved in decision making about the program, whether it be topics for discussion, suggestions, feedback and surveys, community events, or youth moving into leadership roles in the community. This kind of input is key to its success.

For example, youth complete surveys about the facilitation of each 16-week season, and new areas for exploration in the program are taken into consideration. The program is always growing to meet the needs of incoming youth.

Suicide prevention programs need to be culturally competent in their methods and practices. AIRY is grant funded, and able to offer equal opportunity by offering a no-cost program without exclusion, serving the needs of vulnerable groups and eliminating disparities. Over 75 percent of youth in the program identify as LGBTQIA+. Art therapy helps create safe spaces for all youth and their families. We use art therapy to teach communication and relationship-building that is culturally sensitive and focused on nonjudgmental mindfulness of self and others. The environment of the art studio, and the group setting of similar aged peers, increases comfort and accessibility in youth asking for help.

Acknowledging that some populations are at higher risk of suicide than others, the program uses a targeted population-based strategy that is age-appropriate and incorporates expertise in adolescent and young adult development. It models and teaches youth empowerment and leadership skills, increasing resilience. It measures and reduces suicide risk through skills-based learning, self-report, supportive practices, and development of protective factors.

The national and state strategies for suicide prevention emphasize evidence-based practices. AIRY has been formulated with the best evidence available in its planning, designing, and implementing of suicide prevention efforts, and in providing measurable outcomes of what works.

In addition to the foregoing, AIRY's wrap-around model includes consistent caring contact and availability for skills coaching outside of the sessions. This serves to integrate new skills with life experiences in the outside world. Through therapeutic alliance and ongoing peer support, the program functions beyond the scope of its weekly groups and helps youth transition as they go forward from a place of high risk to recovery, stability, and transformation.

With regard to funding, AIRY partners with multiple organizations including its local suicide prevention coalition, area arts organizations, local cultural councils, and private donors in an effort to gain diversified support and further integrate into the community. It continues to seek help to ensure sustainability through advocacy for diversification of funding.

Best practices in suicide prevention

Best practices in suicide prevention can be introduced to any professional or lay person through regional, state, and federal suicide prevention organizations that are working to inform, educate, and train the public. Knowledge of suicidology works alongside safety practices.

Safe talk

Many therapists have experienced youth who have become triggered by talk about suicide, and for this and other reasons may feel hesitant to talk about it. There are some simple parameters every clinician should learn, as well as parents and anyone working with youth. Safe talk involves monitoring how we speak about it. We teach youth and others to refrain from sharing any explicit details, particularly around means or methods of suicide. Studies have found that hearing explicit details of suicide deaths or attempts can trigger destructive urges and suicidal ideation in people. In some ways this is a phenomenon that is much broader than suicide prevention. It speaks to how we as humans process incoming information, particularly when we are vulnerable or have a history of trauma.

In order to help young people who are feeling suicidal, we have a conversation about safety. The most immediate task is reducing access to lethal means, such as removing guns from the house and locking up sharp objects and medications. We find out if they have thoughts of a plan to kill themselves or if they have already taken any harmful measures. We make art about safety, such as safety kits, roads to safety, safe space dioramas, and safe place journal covers.

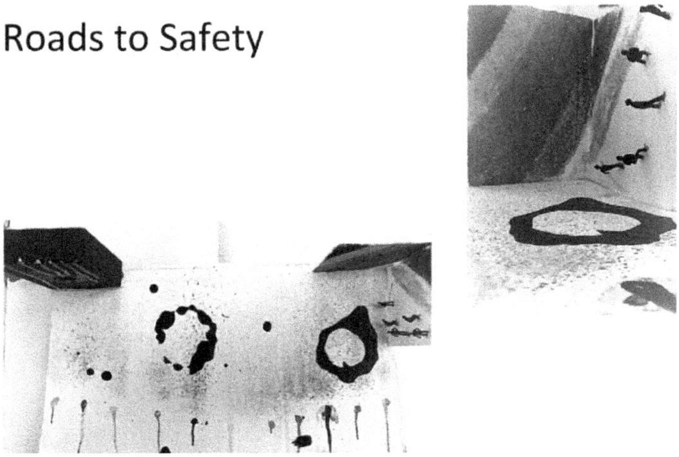

Figure 8.1 Roads to safety

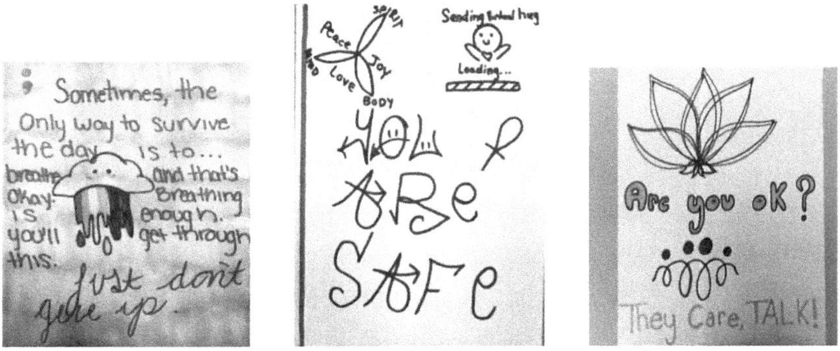

Figure 8.2 Art in the studio: we make safe place journals

In the studio, ground rules are given for how to talk about feeling suicidal or one's history with suicidality. By teaching youth, they can in turn teach parents and peers. We teach youth how to help others who feel suicidal in safe and responsible ways. They are not burdened with confusion or fear, because they have reviewed what to do in advance, and know who to contact for support. Additionally, guidelines for parents and loved ones for talking about suicide are provided (see Appendix B).

Oftentimes, I meet people who have never had a conversation about suicide. It has been a taboo for a long time in our culture. Many myths must be dispelled for others to be productive in helping youth, and reactions to hearing about suicidal thoughts must be re-learned. Toward this end, I have designed a handout which asks people to challenge their bias, stigma, myths, and reactions to hearing about suicide. While change needs to happen on a much more global scale, it starts with the individual (see Appendix C).

Safety plans

The first order of business is always completing a safety plan. The safety plan needs to be practical and accessible. For this reason, youth take screenshots of it on their phones, or they use a suicide prevention app such as MY3. The safety plan is coordinated with their individual clinicians, parents, and supportive friends.

A good safety plan lists resources and phone numbers of people who can be called in times of crisis, as well as places they can go. It contains coping skills of their own choosing to manage distress, from learned skills such as meditation and emotion management, to distracting activities such as listening to music, making art, texting a friend, watching a movie, or playing a video game. We also add to the safety plan supportive statements they would like to hear when they are in crisis, and things people may say that can make it worse.

How you can help

So, what do you do when a young person tells you they are feeling suicidal? It is my goal to leave readers with that information in a practical and specific way. For the general audience, I would recommend, in its simplest form, the five action steps listed on the website for the National

Suicide Prevention Lifeline. These steps are about active, non-judgmental listening, mobilizing support, and following through (Substance Abuse and Mental Health Services Administration n.d.).

1. Ask, then listen.
2. Keep them safe.
3. Be there.
4. Help them connect.
5. Follow up.

Asking the question "Are you thinking about suicide?" communicates that you're open to speaking about suicide in a non-judgmental and supportive way. Studies show that asking at-risk individuals if they are suicidal does not increase suicides or suicidal thoughts. In fact, studies suggest the opposite: acknowledging and talking about suicide may in fact reduce suicidal ideation (Jobes 2016). Other questions you might ask:

"What problems are driving you to feel this way?"
"What is hurting for you right now?"
"How can I help?"

In AIRY we emphasize that we do not ever promise to keep thoughts of suicide a secret. The goal is to keep the individual safe.

> The flip side of the "Ask" step is to "Listen." Make sure you take their answers seriously and not to ignore them, especially if they indicate they are experiencing thoughts of suicide. Listening to their reasons for being in such emotional pain, as well as listening for any potential reasons they want to continue to stay alive, are both incredibly important when they are telling you what's going on. Help them focus on their reasons for living and avoid trying to impose your reasons for them to stay alive. (www.bethe1to.com)

A number of studies such as the Harvard T.H. Chan School of Public Health reinforce the message that removing a suicidal person's access to lethal means directly saves lives and reduces the number of suicides by those means. Research also shows that "method substitution," or choosing an alternate method when the original method is restricted, frequently does not happen. The myth "if someone really wants to kill themselves, they'll find a way to do it" often does not hold true if appropriate safety measures are put into place. The key to keeping youth safe is putting time and distance between the person and their planned method.

Just "being there" for young people as a supportive presence, whether in person or on the phone, can save a life. It can help young people take a moment to self-soothe and better regulate their emotions. As we will discuss in the next chapter, Thomas Joiner's Interpersonal Theory of Suicide highlights human connection as one of its main components to counteract feeling alone or burdensome. In the Three-Step Theory, David Klonsky and Alexis May (2015) also theorize that "connectedness" is a key protective factor, not only against suicide as a whole, but in terms of the escalation of thoughts of suicide to action. Their research has also shown that connectedness acts as a buffer against hopelessness and psychological pain.

Helping someone with thoughts of suicide to connect with ongoing supports can establish a safety net for those moments they find themselves in a crisis. Suicide prevention resources such as the National Lifeline (1-800-273-8255) and the Crisis Text Line (741-741) are listed in Appendix F.

The Impact of Applied Suicide Intervention Skills Training on the National Suicide Prevention Lifeline found that individuals that called the National Suicide Prevention Lifeline were significantly more likely to feel less depressed, less suicidal, less overwhelmed, and more hopeful by the end of calls handled by local counselors. These improvements were linked to listening without judgment, exploring reasons for living, and creating a network of support.

Caroline Kee, BuzzFeed News Reporter, explained in her article what it is like to call the National Suicide Prevention Hotline (Kee 2018). After dialing 1-800-273-8255, callers hear the following automated message:

> You have reached the National Suicide Prevention Lifeline, also servicing the Veterans service line. If you are in emotional distress or suicidal crisis or are concerned about someone who might be, we're here to help. Please remain on the line while we route your call to the nearest crisis center in our network.

The call is routed to a local crisis center. The Lifeline is made up of a network of 161 crisis centers across the country, mostly non-profit and staffed by both professionals and volunteers. There is also a backup network, so if your community doesn't have a crisis center or your crisis center is swamped with calls, you can still reach someone. According to Lifeline, they are able to answer 85 percent of calls within 30 seconds after the greeting, and 97 percent within 75 seconds or less.

Crisis workers are trained to talk comfortably and calmly, use active listening, assess risk, and determine if a person is in danger. They listen in a way that's non-judgmental and comforting so callers feel like they can trust the person on the other end of the line. They do not follow a script or ask a specific set of questions. The caller can start the conversation however they want. People may call to discuss any kind of struggle they are having, whether mental or physical illness, relationship problems, physical or sexual abuse, substance abuse, financial problems, sexual identity, or anxiety.

Crisis workers are trained to share the most effective resources to help. If after talking the caller still feels unsafe or wants to hurt themselves, they brainstorm ways to help, such as having a counselor from the center come to their house, calling a family member or friend, or calling them back later to check in.

Calling the hotline is one way to help create safety. In AIRY, our safety plans connect youth to as many resources as possible. The next action step, and one that is often overlooked, is to follow up and follow through by reaching out to them. We refer to this as caring contact. The simple act of sending a text message inquiring how they are feeling today can go a long way. It helps youth increase their feelings of connectedness and support, and assures them they are not alone. Studies have shown a reduction in the number of deaths by suicide when following up was involved with high-risk populations after they were discharged from acute care services (see National Suicide Prevention Lifeline, www.bethe1to.com/bethe1to-steps-evidence).

Know the warning signs

But what happens when young people do not tell you they are feeling suicidal? Studies have shown that most people who attempt or die by suicide have shown warning signs (National Suicide Prevention Lifeline n.d.).

In my own story which I shared in the Introduction, the warning signs were apparent. I had become increasingly isolated, was sleeping less, and had increased my use of alcohol. I had also left a job, moved, lost a pet, and was in the process of a divorce. I was unable to reach out because I feared burdening my friends and family. If I had not sent a suicide note over e-mail, I would not be alive today to write this book.

Warning signs such as these include new or increased behaviors, painful events, loss, or change. People in suicidal crises often perceive their situation as inescapable and feel an utter loss of control. Some warning signs are more obvious than others. Below is a list of things to take notice of.

- Talking about wanting to die or to kill themselves
- Looking for a way to kill themselves, like searching online or buying a gun
- Talking about feeling hopeless or having no reason to live
- Talking about feeling trapped or in unbearable pain
- Talking about being a burden to others
- Increasing the use of alcohol or drugs
- Acting anxious or agitated; behaving recklessly
- Sleeping too little or too much
- Withdrawing or isolating themselves
- Showing rage or talking about seeking revenge
- Extreme mood swings
- Can't stop the pain
- Can't think clearly
- Can't make decisions
- Can't see any way out
- Can't sleep, eat, or work
- Can't get out of depression
- Can't make the sadness go away

- Can't see a future without pain
- Can't see themselves as worthwhile
- Can't get someone's attention
- Can't seem to get control.

In my experience, feeling suicidal can trigger the fight-flight-freeze-fold mode (Levine 2010). It is a traumatic experience stored in the body. The primal brain has taken over and can shut down access to other parts of our brains, such as executive functioning, reason, and judgment. It can be next to impossible to utilize clear thinking. But as with any crisis, this mental state is temporary and will pass. And it is why human connection is life-saving.

If you suspect someone is struggling, even if you think it is unlikely that they would kill themselves, use direct dialogue about suicide. Breaking the stigma of suicide means being able to talk about it openly. It is now commonly asked in many medical settings if a person has been depressed and experiencing suicidal thoughts. As a public health problem, it is recognized alongside other basic questions about health and medical history.

The best thing we can all do to prevent suicide is to be willing to listen, to learn how to hear and accept others' feelings without judgment. Many people do not know how to talk about suicide and unintentionally stigmatize others for sharing their suicidal thoughts.

When talking to a person who may be feeling suicidal, avoid debating whether suicide is right or wrong, negotiating or making promises, or lecturing on the value of life. I can say firsthand that none of these things work, as rationalizing asks people to use parts of their brain that are simply not functioning during a suicidal crisis. Parents especially can help to avoid punishing or condemning their children for feeling suicidal, and friends can help by not swearing a young person's suicidal thoughts to secrecy.

It may be difficult, but staying calm rather than acting shocked will help a young person to be able to disclose their suicidal thoughts and get the help they need. If collectively we can help one young person at a time to stay safe, we can solve the problem of youth suicide.

References

Bridge, J.A., Greenhouse, J.B., Ruch, D., Stevens, J., *et al.* (2020) Association between the release of Netflix's *13 Reasons Why* and suicide rates in the United States: An interrupted time series analysis. *Journal of the American Academy of Child and Adolescent Psychiatry 59*, 2, 236–243.

Jobes, D.A. (2016) *Managing Suicidal Risk: A Collaborative Approach* (2nd edn). New York: The Guilford Press.

Kee, C. (2018) Here's what happens when you call into a suicide prevention hotline. Retrieved from www.buzzfeednews.com on February 12, 2020.

Klonsky, E.D. and May, A. (2015) The Three-Step Theory (3ST): A new theory of suicide rooted in the "Ideation-to-Action" framework. *International Journal of Cognitive Therapy 8*, 114–129.

Levine, P. (2010) *In an Unspoken Voice: How the Body Releases Trauma and Restores Goodness*. Berkeley, CA: North Atlantic Books.

National Suicide Prevention Lifeline (n.d.) Help someone else. Retrieved from https://suicidepreventionlifeline.org/help-someone-else on February 12, 2020.

Substance Abuse and Mental Health Services Administration (n.d.) How and why the five steps can help. Retrieved from www.bethe1to.com/bethe1to-steps-evidence on February 12, 2020.

Office of the Surgeon General, National Strategy for Suicide Prevention: Goals and Objectives for Action: A Report of the U.S. Surgeon General and of the National Action Alliance for Suicide Prevention, 2012.

Williams, M. (2001) *Suicide and Attempted Suicide: Understanding the Cry of Pain*. London: Penguin Books.

World Health Organization (WHO) (2008) *Guidelines for Reporting Suicide in the Media*. Retrieved from www.who.int/mental_health/prevention/suicide/resource_media.pdf on October 18, 2021.

Chapter 9

Reagan's Story

Reagan was a 15-year-old consumed by thoughts of suicide. After seeing a flyer in the library for our program, their mom had contacted us. While Reagan's family was very supportive, they experienced a lack of available resources in the community and had spent months on a waiting list for an appointment with an adolescent clinician.

Reagan lived with their mother and attended high school as a sophomore. They were an overachieving honor student, with a goal to study art and psychology in college. They enjoyed art, photography, poetry, theatre, and math, and were involved in leadership roles in community youth programs. Reagan participated in wellness activities including use of crystals, Tibetan singing bowls, and in developing a line of all-natural putty using essential oils.

As a child, Reagan endured a good deal of trauma. Their parents divorced after a substantial period of neglect and violence surrounding the father's alcoholism and related behaviors. As I got to know Reagan, I learned that this was a deep source of shame for deeply embedded negative self-beliefs that triggered suicidality and self-injury. Reagan shared memories of feeling trapped and alone, and needed to lock themselves in their bedroom or take long walks out of fear. Reagan was able to acknowledge their feelings about these childhood experiences and how it left them as a withdrawn, confused, and angry teenager.

I learned that Reagan had attempted suicide at 12 years old resulting in an alienating response from their father. This left a good deal of emotional scarring with a fundamental belief that their life did not matter. The father's response to their suicide attempt compounded their feelings of abandonment and being a burden. Reagan was now estranged from their father who lived out of state, but was clearly carrying the psychological gravity of their childhood years. Fortunately, Reagan had a close supportive relationship with their mother and maternal grandmother, with whom they were able to share ongoing thoughts of suicide, leading them to my group after three visits to the emergency room.

During intake Reagan identified feelings of suicidality at a 7 out of 10, with risk for suicide increased by the prior attempt and as an LGBTQIA+ youth with a history of bullying. Reagan identified as a pansexual female, at times leaning toward gender fluidity. They were currently involved in a romantic relationship with a peer that elicited feelings reminiscent of their father's neglect. They described feeling socially awkward and outcast due to repeated bullying at school and a long battle with school administrators for intervention. They had recently switched schools as a result. However, intermittent bullying continued despite their family working very hard to take action against it.

Because of this, Reagan was skeptical of the program and the idea of peer support. They presented as guarded and often responded with sarcasm as a coping mechanism. Reagan agreed to join the group and attended regularly because they enjoyed the art-making process and particularly experimenting with materials in new ways.

Upon joining the group, Reagan and their mother were provided with valuable skills to manage urges to self-harm. Reagan immediately resonated with learning mindfulness strategies to regulate emotions. Together they used the program's number system to identify and measure suicidal thoughts and make plans for safety accordingly. While the suicidal thoughts remained present, they felt more secure that they knew how to handle them.

In the second week of starting the program, Reagan lost a friend in a car accident and had attended their funeral. In art therapy, we made boxes to represent a safe space to hold feelings. Reagan created a purple and teal garden on their box. They did not engage in much conversation but reported feeling soothed by the presence of the other teens in the group.

Reagan struggled with ongoing anxiety related to frustration about society's lack of acceptance of LGBTQIA+ youth. They expressed the desire to move far away and escape, but were also able to rationalize that geography would not solve the problem. That week we introduced the dialectical behavior therapy concept of wise mind—the idea that both our feelings and our logic can inform us in reaching a more intuitive response to problems. Using clay, Reagan was able to conceptualize their wise mind as a state of being which reflected the positive qualities of their grandmother. They sculpted a brain with a heart on top which was finely detailed and well accomplished (Figure 9.1). In another wise mind exercise, they created a painting of a lighthouse inside a light bulb at the ocean and pictures that reflected mindfulness.

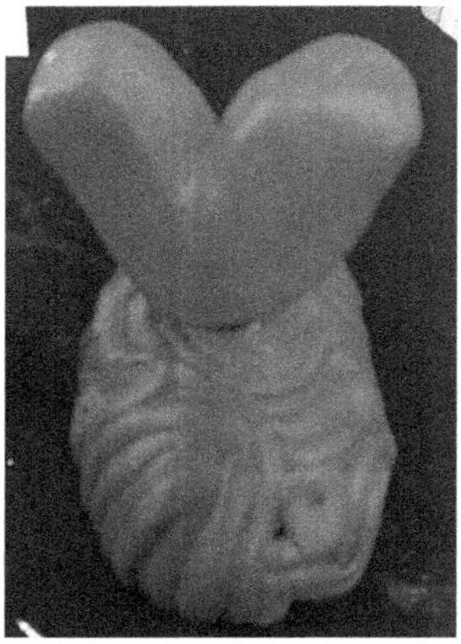

Figure 9.1 Heart and brain sculpture

Reagan's colorful images helped them express a yearning to live life in full color, and to be seen, despite periodic suicidal thoughts. Later, the group was tasked with writing positive affirmations alongside images on poster boards to create grounding mats. Reagan was able to combat negative societal messages about beauty and superficiality through handprints of differing colors and affirmations about authenticity and bravery.

One of their affirmations gave us material to challenge patterns of distorted thinking that contributed to suicidal thoughts, when Reagan expressed wanting to "love myself so no one has to." It was essential to investigate further the perception of being a burden and the idea of people "having" to love Reagan. In the following weeks, we held discussions about the paradox of "feeling" unlovable while at the same time having clear proof of being loved.

In further sessions, Reagan learned skills around having boundaries in romantic relationships and developed strategies for achieving a healthy balance between closeness and separateness. Through image and conversation, we explored sexual consent in great detail, and this began to open doors to healing long-held patterns of secrecy and shame. As an art therapy directive, the group created symbolic pictures of their relationships inside a circle that represented safety and trust. They designed symbols for each person based on qualities of the relationship, and then depicted the boundary style and length of comfortable space within each relationship (i.e. loose, flexible, or rigid; closer or more apart).

Creating these visual symbols inside the circle gave Reagan a map of their feelings in relationships alongside new skills in which to navigate those feelings. Through creative images, Reagan gained a new perspective on their current romantic relationship and began to recognize signs of manipulation and abuse. They gradually came to end a relationship that in many ways mirrored childhood trauma. Reagan began to assert new boundaries going forward in relationships, and a clearer sense of self.

In time, the safe space of the art studio helped Reagan to openly share thoughts and confront feelings related to poor self-concept and feelings of burdensomeness. Guarded and defensive behaviors slowly disappeared. With art materials, Reagan was able to express themselves freely in a judgment-free LGBTQIA+ safe space and come to feel genuinely accepted by the group. Safe and healthy practices of peer support were introduced and practiced over many months, which fostered new possibilities for building relationships based on honesty, respect, and reciprocity. The members of the group formed what were to be long-lasting friendships of mutual support and caring. Outside the program they engaged in distracting activities with group members, such as going to the movies and family barbeques. Four years later, they remain in touch and practice ongoing caring contact.

AIRY helped Reagan to gradually strengthen their sense of identity in addition to their development as a mixed media artist (see Figure 9.2). They began to participate in community arts and experienced a reduction in suicidality and self-harm. Eventually, Reagan stopped self-harming altogether and made a picture about staying strong (see Figure 9.3). They served as a model for their peers to stop as well.

At 17, Reagan was able to leave high school behind to enter an early undergraduate track at a local college. They became more independent and developed more self-esteem, and their suicidal thoughts went into remission for a good length of time. Having respite from long and chronic suicidality helped Reagan build a new sense of hope about their future, and to work toward goals that increased a sense of meaning and purpose in their life. They no longer felt they didn't matter and were able to actively challenge negative thoughts about self-worth.

Figure 9.2 Mixed media art

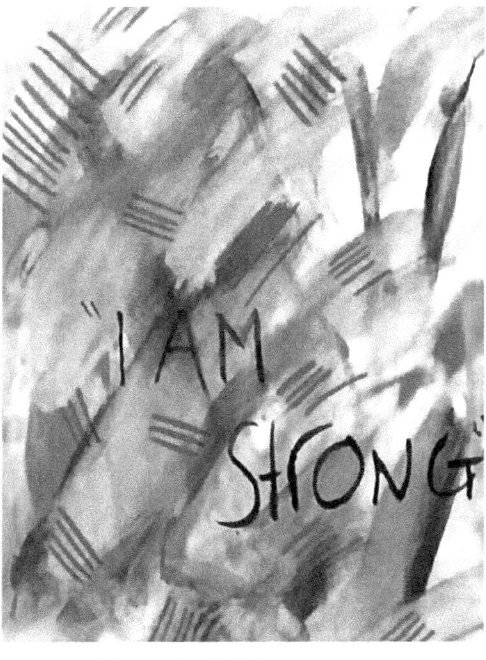

Figure 9.3 Self-harm picture

Reagan felt gratitude and wanted to give back to the program. They became an advocate for suicide prevention and a lived experience speaker at suicide prevention events. They decided to pursue art therapy as a career track and completed a series of internships in the program. After staying connected to the program for four years, Reagan completed training for a skills counselor position, and now co-facilitates teen art therapy groups in the program.

Reagan, like others, is a youth who intermittently battles suicidal thoughts, particularly during times of high emotional distress that may be brought on by environmental circumstances. However, they know what to do when they feel suicidal, and they initiate getting help. They maintain a sense of meaning and purpose that helps them fight the threat of suicidality and stay safe. They do not let suicidal thoughts stop them from living. They are committed to a lifestyle of recovery and find relief in both art-making and peer support.

Chapter 10

The Lived Experience Model

Natalie was 14 years old when she came to the art studio. She was quiet and shaky, and had difficulty speaking. Her mother explained that she suffered from chronic anxiety and social phobias. She had been hospitalized for a suicide attempt after a long history of bullying at school. She was now being homeschooled and had become very isolated from the community. Her mother looked at me with great desperation.

Although the art therapy group was small at the time, Natalie struggled to participate. Most of the time, she kept her head down and drew pictures in her sketchbook. She enjoyed creating characters and was quite skilled at drawing but made it pretty clear that she was not going to talk about her feelings or circumstances. Within a few weeks of starting the group, Natalie experienced two deaths in her family. She subsequently stopped coming to the group but maintained some contact with me.

Naturally I was concerned and wanted to help her and her family. I invited them to visit the art studio during our cooperative's monthly arts walk. To my surprise, Natalie began showing up to meet the artists and to visit with me in my studio. Not long after, she came back to the group. She explained that she felt more ready, and gradually began opening up.

In the program she began learning social and emotional skills while making art with peers. She grew to feel comfortable and safe, and enjoyed talking with peers and showing us her sketches. She made a firm commitment to the group. Through weekly participation, Natalie began to overcome her social phobias and reduce her anxiety through regular self-soothing with art.

In the second year of the program, Natalie decided to share her story on stage before 150 community members. She was proud of her growth. This moment was a turning point that she fully embraced. Soon after, she took on a leadership role in the program, helping newer members experiencing some of the same difficulties she once had. She continued to speak at other community events and performed original music for a live audience. She planned and held her own art exhibition and sold several pieces of her art, which allowed her to buy a new guitar.

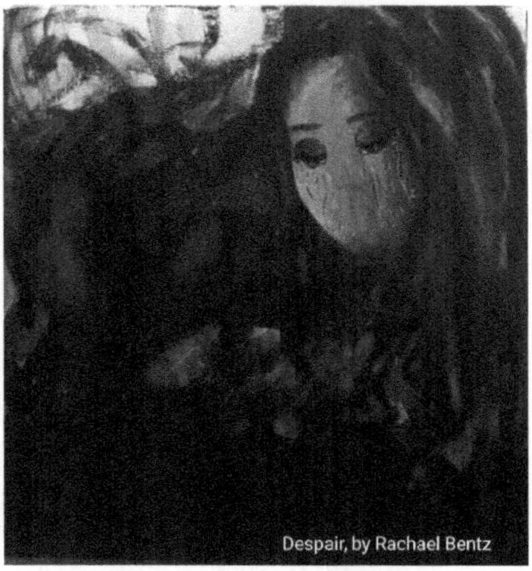

Figure 10.1 Art show pic 1

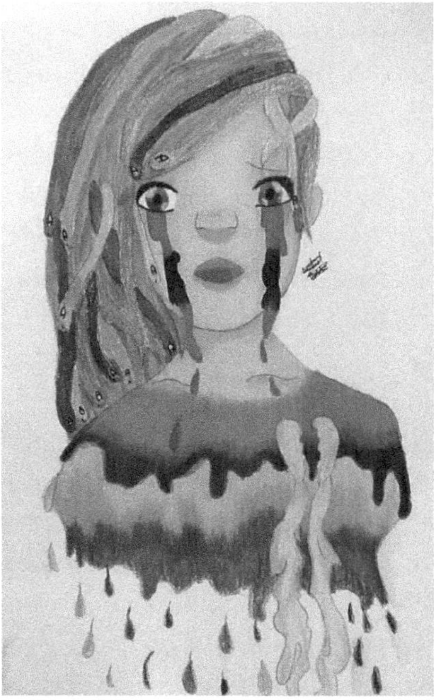

Figure 10.2 Art show pic 2

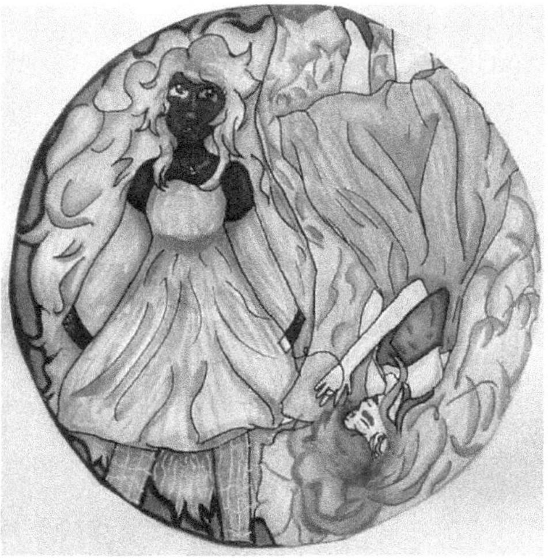

Figure 10.3 Art show pic 3

Natalie's suicidal thoughts have been in full remission for over two years. Using art as a coping mechanism prompted her to become a prolific digital artist. This past year, she designed and produced the program's first short digital film, which was screened for the community at two local performing arts venues. In making the film, she called upon her earlier experiences with bullying and wanted to promote a message of hope for other youth. The theme that emerged was about being true to oneself in the face of adversity.

Currently, Natalie is producing the program's first illustrated comic book derived from characters in the short film. She is in charge of collaborating with three art therapy groups in developing the book and plans to use it to help fundraise for the program. She has expressed that this work in the program has given her a new sense of purpose and she has a strong desire to give back, and to pay it forward. A screen shot from the film is shown in Figure 10.4.

By directly sharing what we have been through, how we survived, and how we are coping now, a message of hope is heard. Youth can identify with common experiences, feelings, and situations that surround them, prompting them to feel less alone and to break isolating habits. Hearing real stories that parallel their own may inspire them to help each other. Focusing on the power of shared experience, they commit to peer support for one another. While there are other resources involved, none have the same effect as hearing another's story.

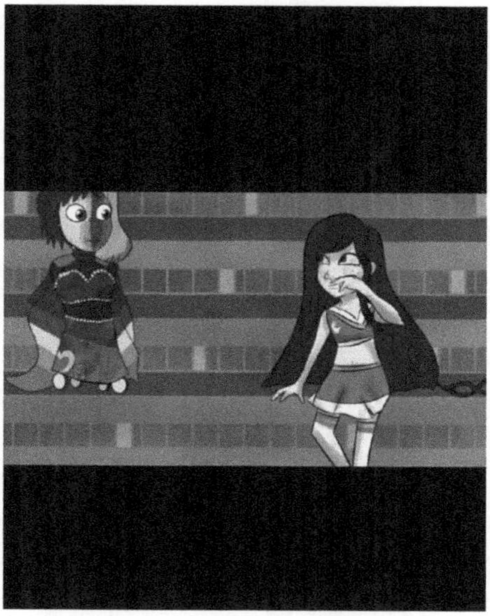

Figure 10.4 Natalie's screenshot from animated film

This is what the lived experience model is about. It has worked for Alcoholic Anonymous since 1935. It has been an ingredient of the peer support movement since the 1960s, which has gained more validity and popularity in the last three decades. Hospitals are finding that the therapeutic milieu, of patients helping one another, is just as effective, if not more, than the treatment and psychotherapy staff provide. The idea of support groups has become a long-held tradition. Infusing those support groups with best practices in suicide prevention, practical skills they can apply right away, guidance from a facilitator, and the expressive arts creates an undeniable mix for success.

The wounded healer: the therapist's lived experience

During graduate school and in the early years of my career, I had terrible fears about other professionals learning that I was a person who struggled with mental illness, let alone someone who had survived attempted suicide. I remember feeling like a double-sided coin, flipping from heads to tails, from patient to professional, back and forth in my day-to-day world. It was very unsettling and as a person I felt split down the center. I did not know how to integrate these two parts of me, so I kept myself hidden for what seemed a very long time.

Since those days, I have learned much about the importance of the personal life of the helping professional, from ancient times to present. Research has revealed that the majority of therapists come from troubled families, most often growing up with a family member with a serious mental illness, and subsequently developing an unusual ability for empathy from surviving these environments (Henry 1971; Burton 1972; O'Connor 2001). Studies by David DeSteno suggest that in many cases such adversity elicits empathy and compassion in those who have experienced it (2015). He states that compassion "while it might appear to be a response to the suffering of others, it is also a strategy for regaining your own footing—for resilience in the face of trauma."

In 1951, Carl Jung introduced the archetype of the wounded healer "whose wounds are both a burden and a driving force in his need to heal the problems of others" (Farber 2017, p.24). Jung adopted the term *wounded healer* from the ancient legend of the physician Asclepius, who learned how to help others from healing his own wounds. Jung asserted that with the therapist, "only what he could put right in himself can he hope to put right in the patient" (Jung 1951, p.116).

Not long after Jung's concept of the wounded healer, the peer recovery movement advocated for a profound shift in how people with mental illness can be helped. They found that healing takes place in sharing our stories of adversity through open and honest self-disclosure, including therapists. This important development launched what was to become popularized as the "support group." But despite the success of support groups, my own journey to integrate the wounded part of me and the healer part of me did not come without strife. In fact, I have found the greatest stigma about sharing my lived experience to be while working alongside mental health professionals themselves.

Susan Farber, in her book *Celebrating the Wounded Healer Psychotherapist*, remarks:

> We ask patients to disclose painful personal experiences so that they can begin to recover. At a time when people are more candidly coming out about their own struggles in life, we in the mental health field have been conspicuously silent for fear of being stigmatized. Therapists are often expected to be immune to the kind of problems that they help clients through and often try to project that persona...recovering from these painful experiences is an ongoing process. Even though our own

> psychotherapy or psychoanalysis helped us heal, disclosing this experience continues the healing process. (2017, p.4)

Farber explains that relational self-disclosure evolved from the concept of a two-person psychology "in which the mind of both patient and therapist are constantly engaged in a cross-fertilization of mutual influence" (p.8).

Kuchuck says:

> As we emerge from hiding and therapeutically reveal more of our true, sometimes less than idealizable selves, we learn—as patients do—that imperfection and mistakes are part of our humanity and in many cases even enhance the work... Learning through experience that we do not have to live up to theoretically antiquated and stifling ego-ideals, that we can have bias, judgment, unresolved issues, and imperfections—some of which might need to be or invariably get communicated through self-disclosure—and still be good-enough, even excellent analysts, can be relieving and healing for all parties. (2009, p.1022)

One of the many psychologists who by sharing their lived experience with mental illness has helped thousands is Marsha Linehan, founder of dialectical behavior therapy. In 2011, Linehan shared for the first time in public what it was like to grow up with borderline personality disorder and to be hospitalized for 26 months, during which time she cut and burned herself and banged her head against the floor and walls, often needing to be physically restrained. After years of therapy, she moved through her adversity, earned her PhD in clinical psychology, and developed the groundbreaking new approach to therapy which we explore in this book.

Linehan's story is a story of resilience, another important aspect of self-disclosing lived experience to clients. Therapists can identify with not only their client's trauma and adversity but can model and facilitate post-traumatic growth. Linehan, like me, is a wounded healer. Surviving trauma became an impetus for transforming her experiences of pain into meaningful work in the service of others. What she was able to create as a result of her history has changed the world.

Research in post-traumatic growth shows that "over the last few decades it has been found that with the right circumstances and support, survivors can actually emerge from their trauma stronger, more focused, and with a new and clear vision for the future" (Farber 2017, p.64).

Rendon confirms this in his book *Upside: The New Science of Post-Traumatic Growth*, when he explains that "trauma is a breaking point in a survivor's life. They are left transformed. Part of that change involves anguish, but research increasingly shows that suffering can catalyze life-altering growth. Survivors are forced to think differently about themselves and the world" (2015, p.xiii).

By relating my experience of survival and recovery, I hope to provide my clients with a different narrative—a new perspective that can aid them in their own story. They can learn from suicide attempt survivors like myself that they too can cultivate resilience over time. It is a shared quality, not just about enduring pain and surviving, but about thriving from, and even transcending, such adversity. Because the belief system of the therapist or facilitator is of great importance in working with suicidal adolescents and young adults, the lived experience model assures youth that they are not alone, and that many others have walked in the same shoes and recovered.

The survivor movement

The evolution of the survivor movement is one of the most remarkable developments in suicidology. Beginning in the late 1970s, the survivor movement has helped suicide loss and suicide attempt survivors move from shame and blame to the forefront of suicide prevention (Bergman, Jobes, and Silverman 2006). Efforts in the survivor movement between 1977 and 2000 focused on developing support groups, as well as committees, advocacy work, conferences, and newsletters for those who had lost a loved one to suicide.

From 1998 to 2000, the Suicide Prevention Advocacy Network (SPAN), with the support of the CDC (Centers for Disease Control and Prevention) and SAMSHA (Substance Abuse and Mental Health Services Administration), convened the first National Suicide Prevention Conference in Reno, Nevada, to develop a national suicide prevention strategy. SPAN's letter-writing campaign and grassroots lobbying efforts on Capitol Hill led to resolutions in both Houses of Congress in support of suicide prevention. In 2004, enactment of the Garrett Lee Smith Memorial Act provided 82 million dollars of federal funding for youth suicide prevention.

But for decades few voices of attempt survivors, and especially youth attempt survivors, were part of the national conversation about suicide and few resources existed online. In a 2014 report called *The Way Forward*, the Suicide Attempt Task Force of the National Action Alliance for Suicide Prevention made groundbreaking recommendations for supporting anyone who has been suicidal.

Since then, support groups and initiatives for suicide attempt survivors have begun to emerge, such as Now Matters Now (an initiative helping those currently experiencing thoughts of suicide and providing skills to cope, maintain, and build resilience; Now Matters Now n.d.) and the Connections Program (an online platform where suicide attempt survivors or those who have experienced suicidal thinking can connect with other suicide attempt survivors to receive support and guidance as they embark upon their journey to recovery; Connections n.d.).

Researchers are beginning to conclude that the lived experience and recovery stories of suicide attempt survivors need to be ingredients in solving the suicide problem. Encouraging youth to be heard in this way is unprecedented, and it is happening now. Attempt survivors are part of the new conversation in the media. For example, *The S Word* is a documentary film featuring attempt survivors. "A Voice at the Table" created a 30-minute video on attempt survivors featuring Craig Miller, Dese'Rae Stage, and Cara Anna. TED Talks by attempt survivors include J.D. Schramm and Kevin Breel. For additional information and resources, please visit the American Association of Suicidology website.

Suicide attempt survivors are also being invited to speak at panels such as the American Association for Suicidology Conference "Can You Hear Me Now? New Voices of Attempt Survivors." In 2018, six teens and young adults from the AIRY program spoke at the Massachusetts Annual Suicide Prevention Conference in Framingham, MA and were very well received.

The lived experience model is an essential component in the success of youth suicide prevention. We are all survivors. In groups, we share not only our hardships, but our stories of hope and recovery, including the story of the therapist. For this reason, we share in this book our experiences, poetry, and art. We hope that readers may pause, listen, and reflect on the real lives of the young people who have pioneered this work with me.

References

Bergman, D.A., Jobes, D.A., and Silverman, M.M. (2006) *Adolescent Suicide: Assessment and Intervention* (2nd edn). Washington, DC: American Psychological Association.

Burton, A. (1972) *Twelve Therapists: How They Live and Actualize Themselves*. San Francisco: Jossey Bass.

Connections (n.d.) https://save.org/peersupport/about.

DeSteno, D. (2015) The Funny Thing about Adversity. *The New York Times*, October 18, 2015.

Farber, S. (2017) *Celebrating the Wounded Healer Psychotherapist: Pain, Post-Traumatic Growth and Self-Disclosure*. New York: Routledge.

Henry, W. (1971) *The Fifth Profession: Becoming a Psychotherapist*. San Francisco: Jossey Bass.

Jung, C. (1951) *Fundamental Questions of Psychotherapy*. Princeton, NJ: Princeton University Press.

Kuchuck, S. (2009) Do ask, do tell? Narcissistic need as a determinant of analyst self-disclosure. *Psychoanalytic Review 96*, 1007–1024.

National Action Alliance for Suicide Prevention: Suicide Attempt Survivors Task Force (2014) *The Way Forward: Pathways to Hope, Recovery, and Wellness with Insights from Lived Experience*. Washington, DC: Author. https://theactionalliance.org/sites/default/files/the-way-forward-final-2014-07-01.pdf.

Now Matters Now (n.d.) https://nowmattersnow.org/skills.

O'Connor, M. (2001) On the etiology and effective management of professional distress and impairment among psychologists. *Professional Psychology: Research and Practice 32*, 4, 345–350.

Rendon, J. (2015) *Upside: The New Science of Post-Traumatic Growth*. New York: Touchstone.

Chapter 11

Social Factors in Suicidology

Society and suicide

With the current trend of rising suicide rates, we as a society must pause and ask ourselves why so many young people are dying by suicide. What is driving them to want to end their lives? What is hurting them so badly that they would rather die? When I first began my search for answers to these questions, I discovered that there is a growing body of research in suicidology which can help us understand what is happening in the lives of our children.

Throughout modern history, suicidality has most often been viewed through the lens of psychiatric disorders. As a culture we have been invested in seeing suicide as related to those "others" who have a serious mental illness, because the idea of suicide is so threatening. But if we are to solve the problem of youth suicide, this attitude must change. The conversation about suicide needs to acknowledge the universal desire of wanting great pain and suffering to end, and our limited threshold as humans for the tolerance of such pain. This is a human condition, not a psychiatric diagnosis. Suicidality is a reaction to the adversity of life in our society.

The most current CDC statistics indicate that more than half of the deaths by suicide are not correlated with any known mental disorder (CDC 2018). As early as 1897, Emile Durkheim rejected the idea of suicidality as solely a psychiatric condition. Instead, he looked at the social causes of suicide. The key to understanding suicide, according to Durkheim, was in its connection to social integration and disintegration.

In the last decade, we can look to several events that evidence social causes of suicide. For example, our many veterans, with all the honor of serving our country, are finding that they cannot survive when they return home. Lack of adequate medical treatment, housing, and employment, and societal attitudes about war, leave them feeling degraded instead of revered for their service. While the trauma of war and resulting brain injuries contribute to their psychological pain and suffering, it is so much more than symptoms of a mental illness that are driving them to self-inflicted death. As hard as it may be to swallow, we, as social creatures, all play a role.

The highest incidence of youth suicide is among the LGBTQIA+ population. They are five times as likely to attempt suicide than their heterosexual peers. According to The Trevor Project (2021), 42 percent of LGBTQ youth seriously considered attempting suicide in the past year, including more than half of transgender and nonbinary youth. That is a frightening number. While we may think that cultural attitudes toward the LGBTQIA+ population are improving, we need only look to the multitude of hate crimes and gun violence in the country, the slander, the bullying, and decisions like the ban on transgender service in the military. It wasn't until the 1970s that homosexuality was removed from the American Psychiatric Association's *Diagnostic and Statistical Manual of Mental Disorders* (DSM) as a mental disorder, and not until recently that being transgender was no longer viewed as a psychiatric condition. Despite advocacy and legislative changes, societal attitudes toward our young LGBTQIA+ continue to deeply wound them. And for this, we are also responsible.

The suicide rate of all populations is highest among white middle-aged males, in part because of access to means, namely guns. Suicide does not discriminate between economic classes or careers. For example, it can be speculated that doctors are at higher risk for suicide because their careers can desensitize them to physical pain and, in doing so, decrease their fear about death.

In examining causes of suicide other than mental illness, evidence shows that there is a gender difference in suicide. Women are more likely to become clinically depressed, and attempt suicide, while men are more likely to die by suicide without reaching out for help. Factors such as poor adaptation to life's stresses, vulnerability to loss and disruptions, and loss of mastery and control are among many drivers for suicide. Cultural expectations about gender are a significant part of the problem.

Durkheim's (1897) main argument was that social facts must be taken into consideration as external realities for the individual.

According to Durkheim, each society has a "collective inclination to suicide" correlated to changes in society. It follows that the more the individual is socially integrated into a social group, the less likely he is to die by suicide. On the flip side, any changes in society that cause greater disintegration will increase the suicide rate.

From this perspective, socio-demographic factors that contribute to suicidality are apparent—increased isolation, unemployment, poor physical health, changes in family structure or in religious beliefs and practices, economic hardship, a poor network of relationships, and a lack of resources especially in rural communities, to name a few. These social factors can create a feeling of entrapment in which the suicidal individual experiences a lack of control over the external factors of their lives, and a subsequent feeling of hopelessness about the future.

In *Suicide and Attempted Suicide* (2001), Mark Williams suggests that suicide is not unique to any particular psychiatric diagnosis, but rather stems from a lack of social support that serves as a protective factor against suicide. He examines vulnerability factors to suicide including parenting, sexual abuse, substance abuse, and employment status. He also takes a look at precipitating factors such as lack of interpersonal problem-solving abilities and public events. Political events are affecting youth more than ever and they often live in a state of fear about the direction of their country.

> People differ widely in the extent to which their mind translates specific stress events into the general feeling that nothing can be done, a sense of helplessness that goes much wider than the original situation… the result is that such people may disengage from thinking about the future…they are less likely to become aware of any future possibilities for happiness or to make plans which could bring about positive events. (Williams 2001, p.92)

Bergman, Jobes, and Silverman (2006) propose that suicidality occurs independent of any diagnosis, and that the old Kraepelinian approach of treating symptoms does not specifically treat suicidality. Effective treatment requires a fundamental understanding that suicidality represents some effort to cope or solve problems. Clinicians should approach this in an empathic, matter-of-fact, and nonjudgmental fashion. This trajectory is different, exploring *what it means to the patient* to feel suicidal.

For centuries we have been afraid as a society to ask such questions.

Cultural myths—like the idea that talking about suicide only makes it worse—have interfered with help-seeking and prevention. Given an opportunity to share their common lived experience of feeling suicidal in a non-judgmental group setting opens the door to destigmatizing the suicidal experience. In the art studio, this kind of direct dialogue with peers fosters important conclusions for youth: they are not unique or alone in their experience; others like them have recovered; and such recovery is evidence that the suicide problem can be resolved. For young people we must also take into account stress associated with school, the impact of social media, peer dynamics such as bullying, circumstances surrounding the development of gender identity and sexual orientation, and the phenomenon of contagion.

Academic pressure and bullying in schools

In our day, adolescents and young adults are feeling increasingly trapped by societal pressures. We must ask ourselves what we are expecting from them when we can barely manage our own feelings of stress. Their feelings of entrapment may become intolerable and create an urgent and intense desire for escape. Their brains are already going through a flux of changes which result in increased impulsivity and lack of judgment. When they are unable to imagine solutions or given tools to control such urges to escape, suicide may feel like the answer.

Young people are especially sensitive to feelings of failure and likely to conclude they are trapped if they fail. In the AIRY program, I have witnessed first-hand how suicidal thoughts and urges increase at the end of the semester when grades are due. I have had to adjust our art therapy directives for that day to offer youth an opportunity to work through their academic stresses and receive much-needed peer support. An example is how the highly competitive nature of the education system is often linked to the rate of suicide amongst teenagers in Japan. The competitive atmosphere in schools can actually encourage the bully until the victim gives up. This increases the risk of suicide (Williams 2001). Williams describes how academic pressure may affect youth:

> The use of exam success as the sole criterion of self-worth produces individuals who feel ashamed of their "weakness" and trapped by their apparent failure. The feeling of humiliation and "weakness" acts as a barrier to sharing the fear of failure with parents or family. The feeling

> of humiliation is exacerbated by feelings of loneliness, and each mood feeds on the other in a vicious spiral of despair. (Williams 2001, p.137)

Moreover, the severity and frequency of bullying between students has warranted a term in suicidology known as "bullicide." After a history of being bullied in school without adequate intervention, children as young as ten years old are killing themselves to escape the accompanying psychological pain. In the AIRY program, over 85 percent of our youth have a history of being bullied at school with little to no intervention. For anti-bullying resources, see Appendix F.

Social rank theory

As humans, we are all vulnerable to signals from our social environment about success or failure. Even on an unconscious level, our social rank within a group, and our acceptance as part of that group, motivates our behavior. Research by Professor Paul Gilbert indicates that there are evolutionary primitive mechanisms at play that cause humans to feel threatened by social rank. "The most important 'unsafe' environment for most humans...is not exposure to predators or physical harm, but exposure to unfavorable social comparison" (Williams 2001, p.141). Like the fight or flight response, when individuals lose rank, their defensive systems of escape become activated.

In his book *Depression: The Evolution of Powerlessness*, Gilbert explains how, as social creatures, we are strongly preoccupied with judgments about sameness and difference in groups. He refers to this as our "social attention holding power," which generates the need to give attention and receive attention from others. For some, the drive to be needed by others becomes the sole source of satisfaction in life. We see this often with people in helping roles. When it is made known to them that their help is no longer needed, they may in turn feel depressed and develop feelings of burdensomeness. Youth especially are prone to black and white thinking. They begin to think "They would be better off without me." They conclude that there are only two possibilities: either they are a help to others or they are a burden to them (Williams 2001).

As in the animal kingdom, social rank theory explains the experience of being involuntarily defeated by an animal with greater power or strength. For humans, this may result in an individual feeling they have no alternative but to submit, which is an important aspect of depression. According to Gilbert, an evolutionary primitive inhibitory system gives rise to symptoms we know as a depressive state. Suicide following bullying can be seen as an example of the long-lasting stress of submission or defeat, and an extreme form of escape.

Negative social comparison and an accompanying feeling of subordination translate to low self-esteem. Such a feeling may be prolonged when a young person grows up in an environment where they can exercise little control, where others have all the power. This may make them even more sensitive to social threats with few, if any, alternatives. Gilbert calls this an "arrested flight" response—that is, a long-term demobilization involving biological and chemical changes such as a decrease in serotonin, feelings of worthlessness, uselessness, and powerlessness, and a lack of interest in engaging in social behavior and inability to mobilize resources.

An interpersonal theory of suicide

The groundbreaking work of suicidology expert Thomas Joiner gives us a more in-depth look at the social factors involved in suicidality. In *The Interpersonal Theory of Suicide*, he proposes three core risk factors that cause people to die by suicide: a sense of thwarted belongingness, a perceived burdensomeness on others, and an acquired capability for completing a suicide (Joiner 2005; Joiner *et al.* 2009).

The first of the three risk factors centers around the fact that humans have a fundamental need to belong found across all cultures and societies. From an evolutionary perspective, human beings are social animals that depend on belongingness for safety, survival, and reproduction. Given the negative consequences of social exclusion and social rejection, humans developed traits that function to prevent rejection and encourage acceptance (Baumeister and Leary 1995; Stillman and Baumeister 2009; DeWall *et al.* 2011).

From a developmental psychology perspective, Abraham Maslow introduced a theory in developmental psychology known as the hierarchy of needs. While Maslow believed that each level of human need was to be satisfied before moving on to the next, scholars now prefer to think of these levels as continuously overlapping each other (Nook *et al.* 2018). At the hierarchy's most basic level are the physical needs of every human such as health, food, water, and sleep, followed by the need for physical safety. The next level on the hierarchy refers to our social needs. These needs are interpersonal and involve feelings of belongingness with family, friendships, and intimacy. Maslow believed that in the absence of belonging, we become susceptible to loneliness, social anxiety, and clinical depression.

Joiner asserts:

> Social connectedness variables are associated with suicide because they are observable indicators that a fundamental human psychological need is unmet; this need is described by Baumeister and Leary (1995) as the "need to belong" (p.1). According to the theory, when this need is unmet—a state we refer to as thwarted belongingness—a desire for death develops. (Van Orden *et al.* 2010, p.595)

The dimensions of thwarted belongingness include loneliness and the absence of reciprocal care that may occur with loss of friends, family conflict, and social withdrawal (Van Orden *et al.* 2010).

The second risk factor proposed by Joiner is the construct of *perceived burdensomeness*, another facet of social disconnection, more particularly "the incorrect mental calculation that individuals make regarding their death being worth more than their life to others" (Chu *et al.* 2017, p.1313). Perceived burdensomeness correlates with feelings of self-hatred, a flawed self-image, and the notion that they are expendable. Young people may express these in statements such as "I make things worse for the people in my life," or more directly, "I hate myself," or "I am useless."

A perception of burdensomeness on family is a key factor in Sabbath's (1969) family systems theory of adolescent suicidal behavior. According to Sabbath, adolescents who feel suicidal perceive they are expendable members of the family, often attributed to parental attitudes that the adolescent interprets as not being needed in the family, and that the family would be better off if the adolescent were dead. In a direct test of Sabbath's theory, perceptions of expendability in the family were found to be positively correlated with suicidal behavior in adolescents (Woznica and Shapiro 1990).

The component of perceived burdensomeness has led researchers to investigate an emerging biobehavioral account of suicidal behavior—the *eusocial theory of suicide* (Joiner *et al.* 2016). In this theory, suicide may link to an evolutionarily adaptive set of behaviors such as sacrificing oneself for the protection of others, often observed among rats and honeybees, as well as humans. Joiner *et al.* assert that for some individuals, they may see suicide as a need to sacrifice themselves.

According to Joiner, people die by suicide when there is a simultaneous presence of thwarted belongingness, perceived burdensomeness, reduced fear of suicide, and elevated physical pain tolerance.

The AIRY program works to reduce these risk factors through specific expressive arts directives that teach interpersonal skills. Writing and art-making components challenge social perceptions and require face-to-face interaction with others in similar situations. A key ingredient in the program is building a wider net of suicide-specific peer support as well as social connectedness inside and outside the program. This is enhanced by community engagement in the form of culturally enriching participant events often planned by youth, such as art shows, poetry readings, open mic nights, music and fashion events, and more. In reducing interpersonal risk factors, both an increased sense of belonging and reduced feelings of burdensomeness are achieved.

In recent decades the peer support movement has gained popularity in combating the social factors that contribute to suicidality. There are many reasons the peer support model is effective. First, it focuses on commonalities rather than differences, which reduces the sense of competition experienced in other settings in and out of school. Second, it creates a sense of belonging that signals to youth that they matter and are needed for their group to thrive. This collective sense of interdependent wellness focuses on strengths rather than symptoms, securing a stronger sense of identity which is at the crux of adolescent and young adult development. Lastly, peer support teaches young people how to navigate social relationships in a productive and cooperative manner. Our suicide prevention program teaches, models, and expands peer support. It supports the idea that human connection is the most powerful force for healing and moving forward.

In the AIRY program, when youth complete the initial group, they are invited to move into a transitional step-up model with peer leadership roles, internships, volunteer work, and employment related to future goals. They are guided with a new way of learning, adaptive skills, and a web of support and resiliency.

Interpersonal skills are further developed through the hands-on practice of dialectical behavior therapy, a skills program developed by Marsha Linehan in 1993, which will be explored in depth in later chapters. It focuses on learning to negotiate interpersonal dynamics, as well as stress reduction through mindfulness and regulation of emotional pain.

References

Baumeister, R.F. and Leary, M.R. (1995) The need to belong: Desire for interpersonal attachments as a fundamental human motivation. *Psychological Bulletin 117*, 3, 497–529.

Bergman, D.A., Jobes, D.A., and Silverman, M.M. (2006) *Adolescent Suicide: Assessment and Intervention* (2nd edn). Washington, DC: American Psychological Association.

Centers for Disease Control and Prevention (CDC) (2018) Suicide prevention: Risk and protective factors. www.cdc.gov/violenceprevention/suicide/riskprotectivefactors.html.

Chu, C., Buchman-Schmitt, J.M., Stanley, I.H., Hom, M.A., *et al.* (2017) The interpersonal theory of suicide: A systematic review and meta-analysis of a decade of cross-national research. *Psychological Bulletin 143*, 12, 1313–1345.

DeWall, C., Deckman, T., Pond, R.S., and Bonser, I. (2011) Belongingness as a core personality trait: How social exclusion influences social functioning and personality expression. *Journal of Personality 79*, 6, 979–1012.

Durkheim, E. (1897) *Le Suicide: Etude de Sociologie*. Paris: F. Alcan.

Joiner, T. (2005) *Why People Die by Suicide*. Cambridge, MA: Harvard University Press.

Joiner, T., Van Orden, K., Witte, T., and Rudd, M.D. (2009) *The Interpersonal Theory of Suicide: Guidance for Working with Suicidal Clients*. Washington, DC: American Psychological Association.

Joiner, T.E., Hom, M.A., Hagan, C.R., and Silva, C. (2016) Suicide as a derangement of the self-sacrificial aspect of eusociality. *Psychological Review 123*, 3, 235–254.

Linehan, M. (1993) *Cognitive Behavioral Treatment of Borderline Personality Disorder*. New York: Guilford.

Nook, E.C., Sasse, S.F., Lambert, H.K., McLaughlin, K.A., and Somerville, L.H. (2018) The nonlinear development of emotion differentiation: Granular emotional experience is low in adolescence. *Psychological Science 29*, 8, 1346–1357.

Sabbath, J.C. (1969) The suicidal adolescent—the expendable child. *Journal of the American Academy of Child Psychiatry 8*, 272–285.

Stillman, T.F. and Baumeister, R.F. (2009) Uncertainty, belongingness, and four needs for meaning. *Psychological Inquiry 20*, 4, 249–251.

The Trevor Project (2021) National survey on LGBTQ youth mental health 2021. Retrieved from www.thetrevorproject.org/survey-2021 on October 5, 2021.

Van Orden, K.A., Witte, T.K., Cukrowicz, K.C., Braithwaite, S., Selby, E.A., and Joiner Jr., T.E. (2010) The interpersonal theory of suicide. *Psychological Review 117*, 2, 575–600.

Williams, M. (2001) *Suicide and Attempted Suicide: Understanding the Cry of Pain*. London: Penguin Books.

Woznica, J.G. and Shapiro, J.R. (1990) An analysis of adolescent suicide attempts: The expendable child. *Journal of Pediatric Psychology 15*, 6, 789–796.

Chapter 12

The Role of Emotional and Psychological Pain in Suicidality

Prolonged emotional pain, when it becomes intolerable, is cited by most experts as the most fundamental aspect of suicidality. In Edwin Shneidman's (1996) book *The Suicidal Mind*, he coined the term "psycheache" to describe the experience of negative emotions that have become unbearable, such as deep shame, guilt, loneliness, grief, and anger. After studying hundreds of suicidal patients, he determined that commonalities amongst suicides include thwarted love, acceptance and belonging, a loss of control or autonomy, an assaulted self-image and the avoidance of shame, defeat, humiliation, and disgrace, ruptured key relationships and related grief, and excessive anger, rage, and hostility related to unmet psychological needs. He also cited commonalities of hopelessness or helplessness, ambivalence about living and dying, and the wish to escape as a solution to problems.

Shneidman concluded that psychiatric diagnosis was not at the heart of suicide—not a psychosis, neurosis, or character disorder:

> Our best route to understanding suicide is not through the study of the structure of the brain...nor the study of mental diseases, but directly through the study of human emotions described in plain English, in the words of the suicidal person. The most important question to a potentially suicidal person is not inquiry about family history or laboratory tests of blood or spinal fluid, but "Where do you hurt?" and "How can I help you?" (Shneidman 1996, p.6)

For Shneidman, the common purpose of suicide is to seek a solution. Suicide becomes seemingly the only available answer to solving problems that are generating intense suffering. Every suicidal act reflects some specific unfulfilled human need (Shneidman 1998).

David Jobes, author of *Managing Suicidal Risk: A Collaborative Approach* (2016), outlines five specific psychological drivers for suicide—psychological pain, stress, destructive urges, hopelessness, and self-hate. In his CAMS approach to assessment (Collaborative Assessment and Management of Suicidality), he empowers clients to answer in their own words what is driving them to feel suicidal. Rather than focusing on a clinical diagnosis of a mental disorder, he elicits responses directly related to suicidality.

For example, he asks the suicidal individual point blank, "What are the two biggest problems driving you to feel suicidal?" While it may seem obvious to ask a client *why* he is feeling suicidal, rarely in hospitals or clinicians' offices is such a question asked in a straightforward manner. In the practice of Western medicine, the doctor knows best. Their focus is on gathering diagnostic criteria for symptoms of mental disorders—depression, anxiety, psychosis, dissociation, personality disorders, and the list goes on.

> We seek to have the patient be a "co-author" of their own treatment plan. In terms of CAMS philosophy, the clinician's honesty and forthrightness are key elements. For any patient teetering between life and death, there can be no more important component of care than direct and respectful candor when suicidal risk is present. The CAMS clinician endeavors to understand their patient's suffering from an empathetic, non-judgmental, and intra-subjective perspective. The clinician never shames or blames a suicidal person for being suicidal; we endeavor to understand this struggle through the eyes of the suicidal patient. (CAMS Care 2021)

In this sense, Jobes's collaborative approach is radical. It breaks down the hierarchy between patient and doctor in favor of honesty, empathy, and equality. Imagine that young people already *know why* they are suicidal and *know how* we can help them. With patience and prompting, more often than not they can tell us exactly what their problems are.

One of Jobes's strategies which we have adopted in the AIRY program is consistent monitoring of suicidal thoughts and psychological drivers for suicide. We do this on a scale of 1 to 10 every session, which we call the "weekly check-in."

Initially the idea of a numeric rating scale is daunting for some young people but after a few times it begins to provide them with a sense of being heard and cared for. When they show up to group, they want to do a check-in right away. On a single piece of paper, they look forward to saying what they are experiencing confidentially with the art therapist, who can then help them find a channel for expression. Writing it down becomes a vehicle to convey things that are hard to vocalize. Self-monitoring gives them useful information, stability, and a tool for measuring their progress. They respond to being treated as if they are capable of understanding their suicidality and can take steps to help themselves.

The weekly check-in also provides the art therapist and the program in general with valuable information and evidence-based measurable outcomes. From studying the variables of over a hundred suicidal youth, we have been able to glean what is hurting them the most, what factors have a direct relationship to their feeling suicidal, and how we can help them heal. We can begin to predict what is needed for successful recovery. Suicidality becomes less of a mystery and more of a solvable problem.

The Arts in Recovery for Youth model has adopted the research of both Jobes and Joiner through weekly self-report and skills coaching to reduce or eliminate the problems causing young people to feel suicidal. By directly addressing and supporting their emotional pain and the interpersonal conflicts in their lives, the process of suicide prevention is streamlined. Instead of enduring a long journey towards identifying diagnoses of mental disorders and treating symptoms with various therapies and pharmacology, youth quickly confront what is happening now and what needs to change for them to no longer feel suicidal.

In fact, David Jobes's assessment includes that simple question when he asks, "What is the one thing that would make you no longer feel suicidal?" Not surprisingly, when asked, most youth know the answer. Moreover, this process of a collaborative conversation about suicide *empowers* youth in a way that a hospital visit may not. Oftentimes, traditional treatment of suicidal individuals can reinforce their sense of helplessness and victimization.

Exploring the phenomenology of youth suicide has led experts in the field to surmise that at the heart of suicidal thinking lies an intense need for escape and relief from psychological pain. Specifically, adolescents and young adults feel hopeless, lack problem-solving skills and future thinking, and have a tendency toward impulsivity and presence of psychological pain (Bergman, Jobes, and Silverman 2006). From the work of Bergman *et al.*, we can glean that suicidal individuals, and more particularly young people, appear unable to regulate their own experiences of emotional pain.

For this reason, youth at risk for suicide need to develop skills in emotion regulation, distress tolerance, and interpersonal effectiveness, three of the main components in dialectical behavior therapy. These skills can effectively be taught to young people through the lens of art therapy.

References

Bergman, A.L., Jobes, D.A., and Silverman, M.M. (2006) *Adolescent Suicide: Assessment and Intervention* (2nd edn). Washington, DC: American Psychological Association.

CAMS Care (2021) What is the "Collaborative Assessment and Management of Suicidality" (CAMS)? Retrieved from https://cams-care.com/about-cams on February 12, 2020.

Jobes, D.A. (2016) *Managing Suicidal Risk: A Collaborative Approach* (2nd edn). New York: The Guilford Press.

Shneidman, E.S. (1996) *The Suicidal Mind*. New York: Oxford University Press.

Shneidman, E.S. (1998) Perspectives on suicidology: Further reflections on suicide and psychache. *Suicide and Life-Threatening Behavior 28*, 245–250.

PART 3

DBT-Informed Art Therapy

Chapter 13

DBT-Informed Art Therapy for Youth Suicide Prevention

I am a 46-year-old woman with a long history of chronic suicidality. I have experienced several inpatient hospitalizations and partial treatment programs, and participated dutifully in individual and group psychotherapy for over 30 years—with social workers, psychotherapists, and psychologists. As a teenager I began reading self-help books in an effort to feel better, and I quickly became curious about the field of psychology, going on to pursue my master's degree. I am writing about this because I can attest, hands on, that the most reliable treatment for my suicidality has been my discovery of dialectical behavior therapy, known more popularly as DBT. The effectiveness of DBT in reducing suicidality, including a reduction in self-harm behaviors and suicidal ideation, is supported by evidence in health technology assessments, systematic reviews, meta-analyses, randomized controlled trials, controlled clinical trials, and observational studies (Rathus and Miller 2002; Linehan *et al.* 2006; Miller, Rathus, and Linehan 2006; CADTH 2010; Salsman 2011).

Why DBT? It is practical. Use of DBT skills can save lives in the moment and empowers the individual. While identifying why I became suicidal has been immensely helpful in providing me with insight, use of that knowledge has not been able to coach me through a suicidal episode. Tracing the origins of my mental health struggles back through my family history was useful and at times revelatory, but it could not get me out of bed when I was depressed. It was only when I learned that I had the power to regulate my own emotions and suicidal urges that I could do something about them. When putting together a program for suicidal adolescents and young adults, I was able to tap into this lived experience in developing a DBT-informed art therapy skills curriculum.

DBT is evidence-based. Through research studies, including randomized clinical trials, DBT has developed a successful empirical track record. It has been shown to reduce the incidence, frequency, and medical risk of suicide attempts. Outcomes of DBT research studies with adolescents suggest a 70 percent lower rate of suicide attempts, 68 percent lower rate of non-suicidal self-injury, and 67 percent lower rate of self-harm within a six-month treatment course (Linehan *et al.* 2006).

So, what exactly is DBT and how does it work? While its name may sound complicated, many of its underlying principles are quite simple. It looks at the causes of suicidality from a very practical approach and is backed by science. It recognizes that young people with suicidal behaviors often lack essential skills in self-regulation, navigating relationships, and managing distress. It is based on the idea that when we become emotionally dysregulated, the centers in our brain for clear thinking and judgment are reduced. We cannot solve problems from an intensely emotional state. In order to return to a more grounded mental state, emotional intensity must be reduced. This is done not with psychoanalytic approaches, but instead with basic skills training. Imbued knowledge and application of new skills can strengthen the resilience of youth and give them a sense of control during what is often a time of turmoil.

This chapter and the following chapter will take a look into the core components of DBT and show how they can be adapted for use in group art therapy. We will examine principles of dialectical thinking, techniques for mindfulness, distress tolerance, emotion regulation, and interpersonal effectiveness skills.

In 1993, Marsha Linehan broke new ground with the development of DBT. For the first time in contemporary therapeutic practice, a model was introduced that combined both Eastern philosophies such as Buddhist concepts of mindfulness with Western behavior strategies to create change. While DBT is considered a cognitive behavioral approach (addressing thinking and behavior patterns), it also moves clients into the experience of their bodies through creative and concrete mindfulness practices.

As a therapeutic approach, DBT suggests therapists help their clients to feel accepted and validated for their emotional and physical experiences. At the same time, therapists guide clients toward motivation for changing self-defeating, harmful behaviors. The idea that therapy can elicit both acceptance and change feels holistic. This approach has been very successful in the Arts in Recovery for Youth program.

At its foundation, DBT recognizes that some individuals are predisposed biologically to states of emotional dysregulation. Such states are often accompanied by, or the result of, living in invalidating environments. "The invalidating environment contributes to emotional dysregulation by failing to teach the child to label and modulate arousal, to tolerate distress, or to trust her own emotional responses as valid interpretations of events" (Linehan 1993, p.3).

> DBT theorizes that the problem behaviors of emotionally dysregulated individuals stem from a combination of biological and environmental factors. Specifically these factors are a biological vulnerability to emotional dysregulation and invalidating social environment—hence the term biosocial theory. (Rathus and Miller 2015, p.7)

While the language of DBT is new to adolescents and young adults, they do possess the capacity to learn and apply its concepts. DBT teaches them to accept themselves just as they are, with self-compassion, and to work toward changing unhealthy behaviors. This information is often new but embraced, as they are already practicing a greater capacity for abstract thinking and exploring varying mental states in the formation of an adult identity. They are hungry for solutions to their perceived problems.

Incorporating DBT skills training into an arts-based youth suicide prevention program has required some modification. The Arts in Recovery for Youth program teaches these immensely useful skills yet adds additional components specific to solving the youth suicide problem, such as peer support, direct dialogue, and safety practices. This is done through a lens of art therapy for many reasons, which have been explored in previous chapters—the expressive arts offer accessibility, various learning styles, enjoyment, a container in which to self-regulate, alternative forms of communication, and so on.

There are a few reasons that modification of traditionally prescribed DBT is necessary in our youth suicide prevention program, including addressing the immediacy of suicidality. Although DBT is clearly efficacious and increasingly used in many practice settings, demand for

DBT programs far exceeds existing resources. There is often a waitlist for availability in some geographic areas. The year-long requirements for these groups can conflict with changing schedules, college, and after-school activities of young people. There may be a lack of DBT skills coaches present, and clinicians are finding that they want to include DBT skills training in other settings such as art therapy, to accommodate the rising need.

The use of DBT in the AIRY program maintains the conceptual framework Linehan has established, but teaches abbreviated skill sets to make room for specific suicide prevention skills that have proved efficacious in the field of suicidology. In order to accommodate the number of youth at risk for suicide, initial art therapy groups are offered in 16-week seasons with two-hour programming. When the initial 16-week season is completed, youth may go onto a graduate or step-up group to further develop and maintain skills.

Like DBT, our model for a graduate group helps taper adolescents and young adults through stages of suicidality. When at higher risk they most need crisis intervention strategies. Later, as their risk reduces, they need maintenance of skills to avoid relapse. These groups are more youth driven as the therapist makes room for youth to take more responsibility in active skills teaching and practicing problem solving with peers. According to Rathus and Miller, a graduate group "mirrors the adolescent developmental trajectory toward separation, individuation, greater self-sufficiency, and the importance of peers" (2015, p.30).

Art therapy may alter the style in which young people learn DBT, which makes it available to a wider audience. Much of the content of the original DBT design is taught through memorizing acronyms. This can be a very linear form of learning that doesn't meet the needs of all incoming youth. For example, the acronym DEAR MAN is used to teach interpersonal skills. The acronym stands for "Describe, Express, Assert, Reinforce, (stay) Mindful, Appear Confident, Negotiate" (Linehan 1993). It has been my experience that not all clients are comfortable with this teaching style and can be resistant to it. Because of differences in emerging teens and young adults, it is important to be able to teach DBT skills in a variety of ways. This ensures that the delivery of skills does not create a barrier to learning essential life skills to cope with feeling suicidal.

Instead of acronyms, skills coaching can be taught in other ways, which may include handouts, discussion, role play, and processing information alongside art-making. The peer support component includes conversations and real-life examples of the contemporary challenges young people face—such as body image, emerging sexual orientation and gender identity, the impact of social media, bullying, and other social aspects of school stress. Art therapy works creatively and organically around specific DBT topics. Skills are reinforced more experientially and, for some, can thus be easier to grasp.

Dialectical thinking

Probably the most core component of DBT taught with expressive arts is dialectical thinking. In its most general terms, a dialectic is the idea that two opposing things can be true at the same time. This is extremely useful for youth to learn, as most often their conflicts derive from getting stuck in black and white thinking, or extremes. DBT teaches them how to think in gray areas. In DBT this is known as the middle path, or a mental state called "wise mind."

It may at first seem simplistic that solving the youth suicide problem involves learning to think in gray areas. However, this is a challenge and takes a good deal of practice and reinforcement, especially in more immediate situations that arise for youth. I have found that most youth are up for this challenge and welcome this new perspective for problem solving.

Dialectical thinking originated with philosophers such as Socrates and Plato (Fox 2005). While a historical discourse on the philosophy of the dialectic is beyond the scope of this book, it is helpful to see how it developed. I will illustrate this with an example. According to Hegel (Chalybäus 1837/2019), in the first of three stages, a dialectic contains a thesis. For example, a young person may assert, "I am alone." In the second stage, we look for the antithesis which contradicts or negates the thought, such as "but there are many people in my life." Finally, in the third stage, the tension between the two is resolved with a synthesis—"I have many people in my life and I feel alone."

In the example above, the youth may be driven toward suicidal thoughts by a conclusion in which they cannot see the full context. They can only see that they are alone and may build upon that with more negative conclusions such as "I am alone, I will always be alone. That means I am unlovable or a burden on people, so it would be better if I die." However, when challenged to use dialectical thinking, they can come to understand that they are not *actually* alone. Loneliness is a *feeling*, a temporary state that is likely to pass if they connect with people. If they are challenged, they can remember instances in which they did not feel alone.

In DBT, dialectical thinking centers on accepting the nature of paradox while moving toward a wiser, more intuitive understanding of our inner worlds. It is essentially a union of opposites. Youth are taught that both emotions and logic are valuable sources of information, but that there is an even wiser source of information in the dialectic. This new perspective reduces feelings of conflict between opposing internal states that contribute to their feeling suicidal. They are prompted to find the middle path to solve their dilemma.

> A dialectical therapeutic position is one of constantly combining acceptance with change, flexibility with stability, nurturing with challenging, and a focus on capabilities with a focus on deficits. The goal is to highlight the opposites, both in therapy and in clients' lives, and to provide conditions for syntheses. (Rathus and Miller 2015, p.8)

As dialectical thinking is at the heart of DBT, Linehan created a visual symbol to help clients learn. In AIRY, teens and young adults are very responsive to this image. They are shown the form of a Venn diagram, or mandorla, to represent three mental states—emotional mind, reasonable mind, and wise mind.

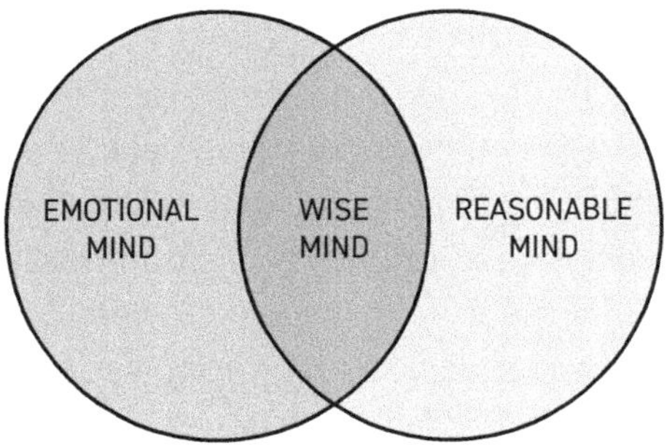

Figure 13.1 Wise mind symbol

Emotional mind is charged by intense feelings and action urges and is sometimes explained as "hot." Reasonable mind is informed by rational thought or logic, and is referred to as "cool." When conflict is present, emotions and logic contradict each other. In the third mental state, wise mind, youth learn to accept both their emotion and logic, and to then integrate them through a deeper, more felt understanding. One youth in the program described the process of wise mind as "You make a deal between your feelings and logic."

Practicing this symbolic shape in art-making reinforces its application in both the right brain and the left. This supports the idea in neuroscience that bilateral integration of the hemispheres of the brain can generate new neuronal pathways for growth. Balancing the brain through expressive arts techniques is a phenomenon that has been introduced into art therapy by authors including Carol McNamee (2003) and Cornelia Elbrecht (2018), and is gaining popularity for treatment of trauma as well.

Visualizing a wise mind symbol and giving it a concrete form with art materials aligns with young people's creative stages of development. In art therapy, teenagers and young adults go further and create wise mind characters and stories—sometimes from the movies they watch, the music they listen to, the comic books they read, the anime they draw, and even in Facebook memes. Art therapy can connect to young people where they are already and make it easier to learn DBT.

In DBT, mindfulness is the first of four skills training modules. Clients are next introduced to the modules of distress tolerance, emotion regulation, and interpersonal effectiveness (Linehan 1993). In this chapter we examine mindfulness, distress tolerance, and emotion regulation. In Chapter 16, we discuss interpersonal effectiveness.

Mindfulness

For centuries, Western medical practice has focused on changing thought and behavior patterns through cognitive strategies and behavior modification but overlooking the idea of intuition (what is known in DBT as wise mind). While at first the idea of using intuition may sound vague or ethereal, new fields in science and psychology are expanding on this premise. For example, support for the idea that we inherently possess and can be guided by "body wisdom" has surfaced in fields related to polyvagal theory, somatic psychology, and sensorimotor therapy. We have come to understand that our most powerful region of the brain for self-regulation—sometimes referred to as our reptilian brains—involves the way we interpret physical sensations in the body to mobilize us for action (Levine 2010; Porges 2012). In DBT, this body wisdom, or intuition, is developed through the practice of mindfulness.

In the Oxford Dictionary "mindfulness" is defined as "the quality or state of being conscious or aware of something" or "a mental state achieved by focusing one's awareness on the present moment, while calmly acknowledging and accepting one's feelings, thoughts, and bodily sensations, used as a therapeutic technique."

Mindfulness, as a form of meditation, has become increasingly popular in the last few decades due to its many health benefits. The practice has moved from a Buddhist concept founded about 2600 years ago to a mainstream psychotherapy construct today.

Davis and Hayes (2012) based their observations about mindfulness on the work of a wide range of researchers who found that mindfulness reduces stress, rumination, and emotional reactivity. People who experience mindfulness-based stress reduction have significantly less anxiety, depression, and somatic distress. Upon MRI, they show less neural reactivity. Mindfulness shifts people's ability to use emotion regulation strategies in a way that enables them to experience emotion more selectively. Mindfulness has also been shown to improve working memory, focus, and cognitive flexibility.

Marsha Linehan defines the DBT skill of mindfulness as "psychological and behavioral versions of meditation practices from Eastern spiritual training" (1993, p.63). They include taking a nonjudgmental stance, focusing on one thing in the moment, and being effective (doing what works).

Fortunately, art-making in itself can be a form of mindfulness. In the studio, mindfulness may be learned with drawing mandalas or zentangles, knitting or weaving fabric strips, drip paintings, collecting nature-based found objects, or building miniature worlds. Mindfulness is also explored in the body through breathwork, movement, and the senses. The rhythm of a paintbrush or the molding of clay can calm anxiety. The meditative aspects of coloring patterns or graffiti, or making and playing with tactile materials like sand, clay, or slime, focus on present experience, while also providing distraction and relief from unwanted thoughts.

Distress tolerance

Distress tolerance is developing the ability to better tolerate a stressful situation. This involves using mindfulness and physiological actions to reduce stress in the moment. It is extremely helpful in crisis situations, where emotions are too intense to be able to problem solve or make decisions and may trigger feelings of suicidality.

According to Linehan, "most approaches to mental health treatment focus on changing distressing events and circumstances. They have paid little attention to accepting, finding meaning for, and tolerating distress" (1993, p.96). The distress tolerance behaviors targeted in DBT skills training are concerned with tolerating and surviving crises. This is not to be confused with accepting unacceptable behavior or abuse, but rather the focus is on accepting life as it is in the moment.

Linehan describes distress tolerance skills as "ways of surviving and doing well in crisis situations without resorting to behaviors that will make the situation worse...when we can't immediately change a situation for the better, or when we can't sort out our feelings well enough to know what changes we want or how to make them" (quoted in Clark 2017, p.420).

Two elements of distress tolerance skills include crisis survival skills and reality acceptance skills. "Crisis survival skills help the person endure extremely painful emotional states in a mindful, nonimpulsive manner" (Clark 2017, p.45). These skills involve reducing impulsiveness, increasing motivation for behavior change, reducing physiological arousal, self-soothing, distraction, and increasing pleasurable moments (Linehan in Clark 2017).

Reality acceptance skills involve the core component known as "radical acceptance"—accepting the facts of reality exactly as they are, in the moment, and with suspending judgment. Radically accepting things that cannot be changed often leads an individual to a feeling of freedom, a liberation from trying to control things that are beyond their scope.

In the AIRY program, practical distress tolerance skills may involve:

- splashing cold water on our face
- squeezing clay or putty
- making sounds
- tapping

- playing music
- taking a shower or bath
- using the senses
- making art
- taking a walk
- being in nature
- reading
- talking to someone.

Distress tolerance with art can be relaxing and quieting or it can be a very physically active practice. With distress tolerance the *content* of the art is not important. It is more about the *process* of making art that reduces stress. It generally involves experimenting with materials in a sensory way. Some of the art therapy directives used for distress tolerance include:

- making a self-soothing or sensory box
- making a 3D safe place
- making a mandala (putting images in a circle)
- adult coloring
- making drip/pour paintings
- using palette knives to scrape paint on canvas
- kneading clay
- making collages
- random painting.

In *DBT-Informed Art Therapy*, Susan Clark (2017) lists suggested art therapy activities for distress tolerance such as creating Zen gardens, pet rocks, flowerpots, personal kaleidoscopes, strength medallions, stress balls, scribbling, and finger painting, among others.

Emotion regulation

According to Linehan (cited in Clark 2017), suicidal individuals report difficulty with identifying their emotions, as they often possess extreme and invalidating core beliefs about their emotional experiences. Emotion regulation skills assist them in naming their emotions and better understanding their function. Skills are learned which enable young people to reduce their susceptibility to highly charged emotional states. These skills teach them that they can change unwanted emotions when necessary and decrease their suffering of emotional pain. Perhaps most significant is the discovery that they can gain a sense of control over their feelings. This in itself provides a hope factor that can tremendously help suicidal inclinations.

In our program, emotion regulation skills are taught in the first few weeks. We focus on learning to notice and accept emotions, and then reduce the intensity of emotions. In plain words, we must acknowledge our feelings in order to dial them down.

Emotions themselves are not the problem driving young people to suicide. Rather it is how we *respond* to our emotions. In AIRY, we define clearly how to work with emotions. DBT teaches that emotion regulation *is not*:

- eliminating or getting rid of emotions
- ignoring emotions
- hiding our emotions or keeping them a secret
- stuffing or repressing emotions
- feeding our emotions by ruminating or obsessing
- acting out on our emotions
- escalating the emotions.

Instead, we teach that emotion regulation is more like balancing them, like getting our feelings to their right size. DBT teaches that emotions are useful and valuable and give us important information.

When working with young people at risk for suicide, "the goal of teaching [DBT] coping skills is to help establish safety, identify emotions, learn grounding techniques, and develop containment strategies in order to reduce maladaptive behaviors and to build a life worth living" (Masino Drass 2015, p.168).

In order to prevent suicide, intense emotional states must be addressed with some immediacy. In AIRY, we teach three initial steps to emotion regulation—Step one: notice the emotion (mindfulness); Step two: measure the emotion's intensity from 0 to 10 (self-monitoring); Step three: focus on regulating the emotion, which means that we save problem solving for later (dysregulated emotions inhibit the capacity to problem solve). Self-monitoring with numbers involves mindfulness, because youth stop and notice their emotions in order to measure them. Once the emotion is measured, they can take small actions to lower the intensity back to a stabilizing size. Then they will be able to solve problems.

In the art studio, we teach emotion regulation skills of metaphor, building mastery, and using an opposite action.

Metaphor

Working with metaphor can help young people reframe their problems dialectically. They are guided toward building a stronger sense of self within the containment of the art therapy environment. Susan Clark (2017) suggests that:

> Both art therapy and DBT regard metaphors as potentially powerful catalysts for change...metaphor facilitates a dialectical worldview by comparing something the client understands with something she does not...the client learns that significantly differing perspectives are possible, and perhaps even desired, as this also suggests the possibility of new behaviors, attitudes and ways of living. (pp.142–143)

Some of our art therapy directives targeted for emotion regulation through metaphor include writing round robin poems based on an emotion, building 3D houses of emotions, and developing emotion characters or creatures with a variety of materials. Other directives consist of personifying emotions with colors and depicting emotions as elements of weather.

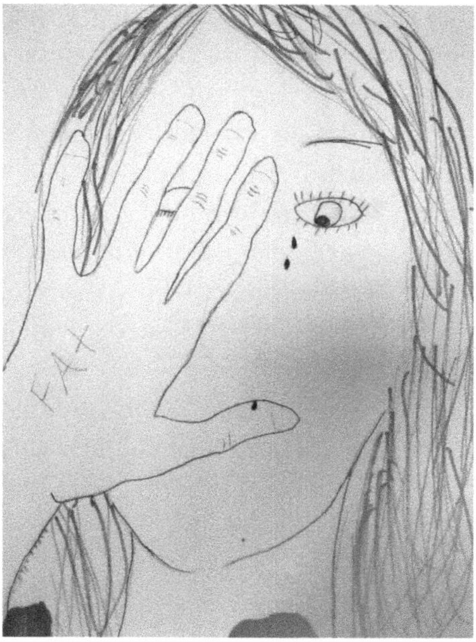

Figure 13.2 Emotion character 1

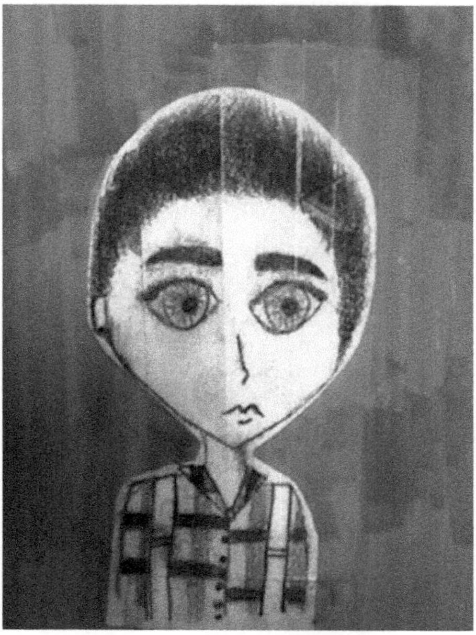

Figure 13.3 Emotion character 2

Mastery

Building mastery is an emotional regulation skill that involves engaging in pleasurable but challenging activities which necessitate decision making and problem solving (Linehan 1993). For example, the act of choosing their own art materials and how they will use them, and then remaining with an artwork from beginning to end, promotes independence and a sense of accomplishment. Completing their unique art products helps young people move toward a stronger self-concept.

Many suicidal youth often present with a history of trauma. Some art therapists suggest that because trauma work is not always processed in a linear manner, it can be helpful for youth to be working on multiple projects at once, and to be able to choose what they would like to work on during that session. This may also help build a sense of control and mastery, as well as help to temper emotional responses that may be evoked by certain materials (Masino Drass 2015).

Opposite action

Another DBT skill for emotion regulation is known as opposite action (Linehan 1993). This generally is an easy skill to learn and use. Once an emotion and its intensity are identified, youth are prompted to think of an action they could take to feel the opposite emotion.

For example, a young person is feeling depressed at an 8 out of 10. When asked what emotion would be opposite to this one, they can choose from many—perhaps joy or humor, or feeling playful, excited, alive, or happy. There is no exact answer, which means there is room to be creative. Let's say they choose to feel silly as the opposite emotion to depression. They are then prompted to brainstorm actions that would elicit feeling silly, such as:

- looking up jokes on their phone
- drawing cartoons
- making funny faces
- watching a comedy
- playing with a pet or a child
- dancing or moving their body in a funny way.

Art-making is used to identify emotion and its opposite in the form of images (e.g. this is how depression feels, this is how being silly feels). An example may be using magazines to create a silly collage. In addition to art-making, group art therapy allows for peer support in arriving at opposite action. A good way to encourage this in the studio is to make opposite action paintings in pairs, where young people share a canvas and find their way to their opposite.

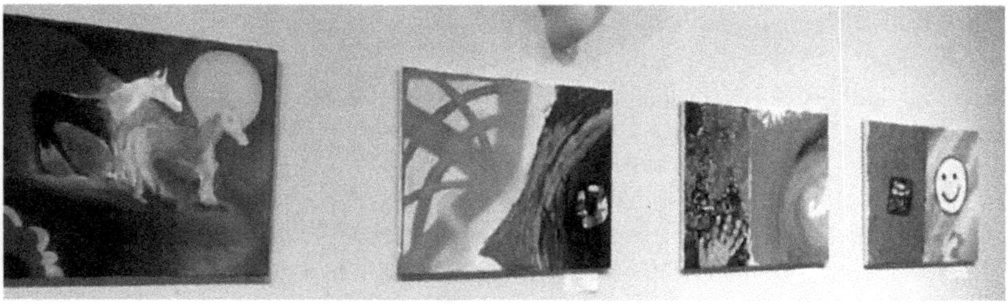

Figure 13.4 Opposite action paintings

Through DBT-informed art therapy, young people can gain a sense of control over their thoughts and emotions during developmental stages of change and growth. Learning to self-regulate is frequently revelatory and liberating. It keeps them present. The desire for escape and feeling trapped is reduced, and suicidality lessened.

Conclusion

DBT through the expressive arts can teach young people in innovative ways how to regulate their own emotions, to better tolerate day-to-day distress, learn and practice mindfulness, and assimilate interpersonal behavior strategies in stressful environments. The expressive arts help young people to understand their own mental and emotional states, as well as provide a source for developing intuition and wisdom. The language of DBT is easily translatable in metaphorical constructs present in art therapy. When verbal expression is difficult, creating personal art helps inform them of what's happening in their minds and bodies. Carefully constructed art therapy directives teach skills necessary to prevent suicide and reduce risk. Expressive arts programs can be eclectic in nature, informed by DBT, and utilize other discoveries in current suicidology.

References

Canadian Agency for Drugs and Technologies in Health (CADTH) (2010) Dialectical behaviour therapy in adolescents for suicide prevention: Systematic review of clinical-effectiveness. *CADTH Technology Overviews 1*, 1, e0104.

Chalybäus, H.M. (2019) *Historical Development of Speculative Philosophy: From Kant to Hegel.* (Trans.). Wentworth Press. (Original work published 1837).

Clark, S. (2017) *DBT-Informed Art Therapy.* London: Jessica Kingsley Publishers.

Davis, D.M. and Hayes, J.A. (2012) What are the benefits of mindfulness? *American Psychological Association 43*, 7, 64. Retrieved from www.apa.org/monitor/2012/07-08/ce-corner on October 18, 2021.

Elbrecht, C. (2018) *Healing Trauma with Guided Drawing.* Berkeley, CA: North Atlantic Books.

Fox, M.A. (2005) *The Accessible Hegel.* Buffalo, NY: Prometheus Books.

Levine, P. (2010) *In an Unspoken Voice: How the Body Releases Trauma and Restores Goodness.* Berkeley, CA: North Atlantic Books.

Linehan, M. (1993) *Skills Training Manual for Treating Borderline Personality Disorder.* New York: The Guilford Press.

Linehan, M.M., Comtois, K.A., Murra, A.M., Brown, M.Z., *et al.* (2006) Two-year randomized controlled trial and follow-up of dialectical behavior therapy vs therapy by experts for suicidal behaviors and borderline personality disorder. *Archives of General Psychiatry 63*, 7, 757–766.

Masino Drass, J. (2015) Art therapy for individuals with borderline personality: Using a dialectical behavior therapy framework. *Art Therapy: Journal of the American Art Therapy Association 32*, 4, 168–176.

McNamee, C. (2003) Bilateral art: Facilitating systemic integration and balance. *The Arts in Psychotherapy 30*, 5, 283–292.

Miller, A.L., Rathus, J.H., and Linehan, M.M. (2006) *Dialectical Behavior Therapy with Suicidal Adolescents.* New York: The Guilford Press.

Porges, S.W. (2012) *The Polyvagal Theory: Neurophysiological Foundations of Emotions, Attachment, Communication, and Self-Regulation.* New York: W.W. Norton.

Rathus, J. and Miller, A. (2002) Dialectical behavior therapy adapted for suicidal adolescents. *Suicide & Life Threatening Behavior 32*, 2, 146–157.

Rathus, J. and Miller, A. (2015) *DBT Skills Manual for Adolescents.* New York: The Guilford Press.

Salsman, N.L. (2011) Adapting dialectical behavior therapy to help suicidal adolescents. *Current Psychiatry 10*, 3, 18–34.

Chapter 14

A DBT-Informed Art Therapy Case Study

THE STORY OF MAYA

Maya was a 16-year-old female referred to the AIRY program after presenting with suicidal thoughts and behaviors including active self-injury (cutting). She attended weekly individual therapy but continued to be consumed by her suicidal thoughts and urges. When I met Maya, she appeared to be carrying a great deal of personal anxiety and stress. She struggled with teen angst somewhere in the middle of making an earnest effort to change her circumstances and rebelling against them. Maya was open and receptive to the group environment and welcomed the company of others her own age in the art studio. She was a natural artist but was very modest about her capabilities.

Maya and the other group members were not accustomed to talking about their feelings of suicidality. In this sense, their shared understanding developed quickly and their direct dialogue about suicide prevention, and exploration of those feelings, was freeing. There was a safe and nonjudgmental atmosphere, in which they could be seen, heard, and validated, and sublimate their urges into productive forms of art-making.

Maya's family history included an estranged relationship with her biological mother and present conflicts with her biological father. She identified current stressors as social problems and academic pressure at school, depression and anxiety, and post-traumatic stress regarding a history of sexual assault within the last year. Sharing about her experiences through ongoing peer support was a new and useful experience.

Using rating scale factors suggested by Jobes, Maya identified high levels of stress (8/10), urges to self-harm (6/10), emotional pain (7/10), and self-hate (5/10) which she described as feeling like a constant disappointment in strained relationships with family, lack of academic success, and unstable romantic relationships. She rated feeling suicidal 7/10.

In group art therapy sessions Maya revealed that her reasons for wanting to die included feeling like a disappointment to her family and lacking meaningful social relationships. Her initial artwork included expressions of feeling isolated and depressed.

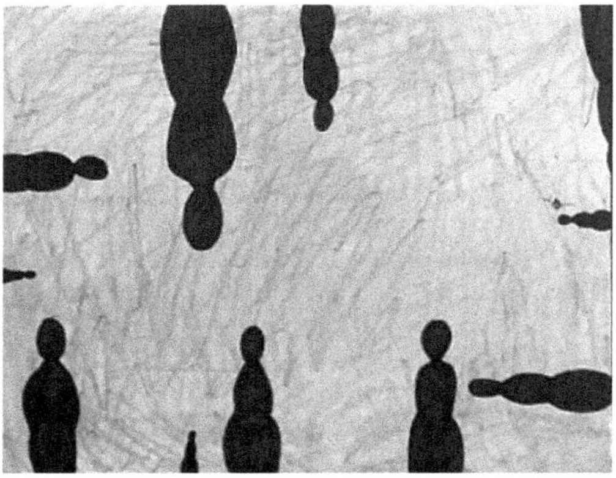

Figure 14.1 Depression picture 1

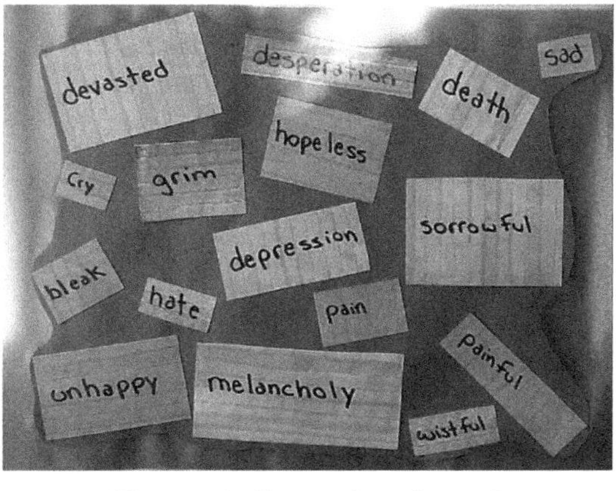

Figure 14.2 Depression picture 2

Maya was introduced to the concept of using mindfulness to regulate her emotions. She enjoyed creating a series of rhythmic paintings with a focus on nature. The space of the studio served to calm her anxieties and allow her to explore mindfulness in a creative way. By practicing painting as a form of therapy, the intensity of her emotions reduced. In addition to painting, she was able to conceptualize additional ways to self-soothe outside of the group and at home.

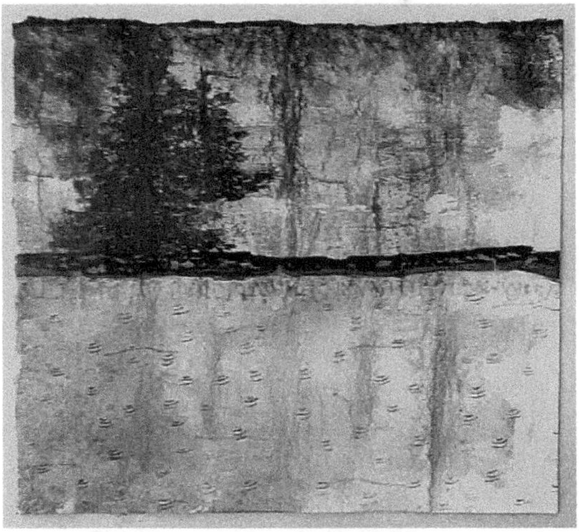

Figure 14.3 Nature watercolor

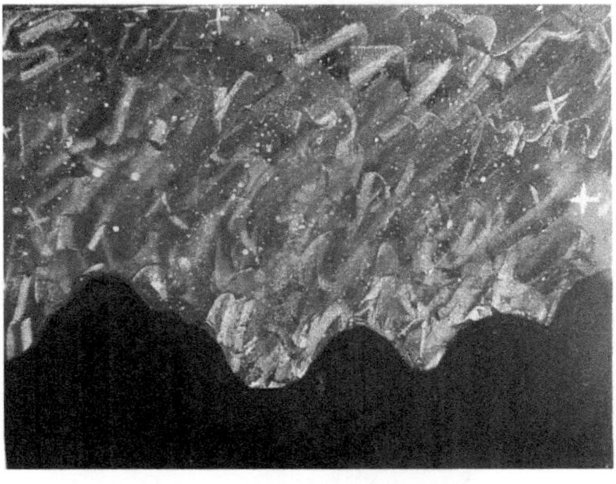

Figure 14.4 Nature acrylic painting

Maya added breathing, walking, and exercise in the outdoors to her practice of mindfulness. In further art therapy sessions, she came to understand the concept of wise mind and created a symbol of it in the form of a pink tree, as she related strongly to nature. She used the symbol of a pink tree to express her desire to move away from self-harm.

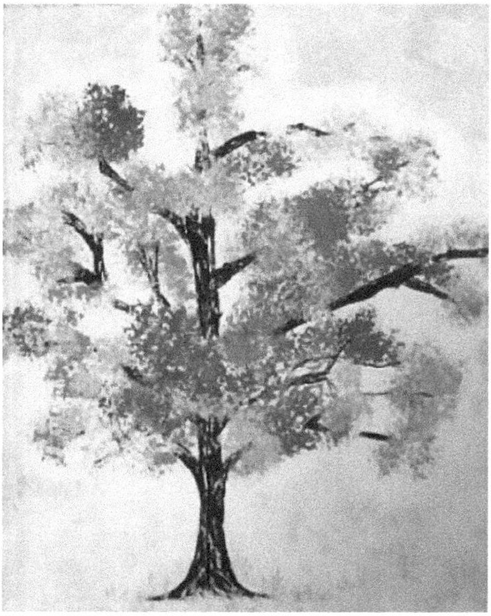

Figure 14.5 Pink tree 1

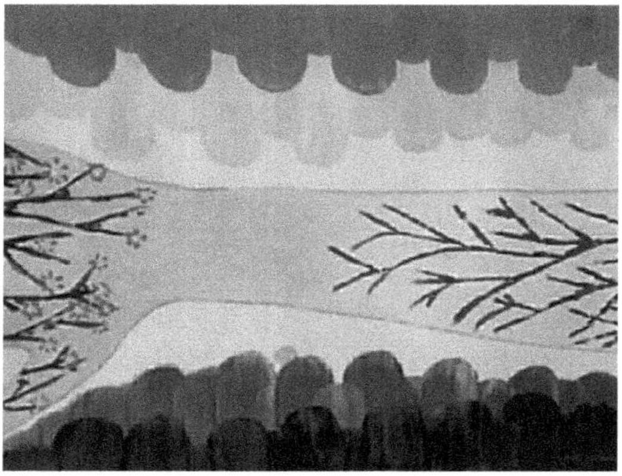

Figure 14.6 Self harm picture

While exploring the image of the pink tree to depict her sense of inherent wisdom, her confidence in her own abilities increased. Dialectical thinking resonated strongly with her and gave her a sense of self-control over chaotic inner states. She became attracted to the DBT symbol of wise mind—the mandorla (Venn diagram). She traced the circles on paper and wrote poetry in them to problem solve emotional conflict in her relationships by balancing her emotions and logic. Poetry became another outlet for her to regulate emotions.

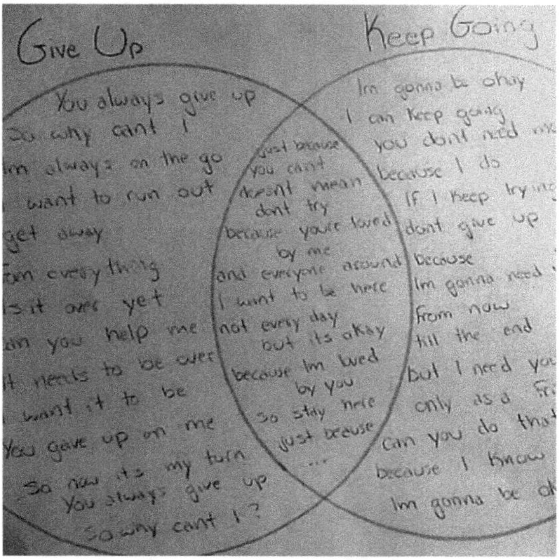

Figure 14.7 Wise mind

I introduced the idea of using self-portrait collage to target feelings of self-hate with DBT's acceptance and change strategies. During the collage-making process, Maya was able to see herself from more than one point of view. This helped her decision-making process in peer and romantic relationships.

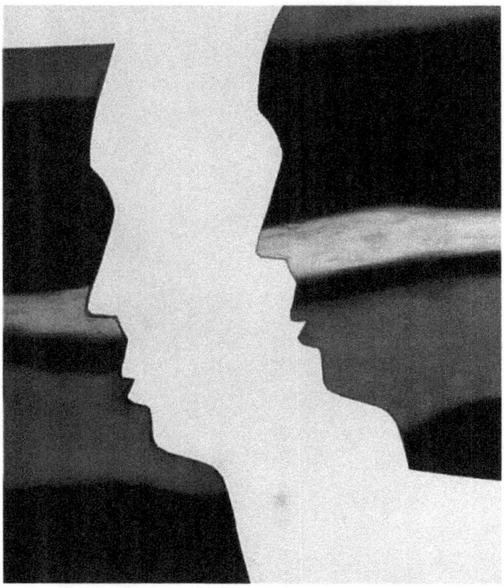

Figure 14.8 Self-portrait collage

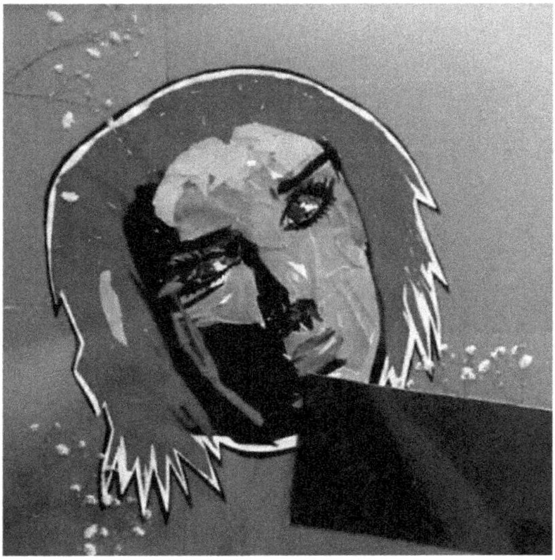

Figure 14.9 Self-portrait collage

Through mask making, Maya came to envision herself as an empowered female in the face of adversity and trauma. She continued to incorporate her love of nature and found a sense of self-preservation.

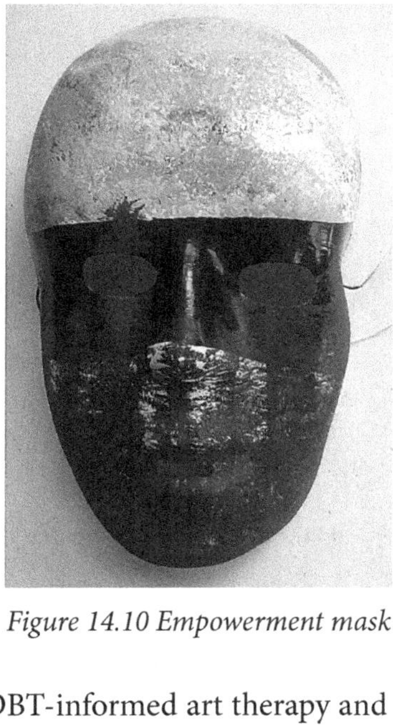

Figure 14.10 Empowerment mask

After 12 weeks of DBT-informed art therapy and peer support, Maya reported lower levels of suicidality, emotional pain, urges, and self-hate.

While her stress levels remained high, she had put effective DBT strategies into place. Her risk level for suicide was reduced from 70 percent to 50 percent.

After 24 weeks Maya reported a continued decrease in suicidal thoughts and abstinence from self-injury. Her risk level was reduced to 30 percent.

Between nine months and one year in the program, Maya maintained no suicidal thoughts and no self-injury. She had identified healthy ways to communicate emotions. Her family relationships improved as well as her self-confidence and academic achievement. She became less preoccupied by anxiety and post-traumatic symptoms became less frequent. She had developed peer relationships in the group and in the community. After one year, she felt ready to graduate from the program.

For Maya's final piece she chose a mindfulness exercise in dripping paint down the canvas to represent all of her multifaceted colors.

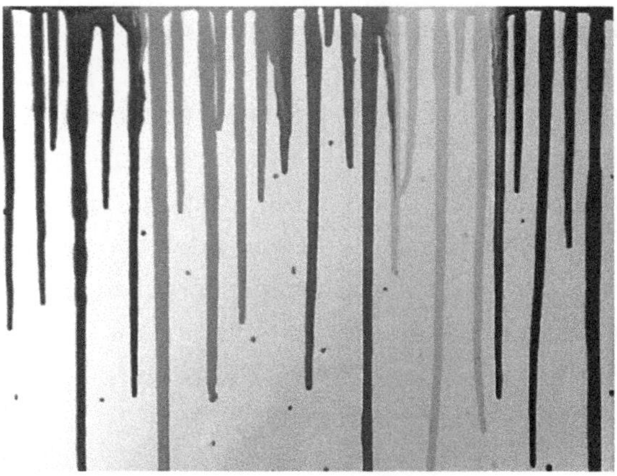

Figure 14.11 Dripping paint

During the second year in my relationship with Maya, we maintained caring contact through text messages and periodic visits to the studio. She continued to write poetry and make art, and she engaged in art projects with her father. She maintained a stable romantic relationship and finished high school early, while concurrently taking college courses.

In our third year of maintaining contact, Maya checked in by self-report. She indicated that she was having mild suicidal ideation triggered by fears related to her family moving out of state. She attended the graduate step-up group for a few weeks to reinforce her DBT skills. Her suicidal thoughts returned to remission shortly thereafter.

In the fourth year of periodically keeping in touch, Maya contacted me with recurring symptoms of anxiety and depression related to moving out of state. Through a few phone sessions, we implemented DBT strategies for reducing anxiety and using dialectical thinking. When asked if she remembered the concept of wise mind, she stated proudly, "How could I forget?" She returned to using the wise mind symbol to help strategize solutions to problems associated with the transitions of young adulthood. In addition, Maya sought out individual therapy to further examine recurrent anxiety. She re-established her skills and her symptoms began to stabilize.

Maya is an example of an emerging young woman who has been able to shift from states of suicidality and inner turmoil to self-compassion, emotional regulation, and mastery, as she moves forward into her future. She continues to make art and write poetry and take walks on the beach to self-soothe during times of distress and as an ongoing practice of mindfulness. She is currently exploring a variety of goals and has a strong desire to increase her sense of purpose and contribution to society. She has stated that she feels a sense of pride about my being able to share her story of success in our program.

Much of what happens in the Arts in Recovery for Youth program involves young people breaking prolonged periods of isolation and making validating and supportive connections with peers. Learning to better navigate relationships during this transitional developmental period is the subject of our next two chapters.

Chapter 15

Gregory's Story

Interpersonal dynamics play a central role in the recovery of youth from suicidality. As discussed earlier, Durkheim proposed that social factors, such as feelings of exclusion from society, are at the heart of suicidal thinking. Our social rank within a group and our acceptance as part of that group often motivates our behavior. The need to give attention and receive attention from others can be a major source of satisfaction in life.

This rang particularly true for a young male who found the program to be life-saving. While Gregory was in his mid 20s when he was referred to Arts in Recovery for Youth, his therapist and I agreed he was a very good fit and that he would get along well with the other young adults in the group, most of whom were struggling with societal expectations and attitudes toward gender roles. This young man experienced the world in an extremely invalidating way—he spoke of feeling persecuted by society and alienated by society's focus on money and beauty. His personal values on anti-fascism, breaking gender norms, and addressing societal needs were part of his daily life. He sought validation and acceptance.

Gregory brought to the forefront of our group the stigma associated with being male and seeking treatment for his symptoms. He talked of the difficulties he experienced with being able to express his emotions among male peers and the level of restriction it presented. I was well aware that the statistics for completed suicides were much higher for males than for females, and that cultural expectations about gender were a significant part of the problem.

Fortunately, Gregory was highly interested in film and wanted to use film to make a difference in the world. He was attending film school while working a full-time job. Despite his history of six suicide attempts within the last year, his passion for film had kept him alive and became his primary protective factor against suicide.

When Gregory reported feelings of suicidality at 80–90 percent, along with engaging in frequent acts of self-harm, I suggested he may need a higher level of treatment, such as that available in a hospital setting. He quickly informed me of his repeated traumatic experiences within systems and institutions, and that he was adamantly against this kind of crisis intervention. We were able to create a safety plan that included the commitment of people he lived with, close monitoring, caring contact, and coordination with his primary therapist.

Gregory's history included family alcoholism, the loss of his father as a teenager, and being victimized in abusive situations. He had survived a good deal of trauma and struggled to find a sense of optimism in life. He defined himself as a nihilist. His drivers for suicidality included feelings of self-hate and burdensomeness, and self-perception of being "never good enough" because of "negative childhood messages." However, he maintained two strong reasons for living—his desire to be a filmmaker and to take care of others, especially in his romantic relationships.

He was drawn to art forms that confronted social issues and expressed himself this way in the studio. His black and white drawings contained subjects such as political and musical references, alcoholism, a gravestone, and a dark shadow of a man dying by suicide. His only color drawing was that of a film director's chair and camera. It was as if he lived in a gray world and only through his self-expression in film could he turn on the color. His art was specific and meaningful, and provided him with a way to discharge his pent-up emotions.

Gregory responded positively to expressive arts and peer support, as well as DBT and interpersonal skills training. After about two months in the program, his feelings of suicidality reduced from 90 percent to 50 percent, as he engaged in filmmaking as therapy. Recognizing that his search for meaning and need to contribute to the world motivated him in a positive way, I offered him the opportunity to film and produce a documentary of the AIRY program. He immediately agreed and began creative collaboration with me and with group members, and in building his own personal crew. Even with a fair degree of self-doubt, he stepped up to the challenge and quickly got to work. With consent from parents, he began interviewing the teens and taking footage of art-making in the studio. He was given the liberty to share his voice in his chosen medium and was well received.

Shortly after we premiered his 24-minute documentary in a theatre of 150 people, he reported to me that his intrusive and constant thoughts of suicide had completely stopped. For the first time in his life, he had found relief. His desire to live increased by 90 percent. He felt alive and transformed.

The film cemented his strong sense of purpose and allowed him to make a deep connection to the community, while expressing his views about society and stigma. In Durkheim's words, he was no longer disintegrated from society—hence his inclination toward suicide had dissolved.

Gregory's increased sense of belonging with peers prompted him to do a film workshop the following summer for our three groups. He also began to mentor younger members. Subsequently, he has become known as the big brother of the program and serves as a role model, especially to younger males. They become excited to see him when he attends our community events or drops by the studio.

After graduating the program, Gregory maintained no thoughts of suicide for nearly a year. He began reaching out when he struggled and put skills into place before things got worse. While he is someone who may struggle with periods of suicidal thinking, he has learned to manage it with supports and to stay safe. His drive to produce more films challenges his old negative beliefs and is helping him to create a new schema for living. He continues to attend therapy and works diligently on his recovery. He now presents as hopeful, optimistic, and well engaged in life. I am proud to know him and to witness both his personal metamorphosis and evolution as a young filmmaker.

Chapter 16

Interpersonal Skills

When Marsha Linehan was studying clients who become suicidal, she noticed that a significant problem among them was a set of belief patterns and uncontrollable emotional responses that inhibited their ability to use skills. Many of her clients struggled with premature termination of relationships. They struggled to tolerate or decrease the intensity of their emotions or to problem solve about what they needed in a given situation. Other barriers in relationships included the client's tendency to go to extremes of belief, complete neediness, feelings of unworthiness, and demanding behavior (1993a). With this in mind, she developed the fourth DBT module of interpersonal effectiveness.

The module of interpersonal effectiveness focuses on "situations where the objective is to change something (e.g. requesting someone do something) or to resist changes someone else is trying to make (e.g. saying no)" (Linehan 1993b, p.71). These skills teach youth to assert themselves in a way that they are taken more seriously, while at the same time not damaging their relationships or losing their self-respect. Specific skill sets relate to developing healthier, reciprocal relationships and improving a sense of mastery and self-respect. Linehan helps clients prioritize and ask for what they want or need and to assert their rights. She also helps them set goals in relationships (Linehan 1993b). Many of these skills are taught with cognitive behavior therapy, giving young people ways to analyze their situations, to reframe their negative thought patterns, and to problem solve.

The priority of interpersonal effectiveness is to do what works. The goal is for both people in the relationship to get what they need. Pitfalls to avoid include escalating the problem, having to be "right," or staying stuck in emotions.

Interpersonal response patterns taught in DBT skills training are very similar to those taught in many assertiveness and interpersonal problem-solving classes. They include effective strategies for asking for what one needs, saying no, and coping with interpersonal conflict (Linehan 1993b, p.70).

Simply put, interpersonal effectiveness skills are designed to improve communication in relationships. Use of these skills involves implementing skills that were previously learned in other modules. Use of mindfulness and nonjudgment in thinking about and dealing with relationship conflict complements assertiveness skills. The ability to tolerate distress and self-regulate emotions are prerequisites to developing stable relationships.

While these skills are immensely useful, they do not work in every situation. Clinicians need to pay particular attention to cases where young people are living in invalidating environments. I have seen this especially with my gender-questioning clients who seek support and acceptance from their families and do not get it. In AIRY it is important to counsel parents in communication strategies, specifically around suicidal thoughts. Parents tend to become so alarmed that their behavior escalates the crisis and interferes with finding solutions. Anyone working with suicidal youth can benefit from examining their own reactions and biases so they can successfully help them.

Thus, an important factor to consider here is that interpersonal effectiveness requires two people to be able to communicate and negotiate. Unfortunately, it does not always work in situations where there are people unwilling to communicate, negotiate, or compromise. "Environmental factors may preclude effectiveness. At times even the most skilled individuals cannot be effective in getting what they want, keeping others liking them, or behaving in ways that they respect" (Linehan 1993b, p.76).

For youth, learned skills such as saying no or insisting on rights with parents can have negative consequences. In some cases, to get basic survival needs met, the client "may have to act in ways that damage her pride or otherwise hurt her self respect" (Linehan 1993b, p.76). In these situations young people often blame themselves when they do not get what they need. This can lead to deeper feelings of shame, burdensomeness, and self-hate, and thereby present increased risk for suicide.

Early on in learning the DBT skill of interpersonal effectiveness,

I recognized these deficits and became frustrated. While it is beneficial for these skills to be practiced in other, more validating relationships until situations improve at home, I found that it was essential to alter and add skills more specific to suicidal youth living in invalidating environments. For this reason, the AIRY model focuses on:

- the strength of peer support within the group
- setting boundaries
- managing anger and communication styles
- increasing a sense of personal power
- challenging feelings of burdensomeness and making contributions to the world.

These help young people develop a greater sense of self, confidence in their own abilities, and a sense of worth and connection. We will review these skills now.

Peer support

While early on group members are often not ready to work on interpersonal effectiveness, there is a social skill that they begin to engage with immediately in the AIRY program: the concept of peer support. Our model teaches peer support strategies in conjunction with interpersonal effectiveness skills, in a non-traditional manner. Whereas most group therapies operate on the premise that forming relationships outside the group can be detrimental to the therapeutic process (i.e. for individuals who engage with peers in ineffective ways), I have found that not to be the case with a guided structure of peer support.

In conventional DBT, limits are restrictive and peers are encouraged not to engage with each other outside of therapy, and especially not in crisis situations. In AIRY, the reverse is true. From day one, youth learn safe skills in how to help each other in crisis and non-crisis situations, and subsequently become empowered when given the confidence to do so. This form of trust in the power of the group to help each other has saved lives. Youth learn and demonstrate how to ask for help and become increasingly more comfortable breaking the silence about their feelings of suicidality. They learn they can rely on each other for basic needs of human connection and understanding. This promotes an attitude of nonjudgment, compassion, and strengths-building.

When teaching peer support strategies, I use a checklist of dos and don'ts to eliminate confusion.

Peer support *is*:

- staying safe
- not getting yourself or others into a harmful situation
- asking an adult for help when needed and when someone is feeling suicidal
- listening without judgment (accepting others as they are)
- sharing your own experience of recovery (what happened and how you got better)
- letting others express their emotions or be vulnerable with you
- letting others know you care and knowing that there is no shame in asking for help
- keeping your own boundaries (e.g. I can't talk after 9 pm) and helping yourself
- staying calm and sharing resources (numbers, hotlines, what works for you)
- helping each other build their support system
- doing distracting activities together
- encouraging others to use their skills
- checking in on others (sending a caring text: "How are you doing today?").

Peer support is *not*:

- talking about explicit details of feeling suicidal/self-harming that may trigger someone
- sharing information about methods to hurt oneself
- solving someone's problems/trying to "fix" things

- rescuing others (you are not a superhero, just one person)
- giving advice, especially on things you don't know about
- lending money
- making promises
- holding others' secrets when it is dangerous
- always worrying about others, becoming obsessed with helping them
- spreading rumors or gossiping
- trying to control the situation
- shaming or judging someone who is different
- overloading someone with too much information
- ignoring someone
- making fun of someone.

In forming a sense of self, youth often turn to peers to find reassurance. The groups that develop in the program are quite diverse, yet all find support amongst their peers. Peer support offers a form of caring contact which also reinforces practical application of day-to-day DBT skills. Maintaining caring contact guides young people towards resilience beyond the scope of the therapy space. Practice of safe talk among peers prevents contagion. They learn to safeguard against sharing details of methods of self-harm and suicide, idealized attitudes, or biased media influence.

Building a wider net of recovery-oriented peer support reduces feelings of burdensomeness and thwarted belongingness, the risk factors for suicide proposed by Thomas Joiner earlier in this book. A young member described the difference between ordinary social connections and peer support on a group mural when he painted the words "We are more than friends."

Figure 16.1 Group mural

As we saw in Gregory's story, positive peer development through the arts increases community engagement. It breaks down long periods of isolation in which youth feel helpless and burdensome. Teaching artists and expressive arts therapists can increase access to the arts and community building when working with youth. They can collaborate with area organizations to offer youth-driven events such as art shows, poetry readings, speaking engagements, open mic nights, music, film, fashion, and more.

This kind of collaboration occurred when working with Gregory. AIRY members participated in the documentary, which introduced film and video therapy in the art studio. They also wrote songs and poetry as part of a community event we called "Love Yourself," hosted by a local performing arts theatre. Engaging with the community in this way fostered greater peer support and social relatedness. It had the effect of normalizing their struggles, and of breaking down barriers of stigma that surround suicidality and mental illness. Benefits to the community included education, awareness, and a new cultural platform for the arts.

Our peer support model has proven to be very successful. This kind of relationship is often brand new to people. Either they have not received support from their peers in a safe, supportive, and healthy way, or they have never been part of a group that uses peer support. They describe their peer support relationships like nothing they have experienced before. They find it helpful during times of distress, and in feeling less alone. With peer support, they become their own skills coaches. They share not only problems but ways to practice skills and stay safe. They use peer support to build healthy relationships with clear boundaries.

Peer support allows for rehearsal of skills through ongoing role play in and out of the art studio. I have found that the experience of peer support provides vital feedback necessary for youth to master interpersonal skills in similar-age settings. Peer support has a positive effect on other relationships as well, addressing the adolescent's need to imitate peers at this stage in their development.

In my experience, peer support works congruently with the DBT concept of radical genuineness. When practiced by both the therapist and peers, youth feel validated and accepted.

Rathus and Miller define radial genuineness as "speaking in a way that conveys your view of the other as an equal and capable of handling direct and honest feedback" (2015, p.54). An example of radical genuineness includes "intermittent and appropriate self-disclosure regarding the skills trainer's personal use of DBT skills in response to life's challenges" (2015, p.54).

Art activities to increase peer support generally involve group projects and projects in pairs. Probably our most popular of these is making "round robin" paintings. Each member of the group gets a canvas and begins working on it. After a few minutes they are instructed to pass their canvas to the person on their right. In turn, they receive a painting begun by another group member and are now tasked with helping to develop it. The paintings continue around the room until they are returned to the original artist. The original artist then makes any needed changes or concluding details. The result is that they can take home a work of art where every member of the group has left their mark.

The round robin painting is an example of a peer support project that serves many functions. It helps encapsulate and memorialize the overall group experience. It expresses each personality in the room. It is a platform for diversity and inclusion. It identifies group members as separate beings functioning together as a cohesive unit. In this way, the artwork becomes a permanent reminder that they belong to something larger than themselves alone. The round robin can also act as a transitional object and assist members as the group comes to an end.

Youth particularly have enjoyed showing their round robin paintings at art shows in the community. They are often proud of their collaboration and creative connectedness. They feel good about representing values of reciprocity, cooperation, and teamwork.

Boundaries

Setting and maintaining boundaries is a very important part of the conversation about interpersonal effectiveness. In AIRY, boundaries are taught by first discussing different types of boundaries, such as physical space boundaries, emotional boundaries, intimacy and body boundaries (including consent), intellectual boundaries, boundaries about money and personal possessions, boundaries about time, and relationship boundaries. Three boundary styles are reviewed and explored—rigid boundaries, flexible boundaries, and loose to no boundaries.

Sharing space and making art together in the studio can often reveal information about boundaries, such as:

- where people choose to sit
- how people share table space and materials
- who comes to group early, who comes late
- whether people want to share or talk about their art
- how people talk to each other
- the volume at which people speak
- body language in and out of the studio.

Teaching teens and young adults to model and maintain boundaries in the group can at times be challenging. Sometimes, a group member may, without realizing it, cross a boundary. Examples are when someone frequently interrupts others, is very loud, asks invasive questions, gives advice in a demanding way, or when someone tries to hug or physically comfort a group member without permission. Such conflict in a group can be used as a learning experience for everyone, and promote the power of the group to govern collectively.

A frequent art activity used to elicit the development of healthy boundaries is a modified version of a symbolic sociogram, which we call a relationship map. When I present this art therapy directive, youth typically engage quickly because their curiosity is piqued. It is new and different. They are eager to discover what they will learn from their relationship maps.

Participants are first asked to trace a large round circle on the page—the boundary line of their relationship map. We use 12- x 12-inch white cardstock and trace a circle from a 10-inch dinner plate. They are next asked to come up with a personal symbol that represents them, and to place this symbol in the center of the circle. Next, they are asked to identify symbols to represent the people in their lives, and to then place these symbols in degrees of closeness and apartness inside or outside the circle.

Sometimes this is a point where the activity ends and youth benefit from just creating the symbols of relationships in their lives and visually representing their feelings about them. It is as if they get to see who is in their world through new eyes. The symbols often show rich and meaningful perceptions of the fullness of their lives.

In some groups, we are able to expand on the relationship maps. Youth are prompted to identify their boundary style with each person on their map. For example, a solid line may represent a close-knit relationship, with healthy and respected boundaries. A dotted line may represent a more distant relationship with a broken boundary. A double line may represent a very rigid boundary, particularly in a relationship that feels less emotionally safe. A zig zag is used to define a conflictual relationship where boundaries feel unsteady. A wavy line may represent an overly loose boundary in a vulnerable relationship.

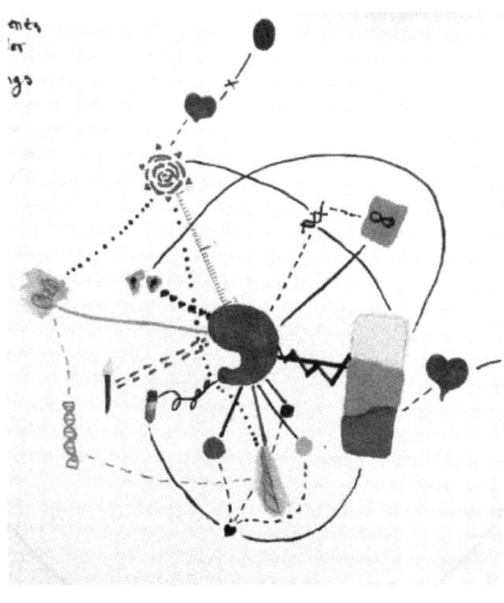

Figure 16.2 Relationship map

When the maps are done, youth are generally quick to want to describe their pictures to the group. As they talk about their relationships, they gain insight and understanding about where they would like to make change. This can also foster a renewed sense of empowerment. They realize they have choices in their relationships. The maps provide fruitful information for further therapy. I often suggest that they share these works with their individual therapists for further exploration.

Managing anger

When teaching skills for managing anger, I usually ask the group how they deal with their anger and whether these ways reduce or increase their anger. The group then brainstorms more effective ways to reduce anger, remembering that the first goal is to lower the intensity of the emotion, then solve problems.

There is a great specific DBT skill set for using interpersonal effectiveness for managing anger. With expressive writing exercises, youth are prompted to challenge thought patterns involved in their conflicts. They are then redirected toward mindfulness via nonjudgmental awareness and cognitive reframing. To simplify the skill set, I adapt DBT concepts into a journaling exercise where they can create their own scripts for conflict resolution.

The journal exercise breaks down the skill into the following six steps:

1. The first step is to write a description of what they are angry about, or in most conflict situations, the story of what happened. For example:

   "My mother really pissed me off because she never understands me. She won't let me stay out for a late movie tonight and it's her fault if my friends get mad at me. She doesn't care if I have friends. I'm so angry I'm just going to ignore her all night."

2. Step two is to identify language in their description that shows any of the following thinking patterns: judging, assuming, blaming, black or white thinking, or ruminating. We generally highlight these words and make notes about the type of thought pattern:

   "My mother really pissed me off because *she never understands me* [assuming, black or white thinking]. She won't let me stay out for a late movie tonight and *it's her fault if my friends get mad at me* [blaming]. *She doesn't care if I have friends* [judging, assuming]. *I'm so angry I'm just going to ignore her all night* [ruminating]."

3. The next step is to rewrite a description of what they are angry about, this time removing all of the identified thinking patterns. They are to reframe their story with just the facts, using objective, non-judgmental language. This helps them learn to express their anger in a non-aggressive tone and demeanor. For example:

   "I'm upset that I can't go to the late movie tonight and I'm worried that my friends will get mad at me. I wish my mother would understand and let me go. It really gets me angry."

4. The fourth step is to identify what they need from the other person, and to write down a way to ask for it. In this "practice conversation" they are also asked to let the other person know how they will benefit from meeting their needs. For example:

   "I need you to understand how important it is that I see my friends and how lonely I feel when I don't get to see them. If you let me go to the movies, we won't have to fight and there will be less stress in the house. Also you'll have some alone time with Dad."

5. Next, they identify any compromises they would be willing to make, as a way of negotiating for an effective outcome.

   "I would be willing to clean the garage for an extended curfew tonight. I can promise to text you from the theatre."

6. Finally, in the last step, they write down a message of self-compassion followed by practicing ways to self-soothe, such as by using sensory objects.

   "I may disagree with my mother but I am still a good person and a good friend. I am proud of myself for being willing to compromise. I will play some music and do some breathing."

When guided through this exercise, youth learn that they may not get what they want but will be okay. They can use their distress tolerance skills to manage intense feelings and then revisit conflicts from a more grounded place.

In art therapy directives for anger management, youth are given the freedom to express their anger in a socially productive way, that is, through art-making. Often they express their anger with metaphors. For example, anger can be depicted with metaphors of nature such as storms, lightning, or fire, or with animals and animal qualities (that we sometimes call spirit animals). They can use any kind of symbol to reflect their emotion, such as a broken heart or a chain.

Another art therapy directive we use for anger management is based on deconstruction and reconstruction. They write down angry words or discharge their emotions with colors on paper. Then they rip up their paper—deconstructing their angry feelings. Then they arrange the pieces into a collage or mosaic—reconstructing their emotion. This can be transformative, turning anger into something positive or beautiful. The remade piece of art can create a new perspective.

In the art studio, we also use the wise mind symbol (Venn diagram or mandorla) to help manage anger. This can be done through writing exercises or art-making to apply dialectical thinking strategies to the dilemmas that are triggering their anger.

Empowerment: being a survivor

Sharing and encouraging each other's survivor stories has been a very effective form of practicing interpersonal skills as well as increasing peer support and renewing a sense of empowerment following feelings of suicidality. Feeling suicidal is scary and traumatizing for most people. When overcome with fear, they may feel small, helpless, afraid, humiliated, and powerless over their lives. They likely feel defeated and even worthless after attempting suicide or experiencing suicidal thoughts. When the dust settles, there are many unprocessed feelings. While it takes time to recover, if feelings are left unprocessed, they may continue to rule over the young person throughout their lives.

In AIRY, we want to make these feelings more manageable. We share our stories and we focus on what we have *survived*. Shifting our perspective from being victimized by feelings of suicidality, to having survived something so difficult, helps us take back our personal power.

One of our most popular art therapy directives for building a sense of empowerment is mask making. Here teens and young adults can transform their adversity into strength and view themselves as powerful. Some youth even recreate themselves as superheroes. A modification of a mask-making exercise is to depict what has happened to them on the inside of the mask and represent their resilience on the outside of the mask.

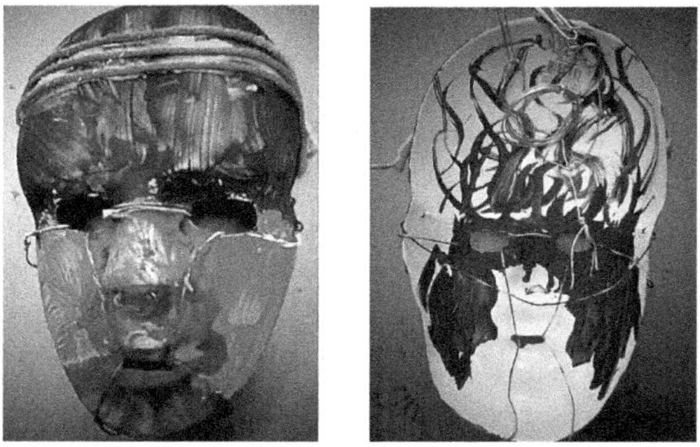

Figure 16.3 Mask 1

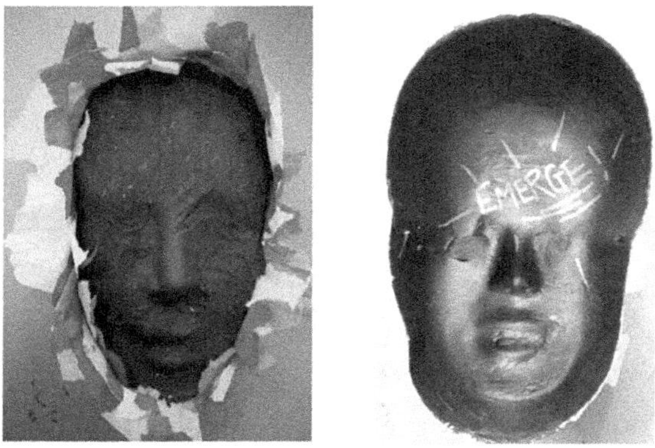

Figure 16.4 Mask 2

Making a difference: challenging perceived burdensomeness

As discussed earlier, Thomas Joiner (Joiner *et al.* 2009) proposes that one of the risk factors for suicide is perceived burdensomeness. Although the person may not be a burden on others, they *perceive* that they are. Feeling like a burden can lead a young person to thinking they may be better off dead. Studies show that people who are depressed are usually unaware that they have cognitive distortions. They need help to reframe their thinking to get well.

There are many things that can contribute to a person feeling like a burden on others. It can be very complex and deeply embedded from experiences throughout their lives, or it can be a temporary passing idea. In AIRY, this thinking is challenged through reframing thoughts and with peer support. Steps are taken to heal these feelings through interpersonal actions. These include recognizing their close relationships as reasons for living, creating meaningful goals, and taking steps toward community engagement. Twice a year, they are invited to contribute to the community through the arts, to raise awareness of suicide prevention through public events, and to help reduce stigma by teaching people how to talk about suicide.

Utilizing peer support in group art therapy provides opportunity for helping others, for taking on leadership and mentor roles, and for carrying a message of hope through sharing lived experience. These aspects involve developing interpersonal skills for success. Building stronger interpersonal skills allows youth to find ways to positively contribute to society and to make a difference in the world. In doing so, feelings of burdensomeness recede.

As discussed in this chapter, interpersonal skills are essential to preventing suicide. Not only do they address the social risk factors for suicide, but they can help young people to feel validated and supported, as they try to navigate a world that is often chaotic, disappointing, and scary. A successful suicide prevention program needs to examine and work toward changing cultural aspects of society which unfortunately contribute to youth suicide. We must acknowledge and address what is happening in the world around us. Our youth carry this weight with them every day. A timely example of this is included in the next chapter, as we take a look at how the global pandemic of Covid-19 has affected young people at risk for suicide.

References

Joiner, T., Van Orden, K., Witte, T., and Rudd, M.D. (2009) *The Interpersonal Theory of Suicide: Guidance for Working with Suicidal Clients.* Washington, DC: American Psychological Association.

Linehan, M. (1993a) *Cognitive–Behavioral Treatment of Borderline Personality Disorder.* New York: The Guilford Press.

Linehan, M. (1993b) *Skills Training Manual for Treating Borderline Personality Disorder.* New York: The Guilford Press.

Rathus, J. and Miller, A. (2015) *DBT Skills Manual for Adolescents.* New York: The Guilford Press.

PART 4

Other Risk Factors for Suicide: Trauma and Addiction

Chapter 17

Art Therapy and Collective Trauma during the Global Pandemic

In the spring of 2020, the entire world just stopped.

AIRY was ready to start its fourth year, with 19 youth signed up for the start of the program, when the quarantine was ordered to stop the spread of Covid-19. For the first few days, I collapsed into despair. I feared that I would spiral down into deep depression, but I was able to pull myself up. I knew on a visceral level that there was important work to do. I knew my kids would suffer. Despite the gravity of a global pandemic, I found that years of working in suicide prevention had helped me develop incredible skills in resilience. I surprised myself. I quickly buckled up and began adapting the program to quarantine. My mission in suicide prevention had become larger than my life. I was never more fully invested.

It was difficult. I learned in the first six weeks of quarantine that an online platform for art therapy was inherently less effective for a number of reasons. First, we lacked the physical safe space youth had co-created in groups over the years. The simple act of showing up to the studio was a step in the direction of hope. The studio had created a certain style of therapeutic milieu. In this space, there was ownership, agency, empowerment. It was their space, protected and safe, away from the stressors of the world and without interruption. The initial minutes of arriving, seeing each other in person, reading each other's faces, and making small talk all provided a peer bonding experience that just couldn't be re-created on Zoom.

Secondly, it was extremely challenging to observe them making art. This is a crucial ingredient to the art therapy process. The art therapist may at times be observer, participant, collaborator, facilitator, and studio assistant to the artists that inhabit the space. The non-verbal language necessary to "read the room" was gone. Little boxes on computer screens and smartphones lacked essential cues that I depended upon to be able to meet them where they were at.

Despite those factors, I worked as creatively as possible, to generate an atmosphere of art and connection. I home delivered bags of art supplies, journals, and handouts. Parents in masks signed consent forms on the steps of their homes. We doubled our outreach by phone and text. We laboriously ironed out technical issues that were constant barriers to communication—setting up video conferencing apps and accounts, adapting to screen time, establishing safe rules for online groups, addressing ethical and privacy concerns, and more.

Initially, there was an optimistic engagement as they met each other for the first time on screen. There was excitement about going through the bag of art supplies and finding a variety of materials. Some members started making art right away, requesting more materials. Second and third rounds of home deliveries were made. Some families asked for help with art supplies and we secured a Covid relief grant to accommodate them.

Sadly, after about six weeks, some members started dropping off. They couldn't tolerate the intensity of a constant virtual life, especially after spending hours online for school. They struggled to connect through the one-inch squares of faces on cell phone screens. They didn't have the ingredients to help them develop new relationships. They became shy and awkward, turning off their cameras. And they became more withdrawn, more isolated, more hopeless. The sadness in their eyes and voices felt so heavy to hold.

Everything about the delivery of the program felt wobbly. We could never quite get a footing. As members left the group, new ones reached out and signed up. Our first three months were marked by a transitional state that was opposite to the sense of grounding they should have received.

And then the feelings of suicidality began to climb, each subsequent week getting higher. A slew of crisis interventions was necessary, and it felt like, all at once, there was an avalanche of psychological pain. They all talked of feeling trapped, riddled with anxiety, and uncertain about their futures. In some cases, because their identity was so related to social connection, they expressed not knowing who they were anymore. Their sense of powerlessness permeated the sessions. Stuck in their bedrooms for hours on end, these young people had nowhere to go. Most were completely isolated and defeated—by the enormity of the pandemic, by the discomfort of quarantine, by frequent loss, death, and just being overtaken in a state of collective trauma.

I felt the pressure like a heavy motor running in my chest and stomach—to keep going, stay resilient, show up, put out fires, and deliver quality services. My anxiety increased alongside theirs. How could it not? Thankfully, I had the foresight to renew my own daily art practice with the extra time I had in quarantine. Art was my primary source of self-care, both personally and professionally. I took all my emotions and fears directly to the materials I set up at my kitchen table. I encouraged them to do the same.

Stuck at home, I made collages about my fear. I painted storms with discordant colors. I constructed a sailboat with upcycled materials. I built a fairy fortress from tree bark and rocks and shells. I painted canvases of pure colors to soothe me. I drew the road of my life to gain perspective. I knew that I would be able to look back and see that this was just one period of time in a full life. I knew that it would pass, and that new roads would emerge. I also started painting pictures of people wearing masks, to process my experience of them. Some were heavy, some were light. Creating works of art helped me escape the daily reminder of the coronavirus.

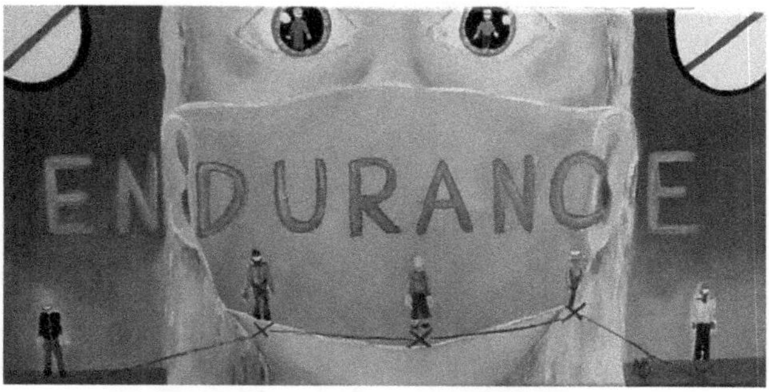

Figure 17.1 (Endurance) mask painting

Quite fast, my kitchen was transformed into an art studio. Behind my computer camera, I hung a tapestry on the wall and lined my shelves with sensory materials to remind them to do the same in their environments. I used candles, essential oils, a colored light box, flower arrangements, and a rock garden with a fountain of water that trickled. I also hung up my art on the walls to show them that the power of art was helping me to cope.

Art and suicide prevention helped me get out of bed and focus every day. I remained on constant alert, embracing my fear and doing the work, no matter what. We had come too far to let Covid win. And so we did what we always do. We kept making art.

By the time we entered Phase one in Massachusetts, I had purchased a flat screen tv, a tv cart on wheels, a microphone, 200 feet of ethernet cable, and upgraded internet for the studio to begin the process of re-opening in a hybrid style, where small groups of two or three could come to the studio on a rotating basis, while the others participated from home on our tv. I shopped for, sanitized, and prepared 18 separate bins of art supplies, a gallon of hand sanitizer, and a host of other cleaning products. Twice a day I wiped down doorknobs, banisters, chairs, tables, and bathrooms.

We also began to hold small gatherings in local parks. Meeting in the outdoors offered a sense of freedom and an outlet to discharge pent-up feelings. I laid tablecloths on the grass with gloves, hand sanitizer, snacks, and bottled water. I arranged beach chairs six feet apart. I set up water guns filled with tempera paints which they squirted on poster boards, making a collective mural that I framed for the studio. The paint was washable and we also used it to color the trunks of trees.

Though my heart was heavy, my body tired and anxious, and my family life in frequent alarm, I am proud to say that I faced this global trauma like a warrior. I had been a survivor most of my life. And in some ways, these circumstances made me thrive. It's hard to articulate. It was just knowing that I must proceed, and that AIRY must prevail. The work was too crucial to stop, and it was needed more now than ever.

I took time for pause, reflection, and self-care as often as I could. And it led me to increase my training in trauma, to further the education of my staff, and to begin incorporating more trauma-informed practices. I edited our curriculum to include ways to process feelings about quarantine and the pandemic, and to weave in body work. This helped them regulate the extremes of overactivation and shutdown that I was witnessing. Because it took twice as long to begin peer bonding experiences, I extended the season for an additional six weeks.

Through this experience I became more well versed in the language of trauma. I revisited Stephen Porges's work with polyvagal theory, Peter Levine's work with somatic experiencing, and Cornelia Elbrecht's guided bilateral drawing (2018), as well as the work of Bessel van der Kolk and the art therapy-based trauma-informed practices of Cathy Malchiodi. I found that we could reinforce the DBT component of mindfulness with body-based exercises to help minimize trauma.

Steele and Malchiodi define trauma-informed practice as:

> a predominantly sensory process for many children and adolescents that cannot be altered by cognitive interventions alone. Because the experience of trauma is often one of terror, and being vulnerable and powerless to do anything about one's situation, trauma-informed care must engage children and adolescents in sensory, neurosequential experiences to help restore a sense of safety and bring about a renewed sense of empowerment. Practices that address individuals' "survival brains" through sensory and somatic (body-oriented) experiences, and enhance self-regulation, trauma integration, and healthy relationships and environments are central to trauma-informed care. (2012, p.xix)

Trauma-informed care directly aligns with best practices in suicide prevention. Our curriculum always addresses safety first and foremost. The development of a safety plan and art directives to restore a sense of safety happen in the first few weeks, alongside developing mindfulness skills to help regulate both the body and brain. In response to the pandemic, I designed additional art activities that could elicit checking in with our nervous systems. I customized use of materials to help create a physical sense of balance and equilibrium.

Because this disease had left us feeling so helpless, I knew I also had to find ways to help the young people feel empowered and maintain a sense of purpose. They made posters for their windows, social action flags, a virtual art show, and videos of their work. They were given more choices in how the groups would be run and what topics they wanted to address. When they could not see their strengths, we created spirit animals to depict them metaphorically. When some of the restrictions started lifting, we were able to turn our focus on developing healthier relationships. Art activities included drawing Covid characters, painting safe places, and imagining with art what life would look like when the pandemic was over.

For us, providers working with youth during this time of collective trauma, it is important to recognize that our work involves witnessing and holding the very heavy stories of young people—stories of great distress, despair, loneliness, entrapment, uncertainty, brain fog and confusion, nervous system imbalance, and more. I have decided to examine some relevant aspects of trauma theory in this chapter, as I cannot see a way to do this work without it. Appendix D includes information about resources for educators on trauma-informed care in the classroom.

The brain-mind-body experience of trauma

Bessel van der Kolk in his groundbreaking book *The Body Keeps the Score* (2014) discusses the impact of trauma and how it alters every aspect of our lives. It affects our bodies, our emotions, and our ability to think and problem solve.

> Overwhelming experiences affect our innermost sensations and our relationship to our physical reality—the core of who we are. We have learned that trauma is not just an event that took place sometime in the past; it is also an imprint left by that experience on mind, body and brain...it changes not only how we think and what we think about, but also our very capacity to think. (p.21)

It is easy to see how we as humans have experienced the global pandemic as traumatic—having become stuck in survival mode with the constant fear of illness or death, with the isolation of quarantine, with the absence of close, meaningful relationships all devastating our lives. Many people have described living through this pandemic as an experience that is "surreal." Covid-19 has generated a completely foreign way of living, turning our daily existence upside down. Subsequently, many youth, in attempting to cope with this collective trauma, found themselves turning to destructive behaviors to cope. van der Kolk describes the urges to turn to unhealthy outlets when we are faced with the profundity of the brain-mind-body experience of ongoing trauma:

> Feeling as if our chest is caving in or we've been punched in the gut is unbearable. We'll do anything to make these awful visceral sensations go away, whether it is clinging desperately to another human being, rendering ourselves insensible with drugs and alcohol, or taking a knife

> to the skin to replace overwhelming emotions with definable sensations. How many mental health problems, from drug addiction, to self-injurious behavior, start as attempts to cope with the unbearable physical pain of our emotions? (p.76)

Fortunately, in the AIRY program, we had begun working with mindfulness of the body's sensations and ways to regulate emotion early on in the quarantine. Reinforcing DBT skills was essential. Becoming aware of physical sensations and ways to soothe them through the five senses helped youth engage in the present moment. Scanning the body for areas that were either pleasant, unpleasant, or neutral helped them gain a sense of control, even if temporarily.

Acknowledging and labeling emotions associated with their experience of the pandemic, then measuring the intensity of those emotional states, was a first step in learning how to manage them. We were also able to look at how those emotions affected their behaviors and their relationship to their bodies. Recognizing that states such as irritability, panic, or numbness were appropriate in the face of trauma helped them avoid feeling shameful. They didn't have to internalize their experience as being "crazy" or doing something "wrong."

Educating youth on trauma is vital when working in suicide prevention. What is happening for them feels like a giant mystery they cannot solve. They feel trapped by their own emotions and behaviors, with no way out. During the pandemic, they have experienced this sense of entrapment virtually everywhere in their lives, from internally in their nervous systems to externally in their quarantined environments.

Reframing traumatic experiences with knowledge of the nervous system drives away the stigma and self-blame often associated with "mental health problems." Many trauma experts have brought our attention to focus on how the nervous system is experienced differently during times of trauma and have proposed new ways of handling it. Many trauma experts have built upon the work of Stephen Porges' polyvagal theory.

The autonomic nervous system and the global pandemic

Stephen Porges is a scientist who first began studying the neurobiological mechanisms of trauma in the laboratory, including heart rate, auditory processes, and facial expressions. His research led him to further examine trauma survivors' emotions and social behavior and the importance of social interactions on health. He studied these through the lens of the autonomic nervous system (Porges 2001, 2009). In describing polyvagal theory, he found that "for these individuals, the theory provided an understanding of how, after experiencing life threat, their neural directions were re-tuned towards a defensive bias and they lost the resilience to return to a sense of safety" (in Dana 2018, Foreword, p.xi).

In simpler terms, trauma affects our ability to understand how we are doing and to respond effectively. Trauma disrupts our nervous systems and makes it difficult to feel safe or to connect in relationships. Since human relationships are the ingredients of restoring a sense of safety, and since trauma impairs our ability to connect with others, we are left in quite a complicated paradox.

I can speak to this personally from both the trauma of the pandemic and from how my childhood experiences of trauma affect me as an adult. Trauma is a web of complexity in the nervous system that remains in the body long after the events that may have elicited it are over. The trauma that has been imprinted in my nervous system for years can be reactivated during times of crisis. Sounds, smells, and images evoke intense sensations in my body which can catch me off guard. I find, in a single moment, that I can become extremely sensitive to an ordinary aspect of life, such as seeing a certain kind of car pass by my home, dropping a plate in my kitchen that creates a smashing sound, or seeing crowds of people in blue masks.

With regard to the pandemic, I may understand rationally that I am safe with my personal protective equipment and being at home in quarantine, but my body memory does not. During Covid we may experience heightened anxiety over minute matters, or periods of shutdown where we feel paralyzed in our ability to reach out to another human being. In moments of complete and raw shock, we may simply freeze up and be unable to make decisions with any clear thought.

I have learned that when working with trauma, we need to focus on the body. *Physical* experiences can restore a sense of control, and we can learn to integrate these experiences into our day-to-day lives. It is vital that we are able to become aware of what is happening in these moments in the body, for the body holds the key to our being able to survive and navigate this trauma. Too often, we bypass what is happening in our bodies, and tune in quickly to our thoughts, sometimes of intense dread, other times of total defeat. I have watched as young people move rapidly from feeling shut down and fatigued in their bodies to being mired in distorted thinking, such as "I am a failure," "I have no future," or "They would be better off if I were dead."

So how can we interrupt the process of developing suicidal or destructive thoughts that are linked to traumatic experiences in our bodies? How can we teach young people to attune to their bodily sensations and safely stay with the experience, without casting judgment upon themselves, or wanting to escape the pain through killing themselves? It is my hope that through this growing body of trauma theory, we can begin to incorporate this work together, as clinicians, parents, teachers, and expressive arts therapists. While it can be daunting to learn the science of trauma, it can be broken down so that we can grasp how to implement its best practices in our work.

Let us return to an explanation of polyvagal theory.

Polyvagal theory explains that our autonomic nervous system is made up of two branches that create three pathways. The two branches are the sympathetic and the parasympathetic. The sympathetic branch elicits our fight or flight response when we feel danger or threat. It mobilizes us for action and triggers the release of adrenaline.

On the other hand, the parasympathetic branch has differing functions. It contains the vagus nerve, which has two ends, the ventral (front) vagus and the dorsal (back) vagus. When the ventral vagus nerve is activated, it can help us calm, feel safe, and engage with others. When the dorsal vagus nerve is activated, it does the opposite. When we feel as though we are trapped and cannot escape, it triggers immobilization and complete shutdown. Porges discovered these multifunctions of the vagus nerve in the 1990s and hence coined the term *poly*vagal.

The sympathetic branch of the autonomic nervous system moves blood to the muscles for quick action, in what we know as the "fight-or-flight" response. The sympathetic nervous system is responsible for arousal, as the adrenal glands flood the system with adrenaline, speed up our heart rate, and increase blood pressure. "In a sympathetic nervous system response, there is too much energy in the system, and the client [can become] flooded" (Dana 2018, p.22). Moving from the sympathetic nervous system into a ventral vagus response is needed to regulate.

The parasympathetic branch of the autonomic nervous system

promotes self-preservative functions like digestion and wound healing. It triggers the release of acetylcholine to "put a brake on arousal," slowing down the heart, relaxing the muscles, and returning breathing to normal (van der Kolk 2014, p.79).

The vagus nerve is part of the parasympathetic nervous system. It starts in our cranial nerves which emerge directly from the brain stem. The vagus nerve is the longest of these cranial nerves and 80 percent of its fibers are sensory. At our diaphragm, the vagus nerve splits—the dorsal (or back of the) vagus nerve travels downward into the lower parts of our body, while the ventral (front) vagus nerve travels upwards, regulating our faces, heart, and breath (Dana 2017).

This splitting of the vagus nerve "in the service of survival" thus creates two distinct pathways—either (1) calmly restoring us to safety and social engagement; or (2) immobilizing us as the body shuts down and collapses into defeat or submission. "When the dorsal vagus comes to the rescue, there is not enough energy to run the system: the system is drained, and the client is numbed" (Dana 2017, p.22). Here, we wait, feeling lost and unable to find our way back to connection.

van der Kolk (2014) suggests there is a simple way to experience the activation of these systems.

Whenever you take a deep breath, you activate the SNS (sympathetic nervous system). The resulting burst of adrenaline speeds up your heart, which explains why many athletes take a few, short breaths before starting a competition. Exhaling, in turn, activates the PNS (parasympathetic nervous system), which slows down the heart. If you take a yoga or meditation class, your instructor will probably urge you to pay particular attention to the exhalation, since long, deep breaths out help calm you down.

In simple terms, the sympathetic branch acts as the body's accelerator, while the parasympathetic branch acts as its brake.

Polyvagal theory recognizes the accompanying states of the three responses as the ventral vagal response, the sympathetic response, and the dorsal vagal response—as socially engaged, mobilized, and immobilized, or in other words, safe, danger, and life threat.

An example of the interplay of these states is provided by Porges. Say we feel threatened by a traumatic event. We may first turn to the level of social engagement—calling out to others for help. If we are in immediate danger and no one comes to our aid, we turn to fight or flight to survive—we fight off our attacker or run to a safe place. If this fails, and we can't get away or feel trapped, we attempt to preserve our lives by shutting down and expending as little energy as possible, in a state of freeze or collapse.

During this time of pandemic, my first response was to shut down—my dorsal vagus nerve was activated. All I wanted to do was stay in bed and hide from the horrible reality "out there." I felt frozen in time and space like I just couldn't face it, and I didn't know what to do. My brain felt in the "off" position. I experienced grief and fear to such a degree that my body collapsed for a short period of time in a state of numbness. And I felt that I couldn't fight it.

But, because I was able to shift—when my nervous system informed me that I must take action—I moved into fight or flight via the sympathetic nervous system. I cannot recall the exact moment when that happened, but I did have the realization that suicide prevention would be needed on perhaps an unprecedented level, and that meant I was needed now. A sense of urgency swept me up and I became driven to action. The adrenaline and cortisol that are created in this mode gave me the energy to regroup and adapt at a fast pace.

Unfortunately, prolonged periods of being in fight or flight mode can take a significant toll on the body and elevate stress levels accompanying things like increased heart rate, blood pressure, appetite changes, headaches, insomnia, and, eventually, body aches and pains. I had previously recovered from back and knee injuries that now flared up. I was losing weight and not sleeping well. My level of anxiety in "fight or flight" mode began to interfere with my daily living activities.

In working with trauma theory, I knew that I needed to regulate my nervous system, and to help my clients do the same, by working with the ventral vagus nerve. I found that the DBT skills I had learned could be used to do this. With intention, I used mindfulness—through art, breathing, body awareness, and meditation practices; and emotion regulation—by journaling, self-soothing with sensory objects, taking more naps, and spending more time with my cat, to calm. I also remembered DBT's interpersonal effectiveness skills and increased my connection to others, albeit mostly on the phone, to share my feelings about the pandemic with friends and colleagues. This activated the social engagement system of the parasympathetic branch. Being mirrored by others helped me feel safe, even during a time when no one was feeling safe.

I cannot say this was a simple or easy process, or that I was left without triggers of unprocessed trauma from my childhood experiences. But the good news is that our autonomic nervous systems continually change in response to experiences and the environment. This means we can learn to effectively engage with our nervous systems and intentionally influence our physiological states (Dana 2018).

The job of the autonomic nervous system is to ensure we survive in moments of danger and thrive in times of safety. Survival requires threat detection and the activation of a survival response. Thriving demands the opposite—the inhibition of a survival response so that social engagement can happen. Without the capacity for activation, inhibition, and flexibility of response, we suffer (Dana 2018).

Most of us didn't know how to respond in the spring of 2020. Indeed, the world just stopped. At the time of writing this book, pandemic-related suicides have been reported in many of the hardest-hit countries in the world. In Italy, for example, the first pandemic-related suicide occurred in March of 2020 when a patient suffering from broncho-pneumonia died by suicide while in the hospital waiting for test results. Numerous other suicides have been reported among people awaiting test results, front-line health workers, and those who have been affected by coronavirus-related bankruptcy. High-profile suicides include a state finance minister in Germany who despaired over the virus's economic impact, and a Manhattan emergency room physician on the front line of treating coronavirus patients.

Thakur and Jain (2020, pp.952–3) comment:

> cases have been reported around the world where people out of fear of getting Covid-19 infection, social stigma, isolation, depression, anxiety, emotional imbalance, economic shutdown, lack and/or improper knowledge, financial and future insecurities took their lives. With recent suicide reports we can anticipate the rippling effect of this virus on worldwide suicide events...the basic psychology and inability of the person and the mass society to deal with the situation are the major factors behind these Covid-19 suicides... One needs to maintain connectedness and solidarity despite the physical distance. Individuals with a previous history of suicidal thoughts, panic and stress disorder, low self-esteem and low self-worth, are easily susceptible to catastrophic thinking like suicide in such viral pandemic.

The latest data available (for 2018) shows the highest suicide rate in the

US since 1941 (Drapeau and McIntosh 2020). It is within this context that the Covid-19 pandemic occurred in the United States. Social distancing and prolonged isolation are risk factors for increased suicide rates particularly among young people. As we become more aware of the mind–body–brain connection, we can help youth and ourselves to take steps toward healing our traumas and reducing suicidality. In the next chapter, we will look at additional art therapy processes to help youth regulate their traumatic responses to the pandemic.

References

Dana, D. (2018) *The Polyvagal Theory in Therapy: Engaging the Rhythm of Regulation.* New York: W.W. Norton.

Drapeau, C.W. and McIntosh, J.L. (for the American Association of Suicidology) (2020) USA. Suicide: 2019 Official Final Data. Washington, DC: American Association of Suicidology, dated December 23, 2020, https://suicidology.org/wp-content/uploads/2020/02/2018datapgsv2_Final.pdf.

Elbrecht, C. (2018) *Healing Trauma with Guided Drawing: A Sensorimotor Art Therapy Approach to Bilateral Body Mapping.* Berkeley, CA: North Atlantic Books.

Porges, S.W. (2001) The polyvagal theory: Phylogenetic substrates of a social nervous system. *International Journal of Psychophysiology 42*, 2, 123–146.

Porges, S.W. (2009) The polyvagal theory: New insights into adaptive reactions of the autonomic nervous system. *Cleveland Clinic Journal of Medicine 76*, 4 suppl. 2, S86–S90.

Steele, W. and Malchiodi, C. (2012) *Trauma-Informed Practices with Children and Adolescents.* New York: Routledge.

Thakur, V. and Jain, A. (2020) Covid 2019-suicides: A global psychological pandemic. *Brain, Behavior, and Immunity 88*, 952–953.

van der Kolk, B. (2014) *The Body Keeps the Score: Brain, Mind and Body in the Healing of Trauma.* New York: Penguin Books.

Chapter 18

Working with the Body

BOTTOM-UP PROCESSES

Since trauma is stored in the body, it is essential that we work with the body to change the response of the autonomic nervous system. We can teach clients how to attune to their bodies, tolerate their physical sensations, and to safely embody that experience. This helps them process what has happened in their body implicitly, without having to relive the details or become re-traumatized. This somatic approach, starting with the body, is referred to as a "bottom-up" process. It does not ask questions about why things happened or assign fault or blame, or even try to problem solve, for these are cognitive processes. A bottom-up approach is the opposite of Freud's "talking cure," which focuses on the mind—a "top-down" process.

> Bottom-up therapeutic approaches focus on the body, the felt sense, and the instinctive responses as they are mediated through the brain stem and move upward to impact the limbic system and cortical areas of the brain. Continuous loops of information travel from the body to the brain and from the brain to the body. (Heller and LaPierre 2012, p.17)

Peter Levine (2010) is a biologist and psychologist who studied animals in their natural environments and was curious about why they did not share the human experience of trauma despite routinely facing terror and fear. He concluded that because animals do not have the higher functions of the human brain, they do not engage with top-down processes. Hence, their minds do not interrupt the flow of physical energy during a traumatic event or divert them from their present experience. In fact, embracing and embodying physical reactions to trauma awakens vitality and we become more alive.

When people are faced with a traumatic event, our minds take over and we become afraid of our sensory experience. This interrupts the expression of physical energy and traps it in our bodies. It becomes encoded with a host of related associations—fragments of sensations—which we are left to interpret cognitively. This often results in emotional suppression and underlying shame.

Levine explains that trauma is an extreme contraction of physical energy that forms a vortex in our system. To release the energy stored in the vortex requires a process he calls "pendulation." This involves gradually moving from the periphery of our stored traumatic experience inward, through a repetition of visceral contraction and expansion.

For example, he demonstrates an activity where the client and therapist use their arms to set up a physical boundary, and then to begin the motion of pushing out, as if swimming, while vocalizing a "roar" or growling sound, much like a tiger. Clients can begin to feel their power and reduce the sense of helplessness they associate with the trauma. Other activities that can be done for this bottom-up process include juggling balls, using contracting and expanding toys such as the "slinky," humming, progressive muscle relaxation, and alternating between active play and quiet play (Levine 2020).

Avoiding this process of experiencing and embodying our sensations leaves us stuck. We relive the traumatic event over and over, such as when triggered by a similar sensory experience, or through flashbacks and nightmares.

Prior to the practice of pendulation, Levine engages his clients in a process he calls "orienting." In an immobilized state, when a client is "underactivated," working with the body can open up pathways to explore blocked emotions. In an "overactivated" state, when the body is flooded with sensations, orienting them to the present, helps clients to calm and regulate.

van der Kolk (2014) also emphasizes how a bottom-up approach can allow the body to have experiences that contradict traumatic reactions such as anxiety, helplessness, entrapment, freezing, or collapse. Heller and LaPierre (2012) discuss how bottom-up approaches can increase a client's capacity for self-regulation, and thereby begin to reduce and dissolve painful identifications and judgments. And, "On the somatic level, to access the felt sense is to retrieve the knowledge and wisdom implicit in bodily experiences" (Heller and LaPierre quoted in Elbrecht 2018, p.50).

The idea of implicit body wisdom is also a cornerstone of dialectical behavioral therapy (DBT), which is practiced in the AIRY program. Drawn from Eastern practices of mindfulness and intuition, DBT sometimes uses a bottom-up approach to help clients develop what Linehan refers to as "wise mind."

Bottom-up work is easily translatable in art therapy by focusing on process instead of product, and on sensations instead of concepts. Kinesthetic use of art materials such as clay, rhythmic painting, and bilateral drawing (using both hands) are among some of the art directives we have used.

In Cornelia Elbrecht's *Healing Trauma with Guided Drawing*, she states:

> The bottom-up approach is essentially kinesthetic, mostly nonverbal, and dominated by motor impulses. Then we move "up" in the body toward sensing, toward sensory awareness. A session will oscillate between drawn motor impulses and sensing the effect they have on the inside. (Elbrecht 2018, p.50)

She goes on to suggest that:

> The role of the art therapist is to encourage the bottom-up approach through supporting trust into the emerging motor impulses and their rhythm, as well as through tracking the sensory impact these motor impulses have in the body. More than perceiving the shapes as images, one deals with the movements it took to create them...looking too soon for images and interpretations will activate the mind and cut off from instinct. Images will become significant at a later stage... In this manner, the drawings "happen" more than they are "done" in accordance with a sense of inner guidance beyond rational control. (Elbrecht 2018, p.50)

Based on my personal and professional experience, I understood how I could help our clients begin to regulate their nervous systems. I provided exercises to calm their bodies when the sympathetic system was overactivated, and at other times, exercises to energize through movement, when the dorsal vagus triggered shutdown. Perhaps most important, was guiding them in co-regulation of their autonomic system, as trauma theories like Porges' polyvagal theory and Peter Levine's "somatic experiencing" suggest that the body needs human connection to restore a sense of safety.

Mirroring, co-regulation, and reciprocity

A fascinating aspect of trauma involves the discovery of mirror neurons by a group of Italian scientists in 1994. How our brains vicariously "mirror" each other explains aspects of the mind such as empathy, imitation, and synchrony—"Because trauma almost invariably involves not being seen, not being mirrored, and not being taken into account, treatment needs to reactivate the capacity to safely mirror, and be mirrored by others" (van der Kolk 2014, p.59).

Connecting during Covid's profound isolation was a struggle. We were persistent and provided a container and virtual safe space for young people to share their emotions and experiences. We increased our outreach, consistently reminding them that we were available to reach out to for support. While quarantine at times prompted a desire to reach out, more often than not it generated unmet social needs and great loneliness. Youth experienced swings between constant overactivation and shutdown—a pattern of "immobilization–mobilization–immobilization" which replayed in a painful autonomic loop (Dana 2018, p.32). According to Eisenberg, social disconnection and social exclusion can activate the same pain pathways as experiences of physical injury (Dana 2018).

Because the restrictions of the pandemic limited our ability to foster in-person connection, we had to focus on creating alternative means of connectedness until we could get back in the studio. We broke into pairs to do peer support by phone calls and text messaging, and sent each other photos of our art. We also made art for each other and mailed it to members of the group, also in pairs. We increased conversation of shared interests. Home deliveries of art supplies increased a sense of comfort and nurturing.

Another technique we used in the AIRY program was to foster feelings of connection by imagining what it would be like when quarantine was over, and more specifically who the young people would look forward to seeing. We also incorporated "remembering" experiences of connectedness in our art activities.

van der Kolk explains the difference between physically being around people and experiencing genuine reciprocity:

> Social support is not the same as merely being in the presence of others. The critical issue is *reciprocity*: being truly heard and seen by the people

> around us, feeling that we are held in someone else's mind and heart. For our physiology to calm down, heal and grow we need a visceral feeling of safety. No doctor can write a prescription for friendship and love. These are complex and hard-earned capacities...many traumatized people find themselves chronically out of sync with the people around them. (2014, p.81)

Deb Dana explains:

> Reciprocity is an important regulator of the nervous system... Remembered reciprocity uses the capacity of the body–mind to re-create an experience taking the memory of a moment of reciprocity and bringing it back to life... Both remembered and imagined reciprocity practices engage the innate drive of the autonomic nervous system to connect and co-regulate. (Dana 2018, pp.47–48)

Attachment: mirroring the sensation of touch

Peter Levine emphasizes the healing power of touch in restoring a sense of safety, as touch is the first sensory experience we acquire from birth. It is our primary means of connection and safety. He suggests that the physical presence of another human can signal to us far more than words. This most primal sense of human touch is five times greater than body language or facial expression (Levine 2020). It is the fundamental ingredient of babies becoming securely attached to their mothers.

Of course, the idea of touch can present a problem for many traumatized youth. They often fear or feel uncomfortable being touched because it may trigger a traumatic reaction. Even at home, it is essential that the touch is welcomed, that consent is given, perhaps beginning with slightly touching a young person on their shoulder to let them know you are there for support, or by placing a blanket on them while watching tv on the couch. Being back in the studio, safely sharing art materials and our created works of art, brought a positive experience that could mirror the feeling of touch, without crossing boundaries.

Oftentimes, adolescents and young adults who present in our work are lacking in secure attachment experiences. The therapist's job may be to help make up for the attachment deficit. They can do this by being fully present, providing a sense of comfort and emotionally attuned communication, as well as by promoting resilience. Kobak *et al.* (2015)

suggest that therapists can also engage adolescents in conversation that directly signals their autonomy needs, monitor the adolescent's safety, and empathize with the adolescent's perspective. "As adolescents' autonomy and engagement in close peer relationships develop, attachment needs are less frequently activated and become more limited to emergency situations and moments of high need or distress" (Kobak *et al.* 2015, p.230).

Levine stresses the importance of the therapist attuning to their own experience and being fully grounded and present in the session before offering their support. Here too, clinicians working with traumatized clients can utilize somatic bottom-up approaches to regulate themselves before, during, and after the session. While this work is useful for our clients, it is also vital for the self-care of those helping them.

As we move forward into transitioning into a new and different future, the expressive arts can provide a medium for us to reflect, review, and make sense of our experiences. One form of the expressive arts which can help us process this global trauma is poetry. For this reason, I am sharing some poetry written by youth in the program about what the experience of the pandemic has been like for them.

Untitled

I.

Elevated heart rate with no motion
Exhaustion from nothing
I would had I started different
Before my get up and go got up and went
I would be spent from spending rather than saving
Than I would have purchased something
An experience, a memory, chemicals swirling
Instead stagnation, stillness, a memory of death
Time stretches forever and stands still
Tomorrow will come
Will it be better?

A memory of spring with the new coming
I was at my mother's, still and stuck and studying
Is this better?
Wherever you go, you bring yourself with you
Best to change the inner worlds.

I am me still.
I have changed.
I remain.

Skin too tight, the inner world bursting
There is too much time and too little
Lack of change causes temporal dilation
A minute stretches an hour
Yesterdays pass like nothing
Tomorrow shifts little so never really comes.

II.
Tomorrow is a new day.
This moment is a new one too.
A day, a second, what's the difference?
A sleep and a blink are the same but for time.

I can reset now.
I can take a breath, take a moment of rest
Or a minute, or an hour, or a day.
Some need months or years.

And then they find themselves swept forward
Willingly or with strident protests
On they go, into some future they can help to shape
And then they take a breath, a step
And everything changes.

III.
Life is beautiful
And it is sorrow
This too shall pass

Life is tragic
And it is healing
This too shall change

I am here now
And it is so brilliantly lovely
That it almost hurts
This too shall fade

Then burn again
To fade again
Amid shadows falling then
The sun will rise
A new day dawn
And I will see once more

Life is beautiful
Even when it is sorrow
And even more so
When it is Joy.

Anonymous

Irritation, Helplessness, and Uncertainty, an AIRY group poem

Knots in my stomach, racing heart, feeling hot
Much smaller than you are
A recluse of slight apprehension and anger
Pores boiling with restlessness
If my heart fell to the floor I think I'd be too distracted to notice.

I just get plain old frantic
Left with resentful retention
Emerging with a murky madness.
I feel that I cannot fix the situation.
Even if the battle has just begun, I feel defeated.
I reach out to solid ground, maybe a ledge or platform.
It turns to sand in my palm.
I've grabbed a moment that I cannot hold.

Exhaustion sets in and I cry beside my cat
Pockets of pain that I run from.
I look at myself, top to bottom, and find myself
hollow in one place and complete in another.
One final abstract resurrection of an eternal realization
which digs throughout and shatters the collective mind.

Anonymous

References

Dana, D. (2018) *The Polyvagal Theory in Therapy: Engaging the Rhythm of Regulation.* New York: W.W. Norton.

Elbrecht, C. (2018) *Healing Trauma with Guided Drawing: A Sensorimotor Art Therapy Approach to Bilateral Body Mapping.* Berkeley, CA: North Atlantic Books.

Heller, L. and LaPierre, A. (2012) *Healing Developmental Trauma: How Early Trauma Affects Self-Regulation, Self-Image, and the Capacity for Relationship.* Berkeley, CA: North Atlantic Books.

Levine, P. (2010) *In an Unspoken Voice: How the Body Releases Trauma and Restores Goodness.* Berkeley, CA: North Atlantic Books.

Levine, P. (2020) Trauma first aid: Awakening the ordinary miracle of healing. [Training.] Embodied Philosophy LLC, Kajabi. www.embodiedphilosophy.org.

Kobak, R., Zajac, K., Herres, J., and Krauthamer Ewing, E.S. (2015) Attachment-based treatments for adolescents: The secure cycle as a framework for assessment, treatment and evaluation. *Attachment & Human Development 17*, 2, 220–239.

van der Kolk, B. (2014) *The Body Keeps the Score: Brain, Mind and Body in the Healing of Trauma.* New York: Penguin Books.

Chapter 19

Addiction and Suicidality

In this book we have discussed many risk factors for youth suicide. I would like to further explore how many teens and young adults are at risk due to drug and alcohol use, eating disorders, and other forms of addiction.

Belinda was only 15 years old when she started our program. After a suicide attempt resulting in a hospitalization, she had been temporarily removed from her home due to drug use, repeatedly missing school, and explosive behaviors toward her mother. She had experienced sexual assault within the last year and reactive acting-out behaviors.

Belinda was both frightened and angry about being placed in a group residential setting and desperately wanted to return home. She felt misunderstood and reported being bullied by peers at her last school as one of the reasons she was suicidal. She presented as quiet and calm but questionably present.

It didn't take long for me to realize that she was coming to group high. I explained to her that we had a policy about not coming to groups under the influence of alcohol or drugs and how it could trigger other people. For the next few weeks she was able to abide by this. She made an effort toward abstinence and began making progress. She became more alert, focused, and able to learn some skills. Unfortunately, toward the end of the season, she relapsed and dropped out of the program.

Paige was 20 years old when she entered the Arts in Recovery for Youth program. She suffered from chronic anxiety. She had difficulty leaving the house and with talking to new people. She had lost her mother at an early age, had a family history of addiction, and lived with her grandparents who had helped raise her. She presented as soft spoken, underweight, and often very tired.

When asked what was driving her to feel suicidal, she talked about self-hate, her battle with daily anxiety, and feeling out of control. She admitted to ongoing self-harm and an eating disorder in which she was regularly binging and purging, starving herself, and abusing laxatives. Living in a rural community she had struggled to find any resources for help with her eating disorder. It was only when we began to view her struggle through the lens of food addiction that we could find services to help her; however, she had to travel across the state.

In art therapy, Paige made pictures about her desire to recover from her eating disorder and body dysmorphia. She found the rhythmic sensations of watercolors to be self-soothing and she identified her favorite coping skill as self-compassion through positive self-talk.

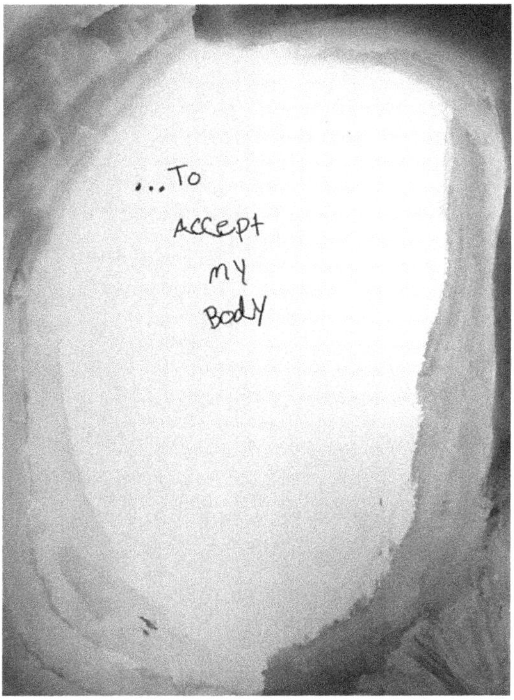

Figure 19.1 Body pic

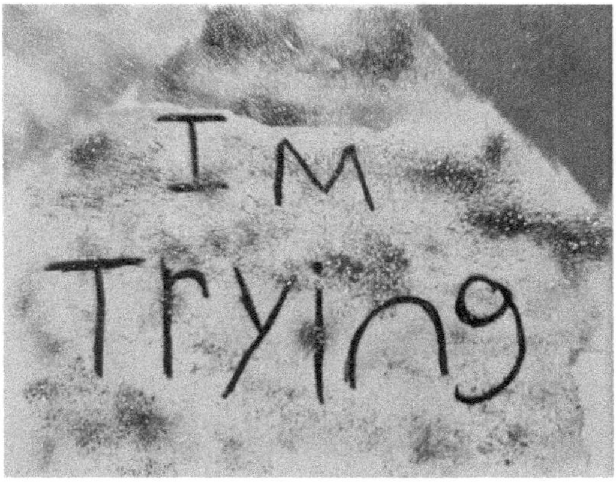

Figure 19.2 I'm trying painting

During her first year in the program, she made incredible progress. She reduced isolating at home and began working part time in the community. She spoke openly about the lack of resources for eating disorders in rural areas. She engaged in new hobbies to help regulate her emotions, and she frequently helped others in group.

As time progressed however, Paige continued to struggle with her eating disorder, self-injury, and breaking through layers of denial about her alcoholism and participation in an abusive romantic relationship. During the pandemic, things got worse. She drove her car into a tree while drinking and was arrested. She began dropping off and distancing herself from the program. While I was concerned, I knew she was engaging in other forms of treatment and remained hopeful.

One early morning I received a message from Paige. She was at the hospital and had a very serious suicide attempt potentially affecting her heart. While I knew Paige struggled with feeling suicidal, it shocked me. Until now she had consistently used skills to manage her urges and to stay safe.

After almost two years in the program, I had developed a close relationship with Paige. I felt her pain and how stuck she had become. I also began to recognize that despite our efforts, the disease of addiction interfered with her taking steps to get better. I feared for her life.

I put on my shoes and mask and met her at the hospital. She cried and expressed how desperate she felt. She began admitting to her alcohol use and the ongoing abuse in her romantic relationship. She talked about her mother's death and the impact this had had on her since adolescence.

She felt she had hit a bottom and became more willing to get the help she needed.

She returned to my young adult group and we agreed to increase our contact by phone. She agreed to stop drinking and attend AA meetings online. She started counting her days of sobriety.

I was shaken up and concerned that I was not doing enough to help these young people. I had put everything I could into a solid and successful suicide prevention program but at the same time I came to realize that these particular youth would not make progress until they got help with their addictions. Addiction was an obstacle to their utilizing DBT skills and they remained at high risk for suicide despite my efforts. It troubled me greatly. It was a difficult situation because I was not an addictions counselor and yet I could see the direct relationship between addiction and suicidality.

While I was able to call upon my lived experience with recovering from my own problematic drinking, and had a deeply felt sense about their battles, it wasn't enough. While I was familiar with 12-step programs such as Alcoholics Anonymous, this didn't equip me for the fight against this powerful disease. So, I buckled down and quickly went to work researching the most efficacious methods of addictions counseling. There had to be a way that I could help them.

This was when I began more in-depth study of the transtheoretical model of behavior change and the method of motivational interviewing (Prochaska and DiClemente 1982; Miller and Rollnick 2002). I found that it could be implemented into our program, alongside DBT skills and best practices in suicide prevention.

At the heart of this counseling style were ways to help motivate young people to want to make change. I also found that motivational interviewing could be facilitated with art therapy directives in the studio. I adopted the methods into our curriculum and found them to be more successful than I had anticipated. While I had lost touch with Belinda and her mother, I was able to help Paige and others who were facing addiction and suicidality. Motivational interviewing helped motivate them to seek the treatment they needed.

Implementing motivational interviewing into our suicide prevention program was particularly helpful when I met Ella. She was in her first year of college at the age of 18 when she enrolled in the program. She was experiencing ongoing periods of deep depression and anxiety. While she had been in therapy for some time, she continued to experience feelings of suicidality and had attempted to kill herself in the previous year.

Although she was a young adult who stayed busy with school and work, Ella felt isolated and alone, and longed for support. She reported continuously feeling suicidal on a scale of 5 out of 10 with a weakened desire to live. She talked about attempts to cope with her feelings by drinking, sometimes alone in her room and sometimes with friends.

Recently it had gotten worse and she recognized that she was having blackouts while engaged in driving, along with other high-risk behaviors. She was able to see that it was a problem but could not connect it to her feeling suicidal. She was ambivalent. She wanted change but did not want to stop drinking for fear of losing her social circle.

In AIRY, I was able to apply a Socratic method of questioning with Ella about what was important to her and what was happening in her life as a result of drinking. I also reinforced the skills of DBT for use prior to drinking, such as learning to tolerate distress and regulate her emotions without picking up a drink, as well as applying dialectical thinking to conflicts before impulsively reacting to them.

Through applied DBT skills, motivational interviewing, and art-making, I was able to help empower both Ella and Paige to see the choices before them, and to make their own decisions about next steps. We used art-making directives about identity and authenticity, and journaling prompts about the stages of change. My goal with these directives was to help these young women recognize that drinking was interfering with the things that mattered most to them, and that they had the power to change that.

For example, to explore what was important to Ella in her life, we made a series of symbolic self-portraits with collage and painting. In the portraits group members could draw, paint, or cut out things that were important to them or that helped them to define themselves. Ella talked about her future career and wanting to excel in school, her love of art-making, and her desire to travel and move across the country one day.

In one painting, she made a beach scene and imagined herself living in California. In a collage, she cut and pasted pictures of elephants that spoke to her as symbolizing strength, power, and leadership. In a watercolor and ink scene, she drew a garden and wrote on it one of her favorite affirmations about being strong, smart, and beautiful.

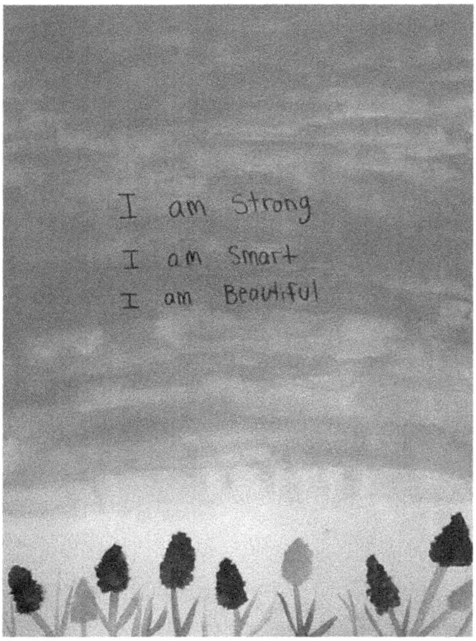

Figure 19.3 Strong, smart, beautiful

While Ella remained uncertain about entering treatment for her drinking, she became willing to engage in harm reduction and tried some online 12-step meetings. She developed for herself a set of "rules about drinking." She stopped drinking and driving, and no longer engaged in drinking when she had to work or go to school the next day. She minimized the number of drinks she would have and subsequently refrained from certain impulsive behaviors, such as text messaging while under the influence of alcohol.

Within a few weeks of implementing harm reduction and practicing strategies in motivation for change in the art studio, Ella began to see a difference in her life. While she struggled with some situations, she did not drink or become suicidal in reaction to them. Instead she practiced her DBT skills and also slowly began reaching out for more support. Her suicidal thoughts decreased and then went into complete remission. She became able to see the direct link between her suicidal thoughts and her drinking patterns. At my suggestion, Ella, Paige, and another group member began to reach out to each other for peer support around staying sober.

Both Paige and Ella enjoyed the therapeutic use of art to help them process their feelings about making change. In group, they enjoyed art as a way to relax and accept themselves in the present moment, while at the same time reflecting about making change. One art directive that we used for these skills was making aboriginal paintings on bark and adorning them with wooden beads and twine for hanging.

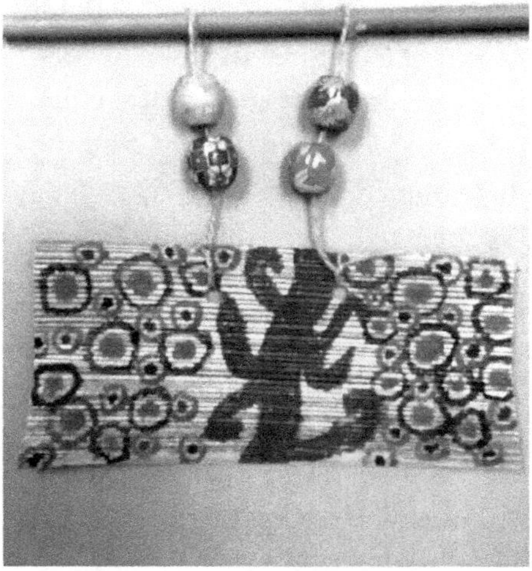

Figure 19.4 Aboriginal bark painting

Motivational interviewing employs the five stages of change model (Prochaska and DiClemente 1982) which I illustrated for our group in a visual as a wheel of change. Each stage was a spoke in the wheel moving in the direction of change. Each stage was identified with a sample comment: precontemplation (I'm not even thinking about it); contemplation (I'm weighing the pros and cons); preparation (I'm making a plan); action (I'm making the change); and maintenance (I'm staying the course and preventing a relapse).

In motivational interviewing, ambivalence is recognized as a factor for change. Often young people are stuck between wanting to make a change but not wanting to make a change. To help them get unstuck, we first encourage their intrinsic motivation, as opposed to external motivators. In the art studio, we construct art directives for reflection about what they value most, what reasons they have for wanting to change, and what their vision for the future looks like.

I have found that motivational interviewing goes hand in hand with DBT. They both utilize dialectical thinking—the idea that two seemingly opposing things can be true at the same time, as with the DBT strategy of "acceptance and change" (Linehan 1993; Miller and Rollnick 2002). This involves accepting ourselves exactly as we are at the present moment, while at the same time becoming willing to change our behaviors. DBT and motivational interviewing also both embrace resistance, so as not to push the client away. Both strategies recognize that pushing a client too hard or taking away their ability to make their own decision will likely result in oppositional and defensive behaviors. In AIRY and with peer support, we encourage youth to think that change is possible and that we all believe in them.

In the program, I adopted the use of open-ended questions designed to elicit positive "change talk." Such questions may include:

- What do you think will happen if you don't change anything?
- How would you like for things to be different?
- What are your strengths that can help you make this change?
- What would you be willing to try?

Through writing and art topics that apply motivational interviewing methods, we can help young people identify their pros and cons for change, their readiness for change, and how to set realistic goals and develop a plan for change. We can listen carefully, reflect, and summarize what they share, and act as mirrors on their journey toward recovery.

Working with addictions can be a demanding and difficult practice for any helping professional. The link between addiction and suicidality may be overlooked and become a major obstacle in preventing suicide. The statistics for youth with addiction issues, particularly the use of alcohol and drugs, remain grave for youth in our society.

As with all the youth I have worked with, I have learned a great deal in my experiences with Belinda, Paige, and Ella. While I continue to challenge our group members in ways that move them forward, they too challenge me to be the best art therapist I can be for them. AIRY acknowledges that as an art-based suicide prevention program we are all works in progress. We continue to grow together. Having an open and empathic attitude is key to helping young people as they face great adversity in an ever-changing world.

References

Linehan, M. (1993) *Skills Training Manual for Treating Borderline Personality Disorder*. New York: The Guilford Press.

Miller, W.R. and Rollnick, S. (2002) *Motivational Interviewing: Preparing People for Change* (2nd edn). New York: The Guilford Press.

Prochaska, J.O. and DiClemente, C.C. (1982) Transtheoretical therapy: Toward a more integrative model of change. *Psychotherapy: Theory, Research, and Practice 19*, 276–288.

PART 5

Resources for Helping Professionals

Chapter 20

Self-Care for Professionals

Karen Saakvitne and Laurie Anne Pearlman, in their book, *Transforming the Pain: A Workbook on Vicarious Traumatization*, discuss the role of self-care for professionals, stating:

> You must love your work or some important aspect of your work. It must be more than a job. This work is too difficult and too personally demanding to do without a sense of mission or conviction. Without a passion for the work, an individual will most likely leave the field and move to a different type of work. In other words, your work must be meaningful to you. Then, paradoxically, your work itself is part of your antidote. (Saakvitne and Pearlman 1996, p.72)

As the quote suggests, our work needs to be inherently rewarding to balance the enormous costs that can come with it. Rarely is there a day that goes by that I don't think about my mission to help prevent suicide and to make the world a better place. For me this work has become so life-affirming. It gives me a sense that I am constantly taking the right action in life, doing good work, and making a difference in the world. It sustains me in mind, body, and spirit.

But the psychological intensity of doing this work, and the physiology of hypervigilance that often accompanies crisis situations, can take its toll on me. I sometimes experience what I call "brain mush"—times when I just need to shut down, rest, and re-set. I am overactivated and need to calm, breathe, and self-nurture. Other times I become overwhelmed by the gravity of youth suicide prevention. There are moments when I feel the weight of the world on my shoulders. I can be prone to experiencing tension, anxiety, agitation, and even physical pain.

What is happening for me in these times is what happens for most helping professionals. The type of work we do by nature makes us vulnerable to what has been called secondary traumatic stress, compassion fatigue, vicarious traumatization, and burnout. Experiencing these things is often an inescapable consequence of our desire to help, our empathic engagement with our clients, our knowing, caring, and facing the reality of trauma and suicide. Addressing the impact of our work on our bodies, minds, and spirits is not only a personal but an ethical consideration. We have an obligation to our clients and to ourselves not to be damaged by the work we do.

Definitions

Let's take a moment to distinguish the terms that have been defined for the impact of our work.

"Compassion fatigue" is a general term applied to anyone who suffers as a result of serving in a helping capacity. It derives from constructivist self-development theory which asserts that our fundamental psychological needs include safety, trust, power, esteem, intimacy, independence, and a cognitive schemata through which life is experienced and interpreted (McCann and Pearlman 1990). Such cognitive schemata are highly individualized and may involve a positive or negative worldview. Clinicians are at risk if they internalize the memories of their clients. They may begin to see the world through their clients' eyes rather than their own.

"Secondary traumatic stress" (STS) involves helping professionals who become overwhelmed with witnessing, whether visually or verbally, the trauma of their clients. Figley (1995) defined STS as "the natural consequent behaviors and emotions resulting from knowing about a traumatizing event experienced by a significant other" (p.7). Symptoms of STS may include re-experiencing the event through recollection, dreams, intrusive thoughts, and reminders of the event. Avoidance and numbness may also be reactions, as well as feeling flat, loss of interest, and in some cases a loss of the sense of a future. The clinician may experience persistent arousal, trouble sleeping or staying asleep, anger, difficulty concentrating, and an exaggerated startle response (Pryce, Shackelford, and Pryce 2007).

Similarly, "vicarious traumatization" occurs when professionals vicariously experience traumatic reactions in their nervous systems. McCann and Pearlman (1990) describe how vicarious traumatization is "a process that alters the inner life of the clinician and ultimately his or her personal and interpersonal behavior" (quoted in Pryce *et al.* 2007, p.14).

"Burnout" happens as an extreme circumstance when a professional's health is suffering as a consequence of their work, or when their outlook on life has turned negative because of the overload of their work. "Burnout is anchored in the organizational culture and is associated with low personal reward and high work-related demand in an unsupportive environment" (Pryce *et al.* 2007, p.12). This person may feel the effects of their work in a way that diminishes their sense of hope and idealism.

Professional self-care

In her book *Art Psychotherapy*, Harriet Wadeson suggests:

> Working with suicidal adolescents may raise profound questions for the therapist. The threat of suicide forces the therapist to face significant existential questions of value in life and responsibility for another. At times a client's longing for the end of a life of suffering may resound in the therapist's own feelings of despair. More so than ordinarily, the therapist's sensitivity to the client is challenged. (Wadeson 1980, p.82)

Restoring and maintaining a sense of hope is essential to our work. For how else can we offer our clients a belief in healing and change? Therefore, for the wellbeing of both the therapist and the client, practitioners need to be able to talk about the emotional stress of their work and become educated about how traumatic stress affects them and their worldview.

However, many work environments still present barriers to adequate supervision for professionals to get help with secondary traumatic stress and support for their professional self-care. Some professionals may feel that others do not understand their work and become socially isolated. They may hide what is happening to them and the effects of their work. This can lead to high incidence of turnover and burnout. Pryce *et al.* suggest that often:

> When practitioners know they are adversely affected by the work and feel helpless, they keep it to themselves, knowing that no one in authority wants to hear about their feelings. It is believed that a mature professional adult isn't supposed to feel helpless. Organizational culture asserts that professional objectivity should keep the practitioner in a cognitive mode and not be emotional about their cases. Agencies expect the practitioner to protect him or herself and not bring additional problems to the organization because he or she isn't capable of adjusting to the stress of the work. (2007, p.19)

To understand the impact of working with trauma and suicide attempt survivors, education and training should be provided to anyone doing work in this field. Training should include theory in traumatology, and its effects on physical and psychological functioning. Learning to effectively cope with stress related to our work involves understanding and accepting our vulnerability to secondary traumatic stress. All helping professionals need to balance their needs with the needs of their clients.

Supervision should be utilized to reduce emotional stress. It is crucial to develop a strong self-care system and to recognize our coping behaviors. Through regular self-assessment we should examine our self-care physically, socially, and emotionally. We should also examine our strengths, vulnerabilities, and personal trauma histories.

Connection at work with colleagues and a supervisor is vital to our being able to take care of ourselves in the midst of suicide prevention work as we negotiate our clients' powerful needs and our own responses. Colleagues and supervisors understand our work, can validate our experiences, and provide social support. Professional support or peer supervision groups can be organized to help restore our connection, hear about others' work and successes, and to help normalize our responses to this work.

Helping professionals can address their stress through self-care (balance, limits, healthy habits, and connection with others). We can engage in nurturing activities (gentleness, a focus on pleasure, comfort, relaxation, and play) and activities that allow us to forget about work, engage in fantasy, and get away from painful feelings.

In Cheryl Richardson's book *Life Makeovers* (2000), she has designed a checklist of basic needs at work as a means of self-care. We may have paid little attention to some of these areas but they can go a long way in helping us reorganize our work lives and manage our stress.

Suggested areas for self-reflection about professional self-care include how many hours you work each week, how much time you allow yourself for things like a lunch break each day and taking vacation and sick time. Also important to consider is where in your schedule you can carve out breathing room for pause and reflection, and whom you can delegate tasks to so that you can free up your time and empower those that work with you. It may be helpful to schedule specific times for tasks such as returning phone calls and checking email.

Another area to evaluate is taking on more work than you can handle or as I once heard from a mentor, trying to do the impossible. You can ask for more time to answer requests and make decisions, so that you don't accept tasks you later regret.

We also need to pay attention to our working environment. It can be difficult to work in an environment that is not free of clutter. Can you make time to clear out the old to make room for the new? How is the lighting in your workspace and the quality of air? Do you need a fan or air purifier? Do you drink enough water throughout the day? What are the comfort items in your workspace? These might include keeping a pair of comfortable slippers under your desk or adding plants or artwork to your room or purchasing a sound machine or playing music. Hanging up a "Do Not Disturb" sign can also allow you more ease with focusing.

Looking at your work–home balance is also essential. Simply asking friends and family to honor and support your work time as well as your time for self-care can be valuable and help eliminate feelings of guilt you may unnecessarily carry. It is vital to have periods of time without distractions and interruptions.

In this chapter we also discuss having adequate supervision and support for our work. It is a good idea to take a look at who you can talk to about your professional life. Mentors, colleagues, spiritual advisors or sometimes co-workers can help us in this area.

Outside of work, developing our personal lives must be front and center—taking care of *you* must be a priority. It's important we have places to be spontaneous, frivolous, silly, carefree, to be completely in control and to have no control, to rest, relax, and play. It is important to discover what restores us. What makes you laugh? What daydreams do you enjoy? Where do you make room for play?

We can do more than just cope with stress. Through awareness we can recognize our vulnerabilities and take steps to strengthen our hearts, minds, and bodies. Feelings such as loss, anger, despair, and cynicism can develop when our work and personal lives are unbalanced. Ignoring these can create a cumulative effect that leads to burnout. Instead, we can work toward *transforming* our secondary traumatic stress by infusing meaning into our lives and participating in community building. To consciously create meaning in our lives may involve reflecting on beauty and nature, connecting with friends, and intentional awareness to reconnect with the spiritual aspects of our experience.

Lee and Waters concluded that spirituality is a protective factor from cumulative traumatic stress (in Pryce *et al.* 2007). As Rogers (2002) pointed out, "A person's spiritual nature produces qualities such as compassion, forgiveness, love, faith, hope, trust, generosity and kindness. [When] these characteristics are affected…[it] produces suffering, leading to stifling or destruction of some aspect of spirit" (quoted in Pryce *et al.* 2007, p.63). Spirituality practices can help clinicians keep their worldview balanced and their belief systems intact in a world of difficult challenges.

I am fortunate that my work as an artist also provides me with respite and relief. I often say to my colleagues when they are stressed, "Take it to the art." I find that if I am not making art, simply put, I am off balance. Art is the most restorative form of self-care that I know. It releases all the pent-up feelings, the worries and the stress. It reinforces spontaneity, freedom, and meaning in my life. Moreover, it provides me with a comforting space for wider reflection, not just about my work but for my identity as a person.

Art is one of my forms of meditation and has many health benefits. I have learned to incorporate other kinds of mindfulness and acceptance strategies as well for use in self-care. "Acceptance goes beyond recognition and awareness; it includes the deeper realization of the fundamental truth and inevitability of our inner changes and pain" (Saakvitne and Pearlman 1996, p.77).

Physiology of secondary traumatic stress

As mentioned earlier, experts in the field of neuroscience suggest that trauma has many effects on physiology and brain functioning. Chronic stress alters one's physiology and contributes to both physical and mental health problems such as vulnerability to heart disease and hypertension, abnormalities in hormones, and alterations in the body's ability to manage pain. Changes in brain chemistry may result in poor coping skills and depression or increased anger and hostility (Pryce *et al.* 2007).

In Babette Rothschild's book *Help for the Helper*, she examines the physiology of the effects of trauma on professionals and what is needed for self-care.

> Therapist self-care requires the proper functioning of at least three neuropsychological systems...the first involves the brain mechanisms that operate interpersonal empathy. The second depends on balance in the autonomic nervous system (ANS) and arousal regulation. The third requires clear thinking that relies, in part, on the balanced functioning of all brain structures. In short for a therapist to minimize risks to her emotional and physical well-being, she needs to be able to find ways to balance her empathic engagement, regulate her ANS arousal, and maintain her ability to think clearly. (Rothschild 2006, p.3)

As helping professionals, empathy is our greatest and most reliable tool. And yet the same tool can threaten our wellbeing. Interestingly, I found while researching for this book that the concept of empathy was first applied to art appreciation. It was considered to be essential to understanding aesthetics—the idea that a person could be deeply affected by the mood of a work of art. Empathy referred to people infusing art with human qualities. Later, researchers began to notice the interpersonal context of empathy, originally defining it as "emotional contagion" (Rothschild 2006).

Experts have opined that empathy is at the root of the survival of the human species, through our tendency to mirror one another—physically such as in facial posture, verbally, as in the development of spoken language, or emotionally. Empathy is activated in the sensory nervous system and through mirror neurons in our brains. It is a highly integrative process involving cognitive, somatic, brain, and body systems.

It is useful for anyone working in suicide prevention to recognize that empathy has somatic manifestations. Through mindfulness, we can increase body and self-awareness, and incorporate strategies for self-care. For example, when we spend countless hours mirroring our clients, it may be useful to take breaks to "unmirror" ourselves. This may involve sitting up straight, crossing or uncrossing our legs, changing our breathing, taking a drink, stretching, doing progressive muscle relaxation, or getting up and moving around.

Recognizing our vulnerabilities by way of ongoing self-assessment and monitoring needs to become part of our regular routine work, not an afterthought. Noticing our arousal patterns, we can regulate ourselves to slow down before a high-risk state is reached. Learning to apply the "therapist brakes" through engagement with the parasympathetic nervous system can help us manage stress. Learning to do boundary work is also a helpful tool, such as paying attention to the physical space between you and your client and making adjustments as needed. Re-examining your workspace is helpful to make room for more comfort.

Rothschild (2006) explores how work stress can compromise rational thought. She suggests taking regular self-inventories and learning to develop "dual awareness" of internal and external sensory information to maintain clear thinking. A therapist must be in touch with both their inner and outer reality to gauge self-regulation and to increase overall feelings of safety. Cleansing and end-of-the-day rituals can also contribute to better self-care.

Art-making in supervision

One of the advantages of working as an art therapist is having a readily available medium for processing work-related feelings. In this section, we will look at how art therapists are using art in this way.

Wadeson opined that art therapists may identify with their clients' struggles, particularly separation and individuation issues experienced by adolescents. Through making their own artwork, therapists can confront and resolve their own feelings in their work with suicidal clients.

Art therapist Tessa Dalley (1987) asserts that contrary to the psychoanalytic view of the past, therapists' countertransference can "incorporate ideas of therapeutic empathy and identification" (p.18). Such feelings may include helplessness, loss, sadness, and confusion. Because the therapeutic relationship in art therapy is formed around images, the instrument of art can serve each stage of therapy. For example, many art therapists find it helpful to create art with a client surrounding termination. This might be a joint picture with the adolescent or the use of a transitional object, in which client and therapist both make pieces of art to exchange and be remembered by. The creative process offers a needed sense of closure.

Art practice that is focused and mindful can be a meaning-making tool. It has been described as:

> an exercise in knowledge construction: a process of coming to know...it allows information to be seen differently, in a fresh, more meaningful, personal, and experiential way (as in art, symbolism, and metaphor). This transformation of concepts through imaging produces new insights and learning. (Marshall 2007, p.23)

Moreover, the art product can help us externalize our experience to aid deeper reflection.

In art therapy supervision, supervisees can share and discuss their response art. Response art can be spontaneous or carefully constructed. It has been defined as "art created...to contain, explore, and express clinical work" (Fish 2008, p.70). For example, an art therapist may make a metaphoric drawing of a case to aid in cognitive synthesizing and emotional process.

Ishiyama developed a procedure that he called the "visual case processing method" (1988) intended to reduce supervisees' anxieties, which involved generating imagery and metaphors, drawing the case, and presenting the case in group supervision. Ishiyama found the majority of supervisees preferred drawing to verbalization as an effective means of processing.

Art therapists often work with art as a form of metaphor, narrative, and story. This can serve to connect emotions and insight, and to influence behavior and action (Robert and Kelly 2010, referred to in Deaver and Shiflett 2011).

Jackson *et al.* (2008) found that mandalas increased supervisees' self-awareness. Drawing within a circle can produce a calming effect. They found that making mandalas helped broaden understanding of complicated cases.

Another art form that can aid in supervision is visual journaling, which pairs experiential art activity with reflective thinking through written response. Ganim and Fox (1999) developed an art therapy supervision method with visual journaling as a way to access and transform negative feelings and then to make a new picture containing different, positive images.

Similar ideas include reproducing client artwork in an effort to empathize with the client's experience or making art that depicts the client.

Art-making, whether in individual or group supervision, has so many useful functions for processing work-related stress. For therapists, it can help to clarify their feelings, explore their subconscious thoughts, differentiate their feelings from the client's, and in general to examine the therapeutic relationship (Kielo 1991).

Another method that can be used in art therapy supervision involves supervisor and supervisee both making art and journaling and then exchanging their entries (Durkin *et al.* 1989). Durkin and colleagues found that it "brought interpersonal richness to [supervisory] relationships, cut through to the core of many issues very quickly, and permitted access to three modes of communication: visual, verbal, and written" (p.392).

Williams (2000, referred to in Deaver and Shiflett 2011) proposed a specific collage-making technique for use in supervision. This involves finding images in magazines that symbolically represent situations to be discussed in supervision.

McNamee and McWey (2004) suggest using bilateral art in the exploration of supervisor–supervisee relationships. Bilateral art is "an art therapy intervention that engages both dominant and non-dominant hands in the process of creating images in response to opposing cognitions or feelings" (p.230).

In summary, effective interventions for secondary traumatic stress need to engage our mind, body, and spirit. Self-care—inside and outside of work—is a necessary ingredient in our work of helping to save young lives. In Appendix E, I have listed the web links to three self-care assessments from different life domains that any helping professional can benefit from doing as well as a way to construct a professional self-care plan. I hope these will be useful to you. It may have been a while since you've been thanked for your work. So, I will ask that you take a minute now, to pause and receive my gratitude. I thank you for being with me on this journey, and I see you and thank you for being so invested. Because it is together that we are making a difference.

References

Dalley, T. (1987) *Images of Art Therapy: New Developments in Theory and Practice.* London: Tavistock Publications.

Deaver, S.P. and Shiflett, C. (2011) Art-based supervision techniques. *The Clinical Supervisor 30*, 2, 257–276.

Durkin, J., Perach, D., Ramseyer, J., and Sontag, E. (1989) A Model for Art Therapy Supervision Enhanced through Art Making and Journal Writing. In H. Wadeson, J. Durkin, and D. Perach (eds) *Advances in Art Therapy*. New York: Wiley.

Figley, C.R. (1995) *Compassion Fatigue: Coping with Secondary Traumatic Stress Disorder in Those Who Treat the Traumatized*. New York: Brunner/Mazel.

Fish, B. (2008) Formative evaluation research of art-based supervision in art therapy training. *Art Therapy 25*, 70–77.

Ganim, B. and Fox, S. (1999) *Visual Journaling: Going Deeper Than Words*. Wheaton, IL: Quest Books.

Ishiyama, F.I. (1988) A model of visual case processing using metaphors and drawings. *Counselor Education and Supervision 28*, 153–161.

Jackson, S., Muro, J., Lee, Y., and DeOrnellas, K. (2008) The Sacred Circle: Using Mandalas in Counselor Supervision. *Journal of Creativity in Mental Health 3*, 201–211.

Kielo, J. (1991) Art therapists' countertransference and post-session therapy imagery. *Art Therapy 8*, 2, 14–19.

Marshall, J. (2007) Image as insight: Visual images in practice-based research. *Studies in Art Education 49*, 23–41.

McCann, I.L. and Pearlman, L.A. (1990) *Psychological Trauma and the Adult Survivor: Theory, Therapy and Transformation*. New York: Brunner/Mazel.

McNamee, C.M. and McWey, L.M. (2004) Bilateral art to facilitate clinical supervision. *The Arts in Psychotherapy 31*, 4, 229–243.

Pryce, J., Shackelford, K., and Pryce, D. (2007) *Secondary Traumatic Stress and the Child Welfare Professional*. Chicago: Lyceum Books.

Rogers, D.F. (2002) *Pastoral Care for Post-Traumatic Stress Disorder: Healing the Shattered Soul*. New York: Haworth Pastoral Press.

Rothschild, B. (2006) *Help for the Helper: Self-Care Strategies for Managing Burnout and Stress*. New York: W.W. Norton.

Saakvitne, K. and Pearlman, L.A. (1996) *Transforming the Pain: A Workbook on Vicarious Traumatization*. New York: W.W. Norton.

Wadeson, H. (1980) *Art Psychotherapy*. New York: John Wiley & Sons.

Chapter 21

Skills-Based Expressive Art Therapy Directives

Below you will find sets of art therapy directives listed according to each skill taught in the Arts in Recovery for Youth program. Suggested materials, the prompt for each directive, and ideas for discussion are also included.

Topics

- Safety
- Mindfulness
- Distress tolerance and self-soothing with the senses
- Self-compassion and self-care
- Emotion regulation
- Anger management
- Opposite action (emotion regulation skill)
- Wise mind
- Interpersonal skills and peer support (sense of belonging)
- Identity
- Empowerment
- Making a difference
- Future goals.

SAFETY

SAFE SPACE JOURNAL COVERS

Materials: Blank journals or notebooks; collage materials, paint, glitter

Prompt: Create a cover for your journal that makes you feel safe

Discussion: Tell us about your safe place

Variation: Use your journal as a place to "dump" your worries; create a cover that soothes you

SAFE PLACE MANDALA

Materials: 12 x 12 inch white paper or cardstock, colored pencils, markers, dinner-size plate or cardboard cake round

Prompt: Trace a circle on the paper. Visualize a safe space and draw it inside the circle

Discussion: Describe your safe place

SAFE SPACE DIORAMA

(This can be a multi-session project)

Materials: Photo boxes or shoeboxes, colored and printed papers, cardboard scraps, foam sheets, scissors or Exacto knife (to be used under supervision), craft paints, tacky glue, recycled materials such as Styrofoam, foam sheets, clothespins, etc.

Prompt: Design a special space all your own using various materials provided (the box is your frame; you can cut windows and doors; paste on wallpaper, hang curtains, build a fence by taking apart clothespins; paint the outside; use your imagination)

Discussion: What makes you feel safe?

YARN DOLLS

Materials: Various yarns, colored duct tape

Prompt: Design a doll or puppet as a reminder that you are safe (shape together various yarns and adhere the shapes with duct tape)

Discussion: Tell us about your doll

BODY FEELING/BODY SCAN DRAWINGS

Materials: Long paper, chalk or oil pastels (variation: colored pencils or markers)

Prompt: Draw a picture of what it feels like to be in your body

Discussion: What does your body need from you right now?

MINDFULNESS

RHYTHMIC COLOR PAINTINGS

Materials: 5 x 7 or 8 x 10 inch canvas panels, acrylic paints and brushes

Prompt: Choose two colors that soothe you; notice how you feel when you look at the colors. Start by painting strokes of one color at one end of the canvas. Then paint the other color at the opposite end. As you draw near the center, begin to blend your colors. Focus on the rhythm of the paintbrush to soothe you

Discussion: Tell us about the colors you chose and how they make you feel

COLOR MEDITATION PAINTINGS

Materials: Acrylic paints and canvas, brushes

Prompt: Choose a color that you are feeling today. Notice how you feel when you look at the color. Paint various shades of that color on your canvas

Discussion: Tell us about the colors you chose and how they make you feel. How does it make you feel to meditate on a certain color of your choosing? What sensations do you notice in your body?

Variation: Paint your shades of the color inside a mandala

ZEN DOODLES

Materials: Black markers or black felt pens, mixed media paper or cardstock, colored pencils and markers

Prompt: Design black and white designs on your paper. Allow yourself to empty your mind as you focus on the lines, dots, doodles, and patterns. When you are done color them in any way you choose

Discussion: How did it feel to make your Zen doodle? Did you notice your mind clearing?

ABORIGINAL DOT PAINTINGS OR BARK PAINTINGS

(This can be a multi-session project)

Materials: Paints, tiny brushes, paper; canvas cloth, stretched canvas, or pieces of bark; sticks or bamboo sticks; wooden beads; pictures of aboriginal dot paintings for reference

Prompt: Notice the patterns in the aboriginal dot paintings. Pick a surface material to work on and create your own patterns with dots. Allow yourself to empty your mind as you focus on the patterns

Discussion: How did it feel to focus on the dots? How do you feel now?

Variation: Use thin pieces of bark to paint on; punch holes in the bark; thread with twine and tie twine to sticks; affix wooden beads

ESCAPE TO THE PERFECT DAY

Materials: Drawing paper, colored pencils or markers

Prompt: Imagine you can escape to the perfect day. Imagine how you feel inside your perfect day. Draw what that looks like

Discussion: Where did you go on your perfect day and what was it like?

FOUND OBJECT SCULPTURE

Materials: Collected objects in nature such as sticks, rocks, bark pieces, shells; plate or lid for base, wire, quick-dry tacky glue, rubber bands

Prompt: Notice all the different textures of the objects you have collected. Hold them in your hands and describe them to yourself. Then create a found object sculpture

Discussion: Describe your found object sculpture

Variation: Paint your found objects, then create a sculpture with them

BILATERAL DRAWINGS

Materials: Large paper, oil pastels

Prompt: Close your eyes and feel the paper with your hands. Notice how the surface of the paper feels. Begin drawing patterns with both hands. Continue to draw, open your eyes, and look at your picture. Decide if you want to develop your picture further

Discussion: How did it feel to draw with both hands? Tell us about your picture

DISTRESS TOLERANCE AND SELF-SOOTHING WITH THE SENSES

MODELING CLAY SCULPTURES

Materials: Plasticine modeling clay

Prompt: Begin by just playing with the modeling clay and notice how it feels. Describe to yourself the qualities of the clay (temperature, texture, etc.). Play with the clay and create a sculpture (real or abstract)

Discussion: What did the modeling clay feel like? What did you make?

DRUMMING CIRCLE

Materials: Hand drums

Prompt: Play with the surface of the drum until you find a beat or a rhythm you like. Notice the sound of the drum and how you feel in your body. See if you can begin to synchronize your rhythm with the rest of the group

Discussion: How did it feel to create your own music with the drums?

SENSORY BOXES

Materials: Fold-up cardboard boxes, collage materials or craft paints and brushes

Prompt: Design a box that you can keep objects in that represent your senses (touch, taste, smell, sound, sight, and movement)

Discussion: Share your self-soothing box. What objects will you put in your sensory bag that can soothe you during times of distress?

SENSORY FABRIC BAGS

Materials: Fabric scraps, sewing needles and thread, scissors, thick string

Prompt: Draw a pattern on the fabric and sew together pieces to create a self-soothing bag that you can keep objects in that represent your senses (touch, taste, smell, sound, sight, and movement). Cut holes one inch apart at the top and pull string through to create a drawstring to close your bag

Discussion: Share your fabric bag. What objects will you put in your sensory bag that can soothe you during times of distress?

SAND, ROCK, OR MOON GARDENS

Materials: Recycled containers or trays; various colored sand or rocks; craft paints and brushes (optional: forks or miniature rakes to play with the sand)

Prompt: Create a garden using rocks or sand. Paint your garden container. Play with the materials and notice how they feel

Discussion: Tell us about your sand, rock, or moon garden

Variations: (1) Add a water fountain to your rock garden with submersible mini water pumps and fill two-thirds of the way with water. Focus on the sound of running water on the rocks. (2) Put a small container with soil in the center of your garden and plant a moonflower seed (which only opens at night). Keep your garden on a windowsill

OTHER SENSORY DIY ART IDEAS

- Scented putty or glitter slime
- Homemade face mask
- Cloth rice bags
- Upcycled wind chimes

SELF-COMPASSION AND SELF-CARE

SELF-CARE WHEEL

Materials: Cardboard cake rounds, plastic spinners, permanent markers, ruler, fine-point pens

Prompt: Make a list of as many self-care activities as you can think of. Then with a ruler, divide your circle into pie pieces and write one self-care activity in each. Affix the spinner in the center. Decorate with markers

Discussion: Tell us about your self-care wheel

POSITIVE AFFIRMATION WATERCOLOR CARDS

Materials: Watercolor paper cut into three 4 x 6 inch squares per person, watercolor paints and brushes, fine-tipped permanent markers

Prompt: Design three watercolor images and, when dry, write positive affirmations on the front or back

Discussion: Share your positive affirmation cards with the group

SELF-COMPASSION LETTER TO MYSELF

Materials: Stationery and envelopes, stamps, writing instrument

Prompt: Whose voice do you find compassionate in your life? Imagine you had a voice of compassion like this for yourself. Imagine what that voice sounds like. Write a letter to yourself from that compassionate voice. When you are done, fill out the envelope and I will mail it to you

Discussion: Tell us about the voice of self-compassion you found. What do you think it would be/feel like if you used this voice and did not judge yourself?

EMOTION REGULATION

EMOTION CHARACTERS

Materials: Drawing or mixed media paper, colored pencils and/or markers such as dual-tipped brush markers

Prompt: Identify a strong emotion you are feeling today. If you could personify this emotion as a character, what would they look like?

Discussion: Tell us about your emotion character. What are they doing in your picture?

ROUND ROBIN EMOTION POEMS

Materials: Writing paper and pencils or pens

Prompt: Choose an emotion that you are feeling strongly today. Write your emotion at the top of the paper. Write a line of poetry about this emotion, and then pass your poetry to the person on your right. Now look at the emotion on the paper you have been given. Add a line of poetry to this person's poem. Then pass it to your left. Continue writing lines of poetry until you receive your poem back. Write a concluding line of poetry to finish your poem

Discussion: Share your poems aloud with the group. How did it feel to express aspects of many emotions in poetry?

EMOTION PAINTINGS

Materials: Small canvas such as 4 x 4, 8 x 8, or 8 x 10 inch, acrylic paints and brushes

Prompt: Identify emotions you are feeling today. What color would those emotions be? Paint your emotions on canvas

Discussion: Share your paintings and tell us about your emotions

"DIRTY POUR"/DRIP POUR PAINTINGS

Materials: Small cups (size of shot glass), craft paints, dish soap, multiple small canvases such as 4 x 4, 8 x 8, or 8 x 10 inch, newspaper or disposable table cloth (optional: canvas holders, toothpicks)

Prompt: Decide what emotions you are feeling and what colors they might be. Choose the colors of your emotions and pour them into the cups. Add a small amount of dish soap. You may want to swirl them a little with a toothpick. Then pour the cups onto canvas. Move your canvas around so that the colors make patterns and fill the space. Variation: swirl the colors around on the canvas with a toothpick

Discussion: Tell us about your emotions and your paintings

Note: These are a favorite in the studio and youth will likely want to create several of these as they are done quickly. They enjoy the freedom to use a lot of paint and to just pour it. Note that these require a good deal of paint. You will need to leave paintings to dry overnight

ANGER MANAGEMENT

REWRITING THE STORY

Materials: Writing paper and pens or pencils

Prompt: Write down a description of what you are angry about. Then review your description and highlight any words that imply judgment, blame, assumptions, black and white thinking (extremes), or rumination. Next, rewrite the description removing these words and use just facts and objective language

Discussion: Share your description and your rewrite. Do you notice any shift in your anger?

TRANSFORMATIVE PAPER MOSAIC

Materials: Paper, paint, glue

Prompt: Today we are going to focus on transforming our anger into a mosaic. First you will paint the colors of your anger on the paper.

Feel free to be as messy as you want. When you are done releasing your anger, you are going to rip these up, so just focus on getting the anger out, and not how it looks. There is no wrong way to do this. Once you are done, begin to rip up your paper into small pieces. Begin to glue these pieces onto another piece of paper in a mosaic

Discussion: How did it feel to just release your anger onto the paper? What does your picture look like now and how do you feel?

FROM ANGER TO COMPASSION WRITING EXERCISE

Materials: Writing paper, rulers, pens or pencils

Prompt: For this exercise, we will write at the top of the page something involving another person that bothered us, or got us angry or upset. Then we will draw a grid of four squares onto the paper. In the upper left square, write down what you were feeling at this moment. In the lower left square write down what you needed at this moment and didn't get. In the upper right corner, write down what you imagine the other person was feeling at this moment. In the lower right corner write down what you imagine the other person needed at this moment and didn't get

Discussion: Did you notice any shift in your anger after this writing exercise? Tell us about what you discovered

OPPOSITE ACTION (EMOTION REGULATION SKILL)

OPPOSITE ACTION PAINTINGS IN PAIRS

Materials: Acrylic paints, larger canvas such as 12 x 12 or 16 x 20 inch, brushes

Prompt: We are going to divide the group to work in pairs for this project. One of you will choose a strong emotion you are feeling. The other person will choose an emotion that is opposite. You will each depict your emotion on a shared canvas and find a way to meet in the middle

Discussion: Share your paintings and tell us how you arrived in the middle

OPPOSITE ME DRAWINGS

Materials: Drawing or mixed media paper, markers and/or colored pencils

Prompt: Identify how you see yourself today. What are you thinking and feeling about yourself? Now imagine the opposite was true. Draw a picture of "opposite you"

Discussion: Share your pictures with the group. How did it feel to imagine the opposite?

WISE MIND

WISE MIND CLAY SCULPTURES

Materials: Air-dry clay, clay tools, water, sealant such as Mod Podge, craft paints and brushes

Prompt: Try to identify your wise mind as a symbol. Then sculpt an image of this symbol using clay. After the clay dries overnight, we will put a seal on it so it doesn't crack, and you can paint it

Discussion: Tell us about your wise mind sculpture

Note: Due to the time it takes for air-dry clay to dry, this is usually a two-week project

WISE MIND DRAWINGS

Materials: Drawing or mixed media paper, markers and/or colored pencils

Prompt: Identify your wise mind as either a symbol or a character and draw it on the paper

Discussion: Tell us about your wise mind

WISE MIND POETRY

Materials: Writing paper and pens or pencils

Prompt: Write a poem about your wise mind (your inner intuitive voice that is self-compassionate and wise)

Discussion: Share your poem

INTERPERSONAL SKILLS AND PEER SUPPORT (SENSE OF BELONGING)

SYMBOLIC RELATIONSHIP MAPS

Materials: 12 x 12 inch paper, dinner plate or other round object to trace, colored pencils and/or markers

Prompt: For this project we are going to draw a map of our relationships. In the center of the circle draw a symbol for yourself. Then begin placing symbols of the people in your life on your map, in distances that show how close you feel to them and whether they are inside or outside the circle

Discussion: Talk about your relationship map and how you feel about it. Who supports you or respects your boundaries? What relationships do you want to improve? What relationships do you want to let go of?

Variation 1: Connect the people on your map to you with a variety of types of lines to show what kind of relationship you have with them. A straight line is a close relationship, a zig zag is a conflictual relationship, a dotted line is a broken or distant relationship

Variation 2: Connect the people on your map to you with a variety of types of lines that show what kind of boundaries are in place in each relationship. A solid and flexible boundary can be represented as a dotted line or a simple straight line, a rigid boundary can be two parallel lines, a lack of boundaries or loose boundaries can be a light and wavy line, and a broken boundary can be a zig zag

PRIDE PAINTINGS, FLAGS, OR SIGNS

Materials: You can choose from a variety of materials such as canvas, paper, poster board or flags, paints or markers

Prompt: Express your feelings of pride about your gender and sexual orientation

Discussion: Share your work and describe your feelings

ROUND ROBIN PAINTINGS

Materials: Paints and canvases size 8 x 8, 8 x 10, or 10 x 10 inch, brushes

Prompt: For this project, we are each going to have a painting to take home that each member of the group has contributed to. This is a good way to remember what the group has meant to you, that has a mark on it by each person in our group. Begin by spending five minutes painting on your canvas. After this time, pass the canvas to the person on your right. Each person's canvas will be going round the group. Every five minutes, pass the canvas you have worked on until your original canvas returns to you. Then make any final changes to your painting

Discussion: Share your group painting

Note: We often do this exercise in the last two weeks of the group as a transitional object of the group experience

GROUP MURAL

Materials: Mural paper, paints, brushes, or markers

Prompt: The group will come up with a theme for a mural. Each person will work on a place on the mural and then decide on the transitions in between. You may also paint words on the mural about your group experience. Please put your initials somewhere on the mural

Discussion: What did the group decide was the theme of this mural? Tell us about your part in the mural and what you like about others' parts

Variation: Use an extra-large canvas placed in the center of the table. Have the group continue to work on it until the canvas is filled

GROUP COMIC BOOK

(This can be digital or on paper)

Materials: Tablets and internet, or paper and drawing materials

Prompt: Work together on creating characters and decide what will happen in the story

Discussion: What do the characters convey about how they see the world?

Variation: Use the characters to tell a story about a social issue that is important to you. How does the story end? What small steps can you take to make a difference in your community about this social issue?

GROUP MASCOT

Materials: Large round pieces of Styrofoam, fabric, paint, mask, a yard stick to hold the pieces together (or choose from a variety of recycled materials)

Prompt: What is important to you in this group? Each group member will participate in designing a mascot that represents the group

Discussion: Tell us about the mannequin and its features. Talk about the group process of creating the mascot

ART MAIL EXCHANGE

Materials: Variety

Prompt: Create an art image for a group member to exchange by mail

Discussion: What was it like to receive art in the mail from another group member?

IDENTITY

SCRIBBLE DRAWINGS

Materials: Paper, colored pencils or markers

Prompt: With eyes open or closed, loosely draw scribbles on the paper. When you are done, look at your picture from all angles and see if you can find an image to develop further

Discussion: Share your image with the group. What might this image say about you or how you are feeling?

SYMBOLIC SELF-PORTRAITS

Materials: Paint, canvas, brushes, water

Prompt: Create a symbol that represents who you are and what is important to you

Discussion: Share your picture with the group and what it says about you

Variation: Create a collage of a symbolic self-portrait using images from magazines, scissors, glue, and paper

EMPOWERMENT

ANIMAL SPIRIT COLLAGES

Materials: Magazines with animals such as *National Geographic*, scissors, paper, glue

Prompt: If you were an animal, or if you could be an animal, what animal would you choose?

Discussion: Share your animal spirit image and tell us about the qualities of that animal. Why did you choose this particular animal?

EMPOWERMENT OR SUPERHERO MASKS

Materials: Masks, paint or permanent markers, tactile materials such as pom-poms, feathers, beads, tacky glue

Prompt: Imagine that you were a superhero. What would your superhero powers be? Create a superhero mask

Discussion: Share and describe your mask with the group

Variation: Design a mask that shows how you feel on the inside of the mask and what you show the world on the outside of the mask

TATTOO DESIGNS

Materials: Paper, colored pencils, markers

Prompt: If you could design a tattoo, what would it be?

Discussion: Tell us about your tattoo and why you chose this image. Why is this image important to you?

MAKING A DIFFERENCE

TELEKINESIS MESSAGES/POSTERS OR SOCIAL ACTION FLAGS

Materials: Paper, writing materials, poster board or blank fabric flags, permanent or fabric markers or paints

Prompt: If you had the power of telekinesis and you could put thoughts into other people's minds, what would you want them to think?

Discussion: Share your telekinesis messages with the group and why these messages are important to you

Variation: Create posters of your messages. Create social action flags of your messages

GUERRILLA ART AND ART ABANDONMENT

Materials: Small pieces of paper and writing instruments, other small art materials

Prompt: Today we are going to create artwork and/or messages to leave behind for people to find. What do you think people in the world need to hear?

Discussion: How did it feel to share your message to the world, knowing someone will randomly find it?

Variation 1: Place the messages inside library books at the public library. Leave messages in public places

Variation 2: Write messages on the sidewalk with chalk

VIRTUAL ART SHOW

Materials: Computer, images taken with cameras on phones

Prompt: Let's create a virtual art show to share on social media. Choose pieces of art to share

Discussion: How does it feel to create your own art show?

FUTURE GOALS

ROAD OF LIFE DRAWINGS

Materials: Large or long paper, colored pencils and markers

Prompt: Draw the road of your life. This can be literal or symbolic. Include things from the past that you have survived as well as your accomplishments

Discussion: What kind of road did you draw? (Is it smooth and straight, winding, bumpy?) What obstacles did you encounter on your path? Where do you see the road taking you in the future?

A DAY IN MY FUTURE

Materials: Paper or canvas, drawing or painting materials

Prompt: Create a picture of a day in your future

Discussion: What are you doing on your day in the future? What did you imagine for yourself?

Variation: Use cardboard boxes to create a diorama of a day in your future

Chapter 22

Measurable Outcomes

Knowing the problem and its causes is the first step in developing an arts-based youth suicide prevention program. It has been a challenging task to define why our young people are dying by suicide.

As cited by Van Orden *et al.* (2010), experts in suicidology have outlined various theoretical approaches to suicidality over the last two centuries. Biological theories propose that suicidal behavior results from the dual presence of a biologically based diathesis (such as dysregulation of the serotonergic system in the ventromedial prefrontal cortex) and an activating psychosocial stressor. Psychodynamic theories argue that suicide is caused by unconscious drives, by existential drives for meaning and attachment problems. Cognitive-behavioralists suggest suicide is driven by hopelessness and emotion dysregulation. Systems models discuss the roles of social forces and family systems.

While multiple theories exist, they are complementary. In summary they inform us that we must address behavioral symptoms, interpersonal and environmental factors, and psychological drivers for why young people become suicidal. A successful suicide prevention program will go beyond addressing these problems and begin to implement working solutions. Our data suggests that group settings are crucial for reparation and recovery of youth suicidality, and in healing interpersonal wounds that lie deep below the surface of symptomatic behaviors. Practical hands-on skills are necessary for youth to overcome existing deficiencies, both inside the mind and in environmental circumstances.

AIRY is informed by the most up-to-date theories in suicidology and best practices in suicide prevention. To further support our work, I have been able to record evidence-based quantitative and qualitative data on participating youth since 2017. With my research and training in suicide prevention I have developed a tangible way to check in with youth and record their progress. The program collects individual outcome studies for every session through numerical self-report. We measure contributing aspects of each member's suicidality and their progress over time.

From the outset of the program, we used this number system. Overall, youth responded in a positive way. Being given the opportunity to consistently record in numbers how they were doing led to a greater sense of control in a world where they often felt powerless. The concrete structure of the number system helped to demystify what they were experiencing. And it gave them a way to acknowledge, contain, and manage their feelings. Recording this data over time served to produce measurable outcomes of solid, evidence-based work, but more importantly, it helped them feel safe.

Several aspects of this data are provided below in a study of 29 participants who completed the AIRY program during a three-year period from September 2017 to September 2020. Studies were conducted with 16 adolescents ages 13–17 and 13 young adults ages 18–26 over a period of four months each in the program. The variables that were measured over a four-month period were:

- individual assessment scores for suicide risk (which included environmental stressors, access to lethal means, and previous history of suicide attempt)
- individual feelings of suicidality by self-report on a numerical scale from 0 to 10
- psychological drivers and interpersonal risk factors for suicide (also recorded by self-report on a numerical scale from 0 to 10). Specifically, this last set of variables measured levels of stress, emotional pain, urges to self-harm or engage in destructive behavior, feelings of hopelessness, self-hate, burdensomeness, and lack of belonging.

Both individual scores and group averages for suicide risk were calculated based on best practices in suicide risk assessment. For example, studies by the National Institute of Mental Health (Bilsen 2018) indicate that youth who had previously attempted suicide were at three times greater risk. Among our participants, the average suicide risk score during the three-year study was 49 percent (63% among the young adults and 34% among the teens). Over half (55%) of the total participants had a history of at least one prior suicide attempt (69% of the young adults and 38% of the teens).

Essentially, one out of every two youth that I met over this three-year period had tried to kill themselves before coming to AIRY. These numbers, when coupled with the knowledge that our county had the highest suicide rate in the state, were grave.

One of the most important things I had learned in my training was to consistently ask youth if they were feeling suicidal. Given their histories, we must not assume that if they don't offer this information, they are no longer at risk. I have learned that if we don't ask, we simply won't know.

At the beginning of every season's programming, we complete individual intakes and assessments for each youth referred. During the intakes, the participants reported on average initial feelings of suicidality at 43 percent. This number fluctuated throughout the four-month period, most specifically in the first two months of the time period measured. During months three and four, this number began to decrease significantly as youth gradually reported feeling less suicidal. By the end of the four-month period, youth reported a reduction in feelings of suicidality on average by 86 percent (89% for teens and 82% for young adults).

As our program grows, these numbers have assured me that we have a well-informed and sound structure for suicide prevention.

The AIRY teen and young adult study measured five main psychological drivers for suicide adapted from David Jobes's Collaborative Assessment and Management of Suicide Risk (CAMS). Youth reported numerical levels of stress, emotional pain, urges to self-harm or engage in destructive behavior, feelings of hopelessness, and self-hate.

During initial assessment, the teen group (ages 13–17) reported the highest of these drivers being stress rated on average at 50 percent, emotional pain on average at 40 percent, and feelings of both hopelessness and self-hate on average at 30 percent. Again, these numbers varied over the course of four months, eventually declining as the period of time progressed. Reduction of the levels of psychological drivers for suicide is reported in the following chart.

Risk factors for suicide in 16 teens ages 13–17	**Percentage reduction after 16 weeks**
Stress	46%
Emotional pain	73%
Urges (to self-harm or behave in a destructive manner)	83%
Hopelessness	72%
Self-hate	64%

In the young adult group (ages 18–26), the scores for the drivers for suicide upon intake were higher. This was congruent with their higher level of suicide risk. They reported levels of stress at an average of 70 percent, emotional pain at 60 percent, feelings of self-hate at 60 percent, and feelings of hopelessness at 50 percent. Reduction of the levels of psychological drivers for suicide among the young adults is reported in the following chart.

Risk factors for suicide in 13 young adults ages 18–26	**Percentage reduction after 16 weeks**
Stress	16%
Emotional pain	27%
Urges (to self-harm or behave in a destructive manner)	33%
Hopelessness	34%
Self-hate	28%

While the young adult group showed progress in all areas, their reported percentages were significantly lower when compared to the teen group. For example, teens reported 46 percent less stress after 16 weeks, while young adults reported only 16 percent less stress. The differences between the teen and young adult data may indicate a few conclusions.

First, the young adults reported a risk level of suicide nearly double the teens upon entering the program. Therefore, progress may have been slower. They simply may have needed more time for the specific drivers measured to decrease.

Second, the young adults showed significantly greater stress levels associated with developmental changes toward emerging adulthood. For example, most of the young adults were taking on a greater level of responsibility with life tasks such as graduating high school and starting college, entering employment for the first time, and moving out of the family home. These major life transitions affected the intensity of their psychological drivers for suicide, and may have also affected the level of support they were receiving (i.e. more time away from family and friends).

Third, additional barriers to change were reported in the young adult group, such as entangled romantic relationships, substance abuse, unsupportive work, school, or living environments, and lack of adult supervision.

Subsequently, a smaller study of 14 participants measured interpersonal risk factors for suicide adapted from Thomas Joiner's (Joiner *et al.* 2009) interpersonal theory of suicide. Specifically, this study measured numerical levels of perceived burdensomeness and thwarted belongingness among seven teens and seven young adults.

Other risk factors (smaller study of 7 teens ages 13–17)	**Percentage reduction after 16 weeks**
Burdensomeness	63%
Lack of belonging	86%

Other risk factors (smaller study of 7 young adults ages 18–26)	**Percentage reduction after 16 weeks**
Burdensomeness	24%
Lack of belonging	31%

Levels of change regarding (1) interpersonal risk factors for suicide and (2) psychological risk factors for suicide were similar in both sets of data. We saw greater reduction in the teen group than with the young adults.

However, despite these differences, the most important factor we measured was consistent across all groups. Reduced levels of suicidality after 16 weeks of programming remained high—89 percent in the teen group and 82 percent in the young adult group. This indicates that the outcomes for reduced suicide risk were the same regardless of fluctuating variables. This also indicates that the program is effective and evidence-based.

In this period we have made changes to the program in efforts to improve our success. We have learned that the length of time in the program directly impacts the level of suicidality of teens and young adults. For example, on average, youth who participated for 8 to 12 weeks had a reduced level of suicidality at 77 percent. Those who completed 16 weeks had a reduced level of suicidality at 86 percent. Finally, youth who remained in the program for a year or more showed 95 percent reduced suicidality, with a large portion achieving full remission. Below, I have provided additional outcomes data for the period 2017–2020.

- Number of youth served: 104
- Number of towns served: 18
- Percentages of youth served by age:

12	1%
13	11%
14	16%
15	17%
16	10%
17	9%
18	13%
19	5%
20	7%
21	6%
22	4%
23	2%
24	1%
25	1%
26	2%

Effects of Covid-19 on AIRY outcomes data

Groups held during Covid began with remote learning during the pandemic and then moved to the studio in small groups within state regulations. Those who completed the program and were able to return to the studio experienced our highest improvement in suicidality to date; this may be in part because we extended the program an additional six weeks (from 16 weeks to 22 weeks) to combat the effects of isolation associated with quarantine. This is consistent with previous data indicating that the longer youth stay in the program or remain connected to the program, the more their suicidality reduces.

I felt it was necessary to record the effects of Covid-19 on our outcomes data and drew the following conclusions:

1. *Change in retention rates during remote programming.* From March to August 2020, the program experienced its lowest retention rate to date (62% of youth left the program early because they could not tolerate an online platform). However, this is countered with a surge in previously served youth reaching out to AIRY for help during the pandemic (18% of youth served were members who returned for help while experiencing difficulties related to Covid, after previously graduating the program). The high rate of returning members speaks to the effectiveness of AIRY to serve youth both short term and long term, within and outside the program. It also speaks to youth feeling comfortable to re-engage with AIRY as needed, and an increase in help-seeking skills.

2. *Need for increased outreach outside of programming time.* Outreach was tripled in frequency, in response to increased risk for suicide (due to risk factors associated with Covid including isolation, traumatization, depression, anxiety, and somatic symptoms). To continue to serve youth and their parents remotely, AIRY hired a part-time outreach assistant/social worker who provided ongoing caring contact outside of groups to both youth and parents. Parents reported feeling supported and helped during the pandemic.

3. *Need for increased trauma-informed applications.* In response to the traumatic effects of Covid, AIRY members received additional training in best trauma-informed methods and practices.

AIRY made alterations in its curricula to include more somatic-based activities aimed at self-regulation. AIRY also adapted its delivery of remote programming by videoconferencing to be increasingly trauma-informed.

4. *Need for in-person contact.* AIRY noticed a marked improvement among members who were able to return to the studio, which suggests that in-person contact is a necessary ingredient for effective suicide prevention. This is supported by evidence in suicidology and traumatology (see Joiner *et al.* 2009; Levine 2010; Porges 2012).

Though Massachusetts has one of the lowest rates of suicide in the country, Berkshire County remains the highest in the state. Arts in Recovery for Youth is gradually having an impact on the youth suicide rate in Berkshire County and spreading to surrounding geographic areas.

References

Bilsen, J. (2018) Suicide and youth: Risk factors. *Frontiers in Psychiatry*, October 30, https://doi.org/10.3389/fpsyt.2018.00540.

Jobes, D. (2016) *Managing Suicidal Risk: A Collaborative Approach* (2nd edn). New York: The Guilford Press.

Joiner, T., Van Orden, K., Witte, T., and Rudd, M.D. (2009) *The Interpersonal Theory of Suicide: Guidance for Working with Suicidal Clients.* Washington, DC: American Psychological Association.

Levine, P. (2010) *In an Unspoken Voice: How the Body Releases Trauma and Restores Goodness.* Berkeley, CA: North Atlantic Books.

Porges, S.W. (2012) *The Polyvagal Theory: Neurophysiological Foundations of Emotions, Attachment, Communication, and Self-Regulation.* New York: W.W. Norton.

Van Orden, K.A., Witte, T.K., Cukrowicz, K.C., Braithwaite, S., Selby, E.A., and Joiner Jr., T.E. (2010) The interpersonal theory of suicide. *Psychological Review 117*, 2, 575–600.

Conclusion

Youth suicide is a storm sweeping across our communities, leaving family, friends, parents, teachers, counselors, churches, schools, and neighborhoods feeling helpless, sad, and confused. Youth suicide matters right now and we are all responsible for stopping it. We know the problem too well. We need to start focusing on the solution. We are failing the next generation.

The good news is that there is hope. Simply put, solving the suicide problem takes human connection. We can learn how to talk and how to listen to what's happening in the minds and hearts of youth who feel suicidal. We can be present, open, and helpful. We can work together to break centuries of stigma. We can take the risk of getting involved in situations that may scare us. Each of us can make a difference one young person at a time. And collectively, we can become stronger, allied in the fight against youth suicide.

This author designed Arts in Recovery for Youth in 2016 by calling upon her own experience as a recovered suicide attempt survivor and art therapist. The success of the program is based on valuing the lived experience of suicide attempt survivors. Young people are not viewed as "patients" but rather as warriors who can learn to mentor others through a restored sense of hope. They can talk about their experiences in a safe, stigma-free, and creative setting where suicidality may be transformed.

Valuing lived experience about suicidality is necessary to reduce youth suicide. As a culture interested in saving young lives, it is imperative that we learn their stories and have open, ongoing dialogue about suicide. Listening to survivors gives us first-hand knowledge and a roadmap for future interventions.

I'm not sure what I expected when I began the program. I just knew

I wanted to do something about the problem of youth suicide all around me. I didn't realize groups of teens and young adults would come forward in droves and be so hungry and so willing to get help. In a rural area, there are slim resources for young people, and even slimmer ones for youth suicide prevention. When I searched around for other resources, combing through book titles and websites, I found very little specific to art therapy and suicide prevention. I realized that while our program is still a work in progress, it is a successful work in progress. It needs to be shared with a larger audience to give people hope and help guide the way for similar programs to develop. Art therapy for youth suicide prevention works.

In order to create an effective design for an art therapy-based model for suicide prevention, I had to start at the very beginning. The statistics from the Centers for Disease Control and Prevention and the Department of Public Health were more than alarming, they were downright terrifying. I was able to get training in suicidology and best practices for suicide prevention, while at the same time implementing therapies which reported the highest efficacy for this population.

As time went on in AIRY, I had to adapt to new situations and circumstances and get feedback from youth about what works for them. We made changes as needed. Today, the statistics continue to rise across the country, and internationally.

It has been an exhaustive effort to design, implement, and fund our program, but it has also imbued my life with great meaning and purpose. The success of the program helps our entire community to rise, and for that I am continually grateful. I believe that our model can be duplicated in other communities and that we can join together in the fight against youth suicide.

While writing this book, I have attempted to provide the reader not only with evidence-based data and a solid theoretical foundation for art therapy as a means to suicide prevention, but also the first-hand stories and artwork of young people who have survived, recovered, and gone on to lead very promising lives. It is my hope that you walk away with an understanding of how AIRY works and a greater sense of hope for the future of arts-based youth suicide prevention. My dream is to inspire us all to work together to solve the youth suicide problem.

For more information about the AIRY program and resources for suicide prevention, please visit www.airyedu.com. Send inquiries to airyberkshires@gmail.com.

Appendices

A. Sample Safety Plan

B. Assessing Suicide Risk at Home: How Parents Can Help

C. Check your Biases, Beliefs, and Reactions

D. Providing Trauma-Informed Care in the Classroom

E. Self-Care Assessments for Professionals

F. Resources for Suicide Prevention

Appendix A

Sample Safety Plan

Safety first

Ways to reduce access to lethal means:

____

____

Ways to make my environment safe:

____

____

Coping

Personally meaningful coping skills I can use to cope when I feel in crisis:

____

____

____

Ways to decrease isolation:

____

____

____

DBT skills I am learning to use:

______________________________ 1. Wise mind 2. Take an opposite action

______________________________ 3. Breathing 4. Finger tapping/counting

______________________________ 5. Ground with the senses/sensory box

People I can call

______________________ National suicide lifeline: 1-800-273-8255

______________________ Text CONNECT to 741741

______________________ Transgender suicide hotline: 877-565-8860

My life or death emergency contact: Emergency: 911

____

Reminders

Things I need to be reminded of in crisis:

____

____

Things I don't want to hear or make it worse:

____

____

My reasons for living (list as many as you can think of):

______________________ ______________________

______________________ ______________________

______________________ ______________________

______________________ ______________________

______________________ ______________________

______________________ ______________________

Appendix B

Assessing Suicide Risk at Home

HOW PARENTS CAN HELP

1. *Check in.* Every child differs. If you don't ask they may not tell you they are struggling. But they have joined this group for a reason, so it's important to check in.

2. *Scale of 1 to 10.* In our groups we use a rating scale from 1 to 10 each week to check in about suicidal thoughts and behaviors. It's a very simple question. On a scale of 1 to 10, how suicidal are you feeling?

3. *Have a plan.* It is recommended that you adopt this scale at home and use it as needed. Write down a plan in advance for what actions you will take when your child tells you what number he/she/they feel on the suicide rating scale. If your child expresses suicidal thoughts do not leave them alone at any time. Just being present may be comforting as these thoughts are very scary.

   For example, if on the *1 to 10* scale they say they feel at a:

   - *1* Put a safety plan in place. Develop a code word if they need one. Remove access to any lethal means. Tell providers. Do distracting activities.
   - *2* Continue to rate suicidal thoughts each day. If they do not decrease, seek help.
   - *3* Contact providers and schedule a medication evaluation.
   - *4* Contact the suicide prevention hotline for advice, your

therapist, or see about a walk-in appointment or a phone consultation. Consult with the local crisis team.

   - *5–6* Contact your area's local crisis team and you may request that they come to the house. Consider the emergency room.
   - *7–10* Bring your child to the emergency room. Do not wait.

4. *Learn how to talk about it.* Direct conversation about suicide without judgment works. We set the model for talking about it. The more comfortable we become with this conversation, the safer the outcome.

5. *Judgment-free zone.* Work towards becoming nonjudgmental about suicide. Recognize that it is part of the universal human condition to want pain and suffering to end.

6. *Ask questions*:
   - When did the thoughts start?
   - How often do they come? (Every day? Every hour?)
   - How long do they last? (Minutes, days?)
   - Do they have a plan? If so, what is it?
   - What is the number one problem they are having? (They usually know what's driving them if you ask...what is their reason for wanting to hurt themselves or die?)
   - What makes it worse?
   - What makes it better?
   - How likely (on a scale of 1 to 10) are they to kill themselves? (This is a hard question but it's an important one.)

7. *Know their coping skills and reasons for living.* Focus on their coping skills. Ask them and reinforce their reasons for living.

8. *Empathy.* In order to increase empathy, imagine having your own suicidal thoughts. What might drive you to feel that way? What would be your reasons for living that would keep you safe? Who would be your supports? Share this with your child to help

them understand they are not alone, they are not a burden, and they are not "going crazy."

9. *Distract and calm.* When your child is distressed, try to focus on distracting activities in the here and now as well as calming the senses (which become overloaded when they feel suicidal).
10. *Make connections.* Social media and our digital world can add to a sense of isolation. Help them make meaningful connections with others who make them feel needed, accepted, and loved, whether family, friends, or mentors.
11. *Work on goals.* Later help them work towards meaningful goals that make them feel a sense of purpose and greater meaning in life.

Appendix C

Check Your Biases, Beliefs, and Reactions

In order to be effective, it is important to check your own beliefs about suicide and your emotional reactions. You will need to not let these interfere with helping a young person. They may be worried they will disappoint you and therefore not tell you what's going on for them. Developing a calm, neutral yet concerned response will help the situation.

Take a moment to examine your own beliefs and emotional reactions to the idea of suicide and challenge the following biases.

- Suicide is irrational.
- Suicide is immoral.
- Suicide is a sin and will be punished by God or send you to Hell.
- Suicide is permissible (if life feels unbearable, one has the right to end it).
- Suicide is a choice (based on free will).
- Feeling suicidal will pass.
- Feeling suicidal means you have a mental disorder.
- Stress creates suicidal thoughts.
- Getting suicidal should have consequences (i.e. punishment/reward).
- If your client is suicidal, you or someone else is to blame.

- Suicidal thinking is contagious.
- Suicide should be kept secret. It's private or shameful.
- Talking about it will make it worse.
- People with suicidal thoughts are just seeking attention.
- Feeling suicidal is just a phase.
- Suicide is a teenage trend/copycat not to be taken seriously.
- People who are suicidal should be left alone to work it out.

Appendix D

Providing Trauma-Informed Care in the Classroom

Recognizing triggers

Triggers are generally sensory, as these memories are the most powerful ones—for example, songs, sights, word phrases, smells.

Cues include changes in behavior, feeling sick, shutting down or being unusually quiet, difficulty vocalizing (as trauma affects the verbalizing part of the brain and most young people cannot talk about it), changes in speech patterns, becoming hot or cold, dizziness, being distracted, awkwardness, being teary-eyed, changes in body language, wanting to leave.

Use simple, straightforward questions like "Are you feeling triggered right now?" "Are you feeling unsafe?" "What do you need?" (They may or may not know what they need.) "Can I help you?"

How can I make my environment trauma sensitive?

- One way to be assured is to get the information you need from your students. Asking the group to write down how the environment could be more trauma sensitive to them could give you ideas.
- We establish our own rules (e.g. some people are germophobic and need wipes to clean their hands often; sound sensitive—we do not raise our voice but raise our hand if needed; body sensitive—we always ask permission to touch, etc.).

- Provide easy access to things that feel safe.
- Consider a quiet area in the back of the room.

How can I teach in a trauma-sensitive way?

- Scan subject matter in a trauma-sensitive way, anticipating reactions and addressing them beforehand. For example, before we begin we are going to ground ourselves and recognize that we are reading a fictional story. How can we stay emotionally safe when we read and respond?
- Be willing to make accommodations for students you know have trauma. For example, we are going to read about a character with a drug addiction today. This may feel triggering to some. If that happens for you, come get a piece of clay. Or raise your hand and come get a bathroom pass. It is okay to need a break. You can also go visit the school counselor or… (depending on resources available).

Helpful ideas

- Grounding and returning to the present are the first goals when someone is triggered.
- Reducing stimulation may be necessary (stepping aside or outside the room). A change of environment may be necessary, especially if the trigger is a person in the room.
- Drinking water, breathing, splashing cold water on the face, getting fresh air, finger tapping (see emotionally focused tapping below), repeating a helpful mantra, making eye contact with the person and assuring they are safe several times, until we know they hear it, and making contact with a familiar voice (being allowed to call home, etc.) can all help.

Sensory exercises

- *One–five sensory exercise*: Name five things you see, four things you hear, three things you can feel in your body, two things you smell, one thing you taste. Breathe. Repeat if necessary.
- *Other anxiety-reducing exercises*: Name things by going through the alphabet (serves as thought distraction and accesses the left brain when the right brain is overstimulated). Counting things you see: how many chairs in the room, cars in the parking lot, tiles on the floor, etc. Name patterns you see in the room.

You can modify this to your curriculum by saying: "Count how many characters are in this story"; "How many metaphors are there in the first chapter?"; "Name five things in the setting," etc. This moves the lesson temporarily from content (which may be too intense) and emotional responses to something neutral and left brain. Temporarily refocusing this way can re-engage students who feel overwhelmed.

Sensory tools

Non-hardening modeling clay (or Play-Doh), yarn, cotton balls, essential oils, drawing utensils, teaching tapping.

I use modeling clay and have it available on the table so kids can come and get a piece and use it to self-soothe—just kneading it helps; or playing with a piece of string, braiding, knitting. These activities help reduce stimulation. Drawing also helps (e.g. doodling while we read aloud or drawing characters). I also use essential oils on cotton balls. Young people can hold the cotton ball and smell it during the class. Peppermint is popular and calming. These sensory aids can be very useful and help people focus and return to the present moment. Essentially we are teaching them to self-regulate or co-regulate with others.

Emotionally focused tapping (EFT)

Tapping seven centers, one at a time (takes about one to two minutes):

1. Top of the head

2. Brow bone
3. Under the eye socket
4. Under the nose
5. Chin right below the lips
6. Collarbone
7. Back of the armpit.

Repeat with opposite hand/side of the body.

Remind yourself of something positive while you do it (e.g. "I'm okay").

Sometimes music can help, but it's tricky since it can provide unwanted memories or difficult lyrics can evoke emotional responses. Picking a neutral, calming song, preferably an instrumental, to warm up can help some re-focus and regulate.

Teaching students to become trauma sensitive

- Don't try to rescue or fix people but just keep them distracted and safe.
- Learn to speak in the "I" and consider others when sharing. (For example: Let's agree not to overgeneralize or stereotype any particular group. Let's recognize the diversity of experiences in the room and that not everyone will have the same response.)
- There is no wrong response to this literature as all have different experiences and all experiences are valuable.
- Teach people that trauma is universal, that it varies from person to person.
- Trauma can be personal, environmental, small, or large. No two people have the same trauma response.
- Trauma happens when a certain part of the brain is activated, and stores memory in a different way than our other memories.
- It is part of the primal brain's response (not our logical brain but

our animal brain), our fight, flight, or freeze part of the brain. (This is a survival response of all animals, that we do not have control over, but can find ways to ground and come back to the present moment. For example: Did you ever try to stop a dog barking at a new person? A cat's tail suddenly fluff up?) These responses were designed to help us survive.

What to expect

- Expect people to have trauma. Allow it to become normalized.
- Expect people to have survival reactions when trauma is triggered. They may experience fear of death and a sense of urgency that does not match the situation. Assure them this is likely a response to trauma, and it will pass after they are able to ground themselves. Do not expect them to be able to verbalize what is happening as they feel frozen in time. However, they may know what they need (or what's effective) and surprise you.
- People with trauma or anxiety may have a difficult time with things that are new, unfamiliar, or surprises and struggle with transitions. They need to feel something familiar to know they are safe and can manage their reactions.
- Making references to things they are familiar with may help: Last week we talked about...this will be like that.
- Explaining what is going to happen in advance is helpful so they can plan what to expect.
- Ending class with an opportunity to relax and distract before transitioning to the next class may be useful.

What not to do

Much research has been done to suggest that talking about the trauma is actually worsening, unless it is done in a safe private setting and the person is helped to close the story and return to the present, assured that they are safe in the here and now. Often talking about the trauma can reactivate it in the brain and later that day, or the next day, create a dysregulating or escalated response, which we aim to avoid. Only trained trauma-informed counselors should do this work, and unfortunately many therapists do not know how.

Appendix E

Self-Care Assessments for Professionals

Instructions for developing a professional self-care plan

Complete these three self-assessments:

- Measuring Life Stress scale
- Checking Your Basic Needs at Work Assessment
- The Professional Quality of Life Scale.

The Social Readjustment Rating Scale "Measuring Life Stress," also known as the Holmes-Rahe Stress Inventory (Holmes and Rahe 1967; Holmes and Holmes 1970; Rahe and Arthur 1978), is available at: www.stress.org/holmes-rahe-stress-inventory. The "Checking Your Basic Needs @ Work" list can be found in Cheryl Richardson's book *Life Makeovers* (2000). The ProQOL 5 Self-Score (English) can be accessed at https://proqol.org/proqol-measure.

When you are done, review the self-assessments and identify areas for which you are at risk. List them in the left column of your professional self-care plan that follows further below.

In the right column choose ways that you can make changes to improve these areas. Be creative. Use the resources listed at the end of this Appendix and the following question to come up with ideas:

- What are some of the things you have done or techniques you have used to reduce your vulnerability to compassion fatigue or assist colleagues experiencing symptoms of compassion fatigue?

Write your ideas here:

Create a plan that is SMART: **S**pecific—**M**easurable—**A**ttainable—**R**ealistic—**T**ime-Based.

Discuss your plan with a supportive friend or co-worker. See if you can develop a buddy system for self-care.

My professional self-care plan

Risk factors/areas where I want to improve	**Changes I can make**

Goals: List three professional self-care goals here. (Example: I will take a 15-minute walk around the building at break time each day for the next week.)

1.

2.

3.

Resources: Identify three resources available to you for the implementation of your work-related goals. (Examples: Walking path around building; friend at work who likes to walk and will go with me.)

1.

2.

3.

Support: Identify a person at work to whom you can turn for support in the implementation of your work-related goals.

Name: ....

Relationship: ....

Identify resistances/obstacles

Are there resistances/obstacles to the implementation of your plan?
[ ] Yes [ ] No

If yes, what are they?
[ ] Time [ ] Money [ ] Lack of Motivation [ ] Fear

[ ] Other. Specify: ....

Strategize to overcome resistances/obstacles

Will any of your identified resources help you overcome the resistances/obstacles? [ ] Yes [ ] No

If yes, which ones?

If not, how will you overcome your obstacles to self-care?

Note: If resistances/obstacles cannot be overcome, then it may be appropriate to seek the assistance of a professional who specializes in compassion fatigue.

How to decrease your vulnerability to stress, burnout, and compassion fatigue

1. Work-related strategies
   - Set realistic self-expectations for yourself and others.
   - Review how you are spending your time.
   - Know your strengths and limitations.
   - Set and keep healthy boundaries for work. Ask yourself, "Would the world fall apart if I step away from my work?"
   - Examine job demands. Are they reasonable? Are they prioritized?
   - Clarify your role and duties.
   - Schedule. Set goals, prioritize tasks, maintain a schedule, and take breaks!
2. Self-awareness and self-care
   - If you are dealing with a community tragedy, learn as much as possible about the event and deal with and articulate the powerful emotions and reactions related to the event.
   - Make a commitment to resolve your own personal issues and continue to monitor your own reactions to others' pain.
   - Have realistic expectations about the rewards as well as limitations of being an educator and set boundaries for yourself.
   - Balance your work with other professional and personal activities that provide opportunities for growth and renewal.
   - Practice mindfulness—keep your attention in the present moment, with full awareness and acceptance and without judgment.
   - Implement positive, rational self-talk.

- Take time where you can reduce interruptions, reflect, stretch, and simply BE.
- Spend some quiet time alone.
- Get up early to make time for yourself.

3. Work toward living a healthy, balanced life
   - Food and sleep are essential for your survival. Don't let them slip out of your control. Don't skip meals nor sacrifice sleep.
   - Something as simple as committing to eating better and stopping all other activities while eating can have an exponential benefit on both your psyche and your physical body. A regular exercise program can reduce stress, help you achieve outer balance, and re-energize you for time with family and friends.
   - Develop and reward a sense of humor. Expose yourself to humorous situations.
   - Check your sleep routine and make any changes needed.
   - Hold one focused, connected, and meaningful conversation each day. This will jump-start even the most depleted batteries. Time with family and friends feeds the soul like nothing else and sadly seems to be the first thing to go when time is scarce.
4. Things to avoid when experiencing compassion fatigue
   - Avoid making big decisions. People experiencing compassion fatigue should not try to make any major life decisions until they've recovered physically, emotionally, and spiritually.
   - Avoid blaming others.
   - Avoid expending energy complaining.
   - Avoid commiserating with discontented co-workers. "Misery loves company." It's easy to fall into the habit of complaining when experiencing compassion fatigue, but it will only make things feel worse. There are other, more constructive

environments to share and express feelings in a more supportive environment.

- Avoid trying a quick fix. Compassion fatigue often makes one vulnerable to addictive behaviors and substance abuse or workaholism. A quick fix usually complicates an already overburdened life, escalating the downward spiral to burnout and depression.

5. Some more ideas for self-care
   - Exercise, garden, walk, clean house
   - Read good novels
   - Watch television
   - Go to church
   - Cook for friends
   - Socialize with family or friends
   - Take vacations
   - Leave work at work
   - Shop
   - Do nothing
   - Meditate/pray
   - Get a massage
   - Turn music up loud.

References

Holmes, T. and Rahe, R. (1967) The Social Readjustment Rating Scale. Retrieved from www.stress.org/holmes-rahe-stress-inventory on January 6, 2022.

Richardson, C. (2000) *Life Makeovers: 52 Practical & Inspiring Ways to Improve Your Life One Week at a Time*. New York: Broadway Books.

Stamm, H., Higson-Smith, C., Hudnall, A., Piland, N., and Hudnall-Stamm, B. (1992) Professional Quality of Life Scale. Retrieved from https://proqol.org/proqol-measure on January 6, 2022.

Appendix F

Resources for Suicide Prevention

Call or text

If you or someone you know may be feeling suicidal, there is help available. You can call these numbers anytime to talk or find out more info:

National Suicide Prevention Lifeline: 1-800-273-8255. 24 hours. Call to talk.

Crisis Text Line: text 741741

Call2Talk—a confidential mental health suicide prevention hotline: 508-532-2255

Trans Lifeline: 877-565-8860—peer support service; www.translifeline.org

The Trevor Project Lifeline: 1-866-488-7386; www.thetrevorproject.org

Veterans Crisis Line: 800-273-8255 (press 1 OR text 838255)

Samaritans 24-Hour Helpline: 877-870-4673

Articles

Information on what it's like to call the suicide prevention lifeline: www.google.com/amp/s/www.buzzfeednews.com/amphtml/carolinekee/what-happens-when-you-call-suicide-hotline

How to talk to a child about a suicide attempt in your family (Rocky Mountain MIRECC): www.mirecc.va.gov/visn19/talk2kids/index.asp

Safety planning

My3 app: https://my3app.org

Safety Planning Interventions: www.suicidesafetyplan.com

Websites

American Association of Suicidology: www.suicidology.org

American Foundation for Suicide Prevention: www.afsp.org

Dougy Center—The National Center for Grieving Children and Families: www.dougy.org

The Jason Foundation: https://jasonfoundation.com

The Jed Foundation: www.jedfoundation.org

National Action Alliance for Suicide Prevention: https://theactionalliance.org

National Suicide Prevention Lifeline: www.suicidepreventionlifeline.org

NOPCAS (National Organization for People of Color Against Suicide): https://nopcas.org

Now Matters Now: www.nowmattersnow.org

Society for the Prevention of Teen Suicide: https://sptsusa.org

Suicide Awareness Voices of Education (SAVE): https://save.org

stopbullying.gov: www.stopbullying.gov

Suicide Prevention Resource Center: www.sprc.org

Guidance

Preventing Suicide: A Resource for Media Professionals (World Health Organization, 2008): www.who.int/mental_health/prevention/suicide/resource_media.pdf

Index

Other JKP books

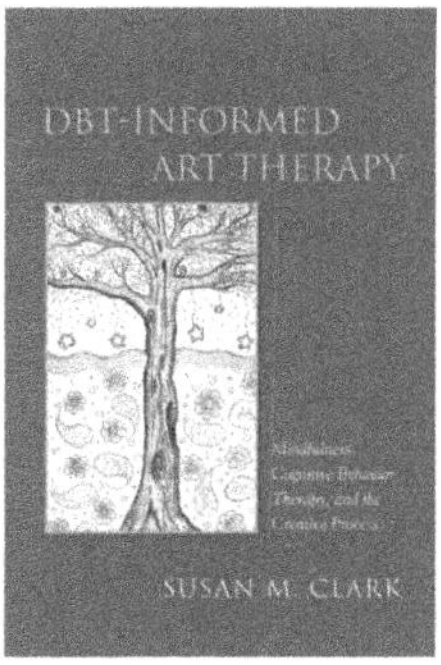

DBT-Informed Art Therapy

Mindfulness, Cognitive Behavior Therapy, and the Creative Process

Susan M. Clark

£26.99 | $45 | PB | 344PP | ISBN 978 1 84905 733 2 | eISBN 978 1 78450 103 7

Understand DBT-informed art therapy and how to apply it to your practice. Dialectical Behavior Therapy (DBT) treats problems with emotion regulation and is especially effective in treating chronic self-harming and suicidal behaviors associated with Borderline Personality Disorder. Combining the structure and skill development of DBT with the creativity and non-verbal communication of art therapy can be a significant advantage when treating patients who are resistant to talking therapy.

This book gives a comprehensive overview of the growing literature and research on DBT-informed art therapy, drawing upon the work of pioneers in the field to explain different types of DBT-informed art therapy and the "Three Ms" at its core: Mindfulness, Metaphor, and Mastery. It also includes creative visual exercises and activities for developing the skills of core mindfulness, interpersonal effectiveness, emotion regulation, distress tolerance, and non-judgmental acceptance among clients.

Susan M. Clark has been an art therapist and counsellor for over 18 years. She possesses extensive experience in leading standard didactic DBT and DBT-informed art therapy skills training groups. Susan is based at The Emily Program in Cleveland, Ohio.

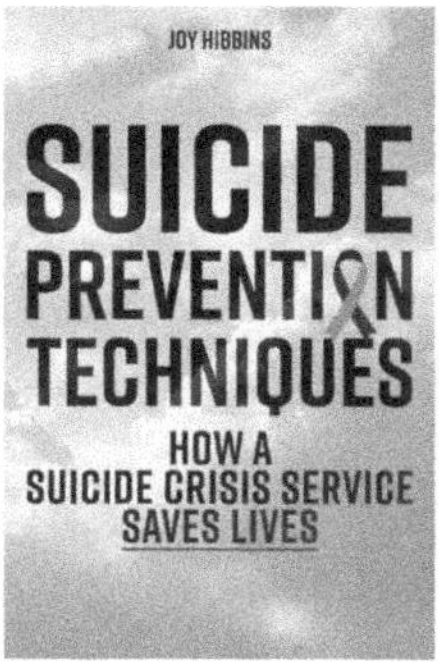

Suicide Prevention Techniques

How a Suicide Crisis Service Saves Lives

Joy Hibbins

£22.99 | $32.95 | PB | 144PP | ISBN 978 1 78592 549 8 | eISBN 978 1 78450 949 1

An unprecedented insight into the approach used by the innovative Suicide Crisis charity, a crisis centre that has so far achieved a zero-suicide rate amongst their clients. This book explains their ethos, how they work, and the ways in which their services operate.

The idea for the service grew out of the author's own lived experience of suicidal crisis, and her inability to find the right kind of help. This experience provides an understanding and awareness of what suicidal clients go through and the kind of help they require, and the success rate of the charity proves that the techniques used are effective. Covering relationship-building, providing intensive support, achieving a balance between protecting clients and giving them control, engaging high-risk men least likely to seek help, assessing risk accurately and more, this groundbreaking approach provides what is needed to save the lives of people in suicidal crisis.

The author's royalties for this book are being donated to the charity Suicide Crisis.

Joy Hibbins is the founder and CEO of Suicide Crisis, a registered charity which runs a Suicide Crisis centre in Cheltenham, UK.

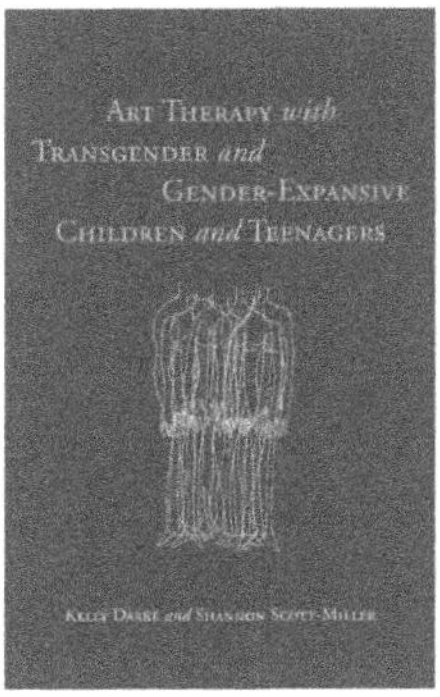

Art Therapy with Transgender and Gender-Expansive Children and Teenagers

Kelly Darke and Shannon Scott-Miller

£22.99 | $32.95 | PB | 176PP | ISBN 978 1 78592 808 6 | eISBN 978 1 78450 847 0

An educational and inspirational book that offers practical guidance for art therapists working with transgender and gender-expansive youth and their families. It provides art therapy goals, recommended treatments, and coping skills to use with this client group.

Each chapter looks at how art therapy can address a different concern or aspect of the experience, such as transitioning, bullying, and recognizing or building a support system. It includes detailed case studies and cutting-edge art therapy interventions, which help young people to express the emotions surrounding the discovery of gender identity, the transition process, and self-care.

Kelly Darke, ATR, MEd, BFA, is an art therapist based in Michigan, USA. She has experience working with gender-expansive children and young people and is the mother of a 17-year-old transgender son.

Shannon Scott-Miller, MA, ATR-BC, has over 20 years' experience in medical art therapy, including working with gender-expansive youth. She has a transgender daughter, and is based in Ohio, USA.